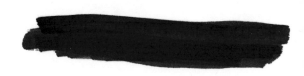

Comparative Endocrinology

COMPARATIVE ENDOCRINOLOGY

AUBREY GORBMAN
University of Washington

WALTON W. DICKHOFF
University of Washington

STEVEN R. VIGNA
University of Oregon

NANCY B. CLARK
University of Connecticut

CHARLES L. RALPH
Colorado State University

A WILEY-INTERSCIENCE PUBLICATION

JOHN WILEY & SONS

New York · Chichester · Brisbane · Toronto · Singapore

Library of Congress Cataloging in Publication Data:

Main entry under title:
Comparative endocrinology.

   "A Wiley-Interscience publication."
   Includes bibliographies and index.
   1. Endocrinology, Comparative. I. Gorbman,
Aubrey, 1914–

QP187.C5966   1982   596′.0142   82-13455
ISBN 0-471-06266-9

Printed in the United States of America

10 9 8 7 6 5 4 3 2 1

We dedicate this textbook to those of our teachers, associates, and friends—pioneers in the young science of comparative endocrinology—who have died in the past 20 years. It was they who inspired our interest and fascination with this remarkable field.

A. Elizabeth Adams
Herbert M. Evans
Irving I. Geschwind
Ernest Scharrer
Philip E. Smith
Emil Witschi

Preface

Comparative endocrinology, like all phases of comparative physiology, has experienced profound quantitative as well as qualitative development since *A Textbook of Comparative Endocrinology* was published nearly 20 years ago. In fact, we could not consider this book a revision of the 1963 version but rather a completely new text, retaining only a few of the original illustrations. Our basic orientation to endocrinology remains the same, however. We consider endocrine mechanisms adaptive systems that play a basic role in making each species fit into its environmental niche.

We have compromised this principle only in Chapter 13, which deals with reproduction. Most college courses in endocrinology or reproductive endocrinology focus on mammalian reproduction, for several good reasons. Mammalian and human reproduction are the most thoroughly understood of all. Endocrine mechanisms regulating reproduction in nonmammalian species are among the most specialized, most specific, and most complexly adapted; at the same time they are the least well understood. Thus we have chosen to emphasize the well-known mechanisms for reproductive regulation in mammals and man and to bring in comparative aspects secondarily.

For all other endocrine systems the comparative approach has been primary. The broad context of the basic biological principles of animal endocrine structure, function, and evolution have motivated the writing of this text. We hope that this orientation will be found as attractive in the future as it has been in the past.

AUBREY GORBMAN
WALTON W. DICKHOFF
STEVEN R. VIGNA
NANCY B. CLARK
CHARLES L. RALPH

Seattle, Washington
November 1982

Contents

Comparative Endocrinology

1

Introduction

MECHANISMS FOR INTEGRATION

The animal body is, after all, a machine, a device that utilizes energy to produce or execute certain functions. It is no accident that physiologists, in speaking of these functions, refer to their "mechanisms." In the literary sense, a machine is "an apparatus for applying mechanical power, consisting of a number of parts, each having a definite function" (*Oxford Universal Dictionary*). The parts of simpler integrated machines generally are connected levers or interlocking geared wheels, or similar contrivances to produce visible motion. In the most complex machines the separate parts are most often integrated by electrical signals that may begin in sensors of various kinds and that are led through a conduction system to appropriate responsive parts of the machine; the signals may be stored in a memory bank, and they may be integrated or modulated in various ways before utilization to provide an element of adaptiveness to the machine.

In animal organisms most of the functions of the living machine are chemical in nature, whether we are dealing with the obvious processing and metabolism of energy-yielding fuels, or the conversion of metabolites into additional organized protoplasmic constituents (growth), or the "mechanism" whereby chemically encoded genetic information is used to regulate cellular processes. This being so, it is not surprising that one of the most effective kinds of agents for integrating the widely distributed chemical functions in the complex organism is itself a chemical rather than an electrical signal. These chemical integrating substances, the focus of this book, are the *hormones*, and typically they are distributed by the blood vascular system. In fact, it is interesting that even when an electric (nervous) signal is used for integrative purposes in the organism, it is transduced into a chemical one when it reaches the target cell (Fig. 1.1).

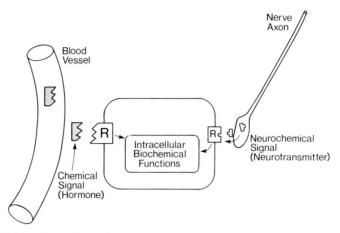

FIGURE 1.1. Comparison of the ways in which hormones and nervous signals interact with target cells to produce their typical actions. Hormones are chemical molecules that are distributed at large through the blood vascular system. When the hormone diffuses out of a blood vessel it may encounter a cell that contains or bears a receptor (R) chemical molecule. The two interact and their interaction sets off a series of intracellular chemical changes that are the "response" to the hormone. Only those cells will respond that have the specific receptor, shown in this diagram by the exact complementary external shapes of the hormonal and receptor molecules. A nervous signal is an electrical one that travels on a prescribed route or "pathway." At its end it causes the release of a chemical "transmitter" which diffuses toward and interacts with the receptor molecule at the target cell surface. The result of this interaction, as with the hormone, is to set off the intracellular chemical processes that comprise the response. The transmitter chemicals may be the same for many different kinds of cells. For nervous responses the specificity of the response depends upon the special route or pathway of the nervous signal.

The mechanism for engaging the chemical integrating signal to the responding intracellular processes involves a *receptor* molecule, whether the signal arrives via the blood or from the end of a nerve. Since hormones are distributed indiscriminately throughout the organism, wherever the blood vascular system extends, the hormone receptor is an important element in the machine because it provides *specificity* to the hormone–target cell relationship. That is, the hormones will be locked into the mechanisms of only those cells that display the receptor which, by virtue of its specific molecular shape, will interact with the hormone molecule. Receptors for neural chemical signals, like hormonal receptors, have the function of coupling the nervous signal to intracellular chemical processes. However, neurochemical receptors are relatively more common (less specific) in their tissue distribution than hormone receptors because their specificity is rendered by the special nervous pathways, as in a complex electrical circuit pattern.

The usefulness of the concept of the organism as a machine, and the hormones as chemical messengers within it, is limited. It is obvious that the organism is different from machines as we know them, being much more complex than any machines so far devised and displaying some properties that no nonliving machine can duplicate. It is useful at this point to better define the nature of hormonal integration, to give some actual examples of physiological processes in which hormones have their typical integrative actions.

Homeostatic Regulation of the Level of Glucose in the Blood

The level of glucose in the blood is subject to considerable variation due to periodic sudden influxes after feeding, and more gradual effluxes due to tissue metabolism (storage in liver or muscle, or breakdown for energy). Yet, it is important that the concentration of glucose in the blood be kept within narrow limits, because the functions of some organs, as the brain, are quite sensitive to changes in glucose levels in their immediate fluid environment.

Several hormonal mechanisms are used to maintain constant blood plasma glucose levels. The insulin-secreting cells in the pancreas are directly sensitive to the plasma glucose concentration. In humans, when glucose levels rise to some value above 100 mg/100 ml, a release into the blood of the hormone insulin is evoked. Insulin is manufactured and stored in specialized (beta) cells in the pancreas (Fig. 1.2). The insulin interacts with receptors in the plasma membranes of muscle and liver cells. These receptors, when "activated" by combination with the insulin, initiate a chain of intracellular chemical processes whose net effect is the uptake of glucose from the blood

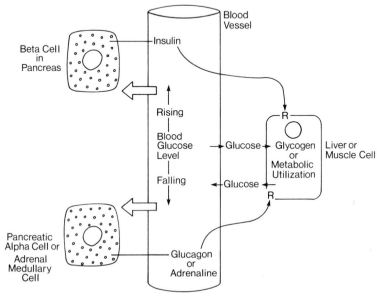

FIGURE 1.2. Diagrammatic representation of the mechanisms for regulating the level of blood glucose. See text for detailed explanation.

by the cells and storage of the glucose as glycogen. The consequent general result is a lowering of plasma glucose to appropriate levels that no longer provoke the beta cell to secrete insulin.

On the other hand, when plasma glucose levels fall significantly *below* the regulated level due to continued glucose utilization between meals (e.g., below 100 mg/100 ml in humans) other glucose-sensitive cells in the pancreas (the alpha cells) release glucagon, and cells in the adrenal gland release adrenaline into the blood. Receptors for these hormones may be found on the same glucose-storing cells that responded to insulin. However, the enzyme-driven chemical system with which glucagon or adrenaline are coupled leads to a release of glucose from glycogen storage. This glucose diffuses back into the blood to raise the plasma glucose level. By interplay of the glucose-lowering (hypoglycemic) and glucose-raising (hyperglycemic) hormones, the plasma glucose level is kept within well-specified limits. This is a simplified description of the blood glucose homeostatic mechanism. This mechanism will be described in greater detail in later parts of this book.

It should be mentioned that similar reciprocal mechanisms exist also for hormonal regulation of blood calcium and phosphate, as well as general ionic or specific ionic (K^+, Na^+) concentrations. In all of these instances the cells that secrete the regulating hormones appear to be directly sensitive to the changing blood plasma levels of the element whose concentration they regulate. The receptors for the hormones, then, are located on cells that, by their action, can appropriately correct the plasma level of the metabolite concerned.

Coordination of Gastric Function During the Digestive Process

When food reaches the stomach after a meal is eaten, the previously quiescent stomach begins to secrete peptic enzyme and hydrochloric acid, and an active phase of muscular activity is triggered. The observable secretory and contractile processes are all responses to a hormone—gastrin—that is secreted by cells in the mucosal layer of the stomach when the meal enters. The gastrin secretion is stimulated by the mechanical presence of the meal in the stomach, as well as by chemical constituents in the food (secretagogues). It is not clear how the mechanical or secretagogue-initiated stimuli are communicated to the gastrin cells. In this instance a hormone messenger is secreted into the blood and is distributed throughout the organism, though its target cells are in the same organ. The target gland and smooth muscle cells of the stomach have been shown to contain gastrin receptors.

It is interesting that the ultimobranchial gland cells also display gastrin receptor activity. This gland is far removed from the stomach and secretes a hormone—calcitonin—whose function, in short, is to reduce blood calcium level. Teleologically, we may suppose that this action of gastrin is in anticipation of the rise in blood calcium that is about to occur as a result of absorption of calcium in the digested meal.

Rapid Maturation of Tissues in Developing Frog Embryos

The metamorphosis of the aquatic tadpole into the terrestrial frog is a remarkable developmental event that appears to be under the control of the thyroid hormone. That is, tadpoles deprived of their thyroid glands fail to metamorphose for prolonged periods. However, if given synthetic thyroid hormone, they quickly resume development and metamorphosis. Although thyroid hormone receptors have been actually identified in relatively few tadpole tissues, it is fairly safe to assume that all of the many thyroid hormone–responsive tissues of the tadpole have such receptors. These tissues include skin, muscle, skeleton, the eye, the brain, the entire digestive tract, mouth parts, etc. In keeping with these facts, it has been found by use of sensitive measuring techniques that the metamorphic climax is preceded by a large surge of thyroid hormone levels in the blood of the tadpole.

How can we account for such a surge in thyroid hormone levels at the precise time when it must be coordinated with a normal developmental event? There is no complete explanation yet available, but we can assume that the hormonal surge is part of the genome-controlled sequence of changes in the developmental program of events. This program would have had to include synthesis of thyroid hormone receptor in time for all of the tadpole's tissues to become responsive to thyroid hormone. The same developmental program should dictate a later disappearance of thyroid hormone receptor in many of the same tissues, since they eventually lose their responsiveness to thyroid hormone.

SURVEY OF THE ENDOCRINE GLANDS

Figure 1.3 represents a summary of most, but not all, vertebrate hormone-secreting tissues. These endocrines are grouped, first of all, with respect to their relationship to the hypothalamus–pituitary–target organ system. Six glandular tissues, which secrete at least ten hormones, can be identified as having no primary or direct relationship to the hypothalamus–pituitary–target organ system. They are the parathyroids, ultimobranchials, gastrointestinal tract, pancreas, liver, and adrenal medulla. It is of interest that secretion of most of the ten hormones in this group is triggered by physical (osmotic pressure or hydrostatic pressure) signals or chemical (glucose or calcium concentrations) signals from the blood itself. The exceptions are the three gastrointestinal hormones whose secretion is triggered by the contents of the gut acting upon the gut wall more or less directly.

The hypothalamus–pituitary–target organ system is large and miscellaneous, but the three anatomical elements in it have a descending hierarchical relationship to each other. That is, the hypothalamus, which is part of the brain, regulates the pituitary by direct nervous connections or by secreting neurohormones whose receptors are located in the pituitary. The pituitary

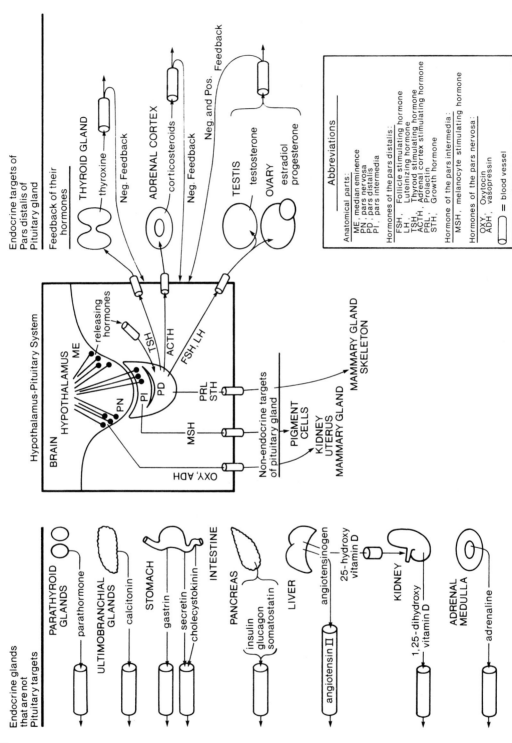

FIGURE 1.3. A summary of most of the hormonal integrators of the vertebrates, organized according to their relationship to the hypothalamo-hypophysial system.

6

then secretes hormones which, in their turn, affect the functions of a variety of target organs (see Fig. 1.3).

The hypothalamus has many other, purely nervous, functions aside from its endocrine regulatory actions. The endocrine actions are exerted in three different ways: (1) by direct secretion of neurohormones, like oxytocin and vasopressin, from the pars nervosa into the general circulation; (2) by direct innervation of the pars intermedia, thus regulating secretion of MSH (see also Fig. 1.4a); and (3) by secreting releasing hormones into short portal vessels in the median eminence, which carry these releasers to the pars distalis. Here the releasers modulate the secretion of the six pars distalis hormones (Fig. 1.4).

It should be noted that the targets of the hypothalamus–pituitary system can be divided into two groups: those that are themselves endocrine glands (thyroid, adrenal cortex, and gonads) and those that are not (kidney, uterus, pigment cells, mammary gland, skeleton). The endocrine targets secrete additional hormones, such as thyroxine or the sex steroids or corticosteroids, which have typical actions on a variety of further targets. However, an important property of thyroxine and the steroid hormones is that they act back upon the hypothalamo-pituitary axis, generally in a negative feedback sense (Fig. 1.3). The significance of the self-regulating brain–pituitary–endocrine feedback mechanisms is that they establish a series of endocrine balances. The details of these interlocked endocrine mechanisms will be dealt with in later sections.

The most important functional property made possible by linking pituitary functional regulation to the brain is that this now permits nervous control over a variety of endocrine functions. That is, certain external changes in temperature, light, odor, sound, or touch, acting through nervous sensory receptors, can be channeled through nervous pathways to the hypothalamus, and thus act upon the pituitary gland. Consequently, it is possible to link certain internal adjustments to environmental changes. Because these complex adaptive responses utilize both nervous and endocrine systems, they can be called neuroendocrine reflexes. Examples of three neuroendocrine reflexes follow.

TYPICAL NEUROENDOCRINE REFLEXES

The Suckling Response

Relatively simpler neuroendocrine reflex responses are those that do not involve the pars distalis. An example is the flow of milk from the mammary gland that is initiated when an infant first begins suckling at the nipple (Fig. 1.4b). At first there is no yield of milk. However, after an interval that is usually less than one minute, continued suckling results in a flow of milk through the nipple. Experimental analysis (to be given in more detail later)

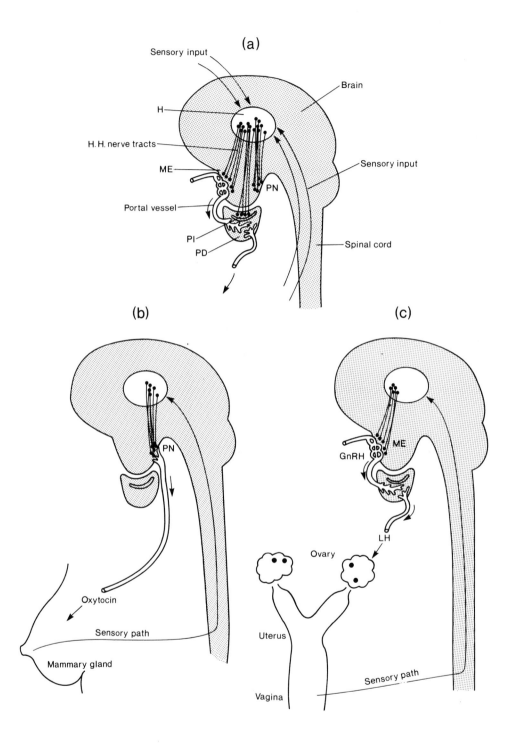

has shown that the first tactile stimuli at the nipple are led to the spinal cord via segmental nerves, and they ascend to the hypothalamus. In the preoptic area the oxytocin-synthesizing neurons are stimulated, and action potentials are propagated toward their endings in the pars nervosa. These secretory nerve endings terminate on blood vessels, and in this sense they differ from most other nerve endings, which terminate at a synapse on another nerve cell or upon an effector cell. A structure like the pars nervosa, where many neurosecretory neurons end upon blood vessels, is called a neurohaemal organ. At this point oxytocin is secreted from the neurosecretory neurons into the blood. When the oxytocin arrives (via the appropriate vascular channels) at the mammary gland, it interacts with receptors on contractile cells that surround the milk-filled alveoli; contraction of these cells initiates the phenomenon of "let-down" of milk. That is, the milk is forced out of the alveoli into the ducts that lead to the nipples. The nervous part of the reflex requires very little time. Most of the 10 to 30 seconds required is taken by the secretion of oxytocin in the pars nervosa, the distribution of the oxytocin by the blood until a physiologically effective concentration is achieved, the contraction of the mammary alveolar elements, and the movement of milk through the mammary ducts to the nipple and thus to the hungry consumer.

The Postcopulatory Ovulation Response in the Rabbit

In the sexually active female rabbit the ovary contains ripe eggs that are ready to be released (ovulate) from the follicular structures in which they form (Fig. 1.4c). They remain in this state until the female mates. Ten hours after copulation, ovulation occurs, and the eggs so released are moved into the oviduct, where spermatozoa by that time are waiting, and fertilization takes place.

In essence, the problem that must be solved by this admirably efficient physiological mechanism is linkage of the release of the egg to the act of copulation. The response is initiated by sensory (tactile) stimulation of the

FIGURE 1.4. Schematic representations of hypothalamo-pituitary regulation. (*a*) The hypothalamus (H) is the site of neuroendocrine integration and linkage of sensory information from the external (e.g., light, sound) and internal (e.g., chemical or physical changes in blood) environments with internal endocrine responses. After appropriate sensory-evoked stimulation, releasing hormones are carried by the hypothalamo-hypophysial (H.H.) nerve tracts to the median eminence (ME), where they are liberated into portal vessels, which carry the hormones to the pars distalis (PD) of the pituitary. Hypothalamic nerves also may end directly on pituitary cells of the pars intermedia (PI), or they may secrete hormones from the pars nervosa (PN) directly into the general circulation. (*b*) Neuroendocrine reflex of the suckling response of mammals. See explanation in text. (*c*) Neuroendocrine pathway of the postcopulatory ovulation response in the rabbit. See explanation in text.

vaginal and cervical surfaces. Such stimulation can be supplied artificially by experimental distention of the rabbit's vagina or by insertion of a glass rod. Local anesthesia of the vagina or cutting of the spinal nerves between the vagina and spinal cord can block the ovulatory response.

The train of nerve impulses, as in the previous illustration, rises in the spinal cord to the hypothalamus, where eventual stimulation of neurons synthesizing gonadotropin-releasing hormone occurs. These neurons extend to the median eminence, where they terminate upon blood sinusoids. Thus the median eminence, like the pars nervosa, is a neurohaemal structure. The sinusoids of the median eminence join to form portal vessels that extend the short distance to the pars distalis. The gonadotropin-releasing hormone (GnRH) interacts with plasma membrane receptors on the LH-secreting cells of the pars distalis. This evokes release of LH, one of whose actions, when it reaches the ovary, is to stimulate ovulation.

Photoperiodic Stimulation of Gonadal Development in Birds

Many vertebrates reproduce seasonally, and their gonads undergo appropriate annual cycles of growth and involution. In birds these cycles involve seemingly enormous fluctuations of over 1000-fold in the size of the testes, for example. For efficient reproduction the annual gonadal cycles must be regulated with sufficient precision so that all or most individuals in a population are in breeding condition at the same time, or else wastage of gametes, for lack of fertilization, would occur. Accordingly, we may ask how the gonad "knows," within narrow time limits, that the season for breeding is at hand, and how growth and ripening of gonads in different individuals, male and female, are so well coordinated that fertile union of gametes is assured.

The clue to the appropriate time of year for breeding, generally the spring, is taken from some cyclical, physical environmental feature. In many temperate-latitude birds this clue is the relative duration of daylight versus darkness during the 24-hour day. Thus, it is possible during the winter, when days are short, to expose birds with involuted testes to artificially lengthened days by the simple expedient of using electric lights. Such an artificial increase in the "photoperiod" results in a rapid increase in the size of the gonad.

Experimental analysis of gonadal stimulation by photoperiod manipulation has shown the following. The light is perceived by a brain photoreceptor (not necessarily the eye) and its *duration* is "measured" by a mechanism called a "biological clock," whose nature is unknown. If the photoperiod so measured is a stimulatory one, there is appropriate nervous activation of a hypothalamic GnRH center. The delivery of GnRH to the pars distalis by portal vessels from the median eminence results in FSH and LH release. These hormones then stimulate gonadal growth and gamete formation.

It should be noted that except for the difference in the nature of the sensory nervous part of the mechanism, the avian photoperiodic neuroendocrine reflex is very similar to that of the mating-evoked ovulation in the rabbit.

Thus a variety of sensory mechanisms, all leading eventually to the hypothalamic GnRH center, can be utilized to serve as triggers for endocrine-regulated reproduction in different vertebrate species. Reproduction is a highly adaptive process in evolution, and it is not surprising to find that there are so many kinds of environmental cues that are characteristically exploited to activate GnRH secretion in different vertebrates. In some species odorants (pheromones) are important in this respect, and in others temperature, auditory signals, or visual stimuli (aside from biological clock-measured photoperiod) affect GnRH release through different afferent pathways to the hypothalamus. These phenomena will be discussed further in Chapter 13.

MORPHOLOGY OF ENDOCRINE TISSUES

We have seen already that there is a large variety of hormone-secreting tissues, each keyed into a specific regulatory function. Common to all of these is the structural need for these tissues to have a rich blood supply and for the constituent gland cells to be located near a blood space. It is only through the blood that endocrine cells can fulfill their mission of chemical integration. Another common structural requirement for endocrine secretory cells is at least a limited hormone storage capacity. Hormones generally must be delivered at specific moments to perform their integrative functions and in amounts that may be greater than the cell could synthesize on demand.

Is there, then, any common feature of histological or cytological structure to serve these common requirements? Generally speaking, but with two exceptions, the histological structural pattern of endocrine organs is in the cell cord–sinusoid pattern. That is, the gland cells are arranged in cords that are no more than two cells thick, and adjacent cell cords are separated by enlarged blood capillary spaces called sinusoids (Fig. 1.5a). In this arrangement every cell makes contact with a blood space, permitting direct secretion of hormone into the blood.

One of the exceptions to the cell cord–sinusoid histological pattern is in the thyroid gland. Here the secretory cells are arranged in a single layer as a hollow sphere. The space in the center of the sphere (thyroid follicle) is filled with stored hormone. To give the secretory cells of the thyroid follicles access to the blood, an extremely dense basketlike pattern of blood capillaries invests each follicle (Fig. 1.6).

The other exceptional histological endocrine pattern is the neurohaemal

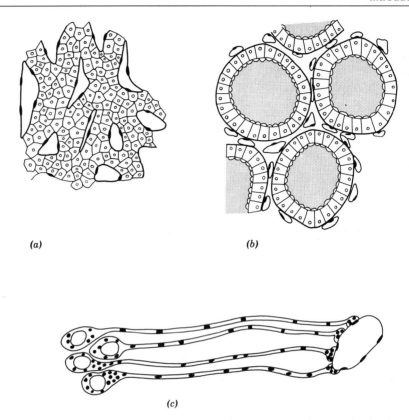

(a)   *(b)*

(c)

FIGURE 1.5. The three most common modes of histological organization of endocrine cells. In each type there is a different relation between the secretory cell and the blood channel into which its hormonal product is released. [From Gorbman and Bern, Wiley, New York, 1962.] *(a)* Cell cord-sinusoid, *(b)* Thyroid follicle, *(c)* Neurosecretory neurons.

one. Here the endings of neurosecretory cells are densely grouped upon the thin-walled blood sinusoids in such structures as the median eminence or pars nervosa.

Storage of peptide hormones in most endocrine cells is in secretory vesicles. Generally, at the electron microscopic level, cytological study shows that in peptide hormone-secreting cells these vesicles are formed in the Golgi apparatus. At times, when there is known to be a very high rate of hormone secretion, these vesicles become depleted in number. Steroid hormones also can be stored to some extent in the secretory cells as droplets. However, generally there seems to be less intracellular accumulation of steroid hormone droplets than of peptide hormone containing vesicles. Storage of hormone in thyroid follicles. as mentioned above, is in the center of the follicular space. Thus, the thyroid gland is the only one in which hormone may be stored in an extracellular position.

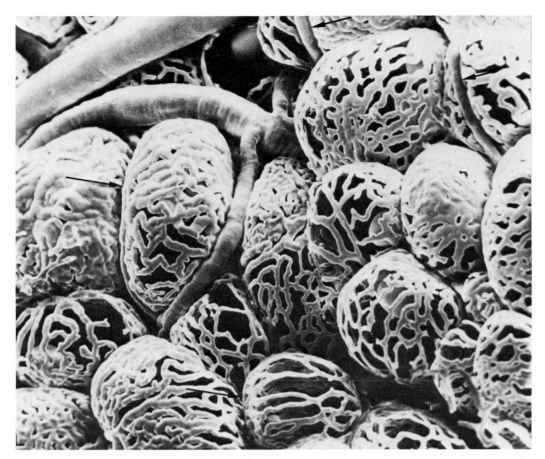

FIGURE 1.6. Scanning electron micrograph of the blood vessel patterns in the monkey thyroid gland. To prepare the tissue for this photograph, a plastic material was injected into the blood vessels. After hardening, all soft tissue was digested away. Only the plastic material remains to indicate where blood vessel spaces existed before. The casts of two larger vessels—one an arteriole and the other a venule—are at the upper left. The rounded units that fill most of the photo are casts of the basketwork of capillaries that surround individual thyroid follicles. On each follicle there is generally one distributing arteriole. Four such arterioles are indicated by arrows. The one at the left can be seen branching from a larger arteriole at its base. From the distributing arteriole capillaries extend in a parallel pattern, with anastomosing connections, to a collecting venule on the opposite side of the follicle. The venules, being shorter and irregular in shape, are not clear in this preparation. [Provided by Professor Hisao Fujita and Dr. Takuro Murakami from their research.]

THE CHEMICAL NATURE OF HORMONES

Since hormones are usually distributed throughout the organism in a mixture with other chemical substances (glucose, CO_2, ions, albumin, fatty acids), the hormone should have a unique molecular shape that can be discriminated exclusively by a specific target cell receptor. One way in which endocrine cells create the unique molecular shapes of hormones is by making chemical modifications of such commonly occurring biochemical substances as amino acids and lipid molecules. Still other endocrine cells synthesize uniquely shaped hormones by producing peptides or proteins containing unique sequences of amino acids. The resulting hormonal structures exhibit a wide range of sizes and complexities of shape. It must be kept in mind, however, that uniqueness of shape does not in itself identify a chemical as a hormone. In order for a unique molecule to qualify as a hormone, it must be delivered via the blood, and all or part of the specially shaped molecules must be able to associate with the specific receptor molecules of the hormonal target cells.

The smallest hormones are produced through chemical modifications of functional groups on amino acids or lipids. The production of the hormone norepinephrine from the amino acid tyrosine in the adrenal medulla is one example of this type of transformation (Fig. 1.7). Through several enzymatic steps, a carboxyl (COOH) group is removed from the amino acid tyrosine, and two hydroxyl (−OH) groups are added. These minor deletions and additions of functional groups to the amino acid result in a sufficient conformational change in the molecule so that the receptor in a target cell of the hormone can recognize norepinephrine as it occurs in the blood, and not confuse it with tyrosine or related molecules. Thus changes in blood concentrations of tyrosine, for example, during digestion of a protein meal and movement of amino acids into the blood will not interfere with the response of target cells to changes in the blood levels of the adrenal medulla's unique chemical signal, norepinephrine.

Synthesis of the hormone progesterone by the ovary is an example of how the widely distributed lipid cholesterol has been modified to produce a unique chemical messenger. Cholesterol is a steroid compound that can be supplied through the diet or synthesized from acetate in the organism. The differences in the chemical structures of cholesterol and progesterone are illustrated in Fig. 1.8*a*. The transformation of cholesterol to progeste-

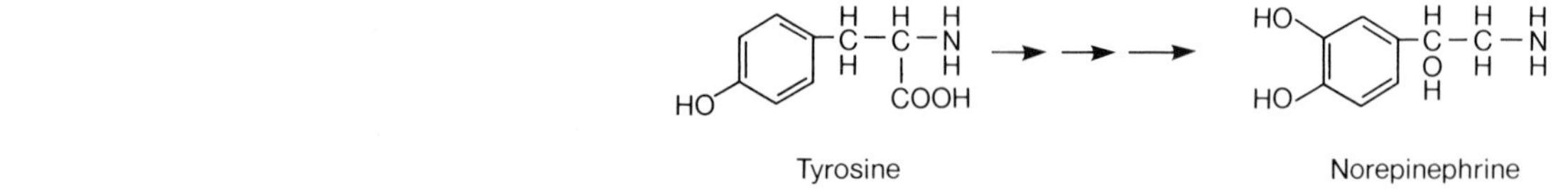

Tyrosine   Norepinephrine

FIGURE 1.7.   Structures of the amino acid tyrosine and the adrenal medullary hormone norepinephrine.

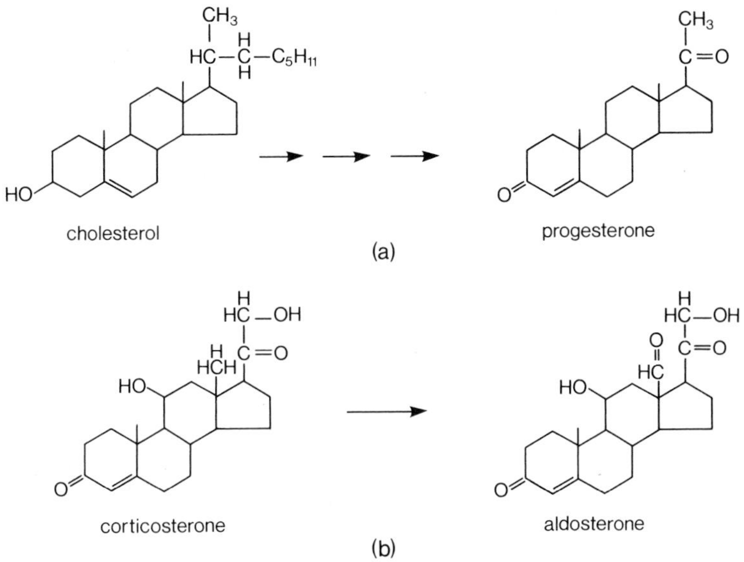

FIGURE 1.8. Structures of steroid molecules. (*a*) Transformation of cholesterol into the steroid hormone progesterone. (*b*) Conversion of corticosterone to aldosterone by oxidation of a methyl group.

rone is accomplished by the enzymatic removal of a six-carbon chain, addition of a keto group (=O), oxidation of a hydroxyl group (–OH), and the movement of a double bond. The relatively minor chemical modifications of cholesterol produce a specific conformational shape that can be recognized as unique among the circulating steroids by the receptor molecule in progesterone target cells.

The examples that we have so far outlined of structurally specialized hormonal compounds and their conformational shapes, which result in a unique "fit" with the receptor molecules of target organ cells are characteristic of all hormone–target cell interrelationships. The shape of the hormone dictates how well it will bind to the receptor. Appropriate binding of the hormone to the cellular receptor must precede the biological response of the target cells. Therefore, in essence, the three-dimensional structure of the hormone, together with the complementary structure of the cellular receptor, determines whether there will or will not be a physiological response of the tissue. This dependence of response on chemical structure of the hormone has been termed by endocrinologists as the "structure–function relationship." An especially striking case of how a structural modification can alter the function of a hormone is that of the steroid hormones corticosterone and aldosterone. These steroids, both produced by the adrenal cortex, differ only in the presence of a keto group (=O) on one carbon (Fig. 1.8*b*); yet they have distinct and separate physiological effects. Corticosterone is involved in carbohydrate metabolism, while aldosterone plays a major role in electrolyte and water metabolism. However, it is important to be aware that the specificity of a hormone binding to its receptor is not absolute. For example, if very large amounts of corticosterone are administered to an animal, the corticosterone will bind to aldosterone receptors and induce a response in target cells that normally respond only to aldosterone. This response is referred to as a "pharmacological effect" of corticosterone, since corticosterone is not normally present in the circulation at high enough concentration for significant binding to aldosterone receptors.

Larger and more complex hormones are synthesized by forming special sequences of amino acids to yield peptides and proteins. Ultimately, the unique conformations of protein hormones are determined by the physical forces that govern all protein structures. The most important element determining the final shape of peptide or protein hormones is the amino acid sequence, or "primary structure." In the tripeptide thyrotropin-releasing hormone (TRH), the sole determinant of the conformation of the molecule is the amino acid sequence, which is: pyro-Glu-His-Pro-NH_2. In larger hormones the three-dimensional structure can be influenced by additional factors. Amino acids in polypeptide chains can interact with each other and form α-helical segments. Other noncovalent interactions of particular amino acids that are far apart in a long peptide sequence can cause the chain to fold over upon itself. Disulfide bonds can be formed between two cysteine residues that may be variable distances apart in the primary sequence of the chain. In some large hormones two separate peptide chains may be linked together either through disulfide bonds, as in the case of insulin, or through weaker, noncovalent bonds, as in the pituitary glycoprotein hormones. Considering all the possible sequences and intramolecular interactions that can occur in proteins, it is obvious that an almost limitless number of unique conformational shapes can be made.

On the other hand, although many very different amino acid sequences of proteins are possible, the genetic mechanisms that determine these sequences have remained somewhat conservative in producing different hormones. Analysis of the amino acid sequences of protein hormones of various types and from different animal species shows that certain hormones share similar or identical sequences in certain regions of their peptide chains. Hormones that show such sequence homology can be grouped together into "hormone families" based on their molecular structural similarities. Such similarities indicate commonness of origin in the evolutionary sense. Inspection of the primary structures of the hormones secretin and glucagon (Fig. 1.9) reveals that the same amino acid is present at 14 of 27 positions in the two molecules. Although a 52% sequence homology might suggest that these two hormones share some physiological activities, in actuality the three-dimensional shapes of secretin and glucagon are quite different and, correspondingly, they have completely separate hormonal functions. Apparently, the amino acid differences at 13 positions in the sequence, along with two additional residues at the end of the glucagon chain, are sufficient

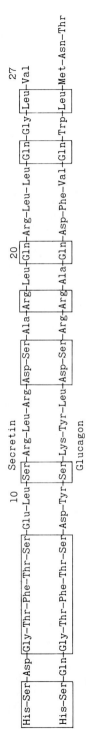

FIGURE 1.9 Amino acid sequences of secretin and glucagon. Rectangles enclose unvarying portions of the molecules.

to cause a significant change in molecular shape conformation. Other peptides that have been isolated from the gut or pancreas have varying lengths and show a degree of sequence homology with secretin and glucagon. These include the vasoactive intestinal peptide (VIP; 28 residues) and the hormone gastric inhibitory peptide (GIP; 43 residues). Since the discovery of these peptides and the deciphering of their amino acid sequences have been relatively recent, their status as hormones is not as well established (see Chapter 8). These peptides do not function like either secretin or glucagon because they do not interact with the same receptors. However, the high degree of sequence homology of these peptides would put them together in the same family with secretin and glucagon. Other families of peptide and protein hormones, are listed in Table 1.1. It should be noted that although there are differing degrees of relatedness among hormones within a family, there are no similarities between families. The fact that most peptide and protein hormones occur in families suggests that modification of existing hormones by amino acid substitution and variation of chain length is a common method by which endocrine cells create new hormones during the process of evolution. The modification of an existing hormone to form a molecule with a distinctly different conformation does not in itself create a new hormone. It must be kept in mind that the shape of the hormone must be such that it will bind with a receptor molecule in a target cell. Thus creation of a new hormone implies either that a receptor for it exists already or that a coinciding change takes place in a receptor molecule already present. In the absence of an appropriate receptor, the new peptide will have no function. There is at present no detailed information regarding the structures of receptor molecules. Therefore, little can be said about the mechanism of creating new receptors, or whether receptors for protein hormones also can be grouped into families.

With the availability of detailed information concerning peptide hormone sequences, it has been possible to synthesize in the laboratory both fragments of a hormone's peptide chain as well as hormone sequences in which only one or a few amino acids have been eliminated or substituted. These laboratory-synthesized peptide chains in which the amino acid sequence differs from that of the naturally occurring hormone at only one or a few positions in the chain are called hormone analogues. Subsequent tests of the biological activity of hormone fragments or analogues have revealed that some of the amino acids in the chain are more important than others for proper hormone action. For example, the pituitary hormone α-melanocyte-stimulating hormone (αMSH) is a peptide which in most animals in which it has been sequenced contains 13 amino acid residues. Biological tests of hormone activity of fragmentary sequences of αMSH show that generally smaller fragments have less biological activity. The smallest fragment that still has measurable activity consists of amino acids in positions 9 through 13 of αMSH. This pentapeptide (His-Phe-Arg-Trp-Gly) is also *essential* for biological activity since larger fragments of αMSH, which do not contain

TABLE 1.1. Hormone and peptide families based on amino acid sequence homologies

Prolactin
Growth hormone
Chorionic somatomammotropin (placental lactogen)

Luteinizing hormone
Follicle stimulating hormone
Thyroid stimulating hormone
Chorionic gonadotropin

Adrenocorticotropin
Melanocyte stimulating hormone
Lipotropin
Endorphin

Oxytocin
Vasopressin
Lysine vasopressin
Arginine vasotocin
Mesotocin
Isotocin
Glumitocin
Valitocin
Aspartocin

Secretin
Glucagon
Gastric inhibitory peptide
Vasoactive intestinal peptide

Cholecystokinin
Gastrin
Caerulein
Bombesin

Insulin
Somatomedin A
Somatomedin C
Insulinlike growth factors I, II
Relaxin

this sequence, have no activity. Accordingly, this sequence in αMSH is referred to as the "active site" of the hormone. Similar studies of the structure–function relationship of other peptide hormones have indicated that these hormones also contain portions or regions in their amino acid sequence that are particularly important for biological activity, in addition to portions that are relatively unimportant. The existence of active sites on peptide hormones implies that the receptor molecule in the target cell binds primarily to only a certain portion of the entire three-dimensional structure of the hormone. Apparently, the configuration of the amino acids making up the active site is the essential conformational shape recognized by the receptor.

Consequential to the evolution of hormone molecules, different vertebrate species show structural diversity of homologous hormones. For example, growth hormone from the pituitary gland of a cow contains a slightly different amino acid sequence than that of sheep growth hormone. Yet these structural differences are of minor significance since either growth hormone is capable of promoting growth in both animals. When the structures of growth hormones from mammals and fish are compared, one can see greater differences that affect the function of the hormone. While injections of mammalian growth hormone can induce growth of fish, injection of fish growth hormone into mammals is without effect. Evidently, the receptors for growth hormone in mammals do not recognize the growth hormone of fish. Comparison of the structures and actions of hormones among vertebrate species continues to be a challenge to comparative endocrinologists, a challenge that sometimes yields surprising results. For example, the hormone calcitonin from the ultimobranchial gland of salmon is approximately 50 times more potent in controlling calcium metabolism than is human calcitonin injected into humans. This has led to the clinical use of salmon calcitonin in treating certain bone diseases of humans (see Chapter 7). In general, however, more distantly related species are more likely to have greater structural and functional differences in their endocrine systems. This fact must be kept in mind when hormones from one animal are tested in an animal of a different species.

Our discussion of the chemical nature of hormones thus far has focused primarily on characteristics of those molecules that have been identified as hormones. However, we have included peptides extractable from blood or tissues that have not been proven to be hormones, but whose function as hormones is suspected since their structures place them in peptide families that include hormones. As has been pointed out, one essential property that a molecule must display to be assigned hormone status is the ability to bind to a receptor in a target cell as a normal physiological chemical mediator. Thus, this criterion is a functional one; it requires that the compound must behave like a hormone by entrainment in an intracellular system that eventually produces a typical response. The substances that endocrinologists call hormones must in a functional sense act as hormones, and at the same time it must be shown that they are naturally occurring biochemical substances. This distinction is important, since some naturally occurring compounds that were originally identified as hormones on a functional basis were later found to serve another physiological role in a different part of the organism. With current sensitive methods of detection and assay of hormonal substances in animal tissues, it has become apparent that at least the smaller hormones often are not limited in their origin and distribution to the classical endocrine organs and endocrine targets alone. Some of the small peptides that were originally isolated from endocrine glandular tissues have been found in minute amounts in neural tissues, and it is believed that these small peptides function here as neurotransmitters or neuromodulators, namely as chemical signals at nerve endings (Fig. 1.1). The idea that the same molecule can function both as a hormone and as a neurotransmitter is not new. It has long been known that the molecule norepinephrine functions as a hormone when it is released into the bloodstream by the adrenal medulla, but it functions as a neurotransmitter within the nervous system when it is released by a nerve ending into the synaptic cleft, the narrow space between the ends of nerve cells. Since it is clear that some small peptide hormones function as neurotransmitters in the nervous system, it would seem futile to insist on a rigid definition of a hormone based on its chemical nature alone.

HORMONOGENESIS

The major "responsibilities" of endocrine cells in the vertebrate organism include the synthesis, storage, and secretion of hormones into the blood in response to particular physiological signals. At any given time the relative effort that the endocrine cell devotes to these various processes will depend on the summation of the signals to either stimulate or inhibit production and release of hormone. Thus, depending on the demand, endocrine tissue can be described as either inactive or at some variable level of activity. Through the use of electron microscopy and sensitive biochemical methods, knowledge of the details of the cellular processes of synthesis, storage, and secretion at the ultrastructural and molecular levels has been greatly advanced. Here we will be concerned with a general view of the dynamic events of hormonogenesis. It has become evident that there are interesting differences in the ways some hormones are produced; the particulars of such differences will be considered in some of the following chapters.

The information for guiding synthesis of a peptide or protein hormone resides in the DNA code of the cell nucleus. It is of interest that the DNAs coding for several peptide hormones, including the human insulin gene, have been isolated and cloned by attaching them to the genome of the bacterial organism *E. coli*. The sequence of DNA nucleotides comprising the gene for the hormone is copied (transcription) into messenger RNA (mRNA). Subsequently, the mRNA molecules are transported out of the nucleus through nuclear pores and into the cytoplasm, where the mRNA associates with the endoplasmic reticulum (ER). The mRNA combines with both ribosomes and transfer RNA (tRNA) molecules, which bring the appropriate amino acids to be covalently linked to form the peptide molecule (translation). Translation of the nucleotide sequence into amino acid chains occurs on many small aggregates of ribosomes called polyribosomes. In electron microscopy the appearance of the ribosomes associated with the outer membranes of the ER is described as granular or rough ER (Figs. 1.10 and 1.11). During protein synthesis a single mRNA molecule is processed consecutively through each of the ribosomes in the aggregate. A peptide chain is

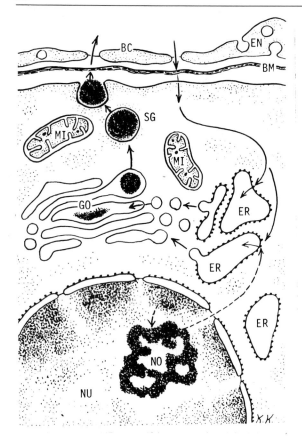

FIGURE 1.10. A diagrammatic representation of a possible mechanism of secretion of a protein hormone. Solid lines indicate the route of uptake of material (amino acids) for synthesis of hormone as well as outward transport of synthesized hormone. Broken lines indicate the route of chemical "information" for guiding eventual synthesis of the hormone from transcription of DNA to translation of mRNA. *NU*, nucleus; *NO*, nucleolus; *ER*, endoplasmic reticulum; *GO*, Golgi apparatus; *MI*, mitochondria; *SG*, hormone-containing secretory granule; *BM*, basement membrane; *BC*, edge of blood capillary; *EN*, endothelium. [From K. Kurosumi and H. Fujita, *An Atlas of Electron Micrographs. Functional Morphology of Endocrine Glands*, Igaku Shoin Ltd., Tokyo, 1974.]

then formed on each ribosome during the translation of the long mRNA molecule. Peptide chains accumulate in the cisternae between ER membranes and are transported to the Golgi apparatus in small, clear vesicles formed, apparently, from the ER membrane. Within the Golgi apparatus the hormonal molecules are concentrated in a manner that results in an increase in their density, as observed in the electron microscope. This condensed hormonal material is then surrounded by a membrane formed from the ends of the Golgi lamellae. The result is a membrane-bound, mature secretory or storage granule that can be retained in the cytoplasm of the cell until the signal for secretory release into the blood.

When the endocrine cells receive the appropriate signal, the secretory granule is moved to the periphery of the cell where the membranes of the granule and the cell fuse to release the contents of the granule into the extracellular space (Fig. 1.10). This process is called exocytosis or emiocytosis (literally meaning "cell vomiting"). Although the ultrastructural details of exocytosis have been well illustrated, the precise sequence of biochemical steps from the stimulus for secretion to the release of the granule

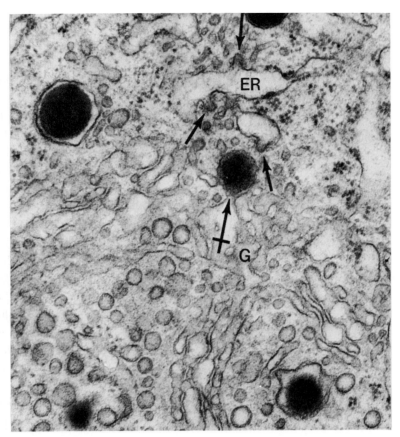

FIGURE 1.11. Electron micrograph of a portion of a growth hormone-secreting cell of a rat pituitary. Arrows indicate the formation of small vesicles from rough endoplasmic reticulum (*ER*). The crossed arrow indicates the formation of a small secretory granule from the Golgi apparatus (*G*). Note the membrane-bound secretory granule at the upper left. Magnification about 50,000. [From K. Kurosumi and H. Fujita, *An Atlas of Electron Micrographs. Functional Morphology of Endocrine Glands*, Igaku Shoin Ltd., Tokyo, 1974.]

contents (stimulation–secretion coupling) is still unclear. Overall, exocytosis is an energy dependent process requiring ATP. Microtubules and microfilaments appear to play roles in transporting secretory granules to the plasma membrane of the cell. In addition, exocytosis depends on an elevation of intracellular Ca^{2+} and production of cyclic nucleotides (cyclic adenosine monophosphate, cAMP, or cyclic guanosine monophosphate, cGMP). The end result of exocytosis is the release of hormone into extracellular spaces from where it is free to diffuse into the bloodstream. Although it is clear that exocytosis is the major means for release of protein hormones, it may not be the only one. There is some evidence that proteins may not necessarily have to be packaged into granules in order to be secreted; in some cases free hormone in the cytoplasm may cross the cell membrane by diffusion. This is particularly true of steroid hormones which, by their chemical nature, are soluble in the lipid environment of the cell membrane.

The biochemical events of synthesis, storage, and secretion of protein hormones have received increasing attention in recent years, and details of the complexity of these processes are beginning to emerge. Protein hormones are not directly synthesized in the form that is the most biologically active. In many cases a protein hormone is synthesized as part of a much larger amino acid chain, which is referred to as the precursor form or *prohormone*. An example of a prohormone is proinsulin (Fig. 1.12), which contains an additional amino acid chain connecting the two peptide chains of insulin. Prohormones can be many times larger than the hormone; they usually have little or no biological activity, since the additional peptide chains apparently interfere with the binding of the hormone sequence with the receptor molecule of the target organ. In most cases the nonhormonal part of the peptide chain is enzymatically cleaved off the prohormone during its transport and packaging within the endocrine cell; accordingly, the "mature" secretory granules contain primarily the most biologically active form of the hormone, which is also the secreted form. However, some hormones (angiotensin and gastrin, for instance) are secreted as prohormones, and high levels of the prohormone can be found circulating in the blood. These circulating prohormones are converted to the active form by extracellular enzymes in the blood.

There are probably many reasons for the synthesis of hormones in precursor forms. In the case of proinsulin, it is suspected that the connecting peptide (C peptide; Fig. 1.12) serves to bring the ends of the long peptide chain into the proper orientation to permit formation of the appropriate disulfide bonds. For other peptide hormones, the additional peptide chain of the prohormone may include small sugar molecules. These glycoprotein portions of the hormone may serve as signals to identify the hormone and

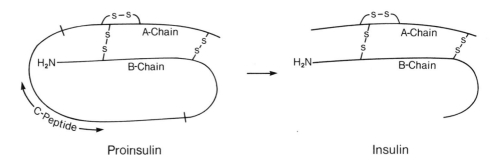

Proinsulin   Insulin

FIGURE 1.12. Diagrammatic representation of the conversion of proinsulin to insulin. A specific enzyme cleaves the single peptide chain at two places to remove the connecting peptide (C peptide). This yields the hormone insulin, which consists of two peptide chains linked by disulfide bonds.

to assure that it is transferred to the Golgi apparatus and packaged into secretion granules.

The mechanisms for the production and secretion of steroid hormones by the gonads and adrenal cortex differ from those of protein hormones. Steroidogenic cells have a well-developed endoplasmic reticulum (ER) that lacks ribosomes and is thus called smooth ER. Small amounts of rough ER can also be found among the elements of the smooth ER. Smooth ER sometimes is observed to be so folded as to form characteristic membranous whorls. Synthesis of cholesterol from acetate and transformation of cholesterol to cholesteryl ester, a storage form of cholesterol, are among the biochemical transformations that take place in smooth ER. Cholesterol is stored with lipids in cytoplasmic droplets probably formed by the Golgi apparatus or smooth ER. Another characteristic of steroidogenic cells is mitochondria with their inner membranes or cristae organized as tubules rather than as the lamellae seen in mitochondria of protein-secreting cells. It is within these tubular mitochondria that some of the steroid transformations take place. Additional enzymatic transformations of steroids occur in the smooth ER. Secretion of steroid hormones is generally believed to occur through simple diffusion of the hormone through the cell membrane and into the blood. However, recent studies of steroid-secreting cells have suggested that some steroid hormones may be released through exocytosis of granules. Steroidogenesis and its control will be discussed in greater detail in Chapter 11.

HORMONE TRANSPORT AND DISTRIBUTION

A distinguishing property of hormones is that they affect target organs at very low concentration. Accordingly, the normal levels of hormones circulating in the blood are low by comparison with other circulating organic compounds (Table 1.2). Even when an endocrine gland is maximally stimulated, the resulting hormonal concentration in the blood rarely achieves levels as high as nonhormonal organic compounds. The typical range of blood levels of insulin, for example, varies from .05 nM (10^{-10}moles/liter) in a fasting person to .5 nM after ingesting a large amount of glucose. It is important to note that, as for almost all other hormones, there is rarely a complete absence of insulin from the blood. Instead, the concentration of hormones is normally maintained at some resting or basal level. Insulin levels do not drop below this level in humans except in pathological states (some cases of diabetes mellitus) in which there is a defect in the ability of pancreatic β cells to produce the hormone.

Concentrations of hormones in blood are controlled by a balance of the rate of secretion by the endocrine gland and the rate of removal or clearance of the hormone from the blood. As we have mentioned, hormonal secretion is determined by the summation of all of the factors stimulating or inhibiting

TABLE 1.2. Comparison of normal concentrations of some organic substances and hormones in human blood[a]

Substance	Concentration (mM)
Glucose	5
Cholesterol	5
Albumin	0.7
Antibodies	0.09
High-density lipoprotein	0.013
Thyroxine	0.00009
Testosterone	0.00002
Insulin	0.00000005

[a] After Altman, P. L. In (1961) *Blood and Other Body Fluids* D. S. Dittmer ed.) *Fed. Am. Soc. Exp. Biol.* 540 pp. and (1979) *Methods of Hormone Radioimmunoassay*, 2nd ed. B. M. Jaffe and H. R. Behrman, eds.) Academic, New York, pp. 1005–1014.

the gland. Once the hormone is in the circulation, it can diffuse into the extracellular space from where it may be picked up by a target cell, combining with a receptor to exert its typical effect, or, alternately, it may be degraded by enzymes in the liver or some other tissue. Another possible fate of a circulating hormone is elimination in intact form through, for example, excretion by the kidney into the urine. The simultaneous ongoing of all these events determines the rate of blood clearance of hormones, which is usually rapid. The biological half-life (time required to clear one-half of the circulating concentration of a hormone from the blood) typically varies in mammals from a few minutes to a few hours. Consequently, in order to maintain a constant low level of hormone in the blood, an endocrine gland must maintain a basal level of secretory activity that equals the rate at which the hormone is cleared from the blood.

Although secreted hormones are diluted in the blood as they are carried throughout the vascular system to be distributed in peripheral tissues, there are some anatomical and biochemical adaptations that assure relatively high concentrations of hormones in certain localized areas of the body. Among these adaptations are portal vascular systems and hormone-binding proteins. The hypothalamo-hypophyseal portal system, for example, conveys releasing hormones from the hypothalamus to the pituitary (Fig. 1.3) before they can be diluted in the general circulation. This system guarantees a high, effective concentration of releasing hormones at the site of the responding pituitary cells. The concentration of releasing hormones in peripheral blood beyond the pituitary is extremely low not only because of dilution of the hormones in the bloodstream, but also because releasing hormones are quickly degraded enzymatically. Another of the factors regulating or influencing the distribution of hormones in the body are specific binding proteins in the blood as well as within the tissues. Generally, these binding proteins associate reversibly with small hormones that have low water solubility (i.e., thyroxine, steroids). Therefore, one of the functions of binding proteins may be to increase the hormonal capacity of the blood. The specific binding proteins in the blood also tend to sequester hormone in the vascular compartment. Bound hormones in blood plasma are not free to diffuse into the extracellular space where they can associate with receptor molecules in target tissue. Both hormone and carrier protein are in a state of reversible equilibrium in which only a small fraction of the hormone in blood is free. Thus, a gradient of hormone concentration is established, with relatively high levels in the blood, mostly protein-bound, and low levels in peripheral tissue. In one sense, binding proteins create a circulating storage pool of hormone. In the example of thyroxine binding to thyroid-binding globulin (TBG), about 99.9% of the total hormone in the blood is bound to carrier proteins, and the minute remaining fraction of the hormone is free to diffuse into the tissue. Yet, that small fraction is large enough to maintain the appropriate effect on target cell metabolism because the target cell hormone receptors are very sensitive to (i.e., they have a high affinity for) low concentrations of thyroxine. The large blood reservoir of thyroxine bound to TBG guarantees that an adequate and even amount of this important hormone will be maintained in the target tissues. Bound hormones are also protected from enzymatic degradation and excretion, and consequently have longer half-lives than hormones without carrier proteins in the blood. As free thyroxine is metabolically degraded or otherwise removed from the circulation, more thyroxine will dissociate from TBG to maintain the blood level of freely diffusible hormone.

Hormone-binding proteins may also play protective roles in situations where it is desirable to prevent the diffusion of the hormone into tissue where it may have a deleterious effect. During pregnancy in some mammals there is a striking increase in the circulating levels of many hormones, including thyroid and steroid hormones. These high levels of hormones are important in maintaining pregnancy, and they promote physiological preparation for lactation by the maternal organism. Diffusion of these high levels of thyroxine and steroids into the developing brain or across the placenta would have adverse effects on the mother or the developing fetus. Fortunately, during pregnancy there are corresponding increases in the blood concentration of both TBG and steroid-binding globulins. Association of the hormones with the high–molecular weight binding proteins minimizes the diffusion of hormones across the blood-brain barrier and placenta. As added protection, the fetus itself has a high level of a steroid (estrogen)–binding protein, α-fetoprotein, which prevents excessively high levels of the free hormone from interfering in the normal processes of fetal development and differentiation.

HORMONE ACTION

Hormone action entails all of the sequential and simultaneous biochemical steps from the binding of hormone to a cellular receptor to the final biochemical or physiological adjustment that is the outcome of the presence of the particular hormone in sufficient amount. As a result of intense research in recent years, study of receptors and the mechanisms of hormone action has emerged as a rapidly growing subdiscipline of endocrinology entering the realms of biochemistry and cell and molecular biology. The importance of hormone receptors in any general consideration of endocrine physiology lies in the fact that tissues that have specific hormone receptors become, almost by definition, the targets of that hormone. In a more dynamic sense, it is now apparent that the number of hormone receptors available to bind to the hormone can vary over time in any given tissue. Hence the capacity of a tissue to respond (be "sensitive") to the hormone must be taken into account, along with changes in blood concentration of hormone, in order to fully understand endocrine control of a physiological process.

Hormone receptor molecules are high-molecular weight proteins that are found associated with the cellular plasma membrane or within the cytoplasm of the target cell. In general, peptide hormones bind to receptors on the surface of a target cell, whereas smaller molecules (steroids), which can pass through the cell membrane, bind with receptors in the cytoplasm. The structural conformation of the binding site on the receptor and the complementary three-dimensional structure of the hormone dictate whether binding will be very specific for one hormone and whether the binding will also be of high affinity. High affinity between receptor and hormone assures that the low concentrations of hormone present in the extracellular spaces will result in adequate binding to produce a response in the target cells. It is generally assumed that the process of a hormone binding to a receptor produces a conformational change in the receptor, which is then activated to initiate the target cell response. Theoretically, the activation of a receptor by hormone binding is analogous to the activation of enzymes by enzyme cofactors or substrates in enzyme-mediated biochemical transformations.

Once the receptor is activated by binding of hormone, a series of biochemical sequelae unfold. Primary events can be categorized into those involved with nuclear phenomena, such as activation of transcription of DNA to yield mRNA, and those concerned with cytoplasmic changes, such as altering transport and permeability.

Steroid hormone action is typical of those hormones that primarily affect the cell nucleus (Fig. 1.13). After steroid binding and activation of the cytoplasmic receptor, the hormone–receptor complex is translocated into the nucleus by a characteristically temperature-dependent process. Once the complex is in the nucleus, it binds to chromatin and activates RNA polymerase. This is followed by a copying of a specific DNA region that contains the code for the sequence of amino acids comprising a specific

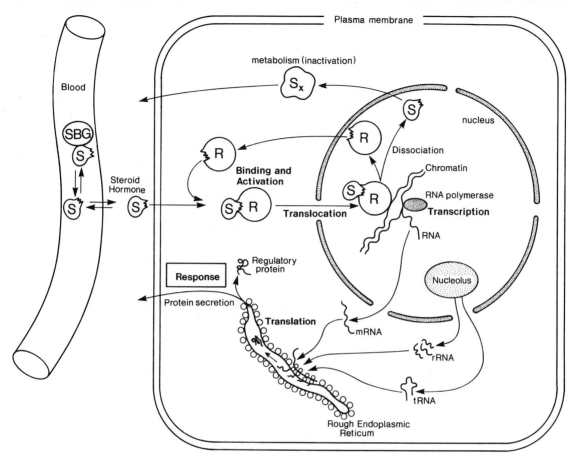

FIGURE 1.13. Schematic diagram of the mechanism of action of steroid hormones. Steroid hormone (*S*), which has dissociated from steroid-binding globulins (*SBG*) in the blood, is free to diffuse into the cell. The steroid binds to a receptor (*R*), resulting in activation and transport of the complex into the nucleus, where it activates transcription. Subsequently, the steroid dissociates from the receptor, leaves the nucleus, and is metabolized to an inactive form (*Sx*). See text for additional description.

protein. This process of transcription is a remarkable coordination of events within the nucleus. The hormone–receptor complex must recognize the specific site on the large DNA molecules that contains the gene for a particular protein and, at the same time, activate the RNA polymerase to initiate transcription of the gene. Once a completed mRNA molecule is produced, the RNA polymerase must return to the initiation site so that many mRNA copies can be produced. The molecular mechanism of transcription is not yet fully understood, although several models of this mechanism have been proposed. In addition to promoting transcription, the steroid–receptor complex may also increase the production of ribosomal and transfer RNA, although this function may be among the secondary responses of the nucleus. The newly formed mRNA is transported out of the nucleus to the rough ER where it participates in protein synthesis. The newly synthesized protein is either incorporated into cellular components, used to activate an intracellular regulatory protein, or it is secreted by the cell. The hormone–receptor complex may remain in the nucleus and exert its effects for several hours before it dissociates and reenters the cytoplasm. The steroid is metabolized to an inactive form and subsequently diffuses out of the cell. The receptor also may be metabolized, or, alternatively, it may recombine with another steroid molecule, become reactivated, and return to the nucleus.

The primary actions of most peptide hormones (and neurotransmitters, incidentally) concern cytoplasmic or cell membrane alterations that are involved with transport and permeability processes (Fig. 1.14). The peptide hormones are hydrophilic, and often they are large molecules that do not readily cross the lipid bilayer of the target cell membrane. Consequently, receptors for peptide hormones are located on the outer side of the cell

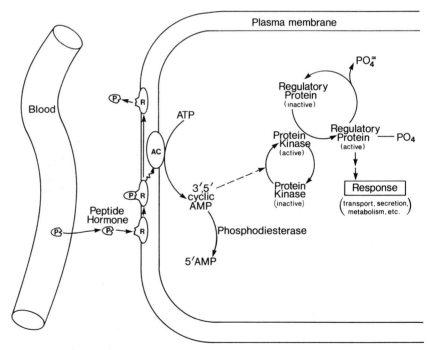

FIGURE 1.14. Schematic diagram of the mechanism of action of a peptide hormone. The peptide hormone (P) diffuses from the blood to the cell plasma membrane where it combines with a membrane receptor (R). The hormone–receptor complex activates the enzyme adenyl cyclase (AC), which converts ATP to $3',5'$ cyclic AMP. Cyclic AMP (cAMP) initiates a sequence of enzyme and regulatory protein activations that produce the cell response. Phosphodiesterase catalyzes the further metabolism of cAMP and removes it from the activating system. Further explanation in the text.

membrane, exposed to the extracellular space. These receptors are also large–molecular weight proteins (10^5 daltons) that appear to be integral parts of the cell membrane, since they can be removed from it only if detergents are used to dissolve the membrane. Peptide hormones diffuse out of the blood and into the extracellular space where they may bind with receptors on target cell membranes. As with steroid hormone receptors, the receptors for peptides show high specificity and affinity for a particular hormone. Once binding is achieved, the receptor is activated in some manner and initiates the function of a closely associated membrane component, the enzyme adenyl cyclase. The catalytic active site of adenyl cyclase faces the interior of the cell, while the hormone binding site of the receptor is on the external surface of the target cell. Thus the hormone can exert its effect on adenyl cyclase through the receptor without entering the cell. In fact, it has been shown that if peptide hormones are exposed to target cells while attached to large Sepharose beads (to eliminate any possibility of their entering the cell), the hormone retains the capacity to bind to the receptor and activate adenyl cyclase. Once activated, adenyl cyclase converts adenosine triphosphate (ATP) into cyclic adenosine -3′,5′-monophosphate (cAMP), a reaction that requires Mg^{2+} or, in some cases, Mn^{2+}. As cAMP accumulates in the cell, it converts a cytoplasmic phosphorylating enzyme, protein kinase, from an inactive form. Protein kinase then goes on to add a phosphate to a regulatory protein, which subsequently induces the appropriate biochemical response of the target cell. When blood levels of the hormone decrease, the amount of hormone binding to receptors falls, adenyl cyclase activity declines, cAMP is degraded to 5′AMP, the protein kinase and regulatory proteins revert to their inactive form, and the particular response of the target cell is no longer expressed.

This has been called the "second messenger" mechanism of peptide hormone action. The hormone constitutes the first message delivered to the cell, while cyclic AMP is the second messenger instructing the cell to respond. This mechanism of action appears to be essentially the same for all peptide hormones. However, there are some minor differences with certain hormones and their target cells. Some hormones (e.g., insulin, growth hormone) elevate intracellular concentrations of cyclic guanosine monophosphate (GMP) rather than cyclic AMP. Other hormones (and particularly neurotransmitters) stimulate the entry of Ca^{2+} into the target cell. In these cases, however, the basic mechanism, as shown in Fig. 1.14, is similar, since both cyclic GMP and Ca^{2+} can act as second messengers and activate appropriate protein kinases to regulate protein phosphorylation and dephosphorylation. An interesting aspect of this model of hormone action is the fact that many different target cells respond to different hormones by producing the same cytoplasmic chemical (e.g., cyclic AMP). This is substantiated by experiments in which the normal hormonal response of the target cell can be mimicked by adding cyclic AMP to cells without adding the hormone. Evidently, the specificity of the cell's response to a hormone depends on the presence of a hormone receptor that will bind the hormone and elevate the intracellular concentration of a second messenger.

Although the schemes for steroid and peptide hormone action have been divided for the purpose of our discussion, these two classes of hormones regulate cell processes in an integrated fashion. Steroid hormones may control the synthesis of regulatory proteins and second messenger dependent protein kinases. Steroids may also regulate the production of peptide hormone receptors and thereby determine whether or not the cell may respond to a peptide hormone. On the other hand, peptide hormones can regulate the general levels of cell metabolism and the rates of synthesis of cell products that are dependent on steroid hormones. In many endocrine-regulated processes the target cells are responsive to several hormones, and it must be kept in mind that changes in the nucleus occur simultaneously with cytoplasmic changes. As more of the details of mechanisms of hormone action become known, we gain a better understanding of how different hormones coordinate the diverse biological responses of cells. Examples of the molecular events of hormone interactions and variations of the two basic mechanisms we have discussed will be presented in later chapters.

One of the most important means of controlling the responsiveness of hormonal target cells is regulation of the number of receptors in the cell. Cells typically contain 10^3 to 10^5 receptors per cell either in the plasma membrane or cytoplasm. This may sound like a large number of receptors, but this amount represents only about 1% of all of the proteins in a cell membrane. The number of receptors in a cell may be controlled by genetic factors, other hormones, or the circulating levels of the receptors' own hormone. There is a deficiency in number of insulin receptors in hormone tissues of a genetic strain (ob/ob) of mice. These mice are both hyperglycemic and obese as a consequence of the tissues' insulin insensitivity. Evidently, there is a genetic defect in such mice that blocks the normal expression of factors governing synthesis of insulin receptors. Insulin can regulate the number of its own receptors (autoregulation) in several responsive tissues. If, for example, fat cells are cultured with insulin, the number of insulin receptors is decreased from the level found in fat cells cultured without the hormone. This property of a hormone to reduce its receptors in target tissues has been termed "down regulation." In addition to regulation of the total number of receptors, the control of tissue responsiveness may also involve the affinity of the receptor. Experimental evidence suggests that treatment of some tissues with glucocorticoid steroid hormones will reduce insulin receptor affinity, so that insulin will less readily bind to its receptor.

ENDOCRINE FACTORS IN ADAPTATION AND EVOLUTION

The study of comparative endocrinology provides the basis for an understanding of the adaptiveness of hormonal control in a wide variety of species. Although the structures of hormones show some variation among vertebrates, overall they are remarkably similar and, in some cases, identical. The comparative anatomy of endocrine glands also shares a fairly conservative evolution, so that it can be said that generally the same or very similar hormones are produced by corresponding glands of different vertebrates. Despite the general similarities, hormones do many different things in different vertebrates. The diverse functions of the pituitary hormone prolactin is perhaps one of the most extreme examples. Prolactin has nearly a hundred clearly recognized functions ranging from control of ion exchange in fish gills to regulation of milk production in mammary glands (Chapter 4). Obviously, since prolactin and most of the other vertebrate hormones appear to have preceded the evolution of modern vertebrates, it follows that the endocrine system has not evolved as much as the capacity of tissues to respond to hormones. A prominent endocrinologist has summarized this situation in the statement, "It is not the hormones that evolve, but the uses to which they are put." Consequently, during evolution tissues that are to come under hormonal control must start producing hormonal receptors in sufficient number. Moreover, these receptors must be functionally linked to the intracellular machinery (e.g., adenyl cyclase, RNA polymerase) that regulates biochemical processes in the cell. The large number of uses to which prolactin has been put in vertebrates indicates that tissues have frequently become responsive to this hormone during evolution. Nothing is known about the molecular mechanisms that are responsible for evolving a cell's capacity to respond to a hormone, although we may surmise that derepression of the genes coding for the particular protein hormone receptor must be involved. Hopefully, comparative studies of hormone action will provide further perspective and understanding of this phenomenon.

HISTORICAL BACKGROUND

Although it can be argued that certain endocrinological concepts originated in ancient Greece, what has developed to the present day as the field of endocrinology has its direct roots in the latter half of the 19th century. The relative youth of this field may be judged from the fact that Starling introduced the word "hormone" in 1905; the term "endocrinology" was not in widespread use until about 1920. The growth of the discipline of endocrinology accelerated through the first half of this century. During the last several decades the field has experienced an explosive growth, so that the concerns of endocrinologists are widely intertwined with other disciplines ranging from biochemistry and molecular biology to behavior and ecology. Looking back, one can see certain key discoveries and general trends that have contributed to the development of endocrinology.

Hippocrates' concept of "humoralism" has been suggested as the first idea that shares some theoretical relationship with endocrinology. Hippocrates (about 400 B.C.) believed that various tissues of the body produced the four "humors": blood, phlegm, black bile, and yellow bile, and that a proper balance of these body fluids was necessary for good health. Humoralism shares with modern endocrine theory the tenet that fluids of the body have an important function. However, it is difficult to say whether Hippocrates' hypothesis had much influence on the thinking of early pioneers in endocrinology. At about the same time in Greece, Aristotle accurately described the effects of castration in men and birds; but nowhere in his description was there any suggestion that the observed effects were due to a lack of blood-borne factor from the testes. It was not until 1775 that Bordeu, in France, suggested that the testes supplied some substance to the blood that was responsible for mating behavior and aggressiveness. Castration removed the source of this substance, and the behaviors were not observed in such animals. Experimental evidence for this idea was provided by Berthold, a German physician, in 1849. Berthold showed that reimplantation of the testis into the body cavity of a castrated rooster reversed the atrophy of the bird's comb. However, this discovery had no impact at the time, since Berthold's valid demonstration of an endocrine function for the testis was ignored for over 50 years. Meanwhile, the foundations of endocrinology were being laid seemingly without benefit either from Berthold's work or Hippocrates' humoral hypothesis.

The French physiologist, Claude Bernard (ca. 1850), introduced the concept of internal secretion based on experiments showing that an organ modifies the chemical composition of the blood that passes through it. He showed, for example, that the liver can release sugar directly into the blood. Although he did no experimental work with hormones, he clearly established a physiological principle basic to endocrinology, as well as the somewhat overworked term "milieu intérieur."

Perhaps the most significant events that stimulated interest in the early development of the field were those surrounding the French physician Brown-Séquard (ca. 1880). While in his seventies, Brown-Séquard attempted to "rejuvenate" himself by giving himself injections of a glycerin extract of animal testes. He claimed the extract contained a substance that produced anatomic, neuromuscular, and metabolic alterations and increased vigor. Although injection of testicular androgen might result in some of these alterations in a human, we now know it is doubtful that Brown-Séquard's extract contained any active substance, and his reported rejuvenation was probably more a result of his imagination than of a hormone in the testicular extract. In any event, Brown-Séquard's claims aroused both the public and the scientific community and focused attention on the biological phenomena that were to become the concerns of endocrinology. It is ironic that the ideas of ancient Greece or Berthold's valid work had less impact than Brown-Séquard's sensationalism.

Much of the early work in endocrinology was of a descriptive nature. Although many of the endocrine glands had been described by anatomists, their functions were not understood. Likewise, many endocrine-related diseases had been described without knowledge of their nature. For example,

Celsus provided a clinical description of diabetes about 10 A.D.; goitrous cretinism was described by Paracelsus in 1526 A.D. The first experimental demonstration of an endocrine basis for diabetes was provided by von Mering and Minkowsky (1889), who reproduced the symptoms (excretion of sugar in the urine) of the disease in a dog after surgical removal of the animal's pancreas. Other significant discoveries in endocrinology to occur before the turn of the century include: substitution therapy using extracts of animal thyroids for human hypothyroidism (Murry, 1891) and the demonstration of pressor activity of adrenal medullary extracts by Syzmonowicz and Cybulski, and by Oliver and Schafer in 1895.

The early part of the 20th century was marked by Bayliss and Starling's excellent series of experiments (1902–1905) demonstrating the hormone secretin by which the duodenum controls the release of pancreatic juices. Gundernatsch accelerated the metamorphosis of tadpoles into frogs by treating them with thyroid tissue in 1912. Banting and Best isolated insulin from dog pancreas in the early 1920's. These and most other studies at this time were principally concerned with crude or partially purified extracts of endocrine glands. Significant advances were achieved when highly purified preparations could be obtained and the structures of hormones could be determined. Takamine and Aldrich, independently, were the first to prepare a crystalline form of the hormone epinephrine (adrenaline) in 1901. Kendall crystallized thyroxine in 1914, and Harrington determined the chemical structure of thyroxine in 1926. The isolation and chemical characterization of steroid hormones occurred for the most part during the 1930's. The more complex peptide and protein hormones were first purified and sequenced in the 1940s and 1950s. The identification and laboratory synthesis of peptide hormones continues today as more sensitive techniques for detecting hormones become available, and the list of hormones and hormone candidates grows. The identification of the chemical nature of hormones and subsequent widespread availability of purified hormone for investigators' experimental use has been a significant stimulus to the advancement of endocrinology during the last several decades. Perhaps the most significant advance in recent times has been the isolation of hormone receptors and the beginning elucidation of the mechanisms of hormone action during the last 10 to 15 years.

BASIC METHODS IN ENDOCRINOLOGY

The rate of development of any field of science frequently is limited by the available methods and techniques of experimentation. Often in endocrinology the introduction of new and particularly powerful laboratory methods has resulted in quantum leaps in experimental design, the amount and type of information gained, and, subsequently, the understanding of endocrine function. Thus, the types of scientific questions that can be asked are dependent, at least in part, on the techniques that are available to the investigator. A broad knowledge of endocrine methodology is also important for the evaluation of information collected by use of different techniques. Some techniques provide more reliable data than others, and this must be kept in mind when judging conflicting information. In this section we shall outline some of the basic methods in endocrinology, including both the classical techniques, which are still used by comparative endocrinologists in particular, and some of the modern methods whose use has permitted the remarkable advances in endocrinology in recent years. Certainly, the most classical approach, used to establish the endocrine function of an organ, involves surgical removal of the investigated organ, observation of the consequences, followed by replacement therapy. After determining the physiological effects of removing the organ, crude extracts of the organ are injected into the animal in an attempt to reverse the physiological changes. This procedure often is followed by successive purifications of the extracts until the hormone is sufficiently pure for its structure to be chemically identified. This technique of replacement therapy after surgical excision is a qualitative method that was used to identify most of the major endocrine organs during the early development of the field. Other primarily qualitative methods involve the use of morphological techniques. Histology of endocrine tissues has relied in part on the use of selective stains for certain cell types. Because of the chemical nature of hormones in storage granules, certain endocrine cells preferentially take up particular stains. By use of the Masson trichrome stain, the prolactin cells of the pituitary are stained red, while gonadotropin or thyrotropin cells take on a blue color. These differential staining methods have been superseded in recent years by the technique of immunohistochemistry, a procedure that combines histology and immunology. As a prerequisite to performing this technique, one must prepare an antiserum that contains antibodies directed against the hormone of interest. Obviously, this technique could not be used in the early phases of endocrine research because it requires the purified hormone for injection. For example, purified rat prolactin may be injected subcutaneously into a rabbit. Over the course of about four to six weeks, the rabbit's immune system responds to the presence of rat prolactin in its circulation, as it would to most other foreign peptide substances (i.e., chemically different from rabbit prolactin), and generates antibodies against the rat prolactin. At this time blood is collected from the rabbit, and if one is fortunate, the serum should contain a high concentration of rabbit anti-rat prolactin antibodies. This procedure for obtaining antiserum to a hormone is also used for developing a hormone radioimmunoassay, which we will describe shortly.

In order to visualize the microscopic distribution in tissue of an antibody, a dye or fluorescent compound can be chemically attached to the antibody. In carrying out this procedure (immunocytochemistry), the tissue suspected of containing the hormone of interest is fixed and sectioned by routine histological procedures. The tissue sections, mounted on a glass slide, are exposed to the chemically-tagged hormonal antisera, allowing the antibodies to attach to any structures in the tissue that contain the hormone. The greatest usefulness of this technique is in detection of very small accumulations of hormones in tissue and in showing in which cells, or even parts of cells, they are located. The most difficult and controversial aspect of the use of immunocytochemistry is in proving that the immunoreaction seen in the tissue sections represents only the hormone of interest, and not some nonspecific cross-reactive substance. Frequently, antisera contain antibodies against not only the hormone in question, but also other components that can be found in biological samples. Thus any procedure using antisera can sometimes give (and often does give) misleading results, and unless the procedure is thoroughly validated, the results must be interpreted with caution.

Other morphological techniques used by endocrinologists include both transmission and scanning electron microscopy, which allow the examination of hormone-producing cells and target tissues at the ultrastructural level. Conclusions concerning the functional state of an endocrine cell can be based on such ultrastructural evidence as the number of secretory granules or mitochondria, the development of the Golgi apparatus, and the proportion of the cell volume taken up by rough or smooth ER. These morphological methods provide valuable qualitative information and are particularly powerful tools when used in conjunction with quantitative biochemical methods.

Of the quantitative methods used by endocrinologists, biological assays played a major role during the last 50 years, and are still in use, particularly in comparative studies. The basis of a bioassay relies on the measurement of an animal's physiological response to a hormone. For example, in one of the bioassays for follicle-stimulating hormone (FSH), immature or hypophysectomized female mice are injected with a sample containing an unknown quantity of FSH several times daily for three days. At the end of the injections the mice are killed, their ovaries are removed and weighed. The weight gain by the ovaries will be in proportion to the content of FSH in the tested material (i.e., blood or tissue extract). The ovarian weight gain in response to an unknown can be compared with the response obtained using a known amount of purified FSH, thus "standardizing" the assay. Sexually immature or hypophysectomized mice must be used in this bioassay so that endogenous FSH from the test mouse's pituitary will not materially interfere with the action of the injected FSH. Although FSH has other actions in addition to ovarian augmentation, ovarian weight gain is used as the endpoint in this particular bioassay, since it is convenient to measure. An advantage of a bioassay is that it measures only the biologically active form of the hormone, not some inactive form (chemically modified hormone) that may be present in the sample. A serious disadvantage of a bioassay is specificity, since other hormones may be present in a sample to be tested.

Also, these bioassays are relatively laborious, expensive to perform, and not sensitive enough to measure the small quantities of hormone in the blood.

The most significant methodological innovation in recent years has been the development of radioimmunoassays (RIA) and related techniques, which allow precise measurement of hormone concentration in small quantities of serum or plasma. The ability to measure circulating levels of hormones, both free and bound, and thereby to determine the amount of hormone available to tissue hormonal receptors, has been of great importance in advancing the development of endocrine concepts. Since the first development of an RIA for insulin by Berson and Yalow in the late 1950s and early 1960s, the technique has been adapted to measure low concentrations of over one hundred hormones and other organic compounds of interest to endocrinologists.

A prerequisite starting material for developing an RIA is a sufficient supply of purified hormone. This is used (1) for generating antisera (see immunohistochemistry technique above), (2) as the basis for labeling some of the hormone with a radioisotope, and (3) for competition with the labeled hormone in constructing a ''standard curve.'' Radiolabeled hormone is usually prepared by reaction with radioactive iodine (^{125}I), which will ''label'' the molecule by adding to tyrosine residues of the peptide or protein

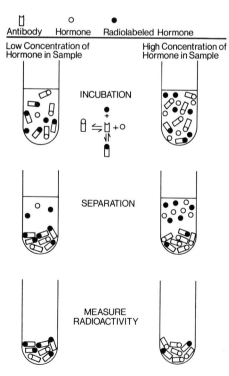

FIGURE 1.15. Diagram of the principal steps in the radioimmunoassay (RIA) procedure. Antiserum containing antibodies to the hormone is added to test tubes containing radiolabeled (radioactive) hormone and known or unknown amounts of unlabeled hormone. This mixture is incubated to allow hormone and antibody to come to binding equilibrium. Antibody-bound and free hormones are separated. The amount of radioactivity bound to antibody is determined. Note that a greater amount of radiolabeled hormone is bound in the tube that contained a small amount of hormone (*left*).

hormone, or by incorporating radioactive tritium (^3H) as the label into a steroid hormone. The basic principle of the assay depends on the competition between radiolabeled and unlabeled hormone for combination with the antibody. A basic assumption is that the antibody will bind equally well to either the labeled or unlabeled hormone. The procedure is best described diagrammatically (Fig. 1.15) with an example of a thyroxine RIA. A reaction mixture containing the sample antiserum (containing thyroxine antibody) and a particular amount of labeled hormone in a buffer solution is prepared; the unlabeled pure hormone is added and allowed to incubate for a sufficient time (usually several hours) to allow the competition between labeled and unlabeled hormone to come to equilibrium. The amounts of antiserum and labeled hormone are kept constant in all assay tubes, while the measured amounts of unlabeled hormone in each tube are varied. When a series of known amounts of unlabeled hormone is used in the competitions, it is possible to construct a standard curve (Fig. 1.16). In tubes containing larger amounts of unlabeled hormone, at equilibrium only a small proportion of labeled hormone will be bound to the antibody. Conversely, when the tubes contain little added known unlabeled hormone, a correspondingly larger proportion of labeled hormone will be bound to antibody at equilibrium. Once binding equilibrium is reached, the antibody-bound and unbound frac-

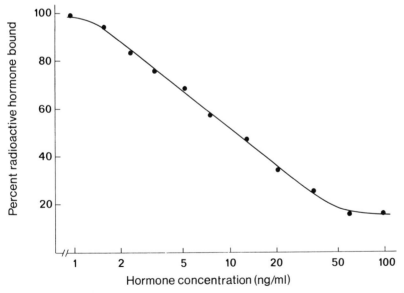

FIGURE 1.16. Representation of a standard RIA curve. As the known concentration of unradioactive hormone increases, the amount of bound radioactive hormone decreases. When a sample containing an unknown amount of hormone is processed through the assay, the amount of radioactivity bound will be measured. The concentration of the hormone in the sample can then be determined using the standard curve by noting what amount of pure, unlabeled hormone will yield a similar radioactivity measurement.

tions are separated by various methods. In the example of the thyroxine RIA a general protein precipitant, saturated ammonium sulfate ($(NH_4)_2SO_4$), is used for this purpose. While free thyroxine is soluble in the presence of $(NH_4)_2SO_4$, thyroxine bound to the antibody is precipitated along with the protein antibody. At this point the assay tubes are centrifuged, bringing the precipitate to the bottom of the tube. The supernatant, containing unbound hormone, is poured off, and the amount of radioactivity remaining in the pellet is determined. The standard curve resulting from these procedures shows the amounts of radioactive hormone bound to antibody in the presence of various known amounts of pure hormone. Once the standard curve is available, "unknowns," such as blood serum samples, can be tested in the same system. The amount of radioactivity in the pellet from an unknown sample is compared with that from the standard curve to determine the corresponding amount of hormone in the sample. Procedures for hormones other than thyroxine vary, particularly in the method of separating bound from free hormone, although the principle is the same.

The greatest advantages of RIA are its sensitivity and precision. A typical RIA for estrogen can be used to measure picogram (10^{-12} gram) quantities of the hormone. This amount represents about one-millionth of the quantity of estrogen in a birth control pill. The normal range of estrogen in a human female ranges from 100 to 800 pg/ml of blood. These assays are also easy to perform, inexpensive, and can be used to measure hormone levels in a large number of samples. However, as we have discussed with regard to immunohistochemistry, there is always a possibility that the antibodies may react with some chemical other than the hormone of interest. Since non-specific cross-reactivity may give misleading results, the investigator is obliged to perform a variety of "control" procedures to be reasonably certain that the RIA is valid.

The need for an appreciable amount of purified hormone to be used for generating antisera and for conducting the RIA is rather limiting to comparative endocrinologists. Although purified hormones and antisera are available for most hormones found in humans and laboratory animals, only a few peptide and protein hormones of nonmammalian vertebrates have yet been purified. It has become clear that an RIA developed for purified rat growth hormone, for example, cannot be used for measuring growth hormones of fish or birds. The chemical structures of fish or bird growth hormones differ sufficiently from those of the rat so that the anti-rat growth hormone antibody does not adequately recognize fish growth hormone. On the other hand, rat growth hormone and anti-rat growth hormone antibodies may be used to assay growth hormone of a closely related rodent species, such as the mouse. Mouse growth hormone may be sufficiently similar to rat growth hormone for the use of a rat growth hormone RIA to be valid. The problem of inappropriate cross-reactivity between species does not always apply. Fortunately, some hormones (steroids, thyroid hormones) are structurally identical in all vertebrates and can be measured by existing RIAs.

Another modern technique worth mentioning is the measurement of hormonal receptors in target tissues. The chemical basis for this procedure is similar to RIA, since receptors bind both radiolabeled and unlabeled hormone in a reversible, competitive fashion, as do antibodies. The first step in the technique is the isolation, by cell disruption and differential centrifugation, of a cell fraction (e.g., cell nuclei or plasma membranes that contain the receptors). Unfortunately, hormones will bind to some extent with many cell components other than receptors. Hormone binding to receptor can be identified according to the criteria that (1) receptors have a high affinity for the hormone and (2) receptors are present in so low a concentration that their capacity for binding hormone also is low. The nonreceptor-binding sites in a cell fraction have a relatively low affinity for the hormone and, because of their abundance, have a high capacity for binding. Therefore, a primary aim of the technique is the separate identification of high-affinity, low-capacity (receptor) binding and low-affinity, high-capacity (nonspecific) binding. This is done by incubating the cell fraction with various amounts of radiolabeled and unlabeled hormone and determining the kinetics of hormone binding and saturation of receptors. For example, in an assay of nuclear receptors, one series of tubes containing a constant amount of nuclei and various concentrations of radiolabeled hormone is incubated for a time sufficient to reach binding equilibrium. In a second series of tubes containing the same amount of nuclei, various concentrations of radiolabeled hormone and unlabeled hormone at 100 times the concentration of radiolabeled hormone are similarly incubated. After equilibrium is reached, the nuclei are separated by centrifugation, and the amounts of radioactivity in the supernatant (free hormone) and nuclear pellet (bound hormone) are measured. Radioactivity in the nuclear pellet in the first series of tubes (nuclei + radiolabeled hormone) represents hormone bound to both receptors and other cellular constituents, while radioactivity in the second series (nuclei + radiolabeled hormone + 100-fold unlabeled hormone) represents binding to nonreceptor components; the large amount of unlabeled hormone saturates the receptors, so that labeled hormone binds only to the low-affinity, high-capacity sites. A saturation binding curve is shown in Fig. 1.17. The graph of bound versus free hormone illustrates the total binding from the first series of tubes and the nonspecific binding from the second series of tubes. The specific binding, which represents hormone binding to receptors, is calculated by subtracting nonspecific binding from total binding. Specific binding is greater at low concentrations of hormone; it increases as hormone concentration in the medium is raised, and then becomes constant when the receptors become saturated.

The specific binding from the binding curve can be analyzed further by methods such as the Scatchard plot (Fig. 1.18). The ratio of bound to free

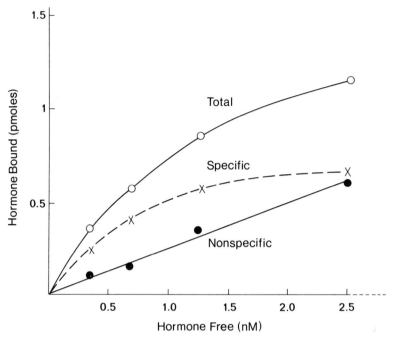

FIGURE 1.17. Kinetics of hormone binding to a cell fraction containing hormone receptors. Nuclei are incubated with various amounts of radiolabeled hormone. The nuclei are centrifuged and the amount of radioactivity bound to the nuclear pellet is determined as a measure of the total binding (○). Similar incubations of nuclei, radiolabeled hormone, and a large amount of unlabeled hormone are used to measure the nonspecific binding (●) which represents hormone bound to parts of nuclei that are not hormone receptors. The reasoning here is that the large excess of unlabeled hormone has fully occupied and saturated all of the specific receptors. If further addition of labeled hormone results in continued binding, then this must be bound to nonspecific, and "unsaturable," proteins which no reasonable amount of hormone can overwhelm. Specific nuclear binding (receptor binding, X) is determined by subtracting the nonspecific binding from the total binding at each concentration of free hormone. The specific binding curve becomes flat at high concentrations of radiolabeled hormone due to saturation of the hormone receptors.

hormone is plotted versus the amount of bound hormone, expressed as pmoles of hormone per mg DNA. The plot shows a straight line with a negative slope. The slope represents the dissociation constant (K_d) of the receptor–hormone complex. A small K_d indicates a high-affinity receptor. The X intercept of the Scatchard plot provides information for calculating the amount of receptor per mg DNA. If one assumes that one hormone molecule binds with one receptor molecule, then the number of receptor molecules, or receptor sites, can be calculated by multiplying the X intercept by Avogadro's number. Thus the saturation binding curve and Scatchard plot analysis indicate the affinity of the receptor for the hormone and the capacity (number of receptors) for hormone binding. Both of these param-

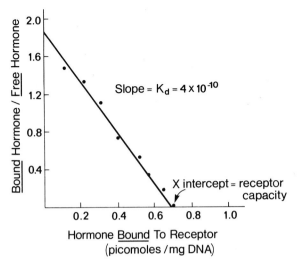

FIGURE 1.18. Scatchard plot of specific hormone binding to nuclear receptors. Data from a saturation binding curve (Fig. 1.17) is plotted, comparing the ratio of specifically bound to free hormone versus the amount of hormone specifically bound to nuclei. This gives a straight line in this example. The slope of the line indicates the dissociation constant (K_d) for the hormone–receptor complex. In this example the K_d is very small, indicating a high affinity of the receptor for the hormone. The X intercept indicates the amount of hormone bound when the ratio of bound over free equals zero (i.e., all hormone is in the bound form). Multiplying the X intercept molar value by Avogadro's number gives the number of receptors per mg DNA.

eters determine the sensitivity of target tissues to circulating hormone concentrations.

ADDITIONAL READING

1. Acher, R. (1980). Molecular evolution of biologically active peptides. *Proc. R. Soc. London* **B210:**21–43.
2. Barrington, E. J. W. (1975). *An Introduction to General and Comparative Endocrinology,* 2nd ed. Clarendon, Oxford.
3. Bentley, P. J. (1976). *Comparative Vertebrate Endocrinology.* Cambridge University Press, Cambridge.
4. Butt, W. R. (1975). *Hormone Chemistry,* 2nd ed. Wiley, New York.
5. Chertow, B. S. (1981). The role of lysosomes and proteases in hormone secretion and degradation. *Endocr. Rev.* **2:**137–173.
6. Frieden, E. H. (1976). *Chemical Endocrinology.* Academic, New York.
7. Gray, C. H., and V. H. T. James (1979). *Hormones in Blood,* 3rd ed. Academic, New York.
8. Katzenellenbogen, B. S. (1980). Dynamics of steroid hormone receptor action. *Ann. Rev. Physiol.* **42:**17–35.
9. Martin, C. R. (1978). *Textbook of Endocrine Physiology.* Williams & Wilkins, Baltimore.

10. Norris, D. O. (1980). *Vertebrate Endocrinology*. Lea & Febiger, Philadelphia.

11. O'Malley, B. W., and L. Birnbaumer, eds. (1977, 1978). *Receptors and Hormone Action*, Vols. 1–3. Academic, New York.

12. Sternberger, L. A. (1979). *Immunochemistry*, 2nd ed. Wiley, New York.

13. Sutherland, E. W. (1972). Studies on the mechanism of hormone action. *Science* **177**:401–408.

14. Tepperman, J. (1980). *Metabolic and Endocrine Physiology*, 4th ed. Year Book Medical Publishers, Chicago.

15. Thorell, J. I., and S. M. Larson (1978). *Radioimmunoassay and Related Techniques*. C. V. Mosby, St. Louis.

16. Turner, C. D., and J. T. Bagnara (1976). *General Endocrinology*, 6th ed. W. B. Saunders, Philadelphia.

2

MORPHOLOGY OF THE PITUITARY GLAND SYSTEM

GENERAL

If we take the mammalian pituitary gland as our model, we find that it is a complex of structures: both nervous and epithelial. The functional significance of pituitary structure has emerged rather gradually over the past 50 years, and it still is not quite settled. Figure 2.1 diagrammatically represents a sagittal section of a mammalian pituitary, showing that one part of the organ, the *neurohypophysis* (*me* and *pn* in Fig. 2.1), is actually a part of the brain floor and is attached to it by a stalk of nervous tissue. The other pituitary structural component, the *adenohypophysis* (*pt*, *pd* and *pi* in Fig. 2.1), is partly wrapped around the free end of the neurohypophysis. The adenohypophysis is composed mostly of cords of secretory cells that by staining techniques and relative position to each other can be further subdivided into characteristic components: the *pars distalis, pars intermedia*, and *pars tuberalis*.

The pars intermedia is that part of the adenohypophysis that characteristically has the closest contact with the lowest, or most distal, part of the neurohypophysis. In mammals, at least, there is often a split, or cleft, between the pars intermedia and the remainder of the adenohypophysis. The pars tuberalis, when present, generally is small, sometimes paired, and characteristically associates with the highest, or most proximal, part of the neurohypophysis. The remainder of the adenohypophysis, the pars distalis, is usually the largest.

The neurohypophysis also becomes regionally differentiated, into a *pars nervosa* and a *median eminence*. The median eminence is distinguished by

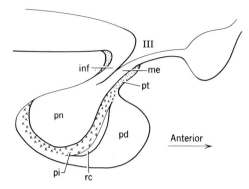

FIGURE 2.1. Diagrammatic sagittal section of a mammalian pituitary. *inf*, Infundibulum; *me*, median eminence; *pd*, pars distalis; *pi*, pars intermedia; *pn*, pars nervosa; *pt*, pars tuberalis; *rc*, residual cleft; *III*, third ventricle of brain extending into the pars nervosa.

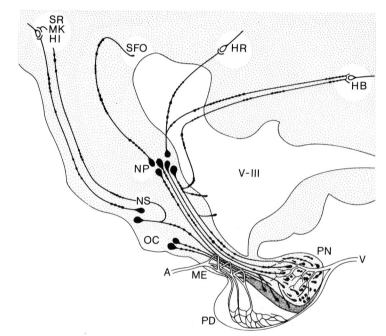

FIGURE 2.2. Diagram of the vertebrate hypothalamic region of the brain showing some typical neurosecretory pathways and some of the afferent innervation of the neurosecretory cells. Cell bodies of neurosecretory neurons are drawn in black; nonneurosecretory cell bodies are white. Gatherings of neurosecretory cell bodies are shown in the paraventricular nucleus (*NP*) and supraoptic nucleus (*NS*); several such cells are just posterior to the optic chiasma (*OC*). Axons carry neurosecretory material to the pars nervosa (*PN*) of the pituitary, where capillaries collect it and carry it to a vein (*V*). Blood from the pars distalis (*PD*) also drains into this vein. Some neurosecretory fibers extend to the septum (*SR*), the amygdala (*MK*), the hippocampus (*HI*), the subfornical organ (*SFO*), the habenular region (*HR*) in the dorsal thalamus, and even as far as the hindbrain (*HB*). A few neurosecretory fibers extend to the third ventricle (*V-III*). Neurosecretory cells that end in the median eminence (*ME*), next to the loops of the primary capillary network, are not included in this diagram. [After G. Sterba, *Neurosecretion and Neuroendocrine Activity, Evolution, Structure, and Function* (W. Bargmann, A. Oksche, and A. Polenov, eds.), Springer-Verlag, Berlin, 1978.]

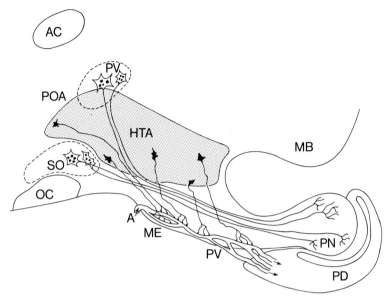

FIGURE 2.3. Diagram of a vertebrate hypothalamus in sagittal section similar to Fig. 2.2, but showing, in addition, the pathways of neurosecretory fibers to the median eminence (*ME*), where they terminate upon capillaries that carry their secretions via portal vessels (*PV*) to the pars distalis (*PD*). These neurosecretory fibers originate in a broad zone, here called the hypophysiotropic area (*HTA*), which extends from the preoptic area (*POA*) to the medial basal hypothalamic area (*MB*). Experimental evidence shows that different releasing and release-inhibiting hormones come from different parts of the hypophysiotropic area. Also shown are the "classical" neurosecretory fibers originating in the supraoptic (*SO*) and paraventricular (*PV*) nuclei and ending in the pars nervosa (*PN*). *OC*, optic chiasma; *A*, artery. [Adapted from L. P. Renaud, in *The Hypothalamus* (S. Reichlin, R. J. Baldessarini, and J. B. Martin, eds.), Raven, New York, 1978.]

having a common blood supply with the pars distalis. That is, the capillaries of the median eminence, instead of joining the general venous drainage of the brain, become gathered into relatively short portal vessels (Figs. 2.2 and 2.3) that extend to the pars distalis and break up again into capillaries. The pars nervosa, which forms the rest of the neurohypophysis, has a blood supply that is mostly independent of the adenohypophysis.

NEUROSECRETORY STRUCTURES OF THE BRAIN AND PITUITARY

The key to the complex structure of the pituitary gland is that it is organized to serve the endocrine function of the brain. That is, there are sets of neurons in the brain that secrete a variety of hormones, usually in response to physical stimuli. For nerve cells to secrete hormones, they must terminate at blood vessels rather than at synapses or motor endings. Structures in which neurosecretory neurons contact blood vessels to enable hormone secretion from their endings are called *neurohaemal*, This process of *neurosecretion*, which is common in the invertebrates, is limited in the vertebrates mostly to the neurohypophysis. Two general types of neurosecretory structures can be distinguished in the neurohypophysis. In one of them, typified by the pars nervosa, neurosecretion takes place into capillaries that lead directly to the head veins and thence to the systemic circulation. The neurohaemal area for oxytocin secretion, for example (see pages 9, 95), is the pars nervosa (Fig. 2.2). The second type of neurosecretion occurs at the median eminence. Here the brain hormones are secreted into specialized capillaries that lead to portal vessels that conduct blood to the pars distalis, where these hormones affect the release of one of the six or more hormones of that organ. The neurohormone in this case is one of the "releasing hormones." An example, given earlier, of this type of mechanism (page 9) is the brain-regulated release of a gonadotropic hormone that is triggered in the female rabbit by copulation.

ENDOCRINE REGIONS OF THE BRAIN

Before it was realized that nerve cells can secrete hormones, it was believed that the relatively few visible cells in the pars nervosa, which do not have the appearance of secretory cells, were responsible for the hormonal activity of this region. However, in the 1930s Ernst and Berta Scharrer published a series of papers in which they claimed that certain hypothalamic nerve cells contained what appear to be secretory granules. Furthermore, they suggested that since such cells end in the pars nervosa, they are responsible for secretion of the hormones of this lobe of the pituitary. This was a novel thought that was not immediately accepted.

However, once the reality of neurosecretion was accepted, it became a prime task to find the locations of the cells whose secretory axons end in the neurohypophysis. Several useful staining procedures quickly established that two regions in the hypothalamus (the ventral part of the diencephalon) are the principal loci for the cells that extend to the pars nervosa in well-defined tracts. These are the *preoptic nucleus* and the *paraventricular nucleus* (Fig. 2.3).

The axons of the neurosecretory cells that terminate in the median eminence of the neurohypophysis proved more difficult to trace back to their cell body origins because they did not stain as did those that terminate in the pars nervosa. However, by a variety of procedures that will be referred to below, they were localized largely in a zone of the hypothalamus that is spoken of as the *hypophysiotropic area* (Fig. 2.3).

Ultimately, by use of immunological methods in which a specific hormonal antibody is coupled to a cytological staining agent (e.g., fluorescent material or a labeling enzyme), it has become possible to localize individual cell bodies and axons containing particular hormones (Fig. 2.4). Such re-

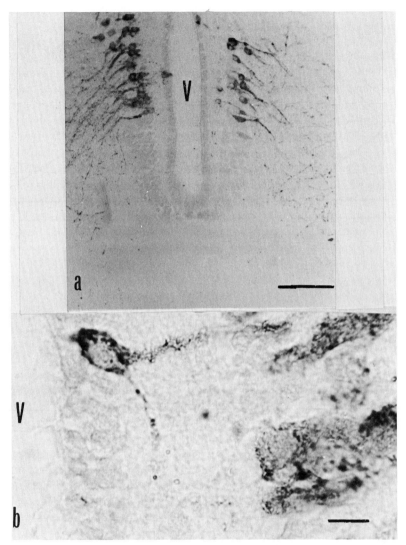

FIGURE 2.4. Lamprey hypothalamus (preoptic region) cross sections treated with anti-LHRH antibody coupled to a cytological staining agent. Neurons containing LHRH are stained black. (*a*) Low-magnification photograph showing LHRH-containing nerve cell bodies on either side of the third ventricle (V). Extending away from the cell bodies are LHRH-containing axons, which have a beaded appearance. (*b*) Photograph at a higher magnification. One LHRH nerve cell is located within the lining-cell (ependyma) layer next to the ventricle (V) and sends axonal or dendritic processes away from this point. A bit deeper there are more numerous LHRH cells, but the reaction is still selective (not all cells are stained even in one region). [Photographs were supplied by Professor J. W. Crim, University of Georgia.]

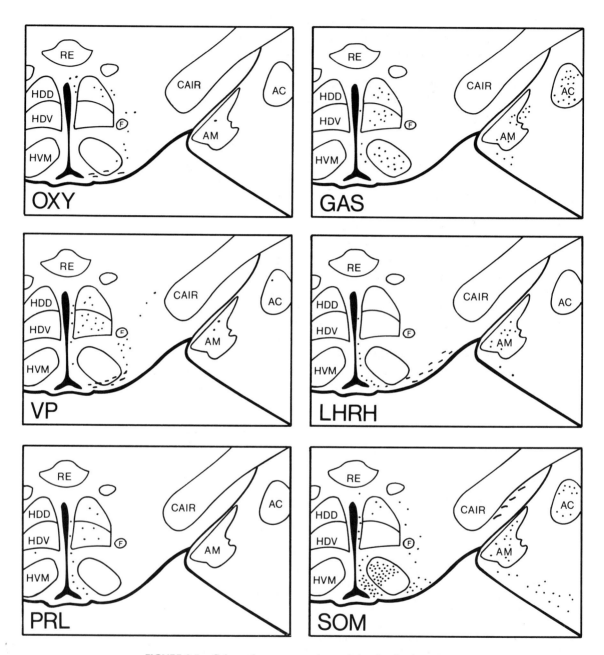

FIGURE 2.5. Schematic representations of the distribution of various hormones in the hypothalamus of the rat. Sites of localization in neuronal cell bodies are indicated by dots, and localization in axons is indicated by short lines. The anatomical locations of various brain nuclei are outlined. The third ventricle is shown in solid black in the center, with the upper end of the pituitary stalk at its ventral (bottom) end. *GAS*, gastrin; *LHRH*, gonadotropin-releasing

search has made it possible to map the distribution of brain nerve cells that contain particular hormones in immunoreactive form. Figure 2.5, for example, summarizes the distribution of a variety of hormones in the hypothalamus of the rat.

It is a remarkable fact that although these sensitive techniques have made it possible to locate the cells that secrete hormones in the neurohaemal areas of the neurohypophysis, they have also revealed several complicated situations. First, those hypophysiotropic releasing hormones for which immunocytochemical techniques have been developed are much more broadly distributed in the brain than in the hypophysiotropic area. TRH (thyrotropin releasing hormone), for example, is found in all regions of the brain and spinal cord. Second, the pars nervosa hormones have a similarly broad distribution and apparently may serve as neurotransmitters. Thus, "oxytocinergic" and "vasotocinergic" neurons have been described (Fig. 2.2). Third, a variety of hormones—gastrin, CCK, prolactin, and others—have been localized in hypothalamic neurons (Fig. 2.5). It is not so surprising to find that neurosecretory hormones may also serve as neurotransmitters since, after all, they are nerve cell products. However, it is more difficult, at this point, to understand the possible significance of gastrointestinal and pituitary hormones localized in certain brain cells. It is possible that immunocytochemical procedures are revealing the small quantities of hormone concentrated by their target receptors while performing a particular function. Gastrin and CCK are known to have central nervous actions (on appetite), and prolactin may be involved in a feedback action, or in an action upon a behavior center.

DEVELOPMENT OF THE PITUITARY GLAND

In view of the relative complexity of the neural, epithelial, and vascular elements that form the adult pituitary, its embryonic development is fairly simple and direct. In all vertebrates the neurohypophysis forms from the floor of the primitive diencephalon as a downgrowth that can vary in shape from broad and shallow to long and stalked. The third ventricle of the brain commonly remains in communication with a space that is included in the neurohypophysis or at least in its stalk.

The adenohypophysis of reptiles, birds, and mammals develops as a fingerlike derivative of the mouth ectoderm that is named *Rathke's pouch*. In

hormone; *OXY*, oxytocin; *PRL*, prolactin; *SOM*, somatostatin; *VP*, vasopressin; *AC*, amygdala; *CAIR*, internal capsule; *F*, fornix; *HDD*, dorsomedial nucleus, dorsal part; *HDV*, dorsomedial nucleus, ventral part; *HVM*, ventromedial nucleus; *RE*, nucleus reuniens. [Adapted from T. Hokfelt et al., *The Hypothalamus* (S. Reichlin, R. Baldasserini, and J. B. Martin, eds.), Raven, New York, 1978.]

such embryos, Rathke's pouch is the apical part of the angle formed by
the folding of the head downward toward the heart (see Fig. 2.6). When
first formed, Rathke's pouch is already close to the diencephalon, which
has begun to form the *infundibulum*, the rudiment of the neurohypophysis
(Figs. 2.6 and 2.7). When the upper end of Rathke's pouch contacts the
infundibulum, it is still connected by a hollow stalk to the oral ectoderm.
The epithelial stalk generally dwindles and disappears. However, it often
remains in the adult in a number of species of birds and fishes. Woerdeman
earlier and Wingstrand more recently have observed that there is a pattern
to the differentiation of the amniote adenohypophysis. The original space
within Rathke's pouch (remnant of the oral cavity) becomes the cleft separating the pars intermedia from the pars distalis. Two lateral projections
(see Fig. 2.8) from Rathke's pouch (the *"lateral lobes"*) differentiate as the
pars tuberalis, which may remain paired or may fuse.

The developing pituitary of cartilaginous fishes generally resembles that
of the amniotes described above. However, the lateral lobes of Rathke's
pouch have been described as bending ventrally, fusing and differentiating
(Fig. 2.9) as the *ventral lobe* of the pars distalis, a lobe that is characteristic

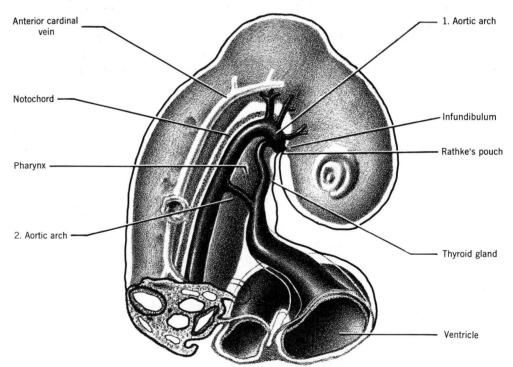

Anterior cardinal vein

Notochord

Pharynx

2. Aortic arch

1. Aortic arch

Infundibulum

Rathke's pouch

Thyroid gland

Ventricle

FIGURE 2.6. Reconstruction of a chick embryo incubated 48 hours. Rudiments of the neurohypophysis and adenohypophysis are indicated as the infundibulum and the Rathke's pouch,
respectively. The thyroid gland anlage is the slight ventral outpocketing in the pharyngeal floor
just anterior to the point where the truncus arterious branches into aortic arches 1 and 2.

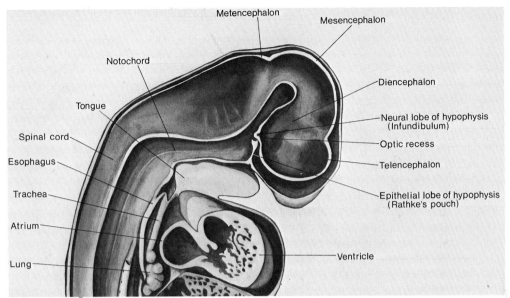

FIGURE 2.7. Reconstruction of the anterior part of a pig embryo representing a slightly later equivalence of development than that of the chick embryo in Fig. 2.6. Rathke's pouch has been closed off from the mouth cavity. A tongue has formed in the floor of the upper gut, the place from where the thyroid was derived, now showing as a slight depression on top of the tongue. The trachea and lung have separated from the foregut, from which they are derived. [Modified from L. B. Arey, *Developmental Anatomy*, W. B. Saunders, Philadelphia, 1954.]

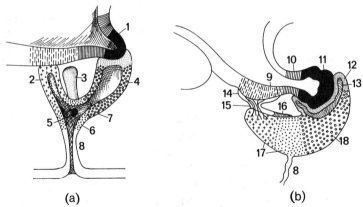

(a)   (b)

FIGURE 2.8. Idealized sagittal sections through a developing (*a*) and fully differentiated (*b*) amniote pituitary gland to show the presumed embryonic origins of more specialized regions of the adult neurohypophysis and adenohypophysis. Equivalent structures at the two stages are suggested by similar patterns of shading (dots, circles, *x*'s, etc.). *1*, Infundibulum; *2*, anterior process of Rathke's pouch; *3*, lateral lobe of Rathke's pouch (becomes *14* and *16*); *4*, aboral lobe of Rathke's pouch; *5*, opening of lateral lobe into Rathke's pouch; *6*, oral lobe of Rathke's pouch; *7*, constriction of Rathke's pouch; *8*, epithelial stalk of Rathke's pouch; *9*, median eminence; *10*, infundibulum; *11*, pars nervosa; *12*, pars intermedia; *13*, hypophyseal cleft; *14*, juxtaneural part of the pars tuberalis; *15*, portal vessels; *16*, internal part of pars tuberalis; *17* and *18*, differentiated zones of the pars distalis. [Modified from K. G. Wingstrand, *The Pituitary Gland* (G. Harris and B. Donovan, eds.), University of California Press, Berkeley, 1966.]

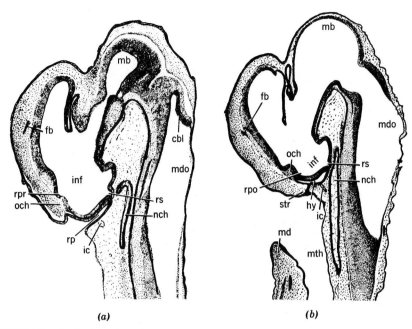

(a)   **(b)**

FIGURE 2.9. Sagittal sections through the anterior parts of two dogfish shark (*Squalus acanthias*) embryos. (*a*) 21-mm embryo (× 20); (*b*) 30-mm embryo (× 12.5). Note that the adenohypophyseal rudiment is formed by two separate folds of head ectoderm and resembles the nasohypophyseal rudiment of the lamprey (Fig. 2.14). *cbl*, Cerebellum; *fb*, forebrain; *hy*, adenohypophyseal rudiment; *ic*, internal carotid artery; *inf*, infundibulum; *mb*, midbrain; *md*, mandible (lower jaw); *mdo*, medulla oblongata; *mth*, mouth; *nch*, notochord; *och*, optic chiasma; *rs*, recess forming saccus vasculosus; *rpr*, preoptic recess; *rpo*, postoptic recess; *rp*, Rathke's pouch; *str*, epithelial stalk. [From H. W. Norris, *The Plagiostome Hypophysis*, copyright 1941, Grinnell, Iowa, p. 57.]

of the elasmobranchs. The pars distalis in this group often contains the space that originally was included in Rathke's pouch (Fig. 2.10).

In birds the pars intermedia never clearly differentiates, and is absent in adults. Furthermore, the pars distalis remains separate from the neurohypophysis. In amphibians the adenohypophyseal ingrowth (Fig. 2.11) is solid and grows in from the front of the head, between the mouth and brain, until it contacts the infundibulum. In teleost fishes the adenohypophyseal ingrowth also tends to be relatively solid and more rounded (Fig. 2.12), and early makes a relatively broad and intimate contact with the neurohypophysis.

In the Agnatha, the most primitive vertebrates, the embryology of the adenohypophysis is known only in the lampreys. Hagfish embryos have never been described adequately with respect to pituitary development. In the lampreys (Fig. 2.13) folds of ectoderm on the lower side of the embryonic head form a nasohypophyseal pit. The posterior part of this pit differentiates

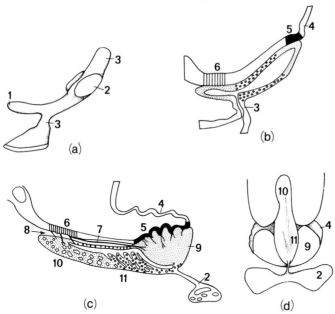

FIGURE 2.10. General structure and development of the elasmobranch pituitary gland. (*a*) Model of Rathke's pouch of a 28-mm dogfish (*Squalus*) embryo (after Baumgartner, 1915); (*b*) median sagittal section of *a* (also after Baumgartner, but with labels added); (*c*) median sagittal section of adult pituitary (based on several authors); (*d*) ventral view of pituitary gland of *Squalus* (after Baumgartner). *1*, Anterior process, Rathke's pouch; *2*, lateral lobe of Rathke's pouch in *a*, ventral lobe of adult in *c* and *d*; *3*, epithelial stalk of pouch; *4*, saccus vasculosus; *5*, pars nervosa; *6*, median eminence; *7*, portal vessel to pars intermedia (according to Meurling, 1960); *8*, portal vessels of usual type to pars distalis; *9*, pars intermedia; *10, 11*, differentiated regions of the pars distalis. [Based on K. G. Wingstrand, *The Pituitary Gland* (G. Harris and B. Donovan, eds.), University of California Press, Berkeley, 1966.]

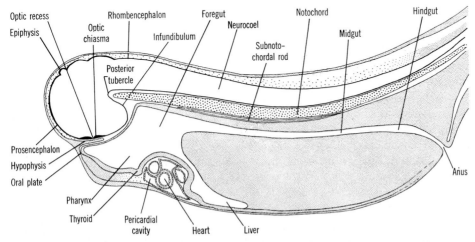

FIGURE 2.11. Median sagittal section of a 5.5-mm frog embryo showing the rudiments of the pituitary and thyroid glands.

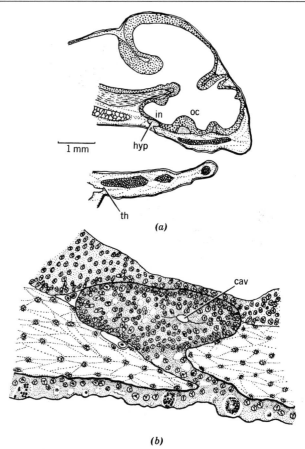

FIGURE 2.12. (*a*) Head of trout (*Salmo trutta*) embryo at hatching showing position of ade-nohypophyseal anlage (*hyp*). *in*, Infundibulum; *oc*, optic chiasma; *th*, thyroid. (*b*) Enlarged pituitary region showing small residual cavity (*cav*) in anlage. [From T. Kerr, *Proc. R. Soc.* (Edinburgh), **60**:224, 1940.]

as the adenohypophysis, the pars intermedia being the part that actually contacts the neurohypophysis at the posterior extremity. The nasohypo-physeal pit never loses its continuity with the outside of the head, and a lip grows between it and the mouth proper (Fig. 2.14). Thus the adult lamprey adenohypophysis remains closely related spatially to the olfactory organ, and the olfactory organ opens to the top of the head through a duct (Fig. 2.14).

Although the adult lamprey pituitary gland (Fig. 2.15) resembles the pi-tuitaries of other vertebrates in its general pattern, its development appears rather different. Some of these apparent differences may be resolved by

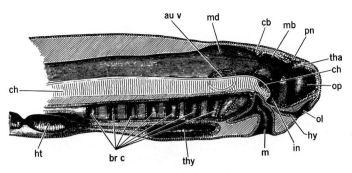

FIGURE 2.13. Schematic sagittal section of a 4.8-mm embryo of the lamprey, *Petromyzon*, showing the rudiments of the pituitary (hy and in) and the thyroid (thy). Abbreviations: au v, auditory vesicle; br c, branchial pouches; cb, cerebellum; ch, notochord; ht, heart; hy, hypophyseal pouch of nasohypophyseal sac; in, infundibulum; m, mouth; mb, midbrain; md, medulla; ol, olfactory pit; op, eye; pn, epiphysis; pn, pineal; tha, thalamus; thy, thyroid, or subpharyngeal gland, or endostyle. [Modified slightly from H. E. Ziegler, *Lehrbuch der vergleichenden Entwicklungsgeschichte*. Gustav Fischer.]

comparative anatomists, who can explain the homology of the upper lip of the lamprey mouth. At present, however, we are faced with the facts that the adenohypophysis of amniotes derives from the ectoderm of the embryonic mouth; in amphibians it derives from the front of the embryonic head near the external olfactory pits (definitively, the nares); in the lamprey its ectodermal origin is even further dorsal and related to the definitive top of the head.

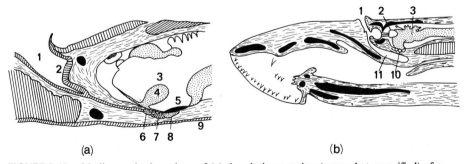

FIGURE 2.14. Median sagittal sections of (*a*) the pituitary region (somewhat magnified) of a larval lamprey (*Petromyzon*) and (*b*) the entire head region of an adult *Petromyzon*. *1*, Nasohypophyseal opening; *2*, olfactory organ; *3*, brain; *4*, optic chiasma; *5*, pars nervosa (colored black); *6, 7*, differentiated regions of the pars distalis; *8*, pars intermedia; *9*, epithelium of roof of mouth; *10*, pituitary; *11*, nasohypophyseal sac. [From K. G. Wingstrand, *The Pituitary Gland* (G. Harris and B. Donovan eds.), University of California Press, Berkeley, 1966.]

bc

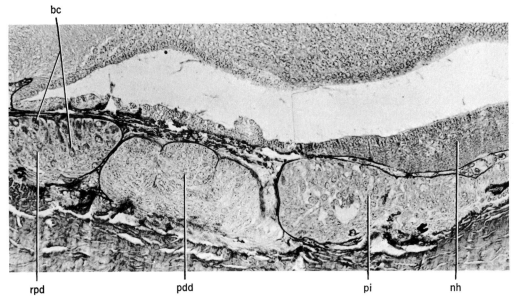

rpd   pdd   pi   nh

FIGURE 2.15. Sagittal section of the pituitary gland of an ammocoete larva of the lamprey *Lampetra planeri*. The space running across the middle of the photograph is the third ventricle. The floor of the third ventricle here is made up entirely of the neurohypophysis. The label *nh* extends to the thickened part of the neurohypophysis, the pars nervosa. The thinner part of the neurohypophysis, to the left, is the supposed equivalent of the median eminence. However, there is a connective tissue septum between the median eminence equivalent and the rostral and proximal pars distalis (*rpd* and *ppd*). Basophilic cells (*bc*) are labeled in the *rpd*. Between the pars intermedia (*pi*) and the neurohypophysis there is a network of blood vessels, here showing some red blood cells. [Photo by J. C. van de Kamer, Zoologisch Laboratorium, Utrecht.]

COMPARATIVE ANATOMY OF THE PITUITARY GLAND

The pituitary gland is found in all vertebrates, but in no invertebrates. Thus there really is no reliable clue as to how the pituitary gland evolved. Perhaps the best apparent homologue of the vertebrate pituitary gland is the cerebral ganglion–subneural gland association seen in a protochordate (Fig. 2.16). This structure has been tested for the presence of vertebratelike hormones without success. Elsewhere among the invertebrates, associations of nervous and epithelial tissues can be found (e.g., the corpus cardiacum–corpus allatum complex in insects; Fig. 2.17), but there is little basis for considering that any of these structures is analogous to the neurohypophysis–adenohypophysis system.

On the other hand, looking at the pituitary glands of vertebrates as a whole, there is remarkably little basic variation to be seen, though distinct animal group–limited characteristics can be recognized. All pituitaries consist of a neurohypophysis apposed to an adenohypophysis. The neurohy-

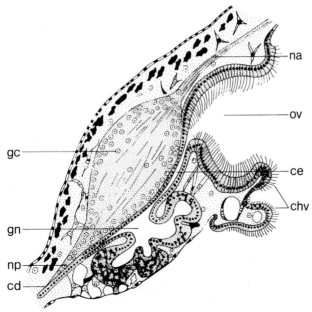

FIGURE 2.16. Vertical section of the neural complex of the tunicate *Clavelina lepadiformis*. *cd*, Dorsal cord (posterior extension of subneural gland); *ce*, duct of the gland; *chv*, ciliated epithelium over the complex that projects as a tubercle into the branchial cavity; *gc*, cerebral ganglion; *gn*, subneural gland (label actually ends in its central cavity); *na*, *np*, anterior and posterior nerves; *ov*, funnel-shaped opening of subneural gland into branchial cavity. [From Grassé (1948), *Traité de Zoologie*, Vol. 11, after Seelinger (1893–1911), in *Bronn's Tierreich*, **3**, *Suppl. Tunicata*.]

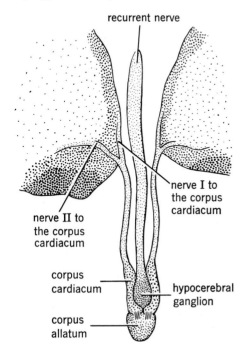

FIGURE 2.17. Diagram of frontal section of brain and endocrine organs of the earwig *Forficula*. On each side, the internal nerve (I) from the medial neurosecretory cells and the external nerve (II) from the lateral neurosecretory cells fuse and proceed to the corpora cardiaca. The ventral portions of the corpora cardiaca surround the hypocerebral ganglion. Nerve fibers from the corpus cardiacum nerves also pass to the corpus allatum. [Redrawn from P. Cazal, *Bull. Biol. France Belg.*, Suppl. 32, 1948.]

pophysis is the most constant in structure, being the neurohaemal terminus of populations of neurosecretory neurons whose cell bodies are in the hypothalamus. The most obvious structural variations in neurohypophyses are with respect to shape, the apparent absence of a median eminence in the most primitive vertebrates, the Agnatha, and in the greater degree of development of the pars nervosa in terrestrial vertebrates. The adenohypophysis is somewhat more variable. Most of the taxon-limited pituitary differences to be described below will involve the adenohypophysis.

The Agnathan Pituitary

To the comparative endocrinologist the greatest theoretical interest is in the pituitary of Agnatha. These eellike animals are descended from the most primitive vertebrates. However, since they diverged from the base of the vertebrate line some 500 million years ago (Fig. 2.18), the Agnatha themselves have had a long time to evolve. Accordingly, to what extent we can consider modern Agnatha representative of the most primitive vertebrates is a question. Nevertheless, we must look to the modern Agnatha for whatever insight we may hope to derive concerning the most primitive pituitary glands (Fig. 2.19).

The two main types of modern Agnatha are the wholly marine hagfishes (Myxinoidea) and the lampreys (Petromyzontia), which may live either wholly in fresh water or have a complex life cycle between fresh water and seawater. The hagfishes have a highly developed flattened saclike neurohypophysis (Fig. 2.20) to which a rather undifferentiated adenohypophysis is applied. The neurohypophysis contains many Gomori-staining neurosecretory endings, especially in the areas that do not face the adenohypophysis. There is a well-developed blood supply that presumably carries neurosecretions out to the general circulation. If there is any blood vessel connection between the neuro- and adenohypophysis, it is at best very poorly developed. Thus modern hagfishes lack a median eminence. The hagfish adenohypophysis consists of a series of relatively undifferentiated follicles separated from the neurohypophysis by connective tissue. There is no recognizable pars intermedia.

In lampreys (Figs. 2.14 and 2.15) the neurohypophysis is not as highly developed as in hagfishes. It consists of a thin anterior section that is really the floor of the diencephalon. The posterior part of the neurohypophysis is slightly thickened and is the terminating neurohaemal structure for neurons whose cell bodies are in the preoptic part of the hypothalamus. It is therefore similar to a pars nervosa. The adenohypophysis is much better differentiated than in hagfishes. There is a distinct pars intermedia in close contact with the ''pars nervosa'' portion of the neurohypophysis (Fig. 2.15). The pars distalis is differentiated into at least two recognizable regions according to histological features. In the lampreys, as well as in hagfishes, there is little or no crossing of blood vessels or neurons between the neurohypophysis

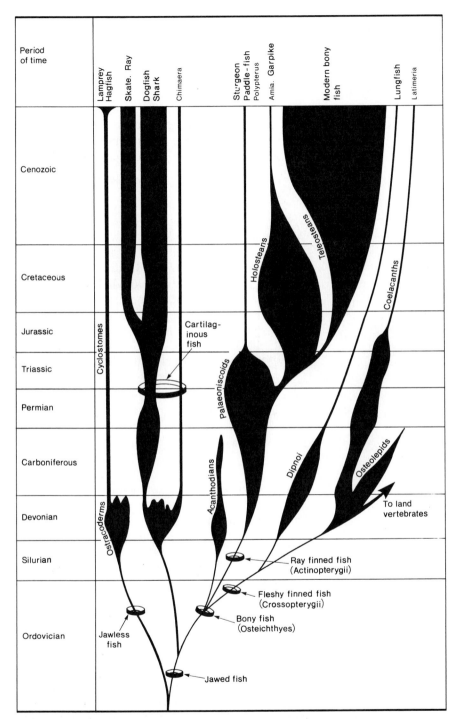

FIGURE 2.18. Phylogenetic tree showing the interrelations of the primitively derived fish groups and their paleontologically estimated times of origin. [From R. Holmes and J. Ball, *The Pituitary Gland*, Cambridge Univ. Press, London, 1974.]

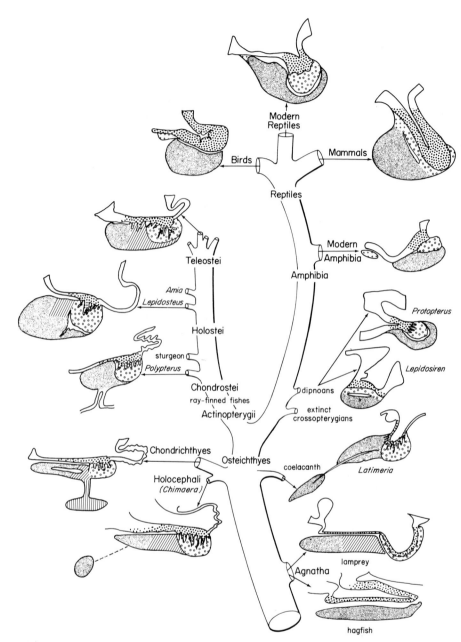

FIGURE 2.19. Phylogenetic tree of all vertebrate groups with superimposed diagrams of sagittal sections of the "typical" pituitary gland in each group. The parts of the pituitary are shaded to show equivalence of structures: *fine stippling and cross-hatching*, zones of the pars distalis; *open circles*, pars intermedia; *plus signs*, pars tuberalis; *coarse dots*, neurohypophysis.

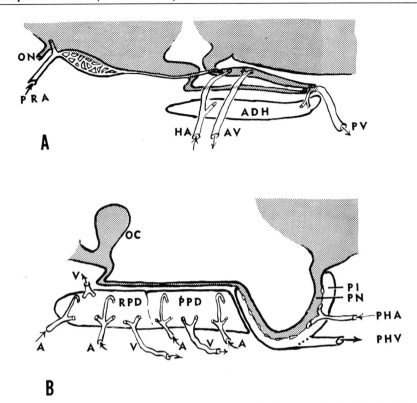

FIGURE 2.20. Comparison of the vascular supplies of the pituitary glands of the hagfish (*A*) and lamprey (*B*). *A*, Artery; *ADH*, adenohypophysis; *AV*, anterior vein draining the dorsal neurohypophysis; *HA*, hypophyseal artery; *OC*, optic chiasma; *ON*, optic nerve; *PHA*, posterior hypophyseal artery; *PHV*, posterior hypophyseal vein; *PI*, pars intermedia; *PN*, pars nervosa; *PPD*, proximal pars distalis; *PRA*, prehypophyseal artery; *PV*, posterior hypophyseal vein; *RPD*, rostral pars distalis; *V*, vein or venule. [From A. Gorbman, *Arch. Anat. Microsc. Morphol. Exp.*, **54**:163–194, 1965.]

and pars distalis (Fig. 2.20). Thus again, a median eminence is structurally absent. The only possible way for the neurohypophysis to regulate secretion by the pars distalis would seem to be by diffusion of the neurosecretions across the connective tissue barrier that separates them. This appears to be an inefficient system at best, and it is dubious whether it is effective at all.

In summary, one agnathan (the lamprey) has an adenohypophysis that is differentiated into the pars intermedia and the pars distalis; the other agnathan type, the hagfish, has an undifferentiated adenohypophysis. We must conclude that the presence of a pars intermedia is a primitive property probably shared by the stem agnathan group and all other vertebrates. The pars intermedia would seem to have been lost by a secondary degenerative process in the hagfishes. Both agnathan groups have a well-developed neurohypophysis innervated by neurosecretory tracts from the anterior hypothalamus (Fig. 2.15). Thus they have the equivalent of a pars nervosa. This conclusion is supported by the finding of vasotocin in the hagfish neurohypophysis (see Chapter 3). However, neither agnathan has the anatomical equivalent of a median eminence, that is, a neurohaemal structure that conveys a neurosecretion to the adenohypophysis via portal blood vessels. Is this a primitive or a degenerate feature? This question will be taken up again in Chapter 4 when the function of the agnathan adenohypophysis is considered.

The Selachian Pituitary

The pituitary of elasmobranch fishes is well developed and presents several puzzling features. The neurohypophysis consists of an anterior thin-walled portion, which resembles that of Amphibia (Figs. 2.21, 2.22, and 2.23). The posterior end of the neurohypophysis is a pars nervosa, which is complexly interdigitated with the pars intermedia. This mixture of pars intermedia and pars nervosa is so completely inseparable that the combined structure is referred to as the "neurointermediate lobe." The thinner part of the neurohypophysis is a true median eminence that is coextensive with the pars

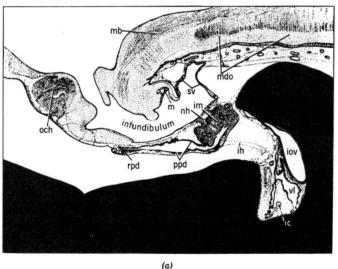

(a)

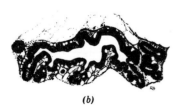

(b)

FIGURE 2.21. The rhinoid type of elasmobranch pituitary gland. (*a*) Sagittal section (× 5) of the brain and pituitary of the shark *Notorhynchus maculatus*. The pars distalis is hollow. (*b*) Cross section (× 20) of the proximal zone of the pars distalis showing its folded saclike character. *ic*, internal carotid artery; *ih*, position of stalk of ventral lobe; *im*, neurointermediate lobe (combined neurohypophysis and pars intermedia); *iov*, pituitary vein; *m*, mammillary body; *mb*, midbrain; *mdo*, medulla oblongata; *nh*, ependymal surface of neurohypophysis; *och*, optic chiasma; *rpd*, rostral pars distalis; *ppd*, proximal pars distalis; *sv*, saccus vasculosus; *vl*, ventral lobe. [From H. W. Norris, *The Plagiostome Hypophysis*, copyright 1941, Grinnell, Iowa, p. 51.]

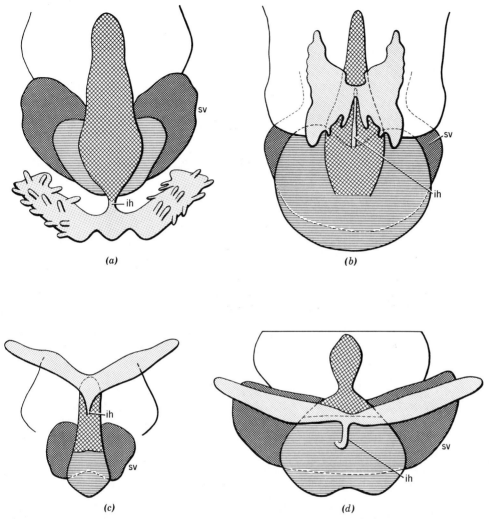

FIGURE 2.22. Ventral view. Outlines of the pituitary glands of four selachians. (*a*) A hexanchoid shark (*Notorhynchus maculatus*); (*b*) the thresher shark *Alopias vulpes*; (*c*) the cow ray *Rhinoptera quadriloba*; (*d*) the barn-door skate *Raia stabuliformis*. *Coarse crosshatch*, pars distalis; *fine crosshatch*, saccus vasculosus (*sv*); *horizontal lines*, pars intermedia; *stippled*, ventral lobe; *ih*, duct connecting ventral lobe. [From H. W. Norris, *The Plagiostome Hypophysis*, copyright 1941, Grinnell, Iowa, pp. 51, 69, 75, and 79.]

distalis (Fig. 2.23). The pars distalis receives portal blood vessels from the parallel median eminence. When a linearly oriented median eminence sends portal vessels to a similarly elongated and differentiated pars distalis, it is possible that this provides the means for separate neurosecretory control of separate types of hormone-secreting cells of the pars distalis.

The developing selachian adenohypophysis does not form a pars tuberalis,

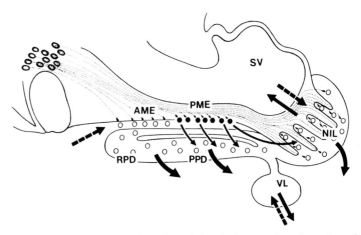

FIGURE 2.23. Diagrammatic sagittal section of the pituitary region of an elasmobranch to show vascular and neurosecretory supply. *RPD*, rostral pars distalis; *PPD*, proximal pars distalis; *NIL*, neurointermediate lobe; *VL*, ventral lobe of pars distalis; *AME*, anterior median eminence; *PME*, posterior median eminence; *SV*, saccus vasculosus. Neurosecretory cells at the left send neurosecretion-bearing axons (dotted lines) to the median eminence and *NIL*. Neurosecretory material (open circles and solid circles) is represented here as moving via portal vessels (lighter arrows) into the adenohypophysis. Heavy arrows indicate nonportal vascular supply, the interrupted arrows being arteries, the solid ones veins. [Modified slightly from R. L. Holmes and J. N. Ball, *The Pituitary Gland*, Cambridge Univ. Press, London, 1974.]

but it does form a structure that is not seen in any other vertebrate: the ventral lobe (Figs. 2.21 and 2.22). The ventral lobe generally hangs from the pars distalis by a short stalk and it has a blood supply completely separate from the median eminence system (Fig. 2.23). Thus, there is a question as to how, if at all, the brain controls hormone secretion from the ventral lobe. This is an important question, since, as is brought out in Chapter 4, the ventral lobe is active in producing gonadotropic and thyrotropic hormones.

The selachian pars intermedia has been known for a long time to be directly innervated by neurons that extend from the hypothalamus through the interdigitating pars nervosa. These neurons, at least some of which are neurosecretory, end upon or near the cells of the pars intermedia (Fig. 2.24).

The Holocephalan Pituitary

There is little known about the holocephalan pituitary beyond its gross structure and vascular supply. Yet, even this limited information answers several important questions concerning earlier evolution of the pituitary complex and presents one additional puzzle. From Figs. 2.18 and 2.19 it can be seen that zoologists consider that the holocephalan vertebrates evolved early from the same stem vertebrate line as the modern elasmobranchs. This

FIGURE 2.24. Section of the neurointermediate lobe of the pituitary of the skate *Raja erinacea* ($\times$ 275), stained with Gomori's chromalum hematoxylin phloxine. The darkest areas in the section are neurosecretory material in endings of axons arranged around blood vessels. The relationship of the neurohypophysis and the pars intermedia here is so intimate that it becomes pointless to question whether the neurosecretory material is actually in the thin neurohypophyseal fingers of connective tissue. It is clear that the adenohypophyseal cells are directly exposed to the neurosecretion and a "hypophyseal portal system" is unnecessary in this case. [Photograph furnished by Ernst Scharrer, Albert Einstein College of Medicine.]

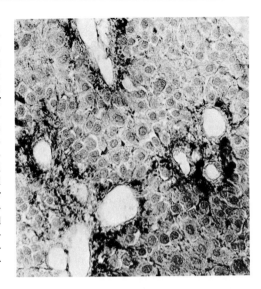

phyletic origin would make them possibly the closest extant vertebrate relatives to the Agnatha, and it might shed some light on the evolution of the median eminence and the ventral lobe of the adenohypophysis.

The holocephalan neurohypophysis is similar to that of elasmobranchs in having a well-developed median eminence and pars nervosa. The pars nervosa is complexed with the pars intermedia, forming a large neurointermediate lobe. The median eminence, like that of elasmobranchs, is coextensive with an elongated pars distalis and sends many short portal vessels into it (Figs. 2.25, 2.26). Part of the median eminence is beyond the anterior tip, so that it must send longer portal vessels to the pars distalis, reminiscent of median eminences of some higher vertebrates. The posterodorsal part of the neurohypophysis balloons out as a saccus vasculosus, a structure that is considered to be sensory, not endocrine, in function (Fig. 2.26).

The elongated pars distalis is recognizably differentiated into rostral and proximal regions, perhaps reflecting segregation of different functions in an anteroposterior pattern. As in many elasmobranchs, the pars distalis contains a cavity. There is no ventral lobe in holocephalans, but there is a unique rounded extracranial structure of still unsettled status, the Rachendachhypophyse (translated: pharyngeal roof pituitary; shown in Fig. 2.19). This structure, on the basis of embryological evidence, develops as an extension from the embryonic pars distalis rudiment, attached to it at first by a stalk, which later disappears. As an adenohypophyseal derivative, the final location of the Rachendachhypophyse is remarkably distant from the remainder of the pituitary: completely outside of the cranium, anterior to the brain and just under the pharyngeal mucosa. Recently Dodd has found high gonadotropic hormonal activity in the Rachendachhypophyse. If this claim

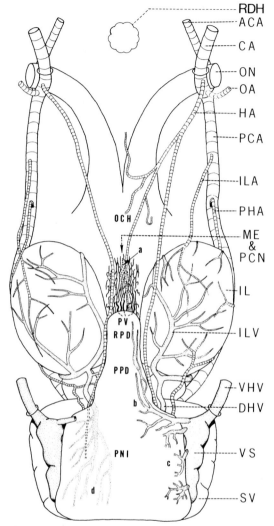

RDH
ACA
CA
ON
OA
HA
PCA
ILA
PHA
ME
&
PCN
IL
ILV
VHV
DHV
VS
SV

OCH
a
PV
RPD
PPD
b
PNI
c
d

FIGURE 2.25. Semidiagrammatic ventral view of the pituitary region of a chimeroid (holocephalan) fish. *ACA*, anterior cerebral artery; *CA*, anterior carotid artery; *DHV*, dorsal hypophyseal vein; *HA*, hypophyseal artery; *IL*, inferior lobe; *ILA*, interior lobar artery; *ILV*, inferior lobar vein; *ME* and *PCN*, median eminence and primary capillary net; *OA*, optic artery; *OCH*, optic chiasma; *ON*, optic nerve; *PCA*, posterior cerebral artery; *PNI*, pars neurointermedia; *PPD*, proximal zone of pars distalis; *PHA*, posterior hypophyseal artery; *PV*, portal veins; *RDH*, Rachendach-hypopyse; *RPD*, rostral zone of pars distalis; *SV*, saccus vasculosus; *VHV*, ventral hypophyseal vein; *VS*, venous sinus between saccus vasculosus and pars neurointermedia; *a (dotted lines)*, branches of hypophyseal artery supplying anterior part of primary capillary net; *b*, fragment of venous net draining the pars distalis; *c*, similar venous drainage from ventrolateral portion of the pars neurointermedia; *d*, venous drainage from the dorsolateral region of the pars neurointermedia. [From A. Jasinski and A. Gorbman, *Gen. Comp. Endocrinol.*, **6**:476–490, 1966.]

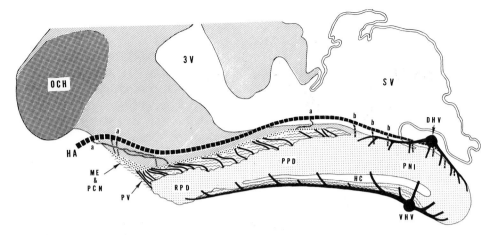

FIGURE 2.26. Schematic representation of the hypothalamo-hypophyseal vascular links in a holocephalan fish. *DHV*, dorsal hypophyseal vein; *HA*, hypophyseal artery; *ME* and *PCN*, median eminence and primary capillary net (dotted area); *HC*, hypophyseal cavity; *OCH*, optic chiasma; *PNI*, pars neurointermedia; *PPD*, proximal zone of pars distalis; *PV*, portal veins; *RPD*, rostral zone of pars distalis; *SV*, saccus vasculosus; *VHV*, ventral hypophyseal vein; *3V*, third ventricle. Small letters indicate the arterial supply of the primary capillary net (*a*) and of the pars neurointermedia (*b*). [From A. Jasinski and A. Gorbman, *Gen. Comp. Endocrinol.*, **6**:476–490, 1966.]

is substantiated, then the Rachendachhypophyse may be equated with the ventral lobe of elasmobranchs.

If the Rachendachhypophyse is the functional equivalent of the elasmobranch ventral lobe, then, like the ventral lobe, it is isolated from a well-developed median eminence and from the possibility of direct hypothalamic control. It may be pointed out that there is one more adenohypophyseal structure that in the adult is relatively removed from the brain, i.e., the rostral pars distalis of the coelacanth fish, *Latimeria* (see Fig. 2.19). Discussion of the homology of these structures is continued in Chapter 4.

The Teleostean Pituitary

Of the ray-finned fishes (actinopterygians), the teleosts form the largest and most diverse group. Their pituitary glands are perhaps the most characteristic and modified in organization of all the vertebrates (see Figs. 2.27*d*, 2.27*e*). The most typical anatomic features of the teleost pituitary are a lack of a median eminence and a rather complete interdigitation of the neurohypophysis with the pars distalis as well as with the pars intermedia. The neurohypophysis forms from the relatively broad and thin floor of the diencephalic ventricle. However, in some teleosts the neurohypophysis is drawn away from the brain, forming a stalk of nervous tissue (Fig. 2.28). That part of the neurohypophysis that invades the pars intermedia contains endings

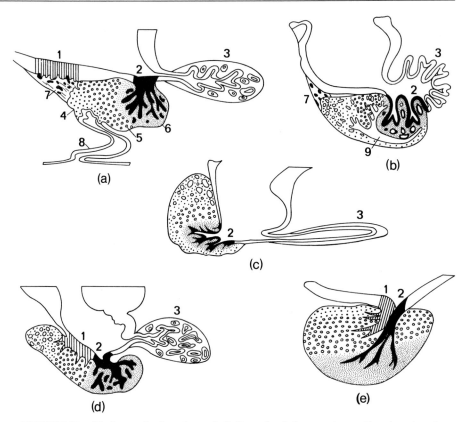

FIGURE 2.27. Median sagittal sections of pituitary glands from various actinopterygians (ray-finned fishes): (*a*) *Polypterus*, the reed fish—a chondrostean and a primitive actinopterygian; (*b*) *Acipenser*, the sturgeon—another primitive type of actinopterygian; (*c*) *Amia*, the bowfin—a holostean, considered a more advanced form toward evolution of the teleosts; (*d*) *Anguilla*, the eel, and (*e*) *Carassius*, the goldfish—both of the latter being modern teleosts. *Vertical shading*, median eminence in *Polypterus*, or its equivalent in the two teleost species; *solid black shading*, part of the neurohypophysis considered analogous to the pars nervosa; fine stippling, pars intermedia; *coarse dots and small circles*, differentiated zones of the pars distalis; *1*, median eminence; *2*, more posterior neurohypophysis; *3*, saccus vasculosus; *4, 5*, zones of the pars distalis; *6*, pars intermedia; *7*, vascularized "ligament"; *8*, duct connecting the pars distalis to the mouth in the adult; *9*, hypophyseal cleft. [From K. G. Wingstrand, *The Pituitary Gland* (G. Harris and B. Donovan, eds.) Univ. of California Press, Berkeley, 1966.]

of neurons from the preoptic area that in histological procedures color with neurosecretory stains (e.g., Gomori stain, aldehyde fuchsin stain). This might be equated with the pars nervosa of other vertebrates. That part of the neurohypophysis that interdigitates with the pars distalis contains endings of neurons that do not stain in this way, and they extend from the nucleus lateralis tuberis and other ventral hypothalamic areas that may be considered a hypophysiotropic area.

Many of the neurons of the neurohypophysis enter the adenohypophysis and terminate either near or upon adenohypophyseal cells in a synaptic fashion. This means that hypothalamic control over adenohypophyseal (pars intermedia and pars distalis) secretion could be exerted through direct action of neurosecretions upon these cells (Fig. 2.29). The neurosecretions in this case would be delivered in a manner analogous to the release of neurotransmitters. There has been much discussion whether there is any structure in the teleost that is equivalent to the median eminence, that is, a means for delivering the regulatory hypothalamic releasing hormones to the pars distalis cells via blood vessels. Since the teleostean pars distalis is directly interwoven with the part of the neurohypophysis that contains neurons from the hypophysiotropic part of the hypothalamus, this question is more or less academic. Blood vessels of the neurohypophysis in teleosts have been found to traverse the pars distalis on the way to the veins near the edge of the gland (Fig. 2.30). Thus, there is a possibility that neurosecretions released into such vessels in the neurohypophysis could in this way reach the cells of the teleost pars distalis. However, it is clear that in teleosts there is no vascular pattern like that in higher vertebrates (Fig. 2.29D) in which a median eminence-like primary capillary plexus leads to a portal vein which leads to a secondary capillary plexus. With neurosecretory cells terminating directly on or near cells of the teleostean pars distalis, vascular transport of hypophysiotropic factors would hardly seem necessary. Most teleost pituitaries have an associated saccus vasculosus (Fig. 2.27), generally believed to serve a sensory function.

The pars intermedia of the teleost pituitary is clearly differentiated, and generally it is the part of the adenohypophysis that is most highly interdigitated with the neurohypophysis (Fig. 2.28). The teleost pars distalis takes many forms (Fig. 2.28), probably reflecting the great diversity of the bony fishes as a group. However, despite this variability in general form, in all teleosts the pars distalis is (1) invaded by tongues of the neurohypophysis and (2) differentiated into at least two recognizably different zones of cells. More careful histological examination shows generally that the several secretory cell types of the pars distalis are unevenly distributed even within these two zones (Fig. 2.30). In some teleosts there is an epithelial stalk or tube connecting the rostral pars distalis to the mouth, an apparent remnant of its embryonic development. In some primitive chondrostean fishes (*Calamoichthys, Polypterus*; see Fig. 2.27) there is also a persistent epithelial duct connecting the pars distalis to the mouth epithelium. In such pituitaries, the prolactin-secreting cells are grouped at the upper (glandular) end of the duct.

Pituitary Glands of Intermediate Fish Groups

We may take Fig. 2.18 as one representation of the phylogenetic relationships of the piscine vertebrates to each other. However, there is not complete agreement among students of vertebrate phylogeny concerning these rela-

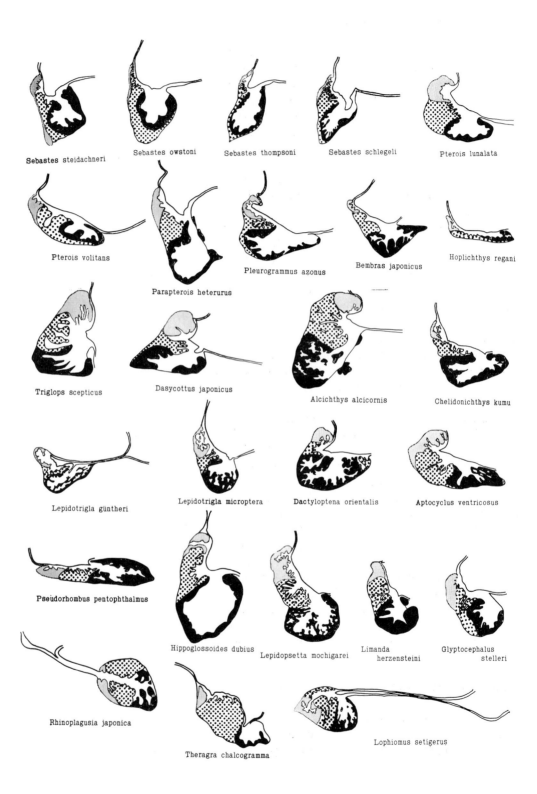

Sebastes steidachneri

Sebastes owstoni

Sebastes thompsoni

Sebastes schlegeli

Pterois lunalata

Pterois volitans

Parapterois heterurus

Pleurogrammus azonus

Bembras japonicus

Hoplichthys regani

Triglops scepticus

Dasycottus japonicus

Alcichthys alcicornis

Chelidonichthys kumu

Lepidotrigla güntheri

Lepidotrigla microptera

Dactyloptena orientalis

Aptocyclus ventricosus

Pseudorhombus pentophthalmus

Hippoglossoides dubius

Lepidopsetta mochigarei

Limanda herzensteini

Glyptocephalus stelleri

Rhinoplagusia japonica

Theragra chalcogramma

Lophiomus setigerus

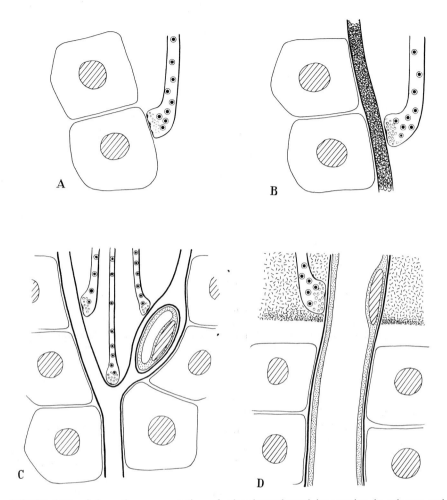

FIGURE 2.29. Schematic representation of adenohypophyseal innervation in teleosts and higher vertebrates. (A) In the sea horse (*Hippocampus*) there is direct synaptic contact between a neurosecretory nerve ending and the endocrine cell. (B) In the tench (*Tinca*) the fibrous basement membrane is interposed between the neurosecretory ending and endocrine cell. (C) In the eel (*Anguilla*) the neurosecretory endings are upon vascular channels among the endocrine cells. (D) In most higher vertebrates there is complete physical separation of the neurosecretory endings from the adenohypophysis; the neurosecretory endings secrete into blood vessels in the hypothalamus (median eminence), and the neurosecretion is transported via hypophyseal portal vessels. [From L. Vollrath, *Zeitschr. Zellforsch.*, **78**:234–260, 1967.]

FIGURE 2.28. Sagittal sections through the pituitary glands of 26 species of teleost fishes to show the variety of organization. Neurohypophysis is white; pars intermedia is black; zones of the pars distalis are shown in fine and coarse dots. Note that various zones of the hypophyseal lobes may be anterior in position. The gland may be flattened and have no stalk (*Hoplichthys*, *Pseudorhombus*), or it may be at the end of a short infundibular stalk (*upper row*) or a long infundibular stalk (*Lepidotriglia*, *Rhinoplagusia*, *Lophiomus*). [From M. Kawamoto, *Arch. Histol. Japon.*, **28**:123–150, 1967.]

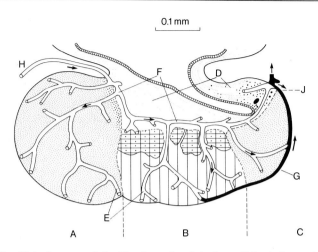

FIGURE 2.30. Main features of the blood supply of the bony fish pituitary. Anterior to the left. *A, B*, differentiated zones of the pars distalis (broken lines mark the boundaries); *C*, pars intermedia; *D*, neurohypophysis. Blood enters the gland from the hypophyseal artery (*H*) and passes to the primary longitudinal distributing plexus (*F*). From here it is distributed to the adenohypophysis in a centrifugal plexus (*E*). It is collected in a superficial venous network (*G*), and proceeds to the hypophyseal vein (*J*). [From R. Holmes and J. Ball, *The Pituitary Gland*, Cambridge Univ. Press, London, 1974.]

tionships. Four new groups of fish appeared almost simultaneously during the Paleozic period (Silurian and Devonian): (1) the ray-finned forms (actinopterygians), which proliferated into the modern teleostean group; (2) the bichirs or reed fish (brachiopterygians), an African group represented today by only about 10 species (*Polypterus* in Fig. 2.18); (3) the dipnoans, or lungfishes; and (4) the lobe-finned fishes (coelacanths), represented today by one species, *Latimeria*. The dipnoans are considered closest to the evolutionary line that led to the amphibians and other tetrapods. It may be noted that in the lungfishes the neurohypophysis is at the end of a narrowed stalk (infundibulum) and it is slightly or not at all (*Lepidosiren*) interdigitated with the pars intermedia. Since there is also no saccus vasculosus, the lungfish neurohypophysis begins to approach fairly closely that of the Amphibia in structure.

If we consider the anatomic patterns of the pituitaries of these "intermediate" fishes (Fig. 2.19), they are reasonably comparable. Excepting, perhaps, *Latimeria*, they have a relatively simple neurohypophysis, which includes a pars nervosa that is less deeply interdigitated with the pars intermedia than that of elasmobranchs or of teleosts. In all of these intermediate groups of fishes, study of vascularization of the pars distalis has shown that there is a median eminence and portal supply to at least part of the pars distalis (Figs. 2.31, 2.32).

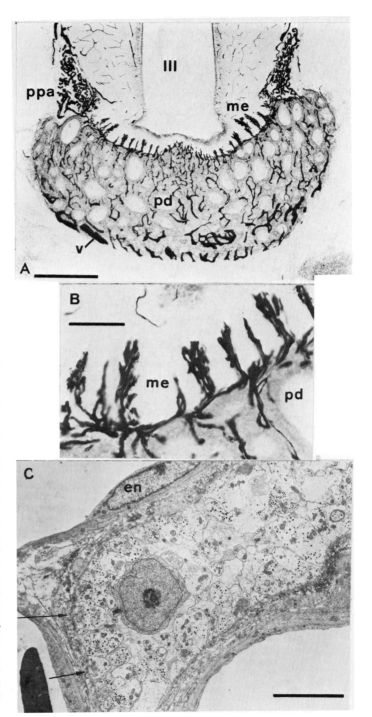

FIGURE 2.31. Sections through the neurohypophysis and adenohypophysis of the holostean fish *Amia calva* after injecting the blood vessels with India ink. (A) Low magnification (bar at lower left equals 0.5 mm); the pars intermedia is not visible. The neurohypophyseal median eminence (*me*) is in contact with the pars distalis (*pd*), which consists of follicular structures. *III*, third ventricle of diencephalon; *ppa*, preportal arterial blood vessels forming a superficial network; *v*, vein draining blood from the pars distalis. Note that the arterioles (at left) lead into the glomerular, tuftlike blood vessel formations that extend into the nervous tissue of the *me* and feed blood directly into the pars distalis. (B) Higher magnification of the glomerular blood vessel tufts in the median eminence. Bar at upper left equals 100 μ. (C) Electron micrograph of median eminence tissue between capillary loops. Capillary spaces are lined by endothelial cells (*en*). Most of the solid area consists of nerve endings that contain granular neurosecretory material. Arrows point to two such nerve endings with synapselike contacts on the connective tissue next to the blood vessels. Bar equals 5 μ. [Photographs supplied by Dr. Michael D. Lagios.]

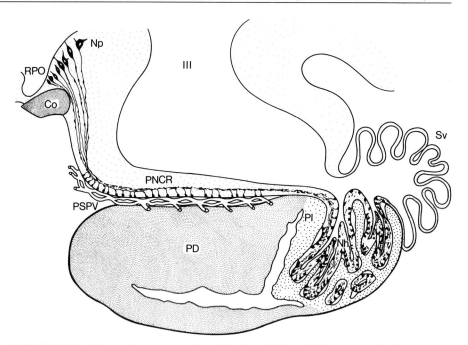

FIGURE 2.32. Schematic reconstruction of the hypothalamo-pituitary system in the sturgeon *Acipenser. Co*, optic chiasma; *Nh*, neurohypophysis; *Np*, preoptic nucleus; *PD*, pars distalis; *PI*, pars intermedia; *PNCR*, primary neurosecretory contact region (median eminence); *PSPV*, loosely organized plexus of hypophyseal portal vessels; *RPO*, preoptic recess of third ventricle; *SV* saccus vasculosus, *III*, third ventricle. [After A. Polenov and P. Garlov, *Zeitschr. Zellforsch.*, **116**:349–374, 1971.]

The exception to the generalizations just made is the pituitary complex of *Latimeria* (Fig. 2.33), which appears at first to be relatively bizarre. It has a fairly conventional neurohypophysis, which forms a neurointermediate lobe with the pars intermedia. However, it also interdigitates with a limited area of the proximal pars distalis. The proximal pars distalis is lobulated, and from it there extends a thin anteriorly and ventrally directed cellular tube. The extreme lower end of this tube forms a rostral pars distalis. Thus there is a long gap between the two principal parts of the pars distalis of *Latimeria*, the attenuated rostral lobe and its thin connecting tube being up to 12 cm in length!

The lower tip of the rostral pars distalis has a direct blood supply from the internal carotid artery. The proximal pars distalis appears to derive its blood supply from the interdigitating fingers of neurohypophyseal tissue and, apparently, from portal vessels. For this reason Lagios speaks of a "median eminence" in referring to this area of neurohypophyseal contact. However, it must be remembered that all conclusions concerning blood supply of the *Latimeria* pars distalis are based on careful dissection and

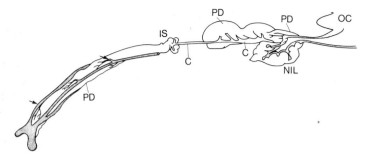

FIGURE 2.33. Pituitary gland of the coelacanth *Latimeria chalumnae* represented schematically. *Right*, brain and infundibulum (stippled); *left*, branches of the internal carotid artery from below (stippled). The pars distalis (*PD*) is divided into several lobes. The more distally located lobe at the left is connected to the more proximal part of the pars distalis by an elongated cellular tube *c* containing an extension of the hypophyseal cavity (*C*). The upper part of the distal pars distalis is generally broken into separate, discontinuous islets of glandular tissue (*IS*). Note that the uppermost part of the pars distalis is penetrated by fingers of vascular and connective tissue from the hypothalamus. *NIL*, neurointermediate lobe; *OC*, optic chiasma; *small arrows*, branches from the internal carotids into the distal pars distalis. [From M. Lagios, *Gen. Comp. Endocrinol.*, **25**:126–146, 1975.]

tissue sections. Vascular injections to trace blood supply have not yet been done.

Millot et al. (1978), authors of the three-volume treatise on the anatomy of *Latimeria*, name the tube connecting the two partes distalis ''canal buccohypophysaire'' and express the belief that it is developed from the embryonic epithelial stalk of Rathke's pouch. Lagios, on the other hand, equates the rostral pars distalis to the ventral lobe and Rachendachhypophyse of cartilaginous fishes. The connecting canal, in this interpretation, is equivalent to the stalk of the ventral lobe of elasmobranchs. This would require that the epithelial tube and rostral pars distalis of *Latimeria* develop from the lateral lobes of Rathke's pouch. It is clear that study of *Latimeria* embryos should settle this intriguing question. Without further evidence, both interpretations are plausible. There is other anatomic evidence of an elasmobranch relationship of the coelacanth fishes. If this is valid, Lagios' interpretation gains (and adds) some support.

Some Speculations Concerning the Early Evolution of the Vertebrate Adenohypophysis

It may be recalled that the Agnatha have no median eminence. Therefore, in the lampreys, at least, if the pars distalis is regulated at all by the neurosecretions of the adjacent anterior neurohypophysis, these secretions would reach the pars distalis by diffusion, not via portal blood vessels. As discussed above, the long history (ca. 500 million years) of the agnathans makes it difficult to decide whether this relatively simple brain–pituitary relationship represents a primitive stage in its evolution or a degeneration from a more advanced form.

However, at this point we can refer once more to Figs. 2.18 and 2.19 to state a pertinent argument. In three groups of primitive fishes (the selachians, the holocephalans, and the coelacanth), only part of the pars distalis is vascularized from the median eminence. The remainder of the pars distalis, like the entire pars distalis of lamprey, is vascularized directly from the internal carotid artery. In all other vertebrates (leaving aside the specialized teleosts), the entire pars distalis is vascularized from the median eminence. It is probably too much to ascribe to coincidence that in three groups of primitive fishes, all having their origins a bit later than the Agnatha (in the Paleozoic period), only a part of the pars distalis is vascularized from a median eminence. It is rational, therefore, to think of the partially developed brain–pituitary relationship in the selachians, holocephalans, and *Latimeria* as intermediate between the lamprey and all other vertebrates. This would argue, in turn, that the lamprey brain–pituitary relationship is primitive, not degenerate.

Another evolutionary issue that can be approached in this speculative manner is the nature of the adaptive force that led to the seemingly complex process of formation of the adenohypophysis from external head ectoderm in the first place. Several isolated facts suggest that the first adaptive value of bringing superficial (glandular) ectoderm into contact with the brain was to make possible regulated pigmentary changes in the skin in response to sense organ-perceived external light stimuli. If the lamprey pituitary is indeed primitive, we can see in its embryonic development something that suggests this. When the rod of ectoderm (equivalent of Rathke's pouch) first grows toward the diencephalon from the nasohypophyseal groove of the lamprey embryo, the presumptive pars intermedia breaks off from its tip prematurely. The pars intermedia quickly associates itself with the posterior neurohypophysis, leaving the stalk that bore it inward in approximate contact with the more anterior part of the floor of the diencephalon, the future anterior neurohypophysis (Fig. 2.14).

Another suggestive recent finding is the common occurrence of a protein, proopicorticotropin, in both the pars intermedia and the pars distalis. This protein contains the amino acid sequences for both ACTH and MSH. In the pars intermedia, enzymatic action releases primarily MSH from this protein, and in the pars distalis another pattern of enzyme action releases mostly ACTH.

The Amphibian Pituitary

In the ascending line of vertebrates, the Amphibia are the first to have a pars tuberalis. Characteristically, the amphibian neurohypophysis consists of a posteriorly directed, thin-walled outpouching of the hypothalamus that ends in a relatively modest thickening, the pars nervosa (see Fig. 2.19). The median eminence forms in the ventral, thin-walled portion of the neurohypophysis, anterior to the pars nervosa. Because the amphibian median eminence is so thin, most of its primary capillary plexus is visible from the ventral view, making it a beautiful sight in the living animal, as well as an attractive photograph or drawing (Fig. 2.34). It even has been reproduced on the cover of a textbook of endocrinology. The primary capillary plexus is drained into a series of portal vessels that proceed to the pars distalis. The neurosecretory neurons that end in the pars nervosa extend mostly from the Gomori-positive preoptic area. The cell bodies of the neurons that extend to the primary capillary plexus of the median eminence are located in a broad hypophysiotropic zone from the preoptic area to the midbrain. As an example, TRH has been found by RIA to be widely distributed not only

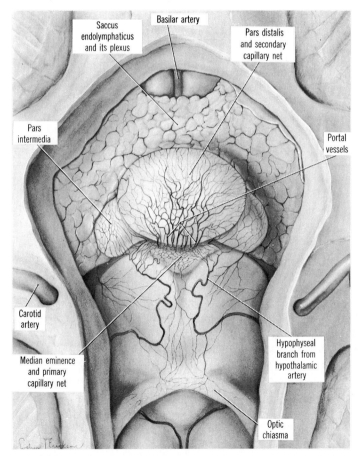

FIGURE 2.34. Ventral view of the brain, pituitary, and hypophyseal portal circulation of the adult bullfrog *Rana catesbeiana*. [Photograph of a drawing supplied by J. D. Green, University of California.]

in the frog hypothalamus but also in all other parts of the frog brain and spinal cord. In fact, TRH can be found by RIA in amphibian skin and gut as well. To add to this confusing picture, TRH has less apparent ability in activating the amphibian thyrotropic–thyroid axis than in higher vertebrates. There are many questions to unravel concerning the structure, distribution, and physiology of hypophysiotropic regulation via the median eminence of amphibians.

The amphibian pars intermedia becomes completely separated from the pars distalis, forming a transverse bar of tissue between the pars distalis and pars nervosa (Figs. 2.34, 2.35). It receives innervation by several types of nerve cells via the adjacent pars nervosa. These neurons make direct synaptic contact with the secretory cells of the pars intermedia. Those neurons that end in the pars intermedia and that are catecholaminergic (judging by electron microscopy and immunofluorescence) come from the hypothalamic preoptic nucleus.

The pars distalis is a rounded or oval structure that is well irrigated by the median eminence portal vessels. Its different secretory cells are fairly well scattered, not tending to segregate in zones as in some other vertebrates. The amphibian pars tuberalis generally is double, often seen as two small

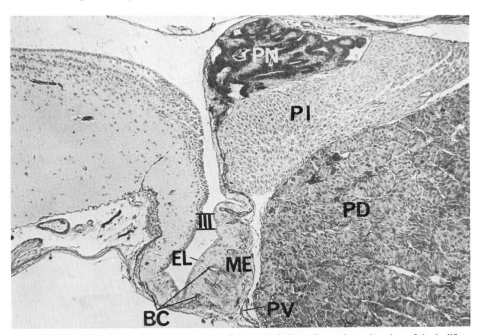

FIGURE 2.35. Sagittal section of a part of the hypothalamo-hypophyseal region of the bullfrog *Rana catesbeiana*. Anterior to the left. The third ventricle (*III*) dips downward, with the median eminence (*ME*) forming part of its floor. Blood capillaries (*BC*) in the median eminence are gathered into hypophyseal partal vessels (*PV*) which carry blood into the pars distalis (*PD*). *EL*, ependymal cellular lining of the third ventricle; *PI*, pars intermedia; *PN*, pars nervosa. [From H. Kobayashi, T. Matsui, and S. Ishii, *Int. Rev. Cytol.*, **29**:288, 1970.]

patches of tissue attached to the infundibulum anterior to the median eminence.

The Reptilian Pituitary

The reptilian pituitary differs from the amphibian in that the intermediate and distal lobes are not so separate; the pars intermedia can be larger than in any other vertebrate group; the pars tuberalis may be lacking in some groups (e.g., snakes); the pars nervosa (as in mammals and birds) is a relatively globular organ at the end of a narrow infundibular stalk.

In development, the reptilian and avian pituitaries are similar. Rathke's pouch, while still attached by an epithelial stalk to the stomodeum, develops an anterior diverticulum and lateral lobes (Fig. 2.36). The top of Rathke's pouch, in contact with the infundibulum, forms (in reptiles only) the pars intermedia; the lower half of Rathke's pouch and the anterior diverticulum

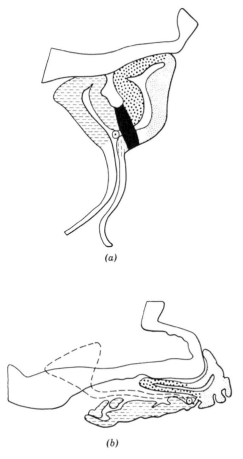

(a)

(b)

FIGURE 2.36. Midsagittal sections through developing pituitaries of two species of reptiles. (a) 4.5-Mm embryo of the lizard *Lacerta muralis* (an early stage, with the epithelial stalk comparable to the chick's adenohypophseal anlage; Fig. 2.39); (b) later stage in the lizard *Anguis fragilis*. The pars tuberalis, since it is out of the median section is shown outlined by broken lines. Corresponding areas are indicated as follows: *white*, infundibulum; *dots*, aboral lobe; *dashes*, oral lobe; *black*, boundary between oral and aboral lobes; *circle and dot*, level from which lateral lobes (pars tuberalis) originate. The pars intermedia in these two species forms from the part of the aboral lobe that is *in contact with the neurohypophysis*. According to Wingstrand, different portions of the aboral lobe (note distribution of large and small dots) form the pars intermedia in these two species. [From K. G. Wingstrand, *The Structure and Development of the Avian Pituitary*, C. W. K. Gleerup, Lund, Sweden, 1951.]

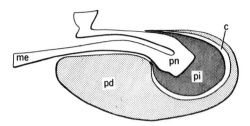

FIGURE 2.37. Sagittal section of the pituitary of a snake. The pars tuberalis in snakes is strongly reduced so it is not shown. *c*, Hypophyseal cleft; *me*, median eminence; *pd*, pars distalis; *pi*, pars intermedia; *pn*, pars nervosa.

(oral lobe of Wingstrand) form the pars distalis. In birds, the pars intermedia never differentiates as such. The lateral lobes grow out at the point of constriction between the original Rathke's pouch and the anterior chamber. The lateral lobes grow toward the infundibulum near the rostral tip of the pars distalis and differentiate as the pars tuberalis. In certain reptiles, particularly lizards and snakes, the pars tuberalis is greatly reduced or absent.

Thus, as in elasmobranchs, the pars distalis arises from two different parts of the embryonic buccal anlage. In the adult pars distalis, zones may be recognized in which the distribution of acidophilic, basophilic, and chromophobic cells is distinctly different. These zones are not given different names as they are in elasmobranchs or teleosts. One may wonder, in the

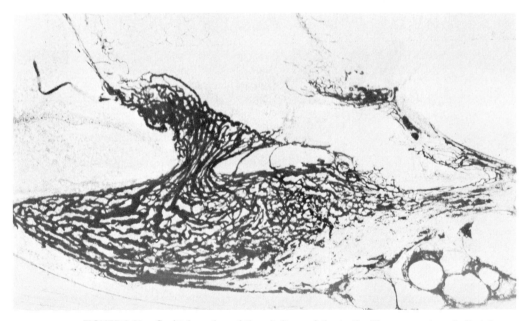

FIGURE 2.38. Sagittal section of the pituitary of the turtle *Chrysemys picta*. India ink was injected through the carotid artery. Its branch, the superior hypophyseal artery, is seen entering the primary capillary net from the upper left. The primary capillary net narrows and extends via the portal vessels into the adenohypophysis below where the large secondary capillary network is visible. [Photograph furnished by J. D. Green, University of California.]

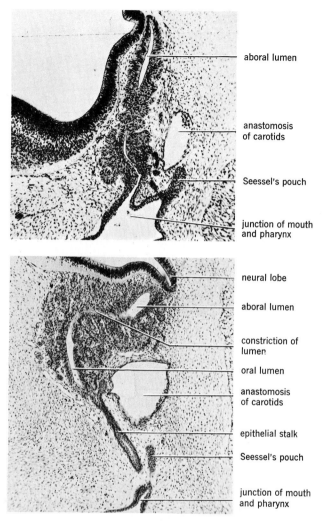

aboral lumen

anastomosis
of carotids

Seessel's pouch

junction of mouth
and pharynx

neural lobe

aboral lumen

constriction of
lumen

oral lumen

anastomosis
of carotids

epithelial stalk

Seessel's pouch

junction of mouth
and pharynx

FIGURE 2.39. Sagittal sections through developing pituitary gland of the chick: *top*, after 5 days of incubation; *bottom*, after 7 days of incubation. Note the lengthening of the epithelial stalk between days 5 and 7. Seessel's pouch, an endodermal structure, remains below and behind the point of anastomosis of the carotid arteries. Note that in the 7-day embryo there is some mesenchymatous connective tissue between the neural lobe of the developing pituitary and the aboral tip of the Rathke's pouch, but not between the constricted (future pars tuberalis) area and the infundibular floor (future median eminence). Proliferation of this mesenchyme into a connective tissue septum is held by some to explain the failure of the bird to develop a pars intermedia. [Photographs prepared by K. G. Wingstrand, University of Copenhagen.]

absence of sufficient information, whether the differentiated zones of the pars distalis of teleosts, for example, are homologous with the zones of the reptilian pars distalis.

The pars distalis of reptiles is distinctive in being curved dorsad so that it makes contact with the anterior wall of the infundibular stalk and the median eminence (Fig. 2.37). Where the pars tuberalis is well developed (e.g., turtles), it usually forms a bridge between the median eminence and the pars distalis. In this bridge run the hypophyseal portal veins.

The reptilian pars intermedia is unusually large in comparison with other vertebrates. As a rule, it may appear small in median sagittal sections, but it is more voluminous laterally. Anteriorly, it may partly surround the pars

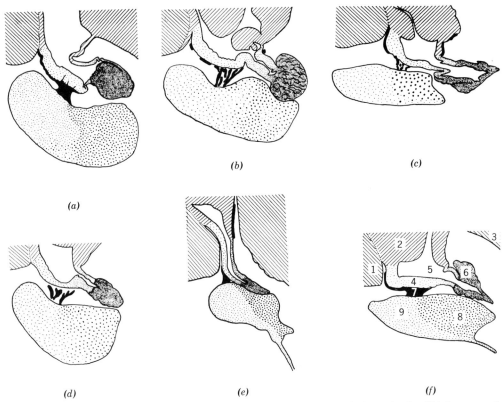

FIGURE 2.40. Variations in the shapes of the lobes of the pituitary glands of birds as seen in the midsagittal plane. (*a*) Ostrich (*Struthio camelus*); (*b*) swan (*Cygnus olor, juv.*); (*c*) grouse (*Lagopus lagopus*); (*d*) pigeon (*Columba livia*); (*e*) swift (*Apus apus*); (*f*) sparrow (*Passer montanus*). The key to the variously shaded parts is included in (*f*): *1*, Optic chiasma; *2*, diencephalon; *3*, medulla oblongata; *4*, median eminence; *5*, lumen of infundibular stem; *6*, pars nervosa; *7*, pars tuberalis; *8*, caudal or proximal zone of the pars distalis; *9*, rostral or cephalic zone of the pars distalis. [From K. G. Wingstrand, *The Structure and Development of the Avian Pituitary*, C. W. K. Gleerup, Lund, Sweden, 1951.]

distalis. The hypophyseal cleft usually persists to separate the pars intermedia from the pars distalis.

The pars nervosa is a bulbous structure at the end of an infundibular stalk most commonly directed in a posterior direction. This feature is shared with the birds and mammals. The infundibular ventricular cavity usually penetrates the pars nervosa. A median eminence is formed on the anterior side of the infundibular stalk near the tip of the pars distalis. In most respects it is similar to that of mammals and birds. It contains a plexus of capillaries derived from a branch of the carotid artery. In some instances the primary capillary plexus consists of vessels that form loops in the median eminence. The portal vessels drain the primary capillary plexus and enter the pars distalis. Here (Fig. 2.38) they distribute blood into the secondary capillary plexus.

The nerve tracts that enter the neurohypophysis are from two secretory hypothalamic centers; the supraoptic nucleus of reptiles, birds, and mammals, alone or together with the paraventricular nucleus, is considered to be the homologue of the preoptic nucleus of the fishes and Amphibia. However, it may be much more lateral in birds and mammals than in fishes or Amphibia. J. D. Green has observed that collateral fibers extend from the supraoptico-hypophyseal tract into the median eminence, where they end near blood vessels of the primary capillary plexus. However, the large ma-

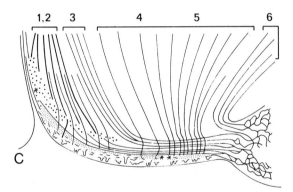

FIGURE 2.41. Simplified representation of the organization of the neurosecretory neuronal pathways between the hypothalamus and the median eminence and pars nervosa of birds. It may be compared, for guidance, with the more detailed schematic representation of such relationships in the white-crowned sparrow, shown in Fig. 2.42. The looped neuronal structures shown in the median eminence (lower left and lower center) are parts of axons of fibers of fairly broad hypothalamic origin, belonging to some of the tracts numbered in the upper part of the figure. Gomori-positive fibers exclusively enter the pars nervosa, but some also end in the anterior median eminence. Anatomical names of the neuronal fiber tracts are *1, 2*, tractus hypophyseus anterior, consisting of both coarse and fine fiber elements; *3*, tractus supraoptico-(paraventriculo-) hypophyseus; *4, 5*, tractus tubero-hypophyseus; *6*, tractus hypophyseus posterior. *C*, edge of optic chiasm. [From A. Oksche and D. Farner, Neurohistological studies of the hypothalamo-hypophysial system of *Zonotrichia leucophrys gambelli*, In *Advances in Anatomy, Embryology and Cell Biology*, Vol. 48, Springer-Verlag, Berlin, 1974.]

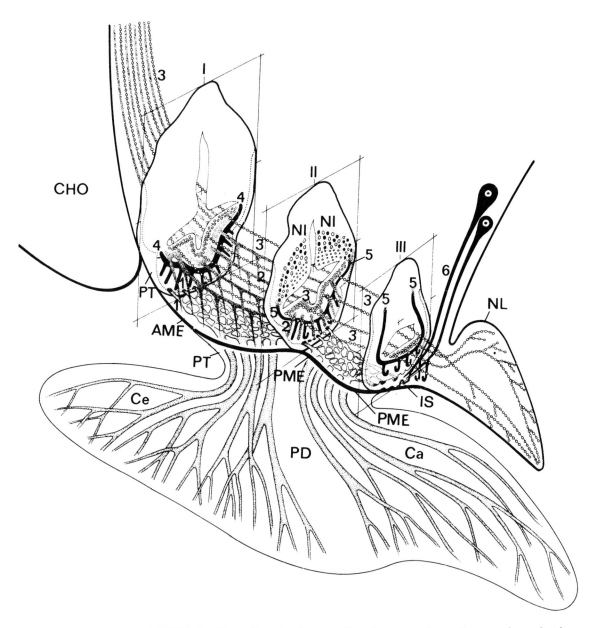

FIGURE 2.42. Three-dimensional organization of neurosecretory pathways and vascular channels in the hypothalamo-hypophyseal system of the white-crowned sparrow. Only blood vessels in the pars distalis (*PD*) are shown. *I, II,* and *III* are cross sections at three levels of the hypothalamus showing the kinds of neurosecretory fibers found at those levels. The beaded-appearing fibers (Gomori-positive) proceed to the pars nervosa. The fine-stippled fiber groups (Gomori-positive and Gomori-negative) are axons going to the median eminence where some of them form the loops illustrated in Fig. 2.41. Fiber groups shown in black are Gomori-negative, mostly going to the median eminence. Numbering of the fiber groups (1 through 6) is the same

jority of fibers in this tract pass directly to the pars nervosa, where their enlarged endings are grouped around blood vessels. The vascular supply of the reptilian pars nervosa is separate from that of the pars distalis.

The Avian Pituitary

The avian pituitary gland consistently lacks a pars intermedia in the adult, but in other respects it closely resembles that of reptiles.

As described earlier (Figs. 2.6 and 2.39), the embryonic adenohypophyseal anlage first forms as a simple, stalked Rathke's pouch. This pouch develops an anterior diverticulum and two lateral lobes. The original aboral part of this complex—part of which in elasmobranchs and reptiles forms the pars intermedia—forms only the pars distalis in the bird (Fig. 2.39). Thus, all parts of the primary anlage of the avian adenohypophysis, except the lateral lobes, form the pars distalis. The lateral lobes move dorsally and adhere to the infundibular stalk in the region of the median eminence to form the pars tuberalis. The epithelial stalk persists in a threadlike state in some birds and may even remain in connection with the buccal epithelium (Fig. 2.40).

In general, the avian pituitary tends to vary within relatively small limits in outline. The pars nervosa is thickened and globular and hangs from an infundibular stalk that usually points, in reptilian fashion, in a posterior direction. The pars distalis is usually ovoid or rounded in shape and is roughly separable into two zones according to the distribution of certain acidophils. These zones correspond to the regions derived originally from the aboral and rostral lobes of Rathke's pouch. The pars tuberalis is usually on the anterior face of the infundibular stalk, but it may be wrapped completely around it.

The avian median eminence is well developed and, in the birds that have been appropriately studied, it is differentiated into two regions. The anterior median eminence is Gomori positive (stains with aldehyde fuchsin), while the posterior median eminence is not. Oksche and Farner's (1974) careful study of the hypothalamo-hypophyseal system of the white-crowned sparrow (Figs. 2.41 and 2.42) shows that these two zones of the median eminence are innervated by different populations of hypophysiotropic neurosecretory neurons. Furthermore, the portal vessels from the two median eminences vascularize different areas of the pars distalis. This suggests that there can

---

as in Fig. 2.41. Note that in the basal infundibular nucleus (NI) there are clusters of neurons of different types. *AME* and *PME*, anterior and posterior median eminence; *Ca* and *Ce*, differentiated zones of the pars distalis; *CHO*, optic chiasma; *IS*, infundibular stalk; *NL*, pars nervosa; *PT*, pars tuberalis. The primary capillary network and hypophyseal portal vessels are shown but are not labeled. [From A. Oksche and D. Farner, Neurohistological studies of the hypothalamo-hypophysial system of *Zonotrichia leucophrys gambelii, In Advances in Anatomy, Embryology and Cell Biology*, Vol. 48, Springer-Verlag, Berlin, 1974.]

be a spatial separation of neurohaemal functions in the avian median eminences that correspond to regulation of separate regions of the pars distalis. Firm proof of this interesting contention is still needed.

As Fig. 2.42 indicates, most of the neurosecretory axons that proceed toward neurohaemal endings in the pars nervosa come from the preoptic area, and they bypass the median eminence en route (Fig. 2.43).

The Mammalian Pituitary

As might be expected, the mammalian pituitary has received more detailed study than any other vertebrate pituitary. The embryonic adenohypophyseal anlage in mammals is a stalked Rathke's pouch (Figs. 2.7 and 2.44). The aboral portion, in contact with the infundibulum, differentiates as the pars intermedia, and the remaining parts of the rudiment, except the lateral lobes, form the pars distalis. The lateral lobes form not in the middle of the anlage,

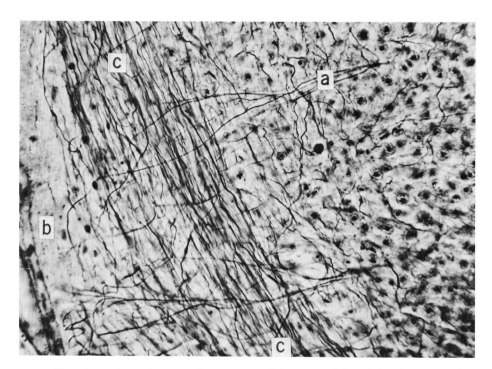

FIGURE 2.43. Fibers in the median eminence of the pigeon. Most of the fibers (c) run in a bundle—the neurosecretory tractus hypophyseus—toward the pars nervosa. However, it may be seen that certain fibers (a) pass through the tractus hypophyseus to the more superficial and vascular part of the median eminence (b), where they form loops. These looping axons originate in the nucleus lateralis tuberis of the hypothalamus. This relation is illustrated diagrammatically in Fig. 2.41. [Photograph provided by K. G. Wingstrand from *The Structure and Development of the Avian Pituitary*, C. W. K. Gleerup, Lund, Sweden, 1951.]

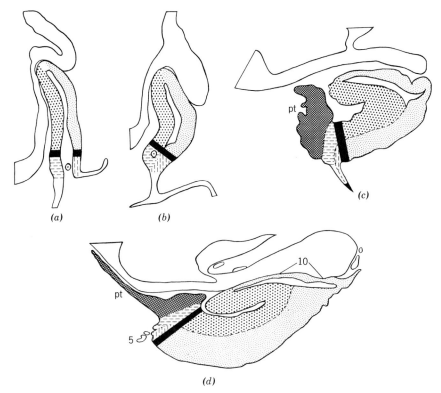

FIGURE 2.44. Development of the pituitary gland in the rabbit *Oryctolagus cuniculus*. These diagrams of sagittal sections of embryos of different ages are based on the work of Atwell, 1918. Wingstrand's interpretation (1951) of the movements and fate of equivalent regions of the original Rathke's pouch is indicated by dots, dashes, and solid black. According to this interpretation, the pars intermedia forms from a small part of the aboral lobe. The oral lobe of birds and reptiles is hardly represented, but forms the rostral tip of the rabbit's pars distalis. The circle-and-dot patterns in *a* and *b* show the level of origin of lateral lobes. These turn anteriorly and attach to the rostral tip of the distalis and the median eminence and become the pars tuberalis (cross-hatched area). (*a*) Embryo of 13 days; (*b*) 14 days; (*c*) 20 days; (*d*) 30 days. *5*, remnants of the epithelial stalk; *10*, pars intermedia; *pt*, pars tuberalis. [After K. G. Wingstrand, *Structure and Development of the Avian Pituitary*, C. W. K. Gleerup, Lund, Sweden, 1951.]

but at the rostral end. This difference in development from other vertebrates led Wingstrand to decide that the mammalian hypophyseal anlage lacks almost completely those elements that correspond to the anterior extension of Rathke's pouch. According to this idea, the pars distalis has a more uniform origin than in those species whose pars distalis forms from both the aboral and rostral lobes of Rathke's pouch. The adult mammalian pars tuberalis, in keeping with this idea, develops at the rostral tip of the pars distalis. The adult mammalian neurohypophysis is well differentiated, and the pars nervosa fairly uniformly forms a bulblike structure at the end of the infundibulum, as in reptiles and birds. The median eminence, however, is particularly well developed, forming a primary capillary plexus around part or most of the circumference of the cylindrical infundibular stalk in a number of species that have been adequately studied (Fig. 2.45). Furthermore, the eminential primary capillary plexus characteristically is made up of long complex capillary loops (Figs. 2.45 and 2.46). These loops, apparently, greatly increase the available neurohaemal contact area for endings of neurons carrying hypophysiotropic hormones.

The well-developed mammalian pars tuberalis often forms a thin collar around the infundibular stalk (Fig. 2.45). As in the reptiles and birds, the mammalian pars tuberalis is commonly the bridge of tissue through which portal vessels pass between the median eminence and the pars distalis.

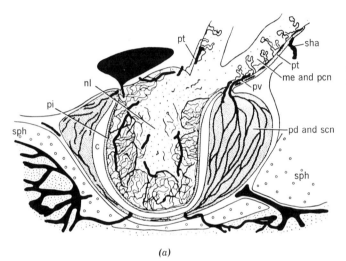

(a)

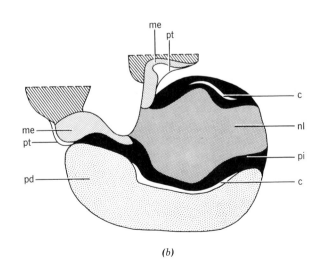

(b)

FIGURE 2.45. (a) Sagittal section of the pituitary gland of the opossum *Didelphis virginiana*. In this mammal the pars distalis is wrapped completely around the pars nervosa so it appears both anterior (right) and posterior (left) to it. The pars intermedia is a thin layer, only one or two cells thick, in contact with the pars nervosa, separated from the distalis by the hypophysial cleft. The pars tuberalis surrounds the median eminence, which in this species is cylindrical, actually the last part of the infundibulum before the pars nervosa. The partes nervosa and distalis have completely separate circulatory supplies. Blood vessels are represented in solid black. The pars distalis receives its blood from the primary capillary plexus in the pars tuberalis via the portal vessels. The pars tuberalis, in turn, is supplied by the superior hypophysial artery, a branch of the internal carotid. Abbreviations: *c*, Hypophyseal cleft; *me*, median eminence; *nl*, pars nervosa; *pcn*, primary capillary net featuring vascular tufts or spikes; *pd*, pars distalis; *pt*, pars tuberalis; *scn*, secondary capillary net; *sha*, superior hypophyseal artery; *sph*, sphenoid bone. [After J. D. Green, *Am. J. Anat.*, **88**:225, 1951.] (b) Sagittal section of the pituitary gland of the wolf. Here the adenohypophysis forms a cylinder around the neurohypophysis, but the pars distalis itself remains rostral. The hypophysial cleft, likewise, is continuous around the pars nervosa. The pars distalis is stippled, and the pars intermedia is represented as black. Other labeling as above. [After B. Hanström, *Kung. Fysiogr. Sällsk. Lund Förh.*, 1955.]

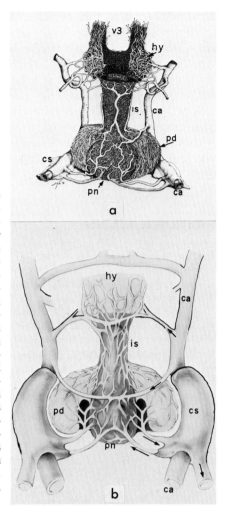

FIGURE 2.46. Drawings of a vascular cast (*a*) and an interpretation (*b*) of the blood vessel connections between the pituitary and hypothalamus of a monkey (viewed from the posterior side). The arterial supply to the pituitary region is mostly from two branches of the carotid arteries (*ca*). The venous drainage is into the cavernous sinuses (*cs*). Directions of flow are indicated in *b*. The vascular spikes of the median eminence would be within the tissue of the infundibular stalk (*is*) and pars nervosa (*pn*). In *b* a network of vessels is shown extending from the neurohypophysis (*is* and *pn*) to the pars distalis (*pd*). (The pars distalis is wrapped around the anterior aspect of the pars nervosa, but extends beyond it at the sides.) However, both figures show that this network is continuous with vessels that extend all the way to the hypothalamus (*hy*). Thus, it is the thesis of Bergland and Page that there is an anatomical basis for some degree of retrograde flow upward from the adenohypophysis toward the hypothalamus. [Drawings were provided by R. M. Bergland, Department of Surgery, Harvard University.]

The pars intermedia, reminiscent of birds, is often absent in adult mammals. In humans the pars intermedia is gradually reduced during the early years, and it is absent in most adults. In the larger mammals (e.g., the elephant), and in aquatic mammals and the armadillo, there is no pars intermedia. It should be noted that it is only in the birds and in some mammals that the pars intermedia is absent among the higher vertebrates. It is also these two groups that lack short-term functional chromatophores in the skin. Unfortunately for this interesting correlation, mammals and birds still form MSH, even though they may lack a pars intermedia.

An interesting issue has arisen recently with respect to the vascular supply of the mammalian pituitary gland. Bergland and Page (1979), as a result of a careful study of the sizes and numbers of blood vessels entering and leaving the various regions of the primate adenohypophysis–median eminence–pars nervosa system (see Fig. 2.46), conclude that some blood must flow from this system, through anastomosing vessels, upward from the pituitary to the hypothalamus. Although this direction is opposite to that usually conceived for this vascular network, it at least appears possible, and it would explain certain phenomena, such as the presence and possible hypothalamic feedback of the pars distalis hormones in the brain. Of particular current interest is the "hormone" β-endorphin, produced in the pars distalis and intermedia and having an analgesic and behavioral action in the brain through interaction with specific receptors. This intriguing suggestion will undoubtedly receive much attention in the near future.

ADDITIONAL READING

1. Assenmacher, I., and D. S. Farner (1978). *Environmental Endocrinology*. Springer-Verlag, Berlin.

2. Baker, B. L. (1974). Functional cytology of the hypophysial pars distalis and pars intermedia. In *Handbook of Physiology*, Sect. 7, Vol. 4, Part 1, Williams & Wilkins, Baltimore, pp. 45–80.

3. Bargmann, W., A. Oksche, A. Polenov, and B. Scharrer, eds. (1978). *Neurosecretion and Neuroendocrine Activity. Evolution, Structure and Function*. Springer, Heidelberg.

4. Barrington, E. J. W. (1978). Evolutionary aspects of hormonal structure and function. In *Comparative Endocrinology* (P. J. Gaillard and H. H. Boer, eds.). Elsevier/North-Holland, Amsterdam, pp. 381–396.

5. Bergland, R. M., and R. B. Page (1979). Pituitary-brain vascular relations: a new paradigm. *Science* **204**:18–24.

6. Fawcett, D. W., J. W. Long, and A. L. Jones (1969). The ultrastructure of endocrine glands. *Recent Progr. Horm. Res.* **23**:315–380.

7. Ferray, L., and B. Vivien-Roels (1975). Etude comparée de l'embryogenèse du complexe diencephalo-hypophysaire de deux cheloniens: *Testudo graeca* L. et *Emys orbicularis* L. *Arch. Biol.* **86**:253–272.

8. Fontaine, M., and M. Olivereau (1975). Aspects of the organization and evolution of the vertebrate pituitary. *Am. Zool.* **15**(Suppl. 1):61–80.

9. Ganong, W., and L. Martini, eds. (1973). *Frontiers in Neuroendocrinology*. Academic, New York.

10. Gorbman, A., and H. A. Bern (1962). *A Textbook of Comparative Endocrinology*. Wiley, New York.

11. Halasz, B., and L. Papp (1965). Hormone secretion of the anterior pituitary gland after physical interruption of all nervous pathways to the hypophysiotropic area. *Endocrinology* **77**:553–562.

12. Harris, G. W., and B. T. Donovan, eds. (1966). *The Pituitary Gland*, Vols. 1–3. University of California Press, Berkeley.

13. Holmes, R. L., and J. N. Ball (1974). *The Pituitary Gland*. Cambridge University Press, London.

14. Jaffe, B. M., and H. L. Behrman (1979). *Methods of Hormone Radioimmunoassay*. Academic, New York.

15. Jasinski, A. (1969). Vascularization of the hypophyseal region in lower vertebrates (cyclostomes and fishes). *Gen. Comp. Endocrinol.*, Suppl. **2**:510–521.

16. Jeffcoate, S. L., and J. S. M. Hutchinson, eds. (1978). *The Endocrine Hypothalamus.* Academic, New York.

17. Kawamoto, M. (1967). Zur Morphologie der Hypophysis cerebri von Teleostiern. *Arch. Histol. Japonicum* **28**:123–150.

18. Krieger, D. T., and J. C. Hughes, eds. (1980). *Neuroendocrinology*, Sinauer Associates, Sunderland, Mass.

19. Lagios, M. D. (1968). Tetrapod-like organization of the pituitary gland of the polypteriformid fishes *Calamoichthys calabaricus* and *Polypterus palmas*. *Gen. Comp. Endocrinol.* **11**:300–315.

20. Lagios, M. D. (1970). The median eminence of the bowfin, *Amia calva* L. *Gen. Comp. Endocrinol.* **15**:453–463.

21. Lagios, M. D. (1975). The pituitary gland of the coelacanth *Latimeria chalumnae* Smith. *Gen. Comp. Endocrinol.* **25**:126–146.

22. Mellinger, J. (1963). Les relations neuro-vasculo-glandulaires dans l'appareil hypophysaire de la Roussette, *Scyliorhinus canicula*. Thesis. Faculté des Sciences, Université de Strasbourg.

23. Meurling, P. (1967). The vascularization of the pituitary in elasmobranchs. *Sarsia* **28**:1–104.

24. Mikami, S. T. Kurosumi, and D. S. Farner (1975). Light- and electron-microscopic studies of the secretory cytology of the adenohypophyses of the Japanese quail, *Coturnix coturnix japonica*. *Cell Tissue Res.* **159**:147–165.

25. Millot, J., J. Anthony, and D. Robineau (1978). *Anatomie de Latimeria Chalumnae*, Vol. 3. Editions Cent. Natl. Res. Scient., Paris, pp. 53–59.

26. Oksche, A., and D. S. Farner (1974). Neurohistological studies of the hypophyseal system of *Zonotrichia leucophrys gambelii* (Aves, Passeriformes). *Advances in Anatomy, Embryology and Cell Biology*, Vol. 48. Springer-Verlag, Berlin, pp. 1–136.

27. Szentagothai, J., B. Flerko, B. Mess, and B. Halasz (1968). *Hypothalamic Control of the Anterior Pituitary*. Akademiai Kiado, Budapest.

3

The Neurohypophysis

The most important functional link between the vertebrate nervous system and the endocrine system is the interrelationship between the basal hypothalamus and the pituitary. As we have shown in the preceding chapter, the close anatomic association of the neurohypophysis and adenohypophysis is a constant feature throughout the vertebrates, although the relative degree or extent of vascular or neural connections between these structures varies among the different vertebrate classes. The functional basis for this association involves the secretion of releasing factors by the median eminence for control of the adenohypophysis. In addition, neurosecretions from the pars nervosa into the general circulation affect target organs at sites that are distant from the pituitary. Therefore, the functions of the neurohypophysis can be classified as having local (hypophysiotropic) and systemic effects (see Fig. 1.4). Hypophysiotropic actions will be considered in detail in later chapters. In this chapter we will concentrate on the systemic actions of the neurohypophysis.

The systemic effects of the hormonal secretions of the neurohypophysis include (1) control of water balance, (2) contraction of uterine muscle, (3) ejection of milk from the mammary gland, and (4) modification of blood pressure (pressor-depressor). The first of these actions is exerted through control of water flow through semipermeable membranes, while the rest are results of contraction or relaxation of certain smooth muscles or other contractile tissue (e.g., myoepithelial cells). The functions of the pars nervosa probably are more recent, in a phyletic sense, than the local hypophysiotropic role of the median eminence. Control of water balance by the neurohypophysis hormones becomes quite important in amphibians. This rise in importance parallels the need for water conservation since vertebrates left the aquatic environment and became terrestrial. Another phylogenetically recent systemic function of the neurohypophysis is the milk ejection reflex, which occurs, of course, only in mammals. Interestingly, the development of a bulbous pars nervosa as a distinct neurohaemal organ (Fig. 2.19) is an anatomic feature that accompanies the rise in physiological importance of the several systemic effects. However, this does not mean that the systemically secreting part of the neurohypophysis lacks importance in the lower aquatic vertebrates. It remains true that no vertebrate group, including the cyclostomes, completely lacks a mechanism for the systemic release of neurohypophyseal secretion. In fact, the neurohypophysis of hagfishes seems particularly well organized anatomically for this purpose, even though we do not know what this purpose is. Furthermore, as we shall discuss next, the same or similar neurohypophyseal peptides are found in all vertebrate groups.

SYSTEMIC HORMONES OF THE NEUROHYPOPHYSIS

The systemic neurohypophyseal hormones are peptides containing eight different amino acids (nine amino acid residues in total). They are generally referred to as octapeptides, if one accepts the convention that two cysteines that are linked by a disulfide bond comprise one cystine molecule. Discussion of their chemical structures is facilitated if we refer to the nine amino acid positions of the hormones as shown in Fig. 3.1 for oxytocin. There are several consistent features in all the naturally occurring peptides. The amino acids at positions 1, 5, and 9 are in the form of amides. The cysteines at positions 1 and 6 are linked by a disulfide bond; this produces a pentapeptide ring structure with a three–amino acid side chain. The structure of oxytocin, isolated from pig and beef neurohypophyses, was first identified and then synthesized by du Vigneaud and collaborators in 1953. This was a significant event, since it was the first time that a peptide hormone was synthesized. Subsequently, Acher, Van Dyke, Sawyer, Chauvet, and others isolated, identified, and synthesized 10 distinct neurohypophyseal hormones from a wide variety of vertebrates (Fig. 3.2).

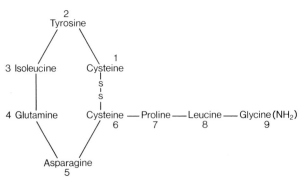

FIGURE 3.1. Structural formula for oxytocin.

Basic peptides	1	2	3	4	5	6	7	8	9

1. Arginine vasotocin (AVT)   Cys–Tyr–Ileu–Gln–Asn–Cys–Pro–Arg– Gly–NH₂

2. Arginine vasopressin (AVP)   Cys–Tyr–Phe– Gln–Asn–Cys–Pro–Arg– Gly–NH₂

3. Lysine vasopressin (LVP)   Cys–Tyr–Phe– Gln–Asn–Cys–Pro–Lys– Gly–NH₂

4. Phenypressin   Cys–Phe–Phe– Gln–Asn–Cys–Pro–Arg– Gly–NH₂

Neutral peptides

1. Oxytocin   Cys–Tyr–Ileu–Gln–Asn–Cys–Pro–Leu– Gly–NH₂

2. Mesotocin   Cys–Tyr–Ileu–Gln–Asn–Cys–Pro–Ileu–Gly–NH₂

3. Valitocin   Cys–Tyr–Ileu–Gln–Asn–Cys–Pro–Val– Gly–NH₂

4. Isotocin   Cys–Tyr–Ileu–Ser–Asn–Cys–Pro–Ileu–Gly–NH₂

5. Glumitocin   Cys–Tyr–Ileu–Ser–Asn–Cys–Pro–Gln– Gly–NH₂

6. Aspartocin   Cys–Tyr–Ileu–Asn–Asn–Cys–Pro–Val– Gly–NH₂

FIGURE 3.2   Structures of the known neurohypophyseal octapeptides.

Note that differences in amino acid sequence occur at amino acid positions 2, 3, 4, and 8. The cysteines at positions 1 and 6 are connected by a disulfide bond.

The naturally occurring neurohypophyseal principles can be divided into two groups: the basic, antidiuretic-vasoactive hormones and the neutral, oxytocinlike principles (Fig. 3.2). The four basic peptides—arginine vasotocin, arginine vasopressin, lysine vasopressin, and phenypressin—are categorized as such because they contain a basic amino acid (Arg or Lys) at position 8 in their structural formulae. The other group contains neutral amino acids at position 8; it includes oxytocin, mesotocin, valitocin, isotocin, glumitocin, and aspartocin. In comparing the structures of the 10 hormones, it can be seen that amino acid substitutions occur only at positions 2, 3, 4, and 8.

PHYLETIC DISTRIBUTION

In general, the neurohypophysis of a given animal species contains at least one basic peptide and at least one neutral peptide. The exception to this rule is the cyclostomes; the existing hagfishes and lampreys have only arginine

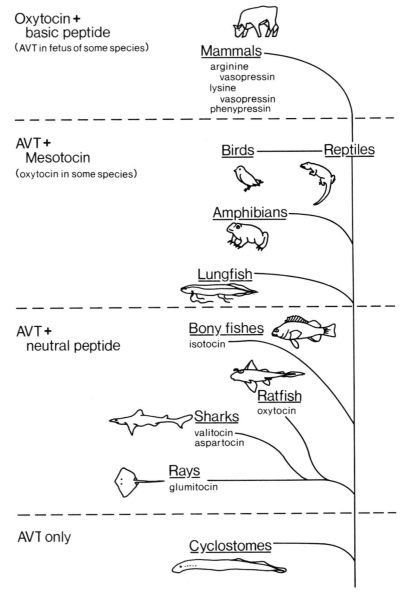

Oxytocin +
basic peptide
(AVT in fetus of some species)

AVT +
Mesotocin
(oxytocin in some species)

AVT +
neutral peptide

AVT only

Mammals
arginine
vasopressin
lysine
vasopressin
phenypressin

Birds ——————— Reptiles

Amphibians

Lungfish

Bony fishes
isotocin

Ratfish
oxytocin

Sharks
valitocin
aspartocin

Rays
glumitocin

Cyclostomes

FIGURE 3.3. Phyletic distribution of the neurohypophyseal octapeptides. Arginine vasotocin (AVT) is the most common peptide among all classes except mammals. Nonmammalian tetrapods and lungfishes usually have mesotocin as the neutral peptide. Most mammals have oxytocin and arginine vasopressin.

vasotocin. The occurrence of the various peptides among the vertebrates is shown in Fig. 3.3. Arginine vasotocin appears to be the most primitive and ubiquitous of the neurohypophyseal peptides, since it is found in representative species of all vertebrate classes. Although arginine vasotocin is replaced by the vasopressins in adult mammals, it is present in the fetal neurohypophysis of some mammals. In Chondrichthyes and bony fishes arginine vasotocin is present along with one or more neutral peptides. Glumitocin is present in rays, while spiny dogfish neurohypophyses contain valitocin and aspartocin. It is not certain at present whether individual dogfishes have both valitocin and aspartocin or whether these are individual differences, since these peptides were isolated from a pool of many individual glands. The ratfish neurohypophysis, like that of mammals, contains oxytocin as its neutral peptide. It is generally accepted that the occurrence of oxytocin in these distantly related groups is an example of convergent biochemical evolution, since oxytocin does not appear to be common in the intermediate phyletic groups. Bony fishes have isotocin, a neutral principle unique to this group.

The sarcopterygian fishes and the nonmammalian tetrapods have arginine vasotocin as their basic neurohypophyseal principle and mesotocin as their neutral peptide. There have been reports that oxytocin may be present in some amphibians, reptiles, and birds, but definitive proof of this has not yet been presented.

The mammals offer an exception to the constancy of arginine vasotocin as the basic neurohypophyseal hormone of vertebrates. All members of this group have oxytocin as the neutral peptide and one of the vasopressins as the basic principle. Most adult mammals have arginine vasopressin; lysine vasopressin is found in members of the suborder Suina, in some marsupials and in the Peru strain of mice. The mutation from arginine to lysine vasopressin probably occurred independently in these latter two groups, since all other strains of mice so far examined have arginine vasopressin. The situation in Suina is interesting because it appears to be an example of genetic polymorphism. While the domestic pig has only lysine vasopressin, wild strains may have either lysine or arginine vasopressin, or both. Thus in such species as the wild European boar, African wild hog, and the hippopotamus there may be an allelic pair of genes, each encoding for either the lysine or the arginine form of the basic hormone. It is not clear what selection pressures are responsible for maintaining the heterozygous condition, since lysine and arginine vasopressins appear to have equal biological activities in pigs. Phenypressin is the most recently discovered neurohypophyseal peptide and has been identified only in marsupials.

Many schemes have been proposed for the evolutionary pathways of amino acid substitution in neurohypophyseal hormones based on their structures and phyletic distributions (Fig. 3.4). In some of these schemes it is argued that arginine vasotocin (AVT) is the primitive or ancestral hormone, since it is the only neurohypophyseal principle found in cyclostomes and its

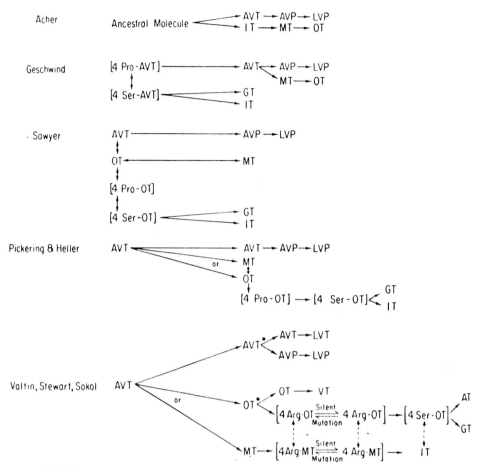

FIGURE 3.4. Proposed schemes for the evolutionary pathways of neurohypophyseal principles. With the exception of the scheme proposed by Acher, each arrow denotes an amino acid substitution that could be accomplished by a single nucleotide base substitution. The models by Geschwind and Sawyer were constructed to accommodate the minimum number of mutations. Compounds in brackets are hypothetical, since these compounds have not been detected in the neurohypophysis of present-day vertebrate species. [From Valtin, Stewart, and Sokol, *Handbook of Physiology*, Vol. 4 (R. O. Greep and E. B. Astwood, eds.), Baltimore, Williams & Wilkins, 1974, p. 156.

occurrence is widespread among vertebrates. Although this is a compelling argument, in other evolutionary schemes it has been proposed that the ancestral peptide was different from any of the neurohypophyseal hormones of present-day vertebrates. Even with the limitation that only single-point mutations (nucleotide substitutions) in the genetic code are observed, several different evolutionary schemes are plausible. However, there is only one path of structural change of octapeptides that must have occurred to result in the phyletic distribution of peptides we observe today. Thus there is a basic problem in attempting to describe the evolution of hormones solely on the basis of their chemical structures. Consideration of evolutionary trends in endocrinology should include both the structure and function of the hormone. In other words, we must have some understanding of how structural changes in hormones may afford an adaptational advantage to an evolving animal species.

Regarding the evolution of neurohypophyseal octapeptides, the parallel evolution of oxytocin and vasopressin and their functions during the emergence of mammals may illustrate a point. In mammals oxytocin (OXY) and other neutral principles have a much greater potency in inducing uterine contraction and milk ejection than in promoting water reabsorption (antidiuresis) by the kidney (Table 3.1). Arginine or lysine vasopressin, on the other hand, are potent antidiuretic factors that have only slight effects on the uterus and mammary gland. AVT, which is not present in the neurohypophysis of adult mammals, has considerable potency in all three responses (Table 3.1) but is less effective than arginine vasopressin (AVP) for antidiuresis and than OXY for uterine contraction or milk ejection. Therefore, in mammals the replacement of AVT by AVP as the basic principle and the evolution of OXY as the neutral principle are associated with a clear separation of regulation by octapeptides of water balance (AVP) and reproductive and mammary function (OXY). Presumably, this separation of octapeptide function has offered mammals some adaptive advantage. Unfortunately, there is not enough information available to speculate on the significance of other vertebrate octapeptides. In any event, this kind of reasoning, which considers the evolution of hormone structures in light of their functions, is useful for speculating about why certain mutations in genes coding for hormones are retained.

TABLE 3.1. Biological properties of some synthetic neurohypophyseal hormones[a]

Hormone	Antidiuretic[b]	Uterine-Contracting[b]	Milk-Ejecting[c]
Arginine vasotocin	260[d]	120	220
Arginine vasopressin	465	17	69
Lysine vasopressin	260	5	63
Oxytocin	5	450	450
Mesotocin	1	291	330
Isotocin	0.18	145	290
Glumitocin	0.41	10	53
Valitocin	0.8	199	308
Aspartocin	0.04	107	298

[a] From R. Acher, *Handbook of Physiology* (R. O. Greep and E. B. Astwood, eds.) Williams & Wilkins, Baltimore (1974).
[b] Measured in the rat.
[c] Measured in the rabbit.
[d] Numbers represent activity measured in international units/μmole.

In some cases the evolution of neurohypophyseal peptides appears to have been associated with an evolution of specificity of hormonal receptors. For example, it has been suggested by La Pointe that during the evolution of mammals from reptiles, there was a parallel development of sensitivity (receptors) to OXY in a new tissue, the mammary gland, and a change in the response specificity of the uterus to octapeptides. Contraction of the uterus of reptiles is much more sensitive to AVT than either to OXY or to mesotocin. The greater uterine-contracting potency of AVT is maintained in birds. However, the mammalian uterus has a greater sensitivity to OXY. Presumably, the uterine receptor for AVT changed during the evolution of mammals to show a higher specificity for OXY.

PRODUCTION AND RELEASE OF NEUROHYPOPHYSEAL HORMONES

As mentioned in Chapter 2, the hormones secreted by the neurosecretory nerve endings of the pars nervosa are synthesized in cell bodies located in the anterior hypothalamus. Because of the large size of the cell bodies of these neurons, they are called "magnocellular neurons." In lower vertebrates these cell bodies are found in the preoptic nucleus, while in birds, reptiles, and mammals the magnocellular neurons are concentrated in two paired structures: the supraoptic nuclei and the paraventricular nuclei (Fig. 2.3). A few magnocellular neurons have been found scattered in the hypothalamic tissue between the supraoptic and paraventricular nuclei.

Ultrastructural studies of the magnocellular neurons of the genetically defective Brattleboro strain of rats, which lack AVP but not OXY, indicate that individual neurons produce only one type of hormone, either AVP or OXY. This one neuron–one hormone hypothesis is supported for the most part by immunohistochemical evidence, which shows that individual magnocellular neurons will react with either anti-vasopressin or anti-oxytocin antisera, but rarely with both. Vasopressin- and oxytocin-containing neurons are found in both hypothalamic nuclei. In rats and humans vasopressinergic nerve cell bodies are concentrated in the ventral portion of the supraoptic and the medial part of the paraventricular nuclei, whereas the oxytocin cells appear concentrated in the dorsal supraoptic and lateral paraventricular nuclei. The functional basis for this distribution of neurosecretory magnocellular neurons is not fully understood.

During the isolation and characterization of neurohypophyseal hormones in the 1950s, Van Dyke and colleagues extracted a protein with a molecular weight of 10,000 from the pars nervosa and the hypothalamus. Subsequently, this cysteine-rich protein, named neurophysin, was found distributed in the brain, along with the neurosecretory magnocellular neurons, and was shown to be the material that was stained by the classical neurosecretory stains (Gomori's chrome alum–hematoxylin or paraldehyde-fuchsin). Furthermore, it was discovered that neurophysin had the property of noncovalently binding the neurohypophyseal hormones. Since no biological function has been associated with neurophysin, it is generally accepted that neurophysin functions as a "carrier protein" for the hormones. Several neurophysins have been identified and appear to occur in a one-to-one molecular ratio with the neurohypophyseal hormones. Throughout the hypothalamo-neurohypophyseal system in mammals, neurophysin I is associated with OXY and neurophysin II is associated with AVP. Additional neurophysins have been detected; however, these may be precursors or breakdown products of neurophysins I and II. With more refined biochemical techniques and RIAs for the neurophysins, it has been shown that these proteins are synthesized, stored, and released into the peripheral circulation along with the hormones. This has stimulated interest in the search for a possible hormonal function for the neurophysins.

The high cysteine content of the neurophysins and hormones made possible the detailed study of the processes of synthesis, transport, and secretion of neurohypophyseal hormones. Sachs and co-workers used radioactive ^{35}S-labeled cysteine to trace the amino acid incorporation and axonal transport of peptides within the magnocellular neurons and their axons. These studies were extended by others to provide a probable model for the production of neurohypophyseal peptides. In the rat the peptide hormones and neurophysin appear to be synthesized in the neurosecretory cell body in the form of a biologically inactive precursor protein within one and a half hours after injection of radiolabeled cysteine into the hypothalamus. Shortly afterward, the peptides are produced by the enzymatic cleavage of the precursor either within the Golgi apparatus or after the material is packaged into neurosecretory granules. Radioactive neurophysin and hormone appear at the neurosecretory endings in the pars nervosa in two to three hours after the injection. Therefore, the rate of transport of secretory granules down the axon can be calculated to be about 3 to 4 mm/hr. Secretory granules are stored in the nerve endings until the signal for secretion arrives and granule contents are released by exocytosis. Although it takes several hours for synthesis and transport of hormone to the neurosecretory nerve ending, the secretion of the hormone in response to a stimulus is rapid. Depolarization of the magnocellular neuron in the hypothalamus is followed by the propagation of action potentials down the axon at a rate of 0.5 to 1.5 m/s. A high frequency (greater than 10 Hz) of experimental electrical stimulation induces maximal secretion of hormone, which elevates the blood level of the hormone within a matter of seconds.

ACTIONS OF THE NEUROHYPOPHYSEAL HORMONES

Water Balance

The major action of AVP in mammals is to promote retention of water at the level of the kidney. Since this water-retaining activity is of greater physiological importance than any blood pressure effects of vasopressin, the hormone is also called "antidiuretic hormone" (ADH). If the pars nervosa is surgically removed, the animal will survive but will produce copious amounts of dilute urine (diuresis) and must drink large amounts of water (polydipsia) in order to replace the water lost through the kidneys. When these animals are injected with AVP, the rate of urine production decreases, and a state of water balance is attained. Inadequate production of AVP is the cause of most cases of the disease *diabetes insipidus*, which in man is associated with an increase of urine production from the normal one to two liters per day to as much as 20 liters per day in extreme cases. In the Brattleboro strain of rats the disease has a hereditary basis; rats that are homozygous for the disease are unable to produce AVP, while the neurohypophysis of heterozygous animals contains about 60% of the amount of AVP found in normal rats. In other cases of the disease (nephrogenic diabetes insipidus), the kidney presumably lacks hormone receptors and is unresponsive to high circulating levels of AVP.

Much work has been done to characterize the mechanism by which ADH reduces renal loss of water in mammals. The possibilities are several: (1) AVP could affect the glomerular filtration rate (by reducing the production of filtrate); (2) it could affect the movement of solutes through the tubular wall (and consequent osmotic movement of water out of the tubule); (3) it could cause passive movement of water out of the tubule by increasing the water permeability of the tubular wall. In mammals the glomerular filtration rate or solute transport are not affected by AVP. The hormone reduces water loss in the mammalian kidney by increasing the water permeability of the tubular wall. In the proximal convoluted tubule of the renal nephron, the majority (about 80%) of the water is reabsorbed, along with solutes, by an AVP-independent mechanism. The proximal tubular wall is freely permeable to water, which follows the solutes out of the tubule. In contrast, the walls of the distal tubule and collecting ducts are much less permeable to water. As the filtrate passes through the distal tubule, some additional solute may be transported out of the tubule, leaving the water behind. The filtrate is then passed on through collecting ducts into the deeper layers of the kidney (renal medulla), where high concentrations of solute are present outside the ducts. In the presence of AVP the relatively water-impermeable walls of the distal tubule and collecting duct become "porous," so that water passes out of the tubule and is reabsorbed in response to the relatively higher osmotic pressure of the blood. It should be noted here that the proximal tubule does the bulk of the work of reabsorbing water and solutes. In most cases only about 20% of the original glomerular filtrate reaches the distal tubule and collecting duct. Thus, in a sense, regulation of water balance by AVP in mammals concerns the "fine tuning" of renal water reabsorption. However, this function of AVP is important for water conservation in the whole animal, and particularly in desert animals, which are faced with a desiccating environment and little available water.

As would be expected, the conditions that are physiological signals for

AVP release are related to the total amount of water in the body. The most important signals are high blood osmolarity (hypertonicity) and low blood pressure or volume (hypovolemia). When an animal loses water without a corresponding loss of solutes, the blood becomes concentrated. Normally, blood osmolarity in humans is maintained within a narrow range (around 280 mosmoles/liter). When it rises above 290 mosmoles/liter, AVP is released into the circulation to increase water reabsorption and dilute the blood. What is the nature of the sensor whose stimulation leads to AVP release when the organism lacks water? Verney and others have hypothesized that there is a cellular "osmoreceptor" sensitive to changes of blood solute concentration in the brain. These sensors have been localized in the anterior hypothalamus, since hypothalamic tissue that has been isolated by surgically cutting nervous connections to the rest of the brain retains the ability to release AVP in response to an injection of hypertonic saline. Moreover, single hypothalamic cells that respond to hypertonic saline by increasing their electrical activity have been detected. However, it is not certain whether these cells are Verney's osmoreceptors.

The release of AVP can also occur when the total blood volume decreases because of a loss of blood (hemorrhage) or following prolonged dehydration. Relatively small (5 to 10%) changes in blood volume are effective modulators of AVP secretion. The body has at least two important sources of information for determining total blood volume. Baroreceptors in the carotid sinus measure the blood pressure in the carotid arteries and send this information to the brain through a nervous pathway. Stretch receptors in the left atrium of the heart measure the distension of the atrium caused by the filling of the heart with blood from the pulmonary circulation. Information on the volume of blood filling the atrium is sent to the brain via the vagus nerve. There probably are other sources of blood volume information (aortic arch baroreceptors, for example); however, the carotid bodies and left atrium have received the greatest attention. It is interesting that these two sensors provide information from the high-pressure (carotid arteries) and low-pressure (left atrium) ends of the blood vascular circulatory system, and both are probably necessary for an accurate assessment of blood volume. The thoracic location of these blood pressure and volume receptors has some interesting consequences. When a person stands up from a recumbent position, blood will at first collect in the large veins in the legs, with a concomitant decrease in upper-body blood pressure. This activates the neuroendocrine reflex, which results in a transient rise in circulating levels of AVP.

Often the blood osmolarity and volume will work together in stimulating or suppressing the secretion of AVP. For example, water loading will increase blood volume and, at the same time, dilute blood solutes; these will both operate to reduce AVP release. On the other hand, loss of blood through hemorrhage has little effect on blood osmolarity. Hermorrhage-induced AVP release will tend to dilute blood by increasing water reabsorption however, this may be preferable to circulatory collapse caused by loss of blood volume. Independent control of AVP by changes in either blood osmolarity or volume suggests separate neural pathways leading to the magnocellular AVP neurons. It is conceivable that many neural pathways influence AVP release, since such stresses as fright, physical pain, or temperature changes may promote AVP secretion. The adaptive advantages of AVP release in these stress situations is not apparent.

In nonmammalian tetrapods, as in mammals, neurohypophyseal peptides promote water conservation; and the basic principle argine vasotocin (AVT) is a more potent antidiuretic factor than either mesotocin or oxytocin.

The present-day amphibian species vary markedly with respect to the proportion of their life history spent in the aquatic versus terrestrial environment. Correspondingly, amphibians show differing degrees of resistance to dehydration and have various physiological mechanisms for water conservation. Therefore, it is not surprising that the importance of neurohypophyseal hormones in controlling water balance in amphibians has some association with the habitat of the particular species. For example, the fully aquatic African clawed toad, *Xenopus laevis*, shows little or no response to AVT or mesotocin. On the other hand, the more terrestrial anuran amphibians have evolved several neurohypophyseal, peptide-evoked mechanisms for water conservation. Injection of neurohypophyseal hormones (AVT in particular) into some frogs or toads that are immersed in water produces a weight gain from water uptake. This phenomenon, called the water balance or Brunn effect, is due to AVT action on the kidney, skin, and urinary bladder. In most urodele amphibians (newts and salamanders), AVT promotes water conservation only through action on the kidney. The renal effects of AVT include an increase in distal renal tubule water reabsorption (as in mammals) and, in addition, a decrease in the glomerular filtration rate. Since amphibians normally do not drink, they must absorb water osmotically through their skin. Anurans have developed AVT-sensitive mechanisms to accelerate water uptake through the skin. It can be shown *in vitro* that AVT-dependent water transfer in skin is due in part to an increase in water permeability of the skin. In other words, AVT will enhance the passive flow of water from the dilute media on the outside of the skin to a hypertonic solution on the inside. Active transport of sodium across the skin is also observed in response to AVT treatment. Therefore, AVT can stimulate osmotic work to allow water uptake against an electrochemical gradient. Certain terrestrial amphibians have a highly vascularized ventral pelvic patch of skin that is a major site of water uptake. In response to AVT, the pelvic patch can absorb water at a rate nearly fivefold that of the adjoining pectoral skin.

The urinary bladder of amphibians and reptiles functions as a reservoir of water to help maintain water balance while the animal is away from environmental sources of water. This structure can be quite large (holding an amount of water equivalent to half the animal's total body weight). While in reptiles and most urodele amphibians the urinary bladder is unresponsive to AVT, it is clearly an AVT target organ in most anurans. In these animals AVT facilitates water transport across the bladder in much the same way as it affects the skin; both passive water flow and water transport coupled to active sodium transport are stimulated.

The physiological stimuli for release of AVT in amphibians are presumably similar to those of mammals; high blood osmolarity and hypovolemia. Recent studies by Pang and Sawyer of circulating levels of AVT in frogs have suggested that loss of blood volume was associated with elevated plasma AVT, whereas infusion of hypertonic saline did not have a consistent effect on AVT. Further studies will be necessary to clarify the regulation of AVT secretion in amphibians.

The water-conserving effects of neurohypophyseal hormones in birds and reptiles are similar to those of mammals in that antidiuresis is produced through water reabsorption in kidney tubules, although an additional effect on decreasing glomerular filtration rate in reptiles appears operative.

The influence of neurohypophyseal hormones on water balance in fishes is not clear. In general, injection of AVT into freshwater fishes produces diuresis, although an antidiuretic effect has been reported in some species. Diuresis would be an appropriate response in freshwater fishes, since they face the problem of water loading because of the influx of water across the gills. However, the physiological significance of AVT-induced diuresis in freshwater fishes cannot be evaluated until circulating levels of the hormone are measured. It might be argued that fishes inhabiting marine waters, in which the salt concentration is hypertonic to body fluids, have a need for water conservation similar to terrestrial animals. However, this is not true, since there is no lack of water *per se* in a marine environment but a need to rid the readily available water of its salt. Marine fishes can do this by swallowing seawater and excreting the salt through the gills.

Blood Pressure Regulation

The rise in blood pressure in mammals in response to hormones of the neurohypophysis was the first observed activity of this gland and, of course, was the basis for naming the vasopressins. Since this original observation by Oliver and Schafer in 1895, the blood pressure effects of neurohypophyseal hormones in vertebrates have received much attention. However, these effects of the various hormones defy simple categorization since the hormones may either raise, lower, or have dual effects, depending on the amount of hormone administered and the species examined. Some of these variable responses in overall blood pressure are due to the selective action of hormones on particular vascular beds in the complex cardiovascular tree. For example, a hormone may constrict the coronary artery, reducing the amount of blood flow to the heart wall and resulting in a lower cardiac contractile force. This decreased cardiac function would contribute to an overall lower blood pressure, since the blood would be pumped with less force. Thus a

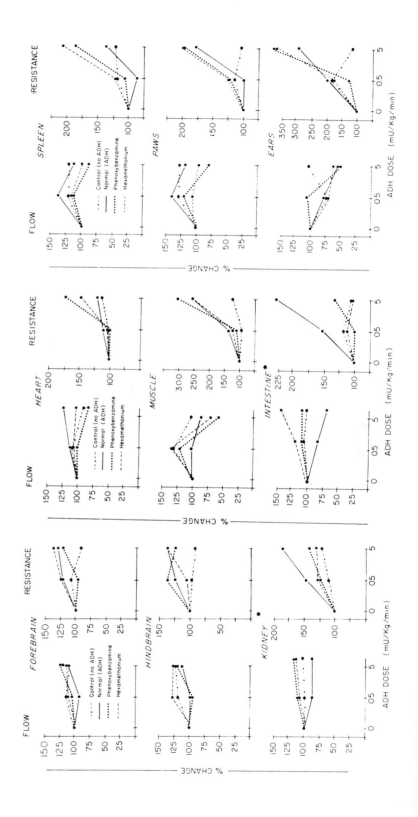

hormone may indirectly reduce systemic blood pressure by acting on small vessels in the heart. In contrast, a hormone may have a general effect on peripheral blood pressure by dilating all the major arteries and arterioles and thereby lowering overall pressure through reduced vascular resistance. It must also be kept in mind that blood pressure is regulated by other hormonal and neural mechanisms, which may antagonize or synergize with neurohypophyseal hormone actions. For example, Hoffman tested the effects of neurohypophyseal hormone on blood flow and vascular resistance in different regional vascular beds of a rat, as shown in Fig. 3.5. Blood flow was measured during infusion of various doses of AVP (ADH) with or without phenoxybenzamine or hexamethonium, drugs that block the activity of the sympathetic nervous system. In this way it could be determined whether the vasopressor or the vasodilator activity of AVP was dependent on the simultaneous activity of the sympathetic system. Infusion of AVP into normal rats caused an increase in the resistance of vascular beds in the kidney, muscle, intestine, spleen, paws, and ears. The increase in the vascular resistance of the kidney, intestine, and ear was sufficient to reduce significantly the blood flow to these tissues. In both kidney and intestine the effect of AVP was reduced when the sympathetic system was blocked. Overall, these results indicate that AVP and the sympathetic nervous system work together to reduce blood flow to the kidney, intestine, muscle, and skin and to maintain blood flow to more vital tissues such as the heart and brain.

A summary of neurohypophyseal hormone action on the systemic blood pressure in vertebrates is shown on Table 3.2. The details of the mechanisms of these hormone effects are too complex to be covered here. Many of the observed effects are probably pharmacological, since the amounts of hormone required to produce detectable changes in blood pressure are so large that it is doubtful whether such amounts would be released by the pituitary under usual "physiological" conditions. The significance of neurohypophyseal blood pressure regulation must await additional knowledge of circulating levels of the hormones. The blood pressure–raising activity of AVT in the fishes, including cyclostomes, has been suggested by Sawyer to be the most primitive or earliest function of this peptide. In bony fishes the pressor effect of AVT on vessels of the systemic circulation is contrasted by the depressor actions of mesotocin and isotocin. In amphibians and reptiles, whether the hormones are pressor or depressor is greatly dependent on the particular species examined. Moving up the evolutionary scale, there appears to have

FIGURE 3.5. Effects of antidiuretic hormone (ADH, arginine vasopressin) on tissue blood flow and vascular resistance changes in various tissues of the rat. Rats received either saline (control) or ADH with or without simultaneous treatment with the sympathetic nervous system blocking agents phenoxybenzamine or hexamethonium. The asterisks indicate that ADH effects were reduced when the sympathetic system was blocked. For a discussion of the data, see the text. [From W. E. Hoffman, *Endocrinology*, **107**:334, 1980.]

TABLE 3.2. Systemic blood pressure responses to neuro-hypophyseal hormones in various vertebrates[a]

	Blood Pressure Response	
Vertebrates	Pressor	Depressor
Mammals	AVP, LVP, AVT	
Birds	(AVT in pigeon)	AVT, MST
Reptiles	AVT, MST	AVT, MST
Amphibians	AVT, MST	MST
Bony fishes	AVT	MST, IST
Cartilaginous fishes	AVT	
Cyclostomes	AVT	

[a] From LaPointe, *Am. Zool.*, **17**:851, 1977.

been a rather clear separation of effects, with predominantly pressor activity in mammals and depressor effects in birds.

Contraction of the Oviduct and Uterus

The strong effect of neurohypophyseal hormone upon uterine muscular contraction was first noted by Dale, in 1906, using the uterus of the cat in early pregnancy. Since that time we have seen the widespread clinical practice of injecting pituitary extract or, more recently, oxytocin for artificial induction of delivery in pregnant women during a difficult labor. Although this control of muscular contraction of the female reproductive tract by neurohypophyseal hormones has been studied most thoroughly in mammals, it is clear that the hormones are involved in live birth or egg laying in most tetrapod vertebrates.

The mammalian uterus is a target of many hormones. During pregnancy estrogen and progesterone induce both hyperplasia and hypertrophy of the uterine myometrium. OXY, given either *in vivo* or *in vitro*, stimulates contraction of the uterus by depolarizing the excitable membrane surrounding the myometrial smooth muscle cell. OXY increases the frequency, force, and duration of contractions and may stimulate local production of prostaglandins, which synergize with OXY. The basic responsiveness of uterine muscle to OXY is modulated during pregnancy by the sex hormones. In mammals it is decreased during most of the gestation period by progesterone and greatly sensitized by estrogens toward term. In addition to these changes in uterine sensitivity to oxytocin, there is evidence that dilation of the cervix stimulates the release of oxytocin at the exact time it is needed for labor contractions.

Control of parturition appears to be a result of the interplay of hormones and tissue responsiveness. The recent measurement of oxytocin receptors in the rat myometrium during pregnancy and labor provide a possible model for this multihormonal phenomenon. Soloff and co-workers showed that the number of oxytocin receptors increases dramatically near the time of labor (Fig. 3.6A), which may explain why the rat uterus is relatively insensitive to oxytocin until six to eight hours before term. Since progesterone blocks the estrogen-induced increase in myometrial sensitivity to oxytocin, high levels of progesterone during the early period of gestation may suppress the number or the activity of oxytocin receptors. Prior to delivery of the fetus, estrogen levels remain high while progesterone levels fall, allowing the expression of oxytocin receptor activity. Additional work is needed to verify this model. Also, the relative importance of oxytocin in the control of parturition has not been established. Hypophysectomized animals retain the ability to give birth, although labor is prolonged and difficult. Perhaps it is safest to say that oxytocin facilitates labor in mammals.

Oxytocin is 10 to 50 times more potent than vasopressin or arginine vasotocin in inducing contractions of the mammalian uterus. In birds, reptiles, and amphibians, however, arginine vasotocin is a more potent stimulator of contraction of the oviduct or uterus than either oxytocin or mesotocin. Evidence is accumulating to show a physiological role of arginine vasotocin in the control of parturition or egg laying in nonmammalian tetrapods. Although isolated oviducts of some fish will contract in response to neurohypophyseal hormones, more work is needed to prove that there is a physiological role for these hormones in fish reproduction.

Egg laying in birds is associated with a depletion in the hypothalamic concentration, and a rise in blood levels, of arginine vasotocin. Injection of

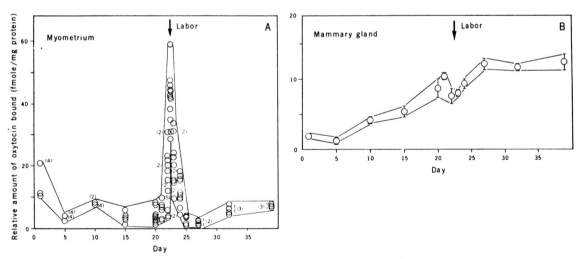

FIGURE 3.6. The relative amount of oxytocin bound specifically by particulate fractions (cell membranes) from (A) the rat uterine myometrium and (B) mammary gland during pregnancy and lactation. Oxytocin binding (receptors) by the myometrium remains low during most of pregnancy and increases sharply near the time of labor. In contrast, oxytocin binding by the mammary gland develops gradually during pregnancy and remains high while the mother lactates. [From M. S. Soloff, M. Alexandrova, and M. J. Fernstrom, *Science,* **204:**1313, 1979.]

the hormone into birds can induce oviposition in 90 seconds in a hen and advance the normal time of laying by as much as a day in some birds. The response of oviducts of some reptiles and amphibians are interesting in that they show some variation in sensitivity, depending on the season or the period of gestation. The isolated oviducts of some iguanid lizards become increasingly sensitive to octapeptide hormone during gestation, with a maximum near term. Although some workers could find no effect of steroid hormones on the hormonal sensitivity of oviducts in some lizard species, Callard and Hirsch found an estrogen-induced increase in oviductal contractions in response to arginine vasotocin in the turtle *Chrysemys picta*. In contrast to the estrogen-induced sensitivity of the oviduct of this turtle and mammals in general, the oviduct of the American chameleon, apparently, is sensitized by progesterone. The oviduct's sensitivity to neurohypophyseal hormones in several species of amphibians is maximal at the time of the year when reproductive activity reaches its peak. Whether this seasonal sensitivity is due to changes in circulating steroid hormone concentrations is not known. However, the above examples of sex steroid modulation of neurohypophyseal hormone action on the female reproductive tract of divergent species suggest that this may be a convenient mechanism for coordination of events during live birth or egg laying.

Milk Ejection

The milk-ejecting or "let-down" effect of oxytocin was recognized in 1910 by Ott and Scott, who found that injections of pituitary extracts induced the mammary gland to release milk in a manner similar to the normal suckling response. Although other neurohypophyseal octapeptides are also effective, oxytocin is by far the most potent. Milk production or secretion into the alveoli is under the control of adenohypophyseal and steroid hormones, and should be distinguished from milk ejection. Oxytocin acts on myoepithelial cells on the alveoli and ducts of the mammary gland to force the stored milk out of the alveoli and into the ducts, which eventually lead to the nipple. The mechanism by which the contractile elements accomplish milk ejection has been clarified by the independent work of Richardson and Linzell. There are two types of myoepithelial cells in the mammary gland: stellate cells, extending over the surface of the alveolus, and spindle-shaped cells along the longitudinal axis of the ducts (Fig. 3.7). When a sufficient level of oxytocin is present, both types of cells contract, reducing the volume of the alveoli and widening and shortening the ducts. In some species the ducts lead to a larger chamber (cistern) that is connected to the nipple, and milk release from the cistern to the nipple is blocked by a smooth muscle sphincter that is not oxytocin sensitive. Mechanical stimulation of the nipple during suckling forces the milk out. On the other hand, other species (the sow, for example) lack a cistern or an effective sphincter, so that oxytocin promotes the free flow of milk from the nipple. Mechanical stimulation of the gland

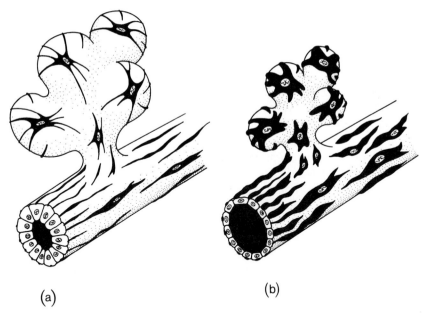

FIGURE 3.7. Disposition of myoepithelial cells (black) around the alveoli and duct of mammary gland tissue. (*a*) When myoepithelial cells are relaxed, the alveoli are full and the duct has a small lumen. (*b*) After exposure to oxytocin, and myoepithelial cells contract and shorten to empty the alveoli and enlarge the lumen of the duct so that milk may flow to the nipple of the gland. [From Linzell; Bisset, *Handbook of Physiology*, Vol. 4 (R. O. Greep and E. B. Astwood, eds.), Williams & Wilkins, Baltimore, 1974, p. 495.]

during suckling plays several roles in milk ejection; there is some evidence that it can directly induce some contraction of myoepithelial cells independent of oxytocin. In addition, as we briefly discussed in Chapter 1, stimulation of nerves in the nipple sends impulses to the central nervous system, which relays this message to the hypothalmus, where the signal for oxytocin release is given. This neuroendocrine reflex is quite rapid; after nipple stimulation, blood levels of oxytocin begin to be elevated in a matter of seconds, and milk ejection often occurs within a minute.

There appears to be a positive correlation between blood levels of oxytocin during suckling and the amount of milk ejected. This fact has some interesting consequences. For example, it has been shown that if only one or two rabbit pups are allowed access to their mother to suckle, blood levels of oxytocin in the mother are lower, and less milk is produced per pup than if the whole litter is allowed to suckle. Presumably, the greater stimulation by the entire litter produces more than a proportionate release of oxytocin and subsequent milk ejection. Higher levels of oxytocin may increase the number of contracting alveoli and the force of their contraction. In lactating women, infusion of low doses of oxytocin produces a single contraction of the alveoli, whereas higher doses result in a series of contractions.

Although the sensitivity of the mammary gland to oxytocin does not appear to vary greatly in women, in some rodents it increases gradually during pregnancy and lactation. Oxytocin receptors in the rat mammary gland have been measured and compared with uterine oxytocin receptors (Fig. 3.6B). In contrast to the large, sharp increases in the number of uterine oxytocin receptors preceding labor, mammary gland oxytocin receptors increase over a longer period of time and to a lesser extent. The mechanism for controlling the number of mammary gland oxytocin receptors is not known, but it is no doubt different from the proposed steroid hormone regulation of uterine receptors, since the pattern of change in receptors differs in the two tissues.

Some details of the neural pathway of the milk-ejection reflex are beginning to emerge. Sterba and co-workers have proposed a scheme for the pathway in the rat (Fig. 1.4b). Nerves from the mammary gland enter the spinal cord and continue either to the thalamus or synapse in the hindbrain. Thalamic nerves project to the magnocellular region where they regulate the activity of oxytocinergic neurons. This proposed scheme also takes into account neurosecretory nerves whose axons project to the hindbrain and not to the pars nervosa. It has been suggested that oxytocinergic neurons ending in the hindbrain modulate the system by reducing oxytocin release by the pars nervosa after blood levels are sufficiently elevated. Additional observations suggest other, as yet unidentified, components of this regulating system. For example, either centrally acting drugs, such as anesthetics, or emotional stress can block the release of oxytocin following a suckling stimulus. Stress, which activates the sympathetic nervous system and elevation of blood catecholamines, can also have an inhibitory effect on milk ejection at the target organ. Catecholamines can reduce blood flow to the mammary gland and thereby decrease the amount of oxytocin getting to the gland. Catecholamines counteract oxytocin action by increasing the resistance of ducts and inhibiting contraction of myoepithelial cells. Thus stress reduces oxytocin release, distribution, and action. This is the basis of the advice frequently given to mothers that they nurse in a quiet, relaxing atmosphere to maximize ocytocin release and milk ejection.

It is useful at this point to discuss briefly a local adenohypophyseal effect of oxytocin on the release of prolactin. As is well known, the mammary gland can be maintained in active lactation for far longer than the normal periods of time by frequent suckling. Conversely, if suckling is interrupted, the mammary gland promptly ceases to *secrete* milk and undergoes involution. Such involution can be delayed in the unsuckled female by repeated injections of oxytocin. Thus it would appear that the oxytocin that is released into the systemic circulation at each suckling is acting upon the pars distalis, leading to release of prolactin. An alternative mechanism for this would involve the hypophyseal portal vessels. The substance transported to the pars distalis in this case would be either oxytocin or some other hypothalamic neurosecretory product. In this way, suckling not only satisfies an immediate requirement—delivery of already manufactured milk to the infant—but also may be the primary stimulus for maintenance of an active state of mammary secretion in the long-term sense.

ADDITIONAL READING

1. Acher, R. (1974). Chemistry of the neurohypophysial hormones: An example of molecular evolution. In *Handbook of Physiology*, Sect. 7 (R. O. Greep and E. B. Astwood, eds.), American Physiological Society, Washington D. C., pp. 103–117.

2. Alexandrova, M., and M. S. Soloff (1980). Oxytocin receptors and parturition in the guinea pig. *Biol. Reprod.* **22**:1106–1111.

3. Babiker, M. M., and J. C. Rankin (1979). Renal and vascular effects of neurohypophysial hormones in the African lungfish *Protopterus annectens* (Owen). *Gen. Comp. Endocrinol.* **37**:26–34.

4. Bentley, P. J. (1980). Evolution of neurohypophysial peptide functions. In *Evolution of Vertebrate Endocrine Systems* (P. K. T. Pang and A. Epple, eds.), Texas Tech Press, Lubbock, pp. 95–106.

5. Bisset, G. W. (1974). Milk ejection. In *Handbook of Physiology*, Sect. 7 (R. O. Greep and E. B. Astwood, eds.), American Physiological Society, Washington, D. C., pp. 493–520.

6. Brownstein, M. J., J. T. Russel, and H. Gainer (1980). Synthesis, transport and release of posterior pituitary hormones. *Science* **207**:373–378.

7. Chan, D. K. O. (1977). Comparative physiology of the vasomotor effects of neurohypophysial peptides in the vertebrates. *Am. Zool.* **17**:751–761.

8. Chauvet, M. T., D. Hurpet, J. Chauvet, and R. Acher (1980). Phenypressin (Phe^2-Arg^8-vasopressin), a new neurohypophysial peptide found in marsupials. *Nature* **287**:640–642.

9. Gibbens, G. L. D., and T. Chard (1976). Observations on maternal oxytocin release during human labor and the effect of intravenous alcohol administration. *Am. J. Obstet. Gynecol.* **126**:243–246.

10. Guillette, L. J., Jr. (1979). Stimulation of parturition in a viviparous lizard (*Sceloporus jarrovi*) by arginine vasotocin. *Gen. Comp. Endocrinol.* **38**:457–460.

11. Kent, W., and L. L. McClanahan (1980). The effects of arginine vasotocin and various microtubular poisons on water transfer and sodium transport across the pelvic skin of the toad *Bufo boreas in vitro. Gen. Comp. Endocrinol.* **40**:161–167.

12. Kleeman, C. R., and T. Berl (1979). The neurohypophysial hormones: vasopressin. In *Endocrinology* (L. J. DeGroot, G. F. Cahill, Jr., L. Martini, D. H. Nelson, W. D. Odell, J. T. Potts, Jr., E. Steinberger, and A. I. Winegrad, eds.), Grune & Stratton, New York, pp. 253–275.

13. Koike, T. I., L. R. Pryor, and H. L. Neldon (1979). Effect of saline infusion on plasma immunoreactive vasotocin in conscious chickens (*Gallus domesticus*). *Gen. Comp. Endocrinol.* **37**:451–458.

14. Kuyala, G. A. (1978). Corticosteroid and neurohypophyseal hormone control of parturition in the guppy, *Poecilia reticulata. Gen. Comp. Endocrinol.* **36**:286–296.

15. La Pointe, J. (1977). Comparative physiology of neurohypophysial hormone action on the vertebrate oviduct-uterus. *Am. Zool.* **17**:763–773.

16. Marshall, J. M. (1974). Effects of neurohypophysial hormones on the myometrium. In *Handbook of Physiology*, Sect. 7 (R. O. Greep and E. B. Astwood, eds.), American Physiological Society, Washington, D. C., pp. 469–492.

17. Pang, P. K. T. (1977). Osmoregulatory functions of neurohypophysial hormones in fishes and amphibians. *Am. Zool.* **17:**739–749.

18. Pang, P. K. T., S. M. Galli-Gallardo, N. Collie, and W. H. Sawyer (1980). Renal and peripheral vascular responsiveness to arginine vasotocin in bullfrog, *Rana catesbeiana*. *Am. J. Physiol.* **239:**R156–R160.

19. Robinson, A. G. (1978). Neurophysins, an aid to understanding the structure and function of neurohypophysis. In *Frontiers in Neuroendocrinology* (W. F. Ganong and L. Martini, eds.), Raven, New York, pp. 35–59.

20. Russell, J. T., M. J. Brownstein, and H. Gainer (1981). Time course of appearance and release of [$^{-35}$S]cysteine labelled neurophysins and peptides in the neurohypophysis. *Brain Res.* **205:**299–311.

21. Sachs, H., P. Fawcett, Y. Takabatake, and R. Portanova (1969). Biosynthesis and release of vasopressin and neurophysin. *Recent Progr. Horm. Res.* **25:**447–491.

22. Sawyer, W. H. (1977). Evolution of active neurohypophysial principles among the vertebrates. *Am. Zool.* **17:**727–737.

23. Schrier, R. W., T. Berl, and R. J. Anderson (1979). Osmotic and nonosmotic control of vasopressin release. *Am. J. Physiol.* **236:**F321–F332.

24. Stiffler, D. F. (1981). The effects of mesotocin on renal function in hypophysectomized *Ambystoma tigrinum* larvae. *Gen. Comp. Endocrinol.* **45:**49–55.

25. Vorherr, H. (1979). Oxytocin. In *Endocrinology* (L. J. DeGroot, G. F. Cahill, Jr., L. Martini, D. H. Nelson, W. D. Odell, J. T. Potts, Jr., E. Steinberger, and A. I. Winegrad, eds.). Grune & Stratton, New York, pp. 277–285.

26. Zucker, A., and H. Nishimura (1981). Renal responses to vasoactive hormones in the aglomerular toadfish, *Opsanus tau*. *Gen. Comp. Endocrinol.* **43:**1–9.

4

The Pars Distalis

It should be clear from the summaries in Chapter 1 that the pars distalis, through its hormones, is involved in the regulation of numerous important functions, including reproduction, growth, behavior, and metabolism. Furthermore, the pars distalis modulates the functions of several other endocrine glands (e.g., thyroid, adrenal cortex) and, thereby, the targets of these glands as well.

Because the effects of surgical removal of the pituitary (hypophysectomy) were so widespread, it was at first difficult to recognize the primary functions of the pituitary gland. The first successful hypophysectomies of dogs and rats showed that although animals can survive after removal of the gland, they are miserable, debilitated creatures, very vulnerable to disease and to stress. Hypophysectomy of frog embryos proved to be easy (compared to the operation in mammals), permitting the preparation of large numbers of relatively healthy pituitaryless specimens. Finally, by combining hypophysectomy with injections of pituitary gland extracts, the puzzles of the functions of this gland were unraveled. The difficulty proved to be due to the fact that the adenohypophyseal part of the pituitary secretes at least six different hormones and the pars intermedia at least one. Ultimately, the improvement of techniques made possible the chemical isolation of the hormones of the adenohypophysis. Use of the purified hormones resulted in the precise definition of the functions of the adenohypophysis, since now the individual hormones could be tested for their actions in hypophysectomized animals.

A summary of the adenohypophysial hormones that have been identified is given in Table 4.1. These hormones are all peptides, and they vary widely in size. MSH (melanocyte stimulating hormone) of the pars intermedia is the smallest. Its physiological properties and its regulation are considered separately in Chapter 5, but its chemistry is dealt with here at least briefly, because it is related to that of a family of peptides from the pars distalis.

TABLE 4.1. Hormones of the adenohypophysis

Hormone and Some of Its Alternate Names	Short Names	Mol. Wt.	Amino Acid Residues	Carbohydrate	Principal Functions
Family I					
Growth hormone	GH				Stimulates somatic growth, bone growth. Specific effects on carbohydrate and amino acid metabolism
Somatotropin	STH				
	hGH[a]	21,500[b]	191	No	
	mGH	23,000	188	"	
	bGH	45,000[c]	191	"	
	pGH	41,500[c]	191	"	
Prolactin	PRL				Stimulates mammary function in mammals, freshwater osmoregulatory function in fishes, modulates thyroxine action on metamorphosis of amphibians, etc.
Lactogenic hormone					
Mammotropin					
Luteotropic hormone	LTH			No	
	hPRL	22,000	199	"	
	oPRL		198	"	
	pPRL		194	"	
	rPRL		195		
Family II					
Thyrotropic hormone	TSH				Stimulates thyroid cells with respect to size, mitotic activity, and all cellular processes leading to production and release of thyroid hormone
	bTSH	28,300	209	Yes	
	bTSHα[d]	13,600	96	"	
	bTSHβ	14,700	113	"	
	hTSH	28,900	201	"	
	hTSHα	14,400	89	"	
	hTSHβ	14,600	112	"	
	rTSH	32,000			
	eel TSH	32,000			
Follicle stimulating hormone	FSH				Stimulates germ cell–forming functions of testis and ovary. Synergistic action with LH
Follitropin					
	hFSH	32,000		Yes	
	hFSHα		92	"	
	hFSHβ		108–115	"	
	eFSH	33,500		"	

Hormone	Symbol	Molecular weight[b]	Amino acids		Biological action
	eFSHα			"	
	eFSHβ			"	
	oFSH	32,000	118	"	
	oFSHα			"	
	oFSHβ			"	
Luteinizing hormone	LH			Yes	Stimulates steroidogenic elements in gonads. Triggers ovulation and corpus luteum formation in ovary
Lutropin				"	
Interstitial cell stimulating hormone	ICSH			"	
	oLH	29,000	215	"	
	b, oLHα		96	"	
	oLHβ		120		
	hLH	28,800	204		
	hLHα		89		
	hLHβ		115		
Family III					
Adrenal corticotropin	ACTH	4,500	39	No	Stimulates growth and multiplication of adrenal cortical cells and all phases of cellular activity for corticosteroid hormone synthesis and secretion
Corticotropic hormone					
α-Melanocyte stimulating hormone	αMSH		13		Dispersion of melanin pigment in melanocytes
β-Melanocyte stimulating hormone	βMSH		19	No	Dispersion of melanin pigment in melanocytes
β-Lipotropin	βLPH	11,700	91	No	Mobilization of fat. Dispersion of melanin pigment. Stimulation of adrenal cortex
β-Endorphin	—	3,000	30	No	Analgesic or opiatelike action on central nervous system
Pro-opiocortin	—	31,000	?	Yes	

[a] Prefixes indicating animal species: h, human; o, ovine (sheep); b, bovine; e, equine (horse); m, monkey; p, porcine (pig); r, rat.

[b] Molecular weight expressed in daltons.

[c] Molecular weight given here is of a double, or dimer molecule. The amino acid number given in the next column is of the monomer.

[d] Greek letter suffixes indicate subunits.

In Table 4.1 three different families of peptide hormones are recognized. These families consist of hormonal molecular types that are sufficiently alike with respect to amino acid sequence that a genetic relationship (i.e., similar DNA derivation) is recognizable. For example, Family I consists of two hormones, both peptides, composed of almost 200 amino acid residues: growth hormone and prolactin. These hormones are generally distinctive in their biological actions, but when the sequences of the constituent amino acids of human growth hormone and prolactin are compared, 16% of them are in identical positions in the series. Between sheep growth hormone and prolactin the similarity is 23%. These resemblances may be relatively small, but they are indicative of a generic relationship, and some biochemists therefore theorize that the two hormones evolved from a common molecular ancestor.

Human chorionic (from the placenta) somatomammotropin is placed in this family despite the fact that it is made by a different (temporary) organ, because its amino acid sequence is 85% like that of human prolactin. It also has some structural similarities to human growth hormone.

Family II in Table 4.1 includes the hormones that have carbohydrate in their molecules (i.e., they are glycoproteins): TSH (thyrotropic hormone), FSH (follicle stimulating hormone), and LH (luteinizing hormone). This group of hormones has another shared property: each hormone is composed of two subunits (designated as α and β) that are noncovalently linked, hence readily separable. The α subunits of TSH, FSH, and LH are almost identical in amino acid sequence. The β subunits differ, and confer the special functional property (e.g., thyroid stimulation, gonad stimulation) to each of the complete hormones. In most instances, the separated subunits have no physiological action when appropriately tested. There is enough similarity in amino acid sequence between the α and the β subunits of the glycoprotein hormones to permit speculation that they may have evolved from a common ancestral molecule. The α subunits of the glycoprotein pituitary hormones are interchangeable. That is, the α subunit of any of them can be exchanged and recombined with the β subunit of any other glycoprotein hormone. The actual functional properties of the new hybrid hormone then depend entirely on the nature of the β subunit component.

As in the case of growth hormone and prolactin, the mammalian placenta can produce pituitary glycoproteinlike hormones. The best known of these is human chorionic gonadotropin, HCG, a glycoprotein composed of α and β subunits. The α subunit is interchangeable with those from the pituitary. Its β subunit strongly resembles hLHβ and endows the whole hormone with an LH-like action on the gonad. Another interesting placental hormone is pregnant mares' serum gonadotropin, PMSG (or eCG). This glycoprotein also is separable into α and β subunits. Its β subunit (when combined with the α) has *both* FSH-like and LH-like actions in the rat. The amino acid sequence of PMSGβ (i.e., eCGβ) has not yet been worked out, but should be of interest in explaining how one molecule can interact with receptors for both kinds of gonadotropic hormone.

The hormones listed as Family III in Table 4.1 appear to be related in a manner that differs from the first two groups. The list includes adrenocorticotropic hormone (ACTH), melanocyte-stimulating hormone (αMSH, βMSH), endorphin, and β-lipotropic hormone (βLPH). Biochemists have

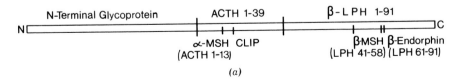

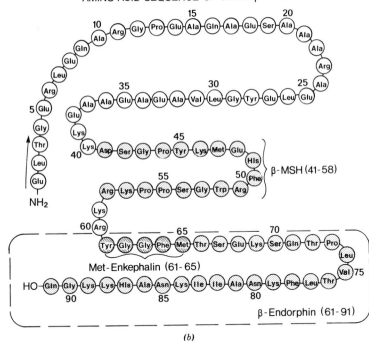

FIGURE 4.1. (*a*) Schematic representation of pro-opiocortin. Different segments of this sequence constitute other, smaller hormones, as shown. Thus, ACTH and βLPH (shown above the pro-opiocortin molecule) consititute more than half of the molecule, at the C-terminal end. These segments, in turn, contain sequences that represent still smaller hormonal peptides, shown below the molecule (αMSH, βMSH, βendorphin). Details of the β-lipotropin sequence are shown in Fig. 4.1*B*, below. Details of the ACTH sequence are shown in Fig. 4.14.(*b*) Detail of the amino acid sequence of ovine βLPH showing the sequences of β-endorphin, met-enkephalin, and βMSH. [After C. H. Li, *Perspectives in Biology and Medicine*, University of Chicago Press, 1978.]

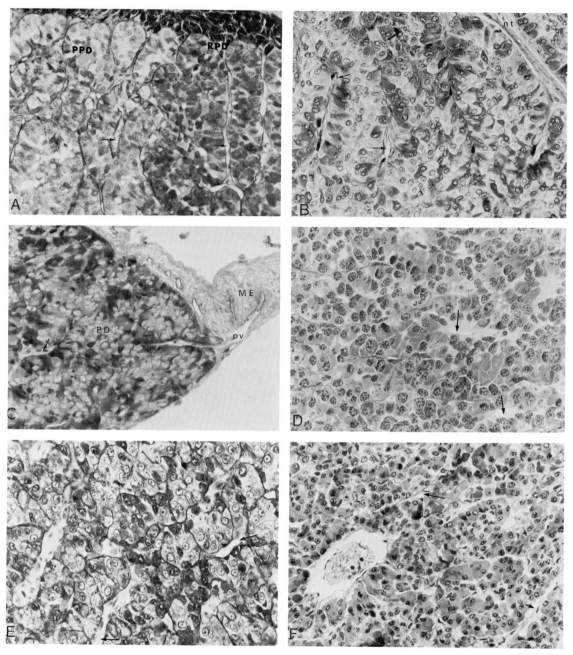

FIGURE 4.2. Sections through the pars distalis of six different vertebrate types showing the basic cell cord–sinusoid histological pattern in each. All are magnified 350 times except *E*, which is magnified 560 times. (*A*) The lamprey (*Lampetra fluviatilis*), Herlant's tetrachrome stain (dorsal is upward). The pars distalis is divided into two recognizably different zones: the rostral (*RPD*) and proximal (*PPD*). The columns of cells are mostly vertical, as are the blood capillaries (arrows). The function of the different cell types is not well established. (*B*) The rainbow trout (*Salmo gairdneri*), iron hematoxylin stain (dorsal is upward). Strands of nerve

found that ACTH, αMSH, βMSH, endorphin, and βLPH all are derived from a protein now named pro-opiocortin, since they are all included in its amino acid sequence (Fig. 4.1). ACTH forms a 39–amino acid sequence that just precedes the N-terminal end of the 91–amino acid molecule of βLPH. β-Endorphin, a 30–amino acid molecule, forms the C-terminal end of the βLPH molecule (Fig. 4.1). αMSH is included within the 39–amino acid sequence of ACTH. β-MSH is a separate sequence within the "interior" of the βLPH molecule. Thus, this family of hormonal substances is related because they are derived by splitting from a larger precursor molecule, pro-opiocortin. Whether βLPH is itself a hormone is a question still under study. The larger molecule of pro-opiocortin (molecular weight about 31,000) has been extracted from the pituitary, and from this molecule βLPH can be split enzymatically.

It is worth mentioning at this point that by use of antibody-labeling techniques, pro-opiocortin and βLPH can be found both in the "ACTH cells" of the pars distalis and the secretory cells of the pars intermedia. Since, after all, these two parts of the adenohypophysis are formed from the same embryological structure, it is not surprising that they can share a biochemical synthetic ability. In this case, we may speculate that evolutionary development was in the provision of different enzymes in the pars distalis and pars intermedia to selectively release MSH from the pars intermedia and ACTH from the pars distalis. Further research should clarify this interesting possibility and explain what happens to the endorphins and other biologically active substances when pro-opiocortin and βLPH are fragmented by enzymatic action.

MICROSCOPIC STRUCTURE OF THE PARS DISTALIS AND THE CELLULAR ORIGIN OF ITS HORMONES

The most usual arrangement of cells in the vertebrate pars distalis is branching cords of cells between which are sinusoidlike blood channels. In a few groups of lower vertebrates, fishes in particular, follicular (hollow, ball-like) cellular groups occur (Fig. 4.2). For many years endocrinologists were con-

tissue penetrate from the neurohypophysis above (*nt*). The arrows indicate places where nerve tissue and blood vessels separate cords of cells. Cells of different shade secrete different hormones. (*C*) The European frog (*Rana temporaria*), sagittal section, Herlant's alcian blue, orange G stain (dorsal is upward, anterior is to the right). A portion of the median eminence (*ME*) is shown. Several hypophyseal portal vessels are cut, but one in particular, labeled *pv*, extends from the median eminence into the pars distalis (*PD*). Cells of different shade and different shape secrete different hormones. (*D*) The African lungfish (*Protopterus dolloi*), Herlant's tetrachrome stain. Blood vessels are not clear, but two are indicated by arrows. Cords of cells are clear, but there is not much differentiation of cell types in this view. (*E*) The raven (*Corvus corax*), Herlant's tetrachrome stain. Arrows indicate blood capillaries. (*F*) The cow (*Bos taurus*), Cleveland-Wolf stain. Arrows indicate blood capillaries. [Photographs were provided by Professor P. G. W. J. van Oordt, Rijksuniversiteit, Utrecht.]

cerned with the question of whether separate types of cells manufacture the different peptide hormones of the pars distalis. They used staining procedures that colored different cell types in a distinctive way and often combined this with experiments in which pituitary endocrine targets (thyroid, adrenal, gonads) were removed or target gland hormones (thyroxine, corticosteroids, sex steroids) were injected. By noting corresponding changes in cells of the pars distalis, it was possible eventually to identify in many species at least six secretory cell types (Fig. 4.3), one for each of the known hormones. As mentioned above, the several hormones of the Family III group or their precursor would all appear to be located in the ACTH cell type.

The use of electron microscopy, and the recognition of six classes of cells in the pars distalis according to the sizes and shapes of the hormone-containing granules (Fig. 4.4), appeared to confirm the conclusions, based on stained histological preparations, that there are the following secretory cell types: STH, PRL, FSH, LH, TSH, ACTH. Most recently, by use of immunocytochemical methods, the definitive identification of the six cell types may have been achieved. This approach utilizes an antibody formed against the pure hormone. The antibody will seek out those cells that contain the antigen (original hormone) against which it was formed. In practice, the antibody is linked to an enzyme that will produce a colored reaction product

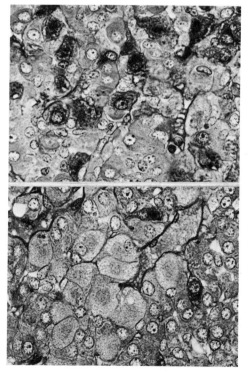

FIGURE 4.3. Sections through the pars distalis of the rat. *Top*, a normal male; *bottom*, a castrated male 30 days after the operation. Both sections were stained with aldehyde fuchsin, which distinguishes between thyrotropic basophils (*T*) and gonadotropic basophils (*G*). *A*, Acidophils; *C*, chromophobes; *S*, blood sinusoid. The gonadotropic cells in the castrate are much enlarged, but not stained. Some of the castrate's gonadotropic basophils are vacuolated (CA). The difference in the number of dark-stained thyrotrophs in the two figures is due to the fact that the lower figure illustrates the anteromedial region, where they are sparse. [Photograph by F. W. Kent from slides of N. W. Halmi, State University of Iowa.]

ERRATA
FOR

Gorbman et al.: COMPARATIVE ENDOCRINOLOGY

The following figure includes the labels that were inadvertently left off the version printed on page 124.

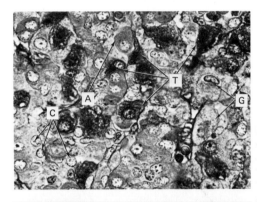
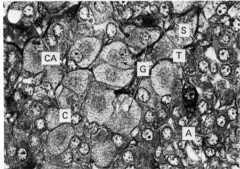

FIGURE 4.3. Sections through the pars distalis of the rat. *Top*, a normal male; *bottom*, a castrated male 30 days after the operation. Both sections were stained with aldehyde fuchsin, which distinguishes between thyrotropic basophils (*T*) and gonadotropic basophils (*G*). *A*, Acidophils; *C*, chromophobes; *S*, blood sinusoid. The gonadotropic cells in the castrate are much enlarged, but not stained. Some of the castrate's gonadotropic basophils are vacuolated (CA). The difference in the number of dark-stained thyrotrophs in the two figures is due to the fact that the lower figure illustrates the anteromedial region, where they are sparse. [Photograph by F. W. Kent from slides of N. W. Halmi, State University of Iowa.]

in the antibody-labeled cell. By this means unequivocal labeling of the STH, PRL, and ACTH cells has been described. However, this technique has revealed what seem to be purely TSH, FSH, or LH cells and other cells that appear to contain two of these glycoprotein hormones. If the antibody were raised against the entire hormone (FSH, LH, or TSH), we might reason that this confusion is due to the common α subunit in these three hormones. However, this apparent multiplicity of glycoprotein hormone content or synthesis is indicated even when antibodies to the pure β subunits are used (Fig. 4.5). If it is true that certain cells in the pars distalis can secrete two, or possibly even three, glycoprotein hormones, how can we explain separate release of only one of them in response to appropriate stimulation?

GROWTH HORMONE (STH)

The Hormonal Molecule

The development of an extraction procedure for isolating a protein hormone such as STH is a trial-and-error process that in some respects resembles certain more complex kitchen maneuvers. In fact, the preparation of Japanese tofu from soy beans has been compared to pituitary hormone extraction procedures! Essentially, pituitaries are ground up in a liquid in which the hormones dissolve. After filtering off the tissue residue, the supernatant liquid can then be treated with reagents that will precipitate out of solution some of the dissolved protein. High concentrations of salts (sodium chloride, ammonium sulfate) or organic solvents such as ethanol or acetone can be used. If the pH of the supernatant is adjusted to a particular value, a partial purification can sometimes be achieved at this step. That is, some of the hormones are selectively precipitated, and others are left in the supernatant. In further purification the problem is to separate the desired hormone from all other substances, taking advantage of whatever distinctive physical properties the hormone may have: solubility, isoelectric point, molecular size or mass, electrical charge of the ionized molecule, and so on. Thus the hormone-containing mixture may be passed through columns of material that selectively adsorbs substances of particular electrical charge; the mixture may be caused to move through an electrical potential field in which substances migrate at different rates (chromatography, electrophoresis), permitting collection of fractions containing maxima or minima of the desired or undesired materials; the mixture may be placed in an ultracentrifuge or in an ultrafilter, in which separation will occur on the basis of molecular size.

At many junctures during the hormone-isolation process the chemist is faced with a need to know into which fraction the hormone has gone after a particular manipulation. This is determined by bioassay; that is, portions of these fractions are administered to test animals, and a biological effect

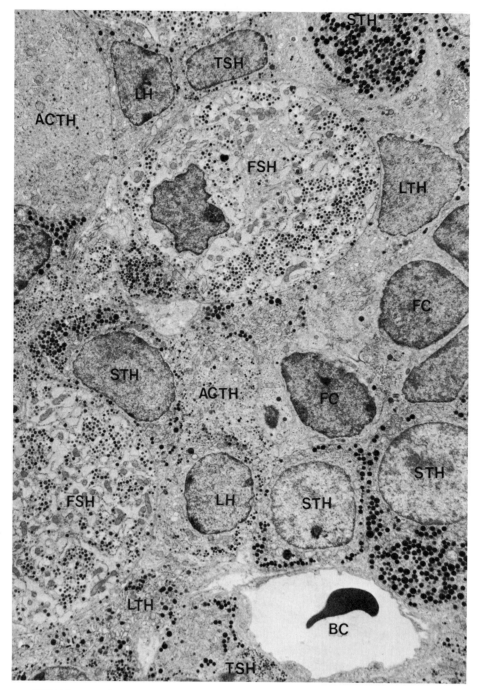

FIGURE 4.4. Electron photomicrograph of the rat pituitary gland. The six basic, hormone-secreting cell types are all visible in this field (*ACTH, STH, LTH, FSH, LH, TSH*). At this magnification (4400 ×), the distinctive features of the hormone-containing specific granules are not apparent, but at least size and density differences are visible. *FC*, Fibroblast; *BC*, red blood cell. [Photo provided by Dr. K. Kurosumi, Endocrine Institute, Gunma University, Maebashi, Japan.]

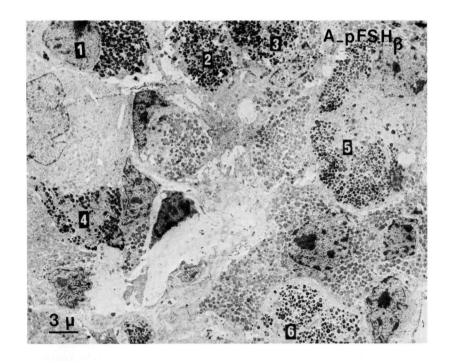

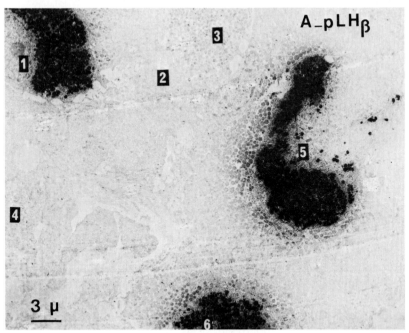

FIGURE 4.5. A section from 2.5% glutaraldehyde-fixed rat pituitary treated with antibody to FSHβ (*above*) and then with antibody to LHβ (*below*). Cell 1 is strongly stained for both FSHβ (*above*) and LHβ (*below*); cells 2, 3, and 4 are positive for FSHβ and negative for LHβ; cells 5 and 6 are strongly stained for LHβ and weakly reactive for FSHβ. [Photographs provided by F. Dacheux, Centre de Recherche de Tours, Nouzilly, France.]

attributable to the hormone is measured. For growth hormone, the bioassay most frequently used at first was measurement of growth in young hypophysectomized rats into which the materials were injected. This was a "wasteful" assay in the sense that so much of the precious hormone was used up in the assay. Because of this, extremely large amounts of pituitary tissue had to be available before efforts to isolate growth hormone could begin. A more efficient assay used later required less growth hormone. This was the so-called rat tibia test, in which one measured the augmenting action of growth hormone on the width of the epiphyseal disc, a cartilaginous structure near the ends of the long bones. It is from these discs that growth in bone length occurs. Currently, extremely sensitive RIAs for growth hormone (see Chapter 1) are available, but, of course, the pure hormone had to be at hand *before* the radioimmunoassay could be developed.

Using such procedures, growth hormones have been isolated from pituitary tissue of some members of each of the vertebrate classes excepting the Agnatha. The first growth hormones were isolated from pituitaries of large mammals (cows, sheep), as might be expected. The procedures developed in this way then permitted the preparation of pure STH from humans, monkeys, whales, rats, and others, and then from the limited available amounts of pituitary tissues of small lower-vertebrate forms such as birds, reptiles, amphibians, and fishes.

The amino acid sequences of only a few mammalian STHs have been worked out, so that only limited comparisons can be made between them. For this reason, not much can be said about the molecular evolution of the growth hormones. What speculations are made at this time are based on total amino acid composition or on the immunological cross-reaction of growth hormone of one species with the antibody prepared against the growth hormone of another species. Table 4.2 compares the total amino acid compositions of growth hormones and prolactins from a variety of vertebrates. According to S. W. Farmer, all of the hormones listed resemble each other in chemical "behavior" during the extraction and purification process; all have two cystine (4 cysteine) residues, a single tryptophan, a relatively low histidine and methionine content, and a high glutamic acid and leucine content. Frog and fish (*Tilapia*) STHs differ most in composition from the mammalian. All STHs cross-reacted immunologically with anti-rat STH antibody and were able to compete to some extent with rat STH in binding to the antibody. Frog and fish STHs, phylogenetically the most "distant" hormones, competed most poorly with homologous rat STH for binding to the anti-rat STH antibody. It is interesting that despite its molecular differences from mammalian STH, frog STH is still quite active in the rat tibia test. Yet bovine or ovine STHs are useless in treating human dwarfism (though human or monkey STH is effective).

We may conclude from all this that the differentiation of STH and prolactin (PRL) from a common "mother molecule" took place early in vertebrate phylogenesis, since both hormones already exist in the fishes. It is

TABLE 4.2.   Amino acid composition of growth hormone (GH) and prolactin (PRL) from various species[a]

Amino Acid	Sheep GH[b]	Duck GH	Snapping Turtle GH	Bullfrog GH	*Tilapia* GH	*Tilapia* PRL[c]	Sheep PRL[d]
Lys	11	12	12	11	8	9	9
His	3	5	4	6	5	5	8
Arg	13	10	13	17	11	7	11
Asp	16	21	20	30	19	16	22
Thr	12	10	9	12	12	9	9
Ser	13	12	14	12	21	22	15
Glu	24	25	24	18	29	17	22
Pro	6	10	7	6	7	11	11
Gly	10	10	9	7	7	8	11
Ala	15	11	11	6	8	10	9
½ Cys	4	4	4	4	4	4	6
Val	6	8	8	11	6	7	10
Met	4	4	4	4	1	5	7
Ile	7	6	7	8	9	9	11
Leu	27	26	26	18	27	24	23
Tyr	6	6	7	10	7	3	7
Phe	13	10	12	11	7	5	6
Trp	1	1	1	1	1	1	2

[a] From S. W. Farmer, *Comparative Endocrinology* (P. J. Gaillard and H. H. Boer, eds.), Elsevier/North-Holland, Amsterdam (1978).
[b] Growth hormones were calculated on the basis of 191 residues per mole.
[c] Calculated on the basis of a molecular weight of 19,400 daltons.
[d] Obtained from structural analysis.

unfortunate that at this time there is no information whatsoever about the most primitive vertebrates, the Agnatha, concerning STH and PRL (their presence and their physical and biological properties).

At the textbook level, there is not much that is instructive about a diagram of the amino acid sequence of a large molecule such as growth hormone. Figure 4.6 is a popular diagram of human STH by C. H. Li. Figure 4.7 compares the sequences of STHs from sheep, cows, horses, and humans with each other and with the sequence of human PRL. This comparison shows that human STH, despite the similarities to other mammalian STHs, is somewhat different from the STHs of the ungulates, probably explaining why beef or sheep growth hormone is without significant effect in humans or monkeys. On the other hand, human STH and PRL are remarkably similar in amino acid sequence. This degree of similarity between STH and PRL is not seen in the ungulates.

In determining the amino acid composition or sequence of some purified growth hormones, there often has been uncertainty about one or two amino acids. Some of this minor uncertainty has been dispelled by the discovery

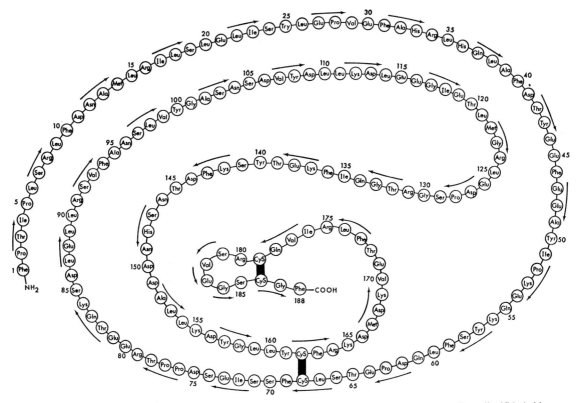

FIGURE 4.6.　The amino acid sequence of human growth hormone. Two disulfide bridges are indicated in black, linking amino acids 68 and 162, and 179 and 186. Arrows indicate the direction of numbering of the amino acids, from the amino (—NH₂) end to the carboxyl (—COOH) end. [From C. H. Li, *Perspect. Biol. Med.*, **11**:498–521, 1968.]

that in some species STH is "polymorphic." That is, when pituitary glands of individual cows are appropriately studied, the STH molecules may have either a valine or a leucine in a particular position, or a given pituitary might contain both valine-STH and leucine-STH in a 1:1 ratio. This is what one might expect if the placement of one or another of these amino acids in a particular position in the STH molecule were a simple, allelic, Mendelian genetic factor. In sheep STH there is similar polymorphism, with glycine and valine as the two possibilities.

Actions of STH

In considering the biological actions of growth hormone, the first and most obvious is the stimulation of somatic growth, both skeletal and of the soft tissues. It is true that body growth ceases in young hypophysectomized rats and that it resumes, though to a limited degree, upon injection of STH.

Furthermore, STH stimulates the transport of amino acids into cells and the incorporation of these amino acids into structural protein, increasing the levels of cytoplasmic mRNA at this time. STH has still other metabolic actions—to be discussed below—that can be interpreted as favoring somatic growth. However, growth is a complex metabolic process, or a complex of metabolic processes, involving a variety of other hormones and even the central nervous system. For example, it has long been known that thyroid hormone, which by itself has only a slight effect on growth in hypophysectomized rats, greatly amplifies the action of STH in such test animals (Fig. 4.8). Other hormones that have a positive or negative effect on growth, or that amplify or reduce the growth action of STH, are the adrenal steroids, insulin, sex steroids, catecholamine hormones, and probably still others.

Another caution must be inserted at this point concerning the interpretation of the somatic growth actions of STH. Most of the studies of hormonal control of growth have been done in mammals. Even among mammals there is variation in the relative roles of different hormones in the growth process. This is to be expected because there is so much variation in diet, intervals between feeding, seasonal limitations in external conditions favorable for growth (temperature, food availability, and other ecological factors), and parental care and feeding during the early growth period. Thus, general patterns of metabolic control will vary, and integrated with these patterns will be the possiblility of different roles for hormones in metabolism, growth, and development. What follows, therefore, will be a discussion based largely on mammalian studies.

Somatomedin

Since it was observed early that STH stimulates cartilage growth (chondrogenesis), it was surprising that it did not do so *in vitro*. Salmon and Daughaday found that incorporation of radioisotope-labeled sulfate into cultured rat cartilage would occur in response to STH only if a factor in normal rat serum was added to the culture. Accordingly, this element was named "sulfation factor." Sulfation factor, later called somatomedin because it had more general actions, is absent from the serum of hypophysectomized rats, and it appears to be produced, at least in part, by the liver and by muscle as an early action (within one hour after injection) of STH. Once in the serum, somatomedin itself can stimulate processes attributed to STH. It is, therefore, a mediator of STH action. It stimulates various phases of protein synthesis associated with chondrogenesis, but this action does not require prior RNA transcription. It also stimulates amino acid incorporation into protein, at least in some tissues. How many other actions of STH are due to mediation by somatomedin is under study.

The nature of somatomedin, beyond the fact that it is a fairly large peptide, is unsettled. Various somatomedins have been isolated, with molecular weights estimated between 3,900 and 12,400. In the blood somatomedin

```
                                                          10                                              20
Bovine GH:  H-Ala-Phe-Pro-Ala-Met-Ser-Leu-Ser-Gly-Leu-Phe-Ala-Asn-Ala-Val-Leu-Arg-Ala-Gln-His-Leu-His-Gln-Leu-Ala-
Ovine  GH:  H ————————————————————————————————————————————————————————————————————————————— – – –
Equine GH:  H ——————— Pro ——————— Ser ——————— – – – Asp ——————— Met ——————— His-Arg — – – –
Human  GH:  H ——————— Thr-Ile-Pro ——————— Arg ——————— – – – Met ——————— Gln ——————— His-Arg-Ala — – – –
Human  PRL: H-Val-Gln-Thr-Val-Pro ——————— Arg ——————— Asp-His ——————— Gln ——————— His-Arg-Ser ——
```

```
                                          30                                          40
Bovine GH:  -Ala-Asp-Thr-Phe-Lys-Glu-Phe-Glu-Arg-Thr-Tyr-Ile-Pro-Glu-Gly-Gln-Arg-Tyr-Ser-  X  -Ile-Gln-Asn-Thr-Gln-
Ovine  GH:                                                                                    X
Equine GH:  – – –    Tyr ———— Ala ——————————    X  – – – – –    Ala – –
Human  GH:  -Phe ———— Tyr-Gln ———— Glu-Ala ———— Lys-Glu ———— Lys ———— Phe-Leu ———— Pro
Human  PRL: -Ile ———— Tyr-Gln ———— Glu ———— Lys-Asp ———— Lys ———— Phe-Leu-His-Asp-Ser ————
```

```
             50                                          60                                          70
Bovine GH:  -Val-Ala-Phe-Cys-Phe-Ser-Glu-Thr-Ile-Pro-Ala-Pro-Thr-Gly-Lys-Asn-Glu-Ala-Gln-Gln-Lys-Ser-Asp-Leu-Glu-
Ovine  GH:  -Ala – –
Equine GH:  -Thr-Ser-Leu ———— Ser ———— Ser-Asn-Arg-Glu ———— Thr ———— Arg ———— Met – –
Human  GH:  -Thr-Ser ———— Asp-Ser ———— Ser-Asn-Met-Glu ———— Thr ———— Asn ———— Gln –
Human  PRL:
```

```
                      80                                          90
Bovine GH:  -Leu-Leu-Arg-Ile-Ser-Leu-Leu-Ile-Gln-Ser-Trp-Leu-Gly-Pro-Leu-Gln-Phe-Leu-Ser-Arg-Val-Phe-Thr-
Ovine  GH:  – –
Equine GH:  Phe ———— Val ———— Arg-Ser ———— – –
Human  GH:  Glu ———— Val ———— Leu ———— Arg-Ser-Met ———— Ala-
Human  PRL: Glu ———— Val-Arg ———— Arg-Ser-Met ———— Ala-
```

```
             100                                          110                                          120
Bovine GH:  -Asn-Ser-Leu-Val-Phe-Gly-Thr-Ser-Asp-  X  -Arg-Val-Tyr-Glu-Lys-Leu-Lys-Asp-Leu-Glu-Glu-Gly-Ile-Leu-Ala-
Ovine  GH:  -Asp
Equine GH:  – – – – –    X    Arg ———— Gln – – –
Human  GH:  Tyr ———— Asn-Ser-Asp ———— Asp-Leu ———— Gln-Thr –
Human  PRL: Asn ———— Tyr-Asp ———— Ser-Asp-Asp ———— His-Leu ———— Gln-Thr –
```

```
                                                    130
Bovine GH:  -Leu-Met-Arg-Glu-Val-Leu-Glu-Asp-Gly-Thr-Pro-Arg-Ala-Gly-Gln-Ile-Leu-Lys-Gln-Thr-Tyr-Asp-Lys-Phe-Asp-Thr-Asn
                                                                                          140

Ovine GH:   ——————— Leu ——— Val ———————————————————————————————————— — — — — —
Equine GH:  ——————— Leu ———————————————————————————————————————————— — — — — —
Human GH:   ——— Gly-Arg-Leu ——— Ser ——————————— Thr ——————— Phe ——— Ser — — — — —
Human PRL:  ——— Gly-Arg-Leu ——— Ser-Arg ——— Thr ——————————————— Ser — — — — —

            150
Bovine GH:  -Met-Arg-Ser-Asp-Asp-Ala-Leu-Leu-Lys-Asn-Tyr-Gly-Leu-Leu-Ser-Cys-Phe-Arg-Lys-Asp-Leu-His-Lys-Thr-
                                                        160                                   170
Ovine GH:   -Leu — — — — — — —
Equine GH:  -Ser-His-Asn ——————— Lys —— Asn —
Human GH:   -Ser-His-Asn ——— Tyr ——— Met-Asp —— Val —
Human PRL:  -Ser-His-Asn-His ——— Tyr ——— Met-Asp —— Val —

            180
Bovine GH:  -Glu-Thr-Tyr-Leu-Arg-Val-Met-Lys-Cys-Arg-Arg-Phe-Gly-Glu-Ala-Ser-Cys-Ala-Phe-OH
                                                                190
Ovine GH:   ——————————————————————————————————————————— OH
Equine GH:  - - - - ——— Ile-Val-Gln ——— Val ——— -X-' Ser-Val ——— Ser ——— OH
Human GH:   ——— Phe ——— Met-Val-Gln ——— -X- Ser-Val ——— Gly ——— OH
Human PRL:  ——— Phe ——— Met-Val-Gln ——— -X- Ser-Val ——— Gly ——— OH
```

FIGURE 4.7. A comparison of the primary structures of growth hormones from several species and human prolactin. The sequence of bovine growth hormone is shown in full. For the other sequences, a solid line indicates identity with bovine growth hormone; differences are written out in full; X's indicate incompletely sequenced regions. [Based on B. M. Wallis, *Biol. Rev.* **50**:35–98, 1975.]

133

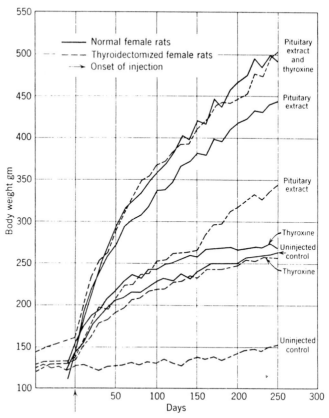

FIGURE 4.8. Growth of normal and thyroidectomized rats that have been given thyroid and pituitary hormones. [From H. M. Evans, M. E. Simpson, and R. Pencharz, *Endocrinology,* **25:**175, 1939.]

appears to be bound to a larger carrier protein. Needless to say, the comparative endocrinology of somatomedin is in a nascent stage.

STH and Carbohydrate, Fat, and Protein Metabolism

The most characteristic effect of STH on carbohydrate metabolism is hyperglycemia ("diabetogenic action"). In rats, at least, the eventual hyperglycemic effect may be preceded by brief hypoglycemia ("insulin-like effect"), but this may be a pharmacologic action requiring higher dosages of STH. The STH hyperglycemia is characterized by a slower rate of clearance of glucose from the blood (contra-insulin effect). A second, and important, consequence of STH treatment is a release of insulin, apparently by direct stimulation of the pancreatic β cells where insulin is synthesized. It may seem illogical that a hormone that is hyperglycemic should stimulate the release of a hormone that is hypoglycemic. However, teleologically it makes sense for STH to recruit insulin in its actions, since insulin is a strong stimulant of transport of free amino acids into cells. Such enrichment of the cellular amino acid supply then supports the synthesis of new protein stimulated by STH. It also makes sense that if STH will recruit insulin for its amino acid transport action, it should create hyperglycemia to offset the hypoglycemic action of the insulin it has caused to be secreted. Teleology is a dangerous tool, but it helps to organize the numerous separate phenomena into an apparently rational system.

A general effect of STH on fat metabolism is indicated by the lipemia that follows STH administration to rats. Together with this, there is a depletion of carcass lipid stores and a movement of fat into the liver. There generally is a decrease in the respiratory quotient (ratio of CO_2 production to O_2 consumption), which indicates increased general body utilization of fat by oxidation. This, in turn, is accompanied by ketosis, which is part of the "diabetogenic" action of STH. The lipolysis (freeing of fat from tissue stores) produced by STH can be countered by insulin, another example of the general opposed action between insulin and STH. Applying the reasoning that was presented above, the opposed insulin–STH action on fat metabolism may be part of the correction that has to be made to achieve normalcy when STH stimulates the secretion of insulin.

As part of the anabolic action of STH, it has been mentioned that this hormone stimulates transport of amino acids and glucose into the intracellular compartment. This can be shown *in vitro* by use of rat diaphragm muscle, as well as in the intact animal. The stimulated transport is not dependent on new RNA transcription. The increased incorporation of the amino acid into muscle protein is a generally observed phenomenon, and it can be stimulated by somatomedin as well as by STH. The net effect of the anabolic state evoked by STH is a "positive nitrogen balance." That is, a larger proportion of ingested protein is resynthesized into new tissue structured protein and a smaller proportion is converted into urea or creatinine, the waste products of nitrogen metabolism. Accordingly, more of the ingested amino acid nitrogen remains in the organism, resulting in true growth.

Control of STH Secretion

The plasma levels of immunoreactive (as determined by RIA) growth hormone are quite labile in mammals, including humans and not at all what one would expect if the sole function of this hormone were the regulation of such a slow, continuous process as body growth. In fact, in nongrowing, older humans or experimental animals, the plasma levels of STH are not appreciably lowered. There is a diurnal cycle of plasma STH, the highest levels occurring during sleep. Superimposed upon this diurnal cycle there are shorter fluctuations, several hours long, of plasma STH. In experimental animals caused to become hypoglycemic or reduced in plasma amino acid level, there is a release of STH from the pars distalis. Violent exercise and stress also lead to a release of STH. Hyperglycemia or injections of glucocorticosteroid hormones evoke a suppression of STH release from the pars distalis and a lowering of plasma levels. Certain neurotransmitters given experimentally, such as dopamine and serotonin, evoke a release of STH.

No clear or common mechanism for regulating STH secretion emerges from all this except that most, if not all, changes in STH secretion are mediated through the brain. Seemingly, they all cause an increase or decrease in the amount of somatostatin, SRIF (somatotropin release–inhibiting factor), secreted into the portal veins from the median eminence to the pars distalis. Since there is some evidence that there may be a growth hormone–releasing factor (GRH), another alternative is that the influences on STH secretion (glycemia, stress, etc.) may be acting through a GRH–SRIF balance. It appears that in the ventromedial nucleus of the rat hypothalamus there is a glucose receptor sensitive to hyper- and hypoglycemia. Deep sleep and administration of opiates such as morphine, which cause release of STH, appear to operate via the limbic system in the hypothalamus, and this in turn projects to the median eminence.

PROLACTIN (PRL)

The name prolactin was first applied in 1928 to a ''factor'' in pituitary extracts that caused lactation to begin in the pseudopregnant rabbit. To comparative endocrinologists, prolactin is easily the most versatile hormone of the pars distalis. It is involved in such a wide variety of phenomena that it must be concluded that receptors for this hormone are very broadly distributed throughout the organism. It acts upon the central nervous system to evoke behavioral phenomena (''water drive'' in Amphibia, brooding in birds); upon the gill and kidney to enable osmoregulatory functions in vertebrates from fish to mammals; on the skin to affect feather growth, molting, mucus secretion (fishes); on visceral growth (birds, reptiles); on body growth (amphibians, mammals); as an antagonist of the metamorphic actions of thyroxine in Amphibia; and on various vertebrate expressions of parental care (milk secretion in mammals, secretion of crop sac milk in birds, multiplication of skin cells and mucus secretion in fish species in which young ''graze'' upon the integument of the mother, nest building in numerous species from fishes to mammals). The list is long and impressive, and the mere listing occupies several pages of a well-known review by Bern and Nicoll.

The Prolactin Molecule

The similarities between STH and prolactin (PRL) were discussed in the previous section. Awareness of these similarities prompted the following rather strong statement from A. G. Frantz in speaking of ovine PRL, human

STH, and human placental somatomammotropin: "These studies leave no doubt that all three proteins arose from a common precursor early in vertebrate evolution, possibly by a process of genetic reduplication of a smaller ancestral peptide."

Most of the known vertebrate PRLs are just under 200 amino acid residues in length, contain at least three internal disulfide linkages (Fig. 4.9), and have a molecular weight in the neighborhood of 23,000 daltons.

Other notable species differences in PRLs are: pig PRL contains seven disulfides instead of the usual three in mammalian PRLs; rat PRL is somewhat shorter than the typical 195 to 198 residues.

Pituitary extracts, in addition to the 23,000-dalton PRL, also contain a "big" PRL of 56,000 daltons. Although this might be a dimer, it is more likely a prohormone of PRL. Some "big" PRLs can be found in human serum, and their proportion to normal PRL varies in certain disease states and during pregnancy.

It will be recalled that human or primate STH receptors will not readily react with STHs of other mammalian groups. However human PRL receptors (as in the mammary gland) will respond to ovine or bovine PRL, or even to human STH. Thus, it would seem that human PRL receptors are not as finely tuned or stereospecific as are human STH receptors. While rat liver will bind (contains receptors) hSTH and bSTH as well as bPRL, rabbit liver will bind only STH. PRL binds also to a variety of tissues in the rat, including mammary gland, adrenal, ovary, prostate, and kidney. A surprising finding is that binding of PRL in rat mammary gland cells is in the cytoplasm and nucleus, not on the plasma membrane (Fig. 4.10). This requires modification of the current concept, which specifies that protein hormone receptors are localized only on the plasma membrane of responsive cells, where the receptors are coupled with the adenyl cyclase system.

Biological Actions of Prolactin

In a review in 1974 Nicoll stated that at that time there were 85 clearly established functions known for PRL within the vertebrate group. This number must be higher at the present time, and the very multiplicity of the actions of PRL defeats any effort to recognize a common or universal factor among them. Nicoll listed the actions of PRL under the following headings: (1) actions related to various phases of reproduction; (2) somatotropic effects; (3) osmoregulatory effects; (4) actions on the integument and its derivatives; (5) steroid hormone synergism. Virtually any tissue in a given vertebrate species may evolve receptors for PRL and so become sensitive to it. Why should receptor evolution for PRL have been so much more frequent than for any other pituitary hormone? There is no obvious answer to such a question.

Perhaps the largest proportion of the actions of PRL is related to some phase of the reproductive process. However, in numerous instances the phenomenon in question is not a direct action of PRL, but one in which it

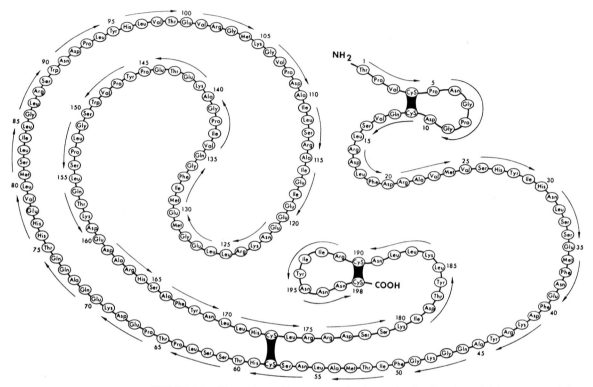

FIGURE 4.9. The amino acid sequence of ovine prolactin. Compare with human growth hormone (Fig. 4.6). [From C. H. Li, *Handbook of Physiology*, Vol. 4 (R. O. Greep, ed.), American Physiological Society, Washington, D.C., 1974.]

modulates, elicits, or synergizes the action of another hormone, most often a steroid hormone. If there is a recurrent theme or rationale characterizing the role of PRL in reproduction, it is the influence that adapts the reproductive process in a given species to the particular specialized pattern that the species has evolved in a particular ecological situation. Often this means that prolactin will have opposite actions in different species, even within the same vertebrate class, or even in the same species. Thus PRL is luteotropic (activates progesterone secretion by the new corpus luteum) in rats and sheep, but luteolytic (destructive) toward older corpora lutea in rats and mice. PRL generally favors progesterone secretion from ovarian structures other than the corpus luteum, sometimes in conjunction with LH. Similar support for the steroidogenic action of LH on rat testes, amplifying the secretion of androgen, has been described. Analogously, PRL acts in conjunction with ACTH in some fishes in stimulating corticosteroid secretion from the interrenal tissue.

On the other hand, PRL may be antigonadal, in birds in particular, actually causing involution of developed gonadal structures. Luteolysis of older cor-

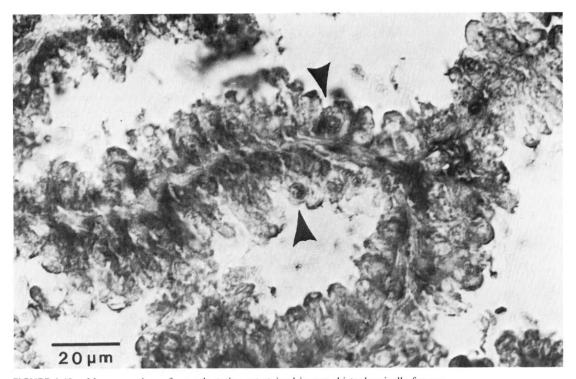

FIGURE 4.10. Mammary tissue from a lactating rat stained immunohistochemically for prolactin (black) that has been secreted in the pars distalis of the same animal. The columnar cells
shown here line milk-secreting alveoli at the onset of a functional cycle. Prolactin is detectable
in milk secreting cells only during the active phases of the secretory (or prolactin-response)
cycle. It is not seen during the resting phase. Prolactin is present in the nuclei (arrows) of milk-
secreting cells, suggesting a direct action of this hormone on the nuclear events that initiate
milk synthesis. [Photograph from J. M. Nolin, *Endocrinology,* **102**:402, 1978, with permission.]

pora lutea can be conceived of as a useful housekeeping action, clearing
away the older structures to prevent their accumulation and to leave space
for growth of corpora lutea involved in a particular cycle. The antigonadal
effect in birds may be though of as a part of a mechanism that insures a
minimun-sized gonad, which costs the bird little energy to carry during the
nonreproductive season.

There are many actions of PRL that control reproductive phenomena
beyond the period of embryonic development. These could be grouped as
"parental" or "care-of-the-young" functions. There are three forms of feeding of maternal secretions that are regulated by PRL. In mammals, of course,
synthesis and secretion of milk is such a function. PRL, together with other
hormones (sex steroids, corticosteroids, insulin), is also involved in the
buildup of the mammary gland, the so-called mammogenic effect. However,
the extent to which PRL is mammogenic seems to vary in different mammals.

Apparently, in humans STH is mammogenic and stimulates lactation, but this is much less true of STHs of other mammals. In the human placenta still another growth hormone-resembling lactogen functions during pregnancy: placental somatomammotropic hormone (HCS). Placental lactogens have been found in other mammals, but their molecular nature is not as well characterized as for HCS. A second type of maternal tissue-derived feeding is seen in the formation of "crop milk" in birds. Under the influence of PRL, the epithelium cells of the crop (an outpocketing of the esophagus) multiply and break free to such an extent that a whitish cheesy mass is formed in the crop. This is regurgitated by the mother into the mouths of the nestlings. A third example of this phenomenon is the feeding of very young fish by allowing them to graze upon mucus secreted near the parent's head in particular. This phenomenon was first studied in *Symphysodon discus*, the "discus fish" that is popular among tropical fish fanciers, but has been observed in some other species as well. Furthermore, integumentary mucus secretion in general appears to be stimulated by PRL in a variety of fish species.

The crop sac response has been utilized as a basis for a very sensitive bioassay for PRL. In this assay small blisters of test solution are carefully injected into the thin tissue layer between the skin and the crop of pigeons. The production of a thickened area of adjacent crop epithelium, visible to the naked eye, is taken as a positive response. By use of such limited areas of local response, many tests can be run at the same time in the same pigeon.

The existence of examples in three vertebrate groups of the phenomenon of infant feeding with secretions from the maternal parent, a common factor being the regulation of the phenomena by PRL, could hardly have failed to excite the interest of comparative endocrinologists, to whom this would appear to be an instance of convergent evolution. The tissues exploited in the three examples have little in common other than that they are epithelial. The crop epithelium is an endodermal gut derivative; the mammary gland is considered to be a modified sweat gland; the feeding of babies on integumentary mucus would seem to be the least specialized of the three mechanisms.

Another series of care-of-the-young phenomena regulated by PRL is behavioral in character. Nest building and protective or incubating behavior in or near the nest form a large series of behaviors individualized by particular species to their own pattern. In a number of instances steroid hormones may be involved along with PRL; in other instances PRL alone can evoke the behavior. In mammals these behaviors take the form of nest construction (rats, rabbits), and PRL-stimulated rabbits pluck hair from their own pelts to line the nest. In both rats and rabbits retrieval of pups that have wandered or that have been removed from the nest is a function of PRL in both sexes. In *Tilapia* and other cichlid "mouth breeder" fish species, PRL apparently regulates the inhibition of feeding in the parent. In such species the young dart in and out of the mouths of the protective parents in dire peril if the feeding response were to occur. Brooding is the complex of behaviors in birds while the eggs are being incubated and the helpless young are fed. It is regulated by PRL, but the extent to which steroids may be involved in the behavior must be determined in individual species. In some species a PRL- and progesterone-regulated phenomenon is the development of the "brood patch." This is a feather-free, highly vascularized area on the breast that is applied to the eggs during incubation.

Brooding behavior in fishes differs greatly in character from that of birds and mammals, and in some species PRL seems not to be involved. However, it has been claimed that "fanning" with the fins in some species, to assure aerated water passing over eggs in the nest, is a function of PRL.

One set of actions of vertebrate PRLs derives from their molecular similarity to growth hormone (STH) and their apparent ability to utilize the same receptors as STH. This area of confusion of action of the two related hormones is quite broad and is summarized in Table 4.3. Thus PRL can stimulate growth in both tadpoles and young metamorphosed amphibians. It leads to splanchnomegaly (hypertrophy of visceral organs) in pigeons, and some PRLs (human, monkey) are active in the rat tibia test. Conversely, some growth hormones (again, monkey and human) are positive in the pigeon crop test. In the early days of pituitary hormone isolation, about 50 years ago, not only were the hormone receptors confused by this situation, but also some well-known endocrinologists were caught up in it. The issue was whether there is a separate growth hormone, or whether PRL can account for all of the growth that is evoked by injection of pituitary extracts. Herbert M. Evans, whose assay was growth in the young hypophysectomized rat, favored the two-hormone idea; Oscar Riddle, whose assay was the pigeon crop sac reaction and who had named prolactin, denied the existence of a separate growth hormone. Both men were dramatic speakers as well as excellent scientists, and "old timers" can still recall very lively scientific meetings at which the two clashed rhetorically.

The antagonism between PRL and thyroid hormones in embryonic amphibians forms another area of interest because the actions are exerted on a developing system. As mentioned before, PRL is somatotrophic in tadpoles. Stimulation of growth of the tail fin is a noticeable phenomenon, since it is the opposite of the response to thyroxine. Since PRL is a general inhibitor of a broad spectrum of metamorphic actions of thyroxine in tadpoles, it may be assumed that many tissues have receptors for both hormones, and that the antagonism between the two is at the tissue level. However, in several species it has been found that PRL also reduces thyroid gland synthesis of thyroxine. In developing salamanders there is an interesting behavioral action of PRL. In some species of urodeles metamorphosis (stimulated by thyroxine, opposed by PRL) results in a terrestrial form. In *Notophthalmus* (*Triturus*) *viridescens*, in which this phenomenon has been studied most, the terrestrial form is known as the "red eft stage." The red eft eventually undergoes a "second metamorphosis," which can be evoked

TABLE 4.3. Effects of purified or partially purified prolactins and growth hormones from different vertebrate species on several physiological processes or target organs[a]

Physiological Response	Prolactins			Growth Hormones				
	Pisces[b]	Amphibians, Reptiles, and Birds	Mammals	Pisces	Amphibians, Reptiles, and Birds	Mammals		Human Placental Lactogen
						Nonprimates	Primates	
Teleosts Osmoregulatory actions	Several species +++[c]	N.I.	Ovine + Bovine + Porcine –	Several species –	N.I.	Ovine – Bovine –	Human + Rhesus +	–
Xanthophore expansion in *Gillichthys*	Several species +++	N.I.	Several species +	Several species –	N.I.	Several species ++	Human +	–
Amphibians Tadpole growth	N.I.	N.I.	Porcine ++ Bovine ++ Ovine ++	N.I.	N.I.	Bovine ± Ovine ±	Human +	–
Antimetamorphic	N.I.	N.I.	Ovine ++ Bovine ++	N.I.	N.I.	Ovine – Bovine –	N.I.	+
Second metamorphic (water-drive)	N.I.	Urodele ++	Ovine ++ Bovine ++	N.I.	N.I.	Ovine – Bovine –	N.I.	+
Toad growth	Several species +	Turtles ++ Other species –	Ovine + Bovine + Rat – Porcine –	Several species ++	Several species +++	Ovine +++ Bovine +++	N.I.	+
Birds Pigeon crop sac	Several species –	Several species ++	Several species +++	Several species –	Several species –	Several species –	Human + Rhesus +	+
Mammals Rat tibia test	Several species –	N.I.	Rat + Porcine – Ovine ± Human +	Several species –	Turtle + Duck +	Several species +++	Human +++ Rhesus +++	±

[a] From C. S. Nicoll, *Handbook of Physiology*, Vol. 4, Sect. 7 (R. O. Greep, ed.) American Physiological Society, Washington, D.C., p. 268 (1974).
[b] Pisces includes the cartilaginous (chondrichthian) and bony (teleostean) fishes.
[c] Number of (+) signs indicates relative effectiveness of the hormone preparation; (–) signs indicate no response and (±) signs indicate possible or marginal effect; N.I., no information.

experimentally by PRL treatment. At this time the eft returns to the water to become a permanently aquatic salamander. There is both a behavioral and a structural aspect to the second metamorphosis. The behavioral element, known as "water drive" is opposed by higher levels of thyroxine. However, it has been claimed that without a minimal level of thyroxine the water drive phenomenon cannot be evoked by PRL.

An important category of actions of PRL, apparently unrelated to those already described, is on those organs (skin, gill, kidney, urinary bladder) in which eletrolyte transport occurs for the purpose of osmoregulation. Some of these actions are listed in Table 4.4. This role of the pituitary gland, and of PRL in particular, was first established when it was found that certain fishes died after hypophysectomy if kept in fresh water. The hormone that

TABLE 4.4. Actions of prolactin involving water and electrolyte balance[a]

Cyclostomes
  Electrolyte metabolism in hagfishes (ACTH-like)
Teleosts
  Survival of hypophysectomized euryhaline freshwater species
  Restoration of water turnover in hypophysectomized *Fundulus kansae*
  Restoration of plasma Na^+ and Ca^{2+} in hypophysectomized eels when given with
    cortisol
  Skin, buccal, and gill mucous secretion
  Reduced gill Na^+ efflux (reduced permeability)
  Reduced gill permeability to water
  Inhibition of gill Na,K-ATPase
  Renotrophic (increased glomerular size)
  Increased urinary water elimination and decreased salt excretion
  Stimulation of renal Na,K-ATPase
  Decreased water absorption and increased Na^+ absorption in flounder bladder
  Decreased salt and water absorption from eel gut
Amphibians
  Skin and electrolyte changes associated with water drive
  Sodium and water transport across toad bladder
  Restoration of plasma Na^+ in hypophysectomized newts
  Possible hypercalcemia in toads
Reptiles
  Restoration of plasma Na^+ levels in hypophysectomized lizard
Birds
  Stimulation of nasal (orbital) salt gland secretion
Mammals
  Lactation
  Increased Na^+ retention at renal level
  Corticotropic

[a] From C. S. Nicoll, *Handbook of Physiology*, Vol. 4 (R. O. Greep, ed.), American Physiology Society (1974).

made possible the survival of hypophysectomized fishes in fresh or diluted waters was known, until identified as PRL, as "freshwater survival factor." Generally, PRL helps maintain minimal ionic concentrations in the blood in hypotonic environments by preventing the loss of such ions through the kidney or gill while promoting water loss through the kidney. This function is obviously very important for aquatic species that alternate between salt and fresh waters. However, some species, such as the eel *Anguilla*, can regulate blood electrolytes independently of PRL in fresh water. This is true also of some permanent freshwater species, such as the goldfish. In fact, in comparing individual fish species there is a puzzling lack of consistency with respect to which ions (Na^+, K^+, Ca^{2+}, Cl^-, etc.) are regulated by PRL and which by corticosteroid hormones. Furthermore, at particular membranes (gill, gut, bladder, skin) there is further variation in whether it is influx or efflux (or both) that are regulated by the hormone. There is additional variability as to which species respond to PRL by changes in ATPase activity. This enzyme is involved in the transport of Na^+ ions.

Although PRL was at first thought of as active only in teleostean osmoregulation, it is now known that this hormone has a similar action—protection against salt loss—in membranes of all vertebrate groups. In mammals, and in humans as well, PRL has a Na^+-retaining action, and in this function it interacts with aldosterone and other corticosteroids to achieve normal plasma levels.

Control of Prolactin Synthesis and Release

Hypothalamic control of secretion of PRL, like that of growth hormone, is by inhibition rather than by stimulation. That is, if lesions are placed in certain parts of the hypothalamus (e.g., the medial basal hypothalamus in the rat), an oversecretion of PRL can be shown to follow if RIA of blood samples is done. Furthermore, the rat pars distalis, successfully transplanted to other regions such as the capsule of the kidney, secretes large amounts of PRL. A female rat with a transplanted pars distalis or with a lesion of the medial basal hypothalamus may become pseudopregnant. That is, the luteotropic action of continuous, unchecked PRL levels can cause the ovary to secrete large amounts of progesterone. Progesterone in turn stimulates pregnancylike growth of the uterus, predisposing it to decidual tissue proliferation.

On the other hand, appropriate injections of extracts of the hypothalamus *reduce* the plasma PRL levels. Figure 4.11 illustrates an experiment in the rat in which rat hypothalamus extracts were injected into a portal vessel between the median eminence and the pars distalis. The result was a reduction in PRL secretion (judged by RIA of circulating blood) proportional to the amount of extract infused.

All of the preceding information is consistent with the existence of a hypothalamic factor that continuously keeps the secretion of PRL in check.

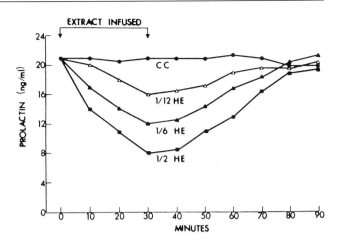

FIGURE 4.11. Direct *in vivo* demonstration of the existence of a hypothalamic prolactin-inhibiting factor in the rat. A microcannula was inserted into a pituitary portal vessel, and the anterior pituitary was infused with an extract of cerebral cortex (*CC*) or increasing concentrations of hypothalamic extract (*HE*). One HE is equivalent to the median eminence removed from a single rat. Prolactin concentrations were measured in peripheral plasma. [Adapted from Kamberi, Mical, and Porter, *Endocrinology,* 88:1294–1299, 1971.]

This factor, PIF (prolactin secretion–inhibiting factor), has not yet been isolated but there is evidence that dopamine may be a PIF. Secretion of PRL appears to be regulated by dopamine from neurons synapsing with the PIF-synthesizing neurons in the hypothalamus or from the PIF neurons directly. There are several kinds of neurogenic systems that reflexively evoke PRL secretion; so they may be considered to send impulses through this nervous mechanism. One is supplied by suckling and the other by stimulation of the cervical region of the uterus during copulation in mammals. It will be remembered that these are both stimuli for the release of oxytocin as well. There are several endocrine manipulations that can affect PRL secretion, possibly through another mechanism. One is a surge of estradiol secretion in the rat. This surge, whether natural during the normal cycle or induced by injection of estradiol, results in a surge of PRL secretion. Another endocrine influence is the injection of PRL itself, which seems to have a negative feedback on pituitary PRL secretion.

PRL secretion also follows a lowering of the ionic concentration of the blood. It was thought at first that this might be in response to an osmoreceptor in the central nervous system that might have afferent input to the PIF center. However, it has been shown that both fish and mammalian pituitary tissues in culture respond directly to a lowering of the osmotic concentration of the culture medium by secreting PRL.

THYROTROPIC HORMONE (TSH)

Two of the three glycoprotein pituitary hormones, TSH and FSH, have been the slowest to be purified and sequenced. Presumably this has been due to the relatively small concentrations of these hormones in the pituitary and to the presence of other glycoprotein substances, which makes the chemical isolation process difficult. Although the presence of thyrotropic activity has

bTSHα: NH$_2$-Phe-Pro-Asp-Gly-Glu-Phe-Thr-Met^8
bTSHβ: NH$_2$-Phe-Cys-Ile-Pro-Thr-Glu-Tyr-Met-Met-His-Val-Glu-Arg^{13}
                    CHO

bLHβ: Acyl-Ser-Arg-Gly-Pro-Leu-Arg-Pro-Leu-Cys-Gln-Pro-Ile-Asn-Ala-Thr-Leu-Ala-Ala-Gln-Lys^{20}

bTSHα: Glx-Gly-Cys-Pro-Gly-Cys-Lys-Leu-Lys-Glu-Asn-Lys-Tyr-Phe-Ser-Lys-Pro-Asx-Ala-Pro^{28}
                                CHO

bTSHβ: Lys-Glu-Cys-Ala-Tyr-Cys-   Leu-Thr-Ile-Asn^{23}
bLHβ: Glu-Ala-Cys-Pro-Val-Cys-   Ile-Thr-Phe-Thr^{30}

bTSHα: Ile-Tyr-Gln-Cys-Met-Gly-Cys-Cys-Phe-Ser-Arg-Ala-Tyr-Pro-Thr-Pro-Ala-Arg-Ser-Lys^{48}
bTSHβ: Thr-Thr-Val-Cys-Ala-Gly-Tyr-Cys-Met-Thr-Arg-Asx-Val-Asx-Gly-Lys-Lys-Leu-Phe-Leu-Pro^{43}
bLHβ: Thr-Ser-Ile-(Cys,Ala,Gly,Tyr)Cys-Pro-Ser-Met-Lys-Arg-Val-Leu-Pro-Val-(Ile,Leu,Pro)^{50}
                    CHO

bTSHα: Lys-Thr-Met-Leu-   Val-Pro-Lys-Asn-Ile-Thr-Ser-Glx-Ala-Thr-Cys-Cys-Val-Ala-Lys^{67}
bTSHβ: Lys-Tyr-Ala-Leu-Ser-Gln-Asp-Val-Cys-Thr-Tyr-Arg-Asp-Phe-Met-Tyr-Lys-Thr-Ala-Glu^{63}
bLHβ: Pro)Pro-Met-Pro-   Gln-Arg-Val-Cys-Thr-Tyr-His-Glu-Leu-Arg-Phe-Ala-Ser-Val-Arg^{69}

bTSHα: Ala-Phe-Thr-   Lys-Ala-Thr-Val-Met-Gly-Asn-Val-Arg-Val-Glx-Asn-His-Thr-Glx-Cys^{86}
bTSHβ: Ile-Pro-Gly-Cys-Pro-Arg-His-Val-Thr-Pro-Tyr-Phe-Ser-Tyr-Pro-Val-Ala-Ile-Ser-Cys^{83}
bLHβ Leu-Pro-Gly-(Cys,Pro,Gly,Val,Asp,Pro)Met-Val-Ser-Phe-Pro-Val-Ala-Leu-Ser-(Cys)^{89}
                    CHO

bTSHα: His-Cys-Ser-Thr-Cys-Tyr-Tyr-His-Lys-Ser-COOH^{96}
bTSHβ: Lys-Cys-Gly-Lys-Cys-Asx-Thr-Asx-Tyr-Ser-Asx-Cys-Ile-His-Glu-Ala-Ile-Lys-Thr-Asn^{103}
bLHβ: His,Cys,Gly,Pro,Cys)Arg-Leu-Ser-Ser-Thr-Asp-Cys-Gly-Pro-Gly-Arg-Thr-Glu-Pro-Leu^{109}

bTSHβ: Tyr-Cys-Thr-Lys-Pro-Gln-Lys-Ser-Tyr-Met-COOH^{113}
bLHβ: Ala-Cys-Asp-His-Pro-Pro-Leu-Pro-Asp-Ile-Leu-COOH^{120}

FIGURE 4.12. Alignment of amino acid chains of bovine TSHα, TSHβ, and LHβ to show maximum homology. In homologous regions the amino acids are underlined whether they are identical or differ by only a single mutation (substitution of a single nucleotide in the triplet codon for that amino acid). CHOs indicate the places where carbohydrate is linked to Asn. Regions in parentheses are not definitely sequenced but the probably homologous amino acids in those regions are indicated. [From J. G. Pierce, T. H. Lian, and R. B. Carlsen. *Hormonal Proteins* (C. H. Li, ed. Academic, New York, 1978.]

been established in crude pituitary preparations of all vertebrate groups, only a few mammalian TSHs have been isolated in quantities that permit determination of the linear sequences of their constituent amino acids.

As mentioned earlier in this chapter, all of the glycoprotein pituitary hormones are composed of an α subunit and a β subunit, each containing about 100 amino acid residues. The subunits are not covalently bound to each other but held in position by hydrogen bonding and van der Waals forces. Simply by placing the hormones in concentrated urea solution at acid pH, the subunits can be readily separated. The separate subunits themselves, if injected into a test animal, have virtually no action. In terms of amino acid sequence, the β subunit of TSH is more like the β subunit of LH than it is like the α subunit of TSH (Fig. 4.12). However, since there is at least some resemblance between the sequences of the α and β subunits they may have evolved from the same parent molecule early, and the separate evolution of different TSH, FSH, and LH β subunits may have occurred relatively more recently. We will return to this interesting question later in discussing the FSH and LH molecules.

TSHs of several nonmammalian vertebrates have been isolated, but not yet purified to an extent that would permit determination of the amino acid sequence. Thus TSHs of teleost fishes, frogs, and domestic fowl have been purified. They are glycoproteins composed of separable α and β subunits.

Functions of TSH

In contrast to the prolactin–growth hormone family of pituitary hormones, which have a broad spectrum of actions on a variety of responsive tissues, the actions of glycoprotein hormones appear to be restricted to single organs. For TSH these actions are upon the thyroid gland, although a few extra-thyroid actions of TSH have been claimed. The actions of TSH encompass a variety of phases of thyroid glandular function, from the stimulation of transport of iodide ions into the thyroid cells to oxidation of the iodide, organic combination of iodine with protein-bound tyrosine molecules, and release of the hormonal iodinated products to the vascular system. These actions will be discussed in greater detail in Chapter 6.

Another typical action of TSH is stimulation of hypertrophy (increase in size of cells) and hyperplasia (increase in numbers of cells) of thyroid follicles. Generally, these morphological thyroid responses to TSH go hand in hand with the metabolic actions upon iodine metabolism and thyroxinogenesis. However, the morphological and metabolic phenomena are separable. For example, when the diet contains little or no iodine, no thyroid hormone can be made. When circulating thyroid hormone levels are thus reduced, there is a lack of negative feedback on the brain–pituitary system, leading to an excessive secretion of pituitary TSH. This increased TSH cannot stimulate thyroxine formation, since iodine is lacking. However, the high level of TSH will in this case stimulate hypertrophy and hyperplasia of thyroid tissue.

An interesting phenomenon was discovered by Y. A. Fontaine in experiments in which glycoprotein hormones were exchanged between fishes and mammals. When mammalian TSH, FSH, or LH were injected into fishes, all were thyrotropic, stimulating thyroxine release by the fish thyroid. It would appear that the fish thyroid "TSH receptor" cannot distinguish between them, and responds to all. This "heterothyrotropic" response by fish thyroid is evoked also by human and equine chorionic gonadotropin (in the killifish, *Fundulus*). Similarly, Licht and Papkoff, who have isolated bullfrog TSH, FSH, and LH, find that the frog thyroid responds only to its own TSH. However, when frog hormones were tested for action upon reptilian thyroid glands (turtle, lizard), frog LH was more thyrotropic than frog TSH! Thus it is quite clear that there has been considerable evolutionary change in the α and β subunits of TSH and the gonadotropins. However, the receptors for these hormones have been evolving too, and Licht and Papkoff's experiments indicate that one cannot predict whether the glycoprotein hormone *receptors* will "see" a given glycoprotein hormone from an alien species as a thyrotropin or as a gonadotropin.

Regulation of TSH Secretion

The level of TSH secretion can be affected via either or both of two mechanisms (Fig. 4.13): (1) a neurogenic release of TRH (thyrotropin-releasing hormone) into the portal vessels of the median eminence or (2) feedback response to the circulating level of thyroid hormone. An example of the first type of control is the response in mammals to the lowering of body temperature. This is followed promptly by the release of TRH, then TSH, followed by release of thyroid hormone. The thyroid hormone, by affecting certain metabolic processes, leads to thermogenesis and adjustment of body temperature. In cold-blooded animals there has been little study of TSH levels in experimentally or naturally cooled animals. However, what has been done in fishes and amphibia tends to indicate that lowered body temperature lowers thyroid activity. In hibernating mammals, in which there is a depression of body temperature during the sleep phase, TSH and T_3-T_4 levels are not necessarily depressed, or may actually be increased. Thus the role of the brain-pituitary-thyroid axis in thermogenesis and in hibernation and reawakening is not fully explained.

An example of feedback regulation of thyroid hormone versus TSH levels in the blood has been given above with respect to hypothyroidism induced by diet (low iodine). Other methods of induction of hypothyroidism will evoke TSH secretion in this way. For example, antithyroid drugs (further discussed in Chapter 6) block the synthesis of thyroid hormone and evoke feedback release of TSH, with consequent thyroid enlargement. Hyperthyroidism (e.g., experimentally induced by injecting thyroxine), conversely,

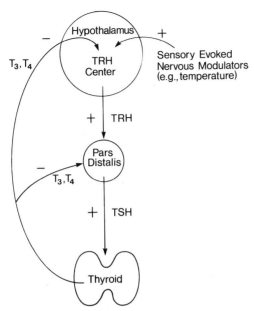

FIGURE 4.13. The sequence of stimulatory actions of TRH and TSH leads to increased secretion of thyroid hormones, T_3 and T_4. These exert a negative feedback action at two levels, the pars distalis and the hypothalamus.

leads to decreased levels of TSH in the blood. The site of feedback sensitivity to blood thyroid hormone levels is of interest. Although there may be some TRH changes in response to altered levels of plasma thyroid hormones, they do not explain the wide fluctuations in TSH secretion that accompany such plasma thyroid hormone changes. Thus, feedback sensitivity of TSH secretion is not located so much in the hypothalamus as in the pituitary itself (Fig. 4.13). One possible mechanism suggested in experimental observations is that thyroid hormones appear to inhibit the stimulatory action of TRH upon the pituitary TSH cell.

The two mechanisms of regulating TSH production by neurogenic (involving TRH) and feedback actions apparently operate simultaneously. If a lesion is made experimentally in the hypophysiotropic area of the hypothalamus of a mammal, circulating TSH levels and thyroid function are lowered. Thus, even if most thyroxine feedback sensitivity in mammals is at the pituitary level, a continuous connection between the pars distalis and the brain is still needed to keep plasma TSH and thyroxine levels up. A related phenomenon is seen in rats injected with large amounts of thyroxine at birth. Such rats, when adult, are permanently hypothyroid, their feedback "thyrostats" having been permanently altered. Whether this altered thyrostat (i.e., sensitivity and adjustment to circulating thyroid hormone levels) is located in the pars distalis or the hypothalamus, or both, is not known.

In fishes and most Amphibia, if the brain-pituitary connection is broken or if the pituitary is transplanted from its normal site, thyroid function may remain normal or may increase. Thus in these vertebrates it would seem that the normal relation of the brain to the secretion of TSH by the pars distalis is *inhibitory*. An exception to this generalization is the toad *Bufo bufo*, in which dissociation of the pituitary from the hypothalamus (e.g., by transplantation) leads to *decreased* thyroid activity. It is probably significant that in some fishes and Amphibia it has been claimed that TRH injections have no effect on thyrotropic function. Again, in the exceptional *Bufo bufo* TRH stimulates thyrotropic activity. In those species in which TRH has no apparent effect on thyrotropic function, it is interesting that the brain contains large amounts of TRH.

GONADOTROPIC HORMONES (LH AND FSH)

The molecules of the other glycoprotein hormones, FSH and LH, have α subunits that are virtually identical with those of TSH, and their β subunits share some primary amino acid sequences with each other and with TSHβ. Thus all have molecular weights in the neighborhood of 31,000. The fact that the three types of α subunits are almost but not absolutely identical has raised some questions as to whether there are separate genes for each of them. The possibility of post-translational modifications of the three α subunits has been raised. The fact that an excess of α subunits over β subunits is usually extractable from the pituitary suggests that they are separately synthesized and assembled within the cell, possibly in the Golgi apparatus. Assembly itself cannot be a simple process, since it may have to be preceded or followed by still other chemical processes. This is suggested by the finding of what appear to be prohormones: ''big FSH'' and ''big LH,'' molecules larger than the usual 31,000 daltons.

Another interesting problem is posed by β subunits that have *both* FSH and LH activities. In teleost pituitaries several laboratories have found only one gonadotropin, which is separable into α and β subunits, the β subunit having both gametogenic and steroidogenic (FSH-like and LH-like) functional properties. There is one claim, as yet unconfirmed, of two teleostean gonadotropins. The single gonadotropic molecule of fishes may be compared with the chorionic gonadotropin of horses (PMSG or eCG; pregnant mares' serum gonadotropin or equine chorionic gonadotropin). This hormone is separable into α and β subunits, the β subunit having both FSH-like and LH-like properties when tested in rats. The β subunit of PMSG has not yet been sequenced, but it should be interesting to compare it with known pituitary FSHβ and LHβ of horses and other species. Separate FSH and LH has been extracted and purified from bullfrog and bird (chicken and turkey) pituitaries. However, duck pituitaries yield only one gonadotropin; this has not yet been analyzed.

The presence of a single gonadotropin in several species of fish pituitaries supports the thesis of Y. A. Fontaine that evolution of separate FSH and LHβ subunits probably occurred in organisms between the fishes and tetrapods. This would have been accompanied by evolutionary differentiation of separate receptors for the two gonadotropins. The occurrence in tetrapods of occasional bipotential β subunits, such as those of PMSG and perhaps of duck gonadotropin, are possible examples of convergent evolution or of retention of a primitive property. There is evidence that there is only one gonadotropin in an elasmobranch fish, the dogfish. This is an obvious field for further research and exploration of gonadotropic function in lower vertebrate species.

Functions of Gonadotropins

Because reproduction takes so many adaptive patterns, it becomes difficult, if not inadvisable, to generalize concerning the roles of the gonadotropic hormones in it. Indeed, even designating *which* hormones are gonadotropic often is difficult. Fortunately, it appears that only the gonads contain receptors for the pituitary gonadotropins, and it is the distribution, relative quantities, and hormonal affinities of these receptors within the gonads that determine their gonadotropic functions.

In a general sense, the gonads perform two basic functions: production and release of gametes and production and secretion of sex steroids. Both functions are under gonadotropic control, gametogenesis being more generally identified with FSH and steroidogenesis with LH. Receptors for FSH in the mammalian testis are primarily in the seminiferous tubules and as radioautographic evidence indicates, mostly in the Sertoli cells. Testicular receptors for LH are principally in the interstitial (or Leydig) cells, which are the principal steroidogenic elements. Ovarian follicular and interstitial structure is more complex, and there is greater variability in the character of ovarian structures, depending upon the phase of the ovarian cycle. Correspondingly, there is a more complex and variable distribution of FSH and LH receptors, and there is evidence that some ovarian gonadotropin receptors are at least in part inducible by one or another of the sex steroids. It is thus more appropriate to consider these details in later chapters of this book where reproduction is considered in greater depth.

At this point we can identify the gonadal functions of FSH as largely gametogenic and those of LH as largely steroidogenic. However, there is major interaction between the two gonadotropins in both of these functions, and between the gonadotropins and sex steroids. For example, testosterone has a major role in spermatogenesis, and it is difficult to separate the direct action of FSH on spermatogenesis from that of testosterone, whose secretion is stimulated by FSH, LH, or both gonadotropins. An important part of oogenesis in many species is the filling of the egg with yolk. In this complex function there is recruitment of the liver to synthesize yolk protein, which is secreted into the blood and finally accumulated by the egg. Yolk synthesis by the liver is evoked principally by estrogenic hormone, the secretion of which is regulated by the gonadotropins. The uptake of yolk by the egg from the blood and the nuclear maturation of the ovum itself are under FSH and LH control, but the precise roles of the pituitary gonadotropins in these events are not completely worked out and may vary considerably in different species. Ovulation, or release of ova from the ovary, seems to be principally under LH control in mammals, but the role of steroids (e.g., progesterone, corticosteroid) in this event is important, and possibly essential in lower vertebrates (teleosts, Amphibia). However, these steroids, too, are secreted under gonadotropic regulation, and in some mammals prolactin may supplement the usual gonadotropins in such regulation. In male mammals final maturation of spermatozoa in testicular and epididymal ducts is at least partly dependent on the presence of testosterone, the level of which, in turn, is regulated by LH.

Control of Gonadotropin Secretion

Control of gonadotropin secretion by the brain appears to be more complex than for any other hormones of the pars distalis. This is because secretion of the two hormones must be related to external events (season, time of day, temperature, presence of a mate, presence of dependent offspring, etc.) and to the stage of the life cycle (puberty, senescence) as well as to the progression of the successive phases of the reproductive cycle itself, mentioned above.

The gonadotropins are released from the pars distalis in response to a decapeptide hypothalamic gonadotropin releaser (LHRH, GnRH). Most of the complexity of the programming of LHRH secretion is in the nervous organization that impinges on the LHRH-secreting cells in the hypothalamus. These nervous structures integrate the activity of the LHRH cells with external influences, phase of the life cycle, and even with feedback sensitivity to circulating levels of steroid hormones. What is remarkable is that only one gonadotropin releasing hormone has been found, despite past and continuing searching for other releasing hormones that might explain how the separate release of FSH or LH can be accomplished. At this time, the only viable explanations of the separate release of *one* gonadotropin (FSH or LH) by a releasing hormone capable of releasing both are based on the modifying actions of a variety of other substances at the level of the pituitary gland. Thus various sex steroids have been found to modify the action of LHRH on FSH and LH secretion. The same has been claimed for prostaglandins, some neurotransmitters, and other, less well defined agents. Unfortunately, none of these has yet been fitted into an acceptable scheme to explain the alternation of gonadotropins in the female rodent cycle, the preovulatory LH surge, or other types of natural cycles in gonadotropin release.

ADRENOCORTICOTROPIC HORMONE (ACTH) AND RELATED
BIOLOGICALLY ACTIVE SUBSTANCES

ACTH, as the smallest of the hormones of the pars distalis, has had the largest amount of attention by peptide chemists. Since it is composed of only 39 amino acids (molecular weight 4500) in linear sequence, it has not only been isolated from pituitaries of various species (Fig. 4.14) but has also been sequenced, synthesized artificially, and analogue variants of the hormone have been synthesized as well. The sequencing of ACTH revealed that the first 13 amino acids of its sequence comprise αMSH, a hormone that affects pigment cells and causes darkening of the skin in lower vertebrates. Artificially synthesized molecules consisting of amino acids 1 to 24 have the full activity of $ACTH_{1-39}$. As Fig. 4.14 suggests, the first 24 amino acids of the ACTH sequence are common to a number of mammals, as are the final eight amino acids. The molecular variations in ACTH in mammals are limited to amino acids 25 to 33. Human ACTH is identical to bovine ACTH. Dogfish ACTH was sequenced and synthesized recently, and it is interesting that its 39–amino acid sequence contains substitutions at positions 13, 15, and 20, that is, within the so-called conservative or heretofore invariable part of the molecule. It is curious that natural dogfish ACTH has been found to be only 15% as effective in the dogfish as is human ACTH. Similarly, synthetic dogfish ACTH has about one-fifth the activity of human synthetic ACTH when tested in the dogfish. Obviously, more study is needed before the relationship between the evolution of molecular structures of vertebrate ACTHs can be understood in terms of their biological actions.

In 1964 a larger peptide with some ACTH-like action, β-lipotropic hormone (βLPH), was isolated from sheep pituitaries in the laboratory of C. H. Li. Its name derives from the fact that, like ACTH, it can stimulate mobilization of fat from adipose tissue. This substance was called a hormone even before it was known whether it is normally secreted as such. Parenthetically, we may say that βLPH was later found (by RIA) in the circulating blood of sheep at a concentration of 10 ng/ml. The same assay shows *no* circulating βLPH in human blood. Thus, this question remains unsettled.

βLPHs of several mammalian species were promptly sequenced by Li and colleagues in 1965 and 1966, and all proved to be peptides composed of 91 amino acid residues, (molecular weight 11,700) (Fig. 4.1). Amino acids 41 to 58, a 19-residue segment, form the middle portion of the βLPH molecule and are identical with βMSH. This strongly suggested that the βLPH molecule is a precursor or prohormone for βMSH. No function at first could be ascribed to the remaining C-terminal portion of βLPH. However, in 1975 the opiate met-enkephalin was isolated from the brain and found, when sequenced, to be identical with a five–amino acid segment (residues 61 to 65) of βLPH. This led, the following year, to the identification of the C-terminal, 30-residue portion of βLPH (residues 61 to 91) as β-endorphin, a

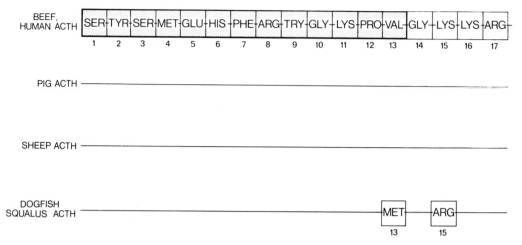

FIGURE 4.14. Amino acid sequences of ACTH molecules of several vertebrate species. The sequence 1–13 comprises the hormone αMSH, identical in many vertebrates, but differing at sequence 13 from the dogfish. Only the human and beef ACTH sequence is shown in full.

powerful opiate, or analgesic substance. Enkephalin and endorphin were found to compete with morphine and other addictive substances for receptor binding in certain parts of the brain. More recently, it was found that ACTH and βLPH are both constituents of a larger peptide, pro-opiocortin. Thus, the pro-opiocortin molecule became a strange assembly of peptides: one that stimulates the adrenal cortex, two that regulate pigment cell function, and one (or more) that has powerful analgesic actions in the brain. As might be expected, this has become an intriguing and active area for research. One of the interesting products of this research is the recent cloning of DNA coding for a major fragment of mouse βLPH from recombinant DNA in a bacterial culture (*E. coli*). The bacterial product of this cloning is a peptide equivalent to residues 44 to 90 of βLPH, comprising most of the βMSH molecule and all but the C-terminal amino acid of β-endorphin.

Pro-opiocortin reacts with antibodies to ACTH and βLPH. Hydrolysis of this larger molecule yields ACTH, MSH, and βLPH. Accordingly, this substance must be considered the prohormone for the entire ACTH family of peptides, including βLPH. Peptides with the immunological properties of βMSH and a portion of the βLPH sequence have been extracted from elasmobranch (dogfish) and teleost pituitaries, in addition to the dogfish ACTH mentioned above. Finally β-endorphin activity has been extracted from both the pars distalis and the pars intermedia (neurointermediate lobe) of trout. Thus βLPH, and possible pro-opiocortin, may be found even in the pituitaries of the more primitive vertebrates. This presents an opportunity to study the evolution of the opiocortin molecule and its complex of functions.

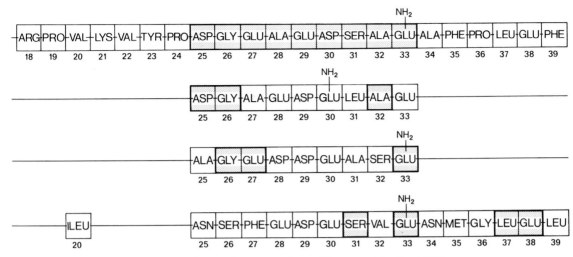

Where the sequences of the other species are the same as those of human and bovine ACTH, a straight line is drawn or the squares are distinctively shaded. [After C. H. Li, *Scientific American*, July, 1963.]

Since ACTH secretion characteristically is a function of the ACTH cells of the pars distalis, while the secretion of MSH is typical of the parenchymal cells of the pars intermedia, and both cell types contain βLPH, how can they be separately secreted? $ACTH_{1-39}$, MSH, as well as βLPH can be extracted both from the pars distalis and from the pars intermedia. Rat pars intermedia cells in tissue culture will release ACTH-like material in response to secretory stimulation, but this is in the form of a molecule larger than $ACTH_{1-39}$, possibly opiocortin. In rats subjected to experimental stress, β-endorphin and ACTH are secreted into the blood in about equal amounts during the same time interval after stress. None of these studies yet settles the question of whether specific enzymes in the pars intermedia and pars distalis can selectively release, or selectively destroy, particular fragments of the opiocortin molecule or whether release of intact βLPH is a normal physiological event.

ADDITIONAL READING

1. Acher, R. (1980). Molecular evolution of biologically active peptides. *Proc. R. Soc. London* **B210:**21–43.

2. Ball, J. N. (1981). Hypothalamic control of the pars distalis in fishes, amphibians and reptiles. *Gen. Comp. Endocrinol.* **44:**135–170.

3. Ball, J. N., T. F. C. Batten, and G. Young (1980). Evolution of hypothalamo-adenohypophysial systems in lower vertebrates. In *Hormones, Adaptation and Evolution* (S. Ishii, T. Hirano, and M. Wada, eds.). Springer-Verlag, Berlin, pp. 45–56.

4. Barraclough, B. A. (1980). Sex differentiation of cyclic gonadotropin secretion. In *Development of Responsiveness to Steroid Hormones* (A. M. Kaye and M. Kaye, eds.) Pergamon, Elmford, New York.

5. Bern, H. A. and C. S. Nicoll (1968). The comparative endocrinology of prolactin. *Recent Prog. Horm. Res.* **24**:681–696.

6. Chan, V., R. N. Clayton, G. Knox, and K. J. Catt (1981). Ontogeny of pituitary GnRH receptors in the rat. *Endocrinology* **108**:2086–2092.

7. Childs, G. V., and D. G. Ellison (1980). A critique of the contributions of immunoperoxidase cytochemistry to our understanding of pituitary cell function as illustrated by our current studies of gonadotropes, corticotropes, and endogenous pituitary GnRH and TRH. *Histochem. J.* **12**:405–418.

8. Clemens, J. A., C. J. Schaar, and E. B. Smalstig (1980). Dopamine, PIF and other regulators of prolactin secretion. *Fed. Proc.* **39**:2907–2911.

9. Daughaday, W. H. (1979). Anterior pituitary. In *Contemporary Endocrinology* (S. H. Ingbar, ed.). Vol. 1 Plenum, New York, pp. 21–76.

10. Dodd, J. M. (1960). Gonadal and gonadotrophic hormones in lower vertebrates. In *Marshall's Physiology of Reproduction* (A. S. Parkes, ed.) Vol. 1. Little, Brown, Boston, pp. 417–582.

11. Fontaine, Y. (1980). Evolution of pituitary gonadotropins and thyrotropins. In *Hormones, Adaptation and Evolution* (S. Ishii, T. Hirano, and M. Wada, eds.). Springer-Verlag, Berlin, pp. 261–270.

12. Gorbman, A. (1965). Vascular relations between the neurohypophysis and adenohypophysis of cyclostomes and the problem of evolution of hypothalamic neuroendocrine control. *Arch. Anat. Microsc. Morphol. Exp.* **54**:163–194.

13. Greep, R. O. (1961). Physiology of the anterior hypophysis in relation to reproduction. In *Sex and Internal Secretions* (W. C. Young and G. W. Corner, eds.) Vol. 1. Williams & Wilkins, Baltimore, pp. 240–301.

14. Harris, G. W., and B. T. Donovan, eds. (1966). *The Pituitary Gland*, Vols. 1 and 2. University of California Press, Berkeley.

15. Hayashida, T., and M. D. Lagios (1969). Fish growth hormone: a biological, immunochemical and ultrastructural study of sturgeon and paddlefish pituitaries. *Gen. Comp. Endocrinol.* **13**:403–411.

16. Hayashida, T., S. W. Farmer, and H. Papkoff (1975). Pituitary growth hormones: further evidence for evolutionary conservation based on immunochemical studies. *Proc. Natl. Acad. Sci. USA* **72**:4322–4326.

17. Holmes, R. L., and J. N. Ball (1974). *The Pituitary Gland. A Comparative Account.* Cambridge University Press, London.

18. Honma, Y. (1969). Some evolutionary aspects of the morphology and role of the adenohypophysis in fishes. *Gunma Symp. Endocrinol.* **6**:19–37.

19. Imura, H., and Y. Nakai (1981). Endorphins in pituitary and other tissues. *Ann. Rev. Physiol.* **43**:265–278.

20. Justisz, M., A. Berault, L. Debeljuk, B. Kerdelhue, and M. Theoleyre (1979). Gonadoliberin. In *Hormonal Proteins and Peptides* (C. H. Li, ed.) Vol. 7. Academic, New York, pp. 56–122.

21. Kawamoto, M. (1967). Zur Morphologie der Hypophysis cerebri von Teleostiern. *Arch. Histol. Japonicum* **28**:123–150.

22. Knobil, E. (1980). The neuroendocrine control of the menstrual cycle. *Recent Prog. Horm. Res.* **36**:55–83.

23. Knobil, E. (1981). Patterns of hypophysiotropic signals and gonadotropin secretion in the rhesus monkey. *Biol. Reprod.* **24**:44–49.

24. Knowles, F., and L. Vollrath (1975). Cytology and neuroendocrine relations of the pituitary of the dogfish *Scyliorhinus canicula. Proc. R. Soc. London* **B191:**507–525.

25. Koide, S. S., T. Maruo, H. Cohen, and S. J. Segal (1980). Choriogonadotropin in evolution. In *Hormones, Adaptation and Evolution* (S. Ishii, T. Hirano, and M. Wada, eds.). Springer-Verlag, Berlin, pp. 253–260.

26. Lagios, M. D. (1975). The pituitary gland of the coelacanth *Latimeria chalumnae. Gen. Comp. Endocrinol.* **25:**126–146.

27. Licht, P. (1979). Reproductive endocrinology of reptiles and amphibians: gonadotropins. *Ann. Rev. Physiol.* **41:**337–351.

28. Pang, P. K. T., and A. Epple, eds. (1980). *Evolution of Vertebrate Endocrine Systems.* Texas Tech Press, Lubbock.

29. Papkoff, H. (1972). Subunit interrelationships among the pituitary glycoprotein hormones. *Gen. Comp. Endocrinol.* , Suppl. **3:**609–616.

30. Peter, R. E., and L. W. Crim (1979). Reproductive endocrinology of fishes: gonadal cycles and gonadotropins in teleosts. *Ann. Rev. Physiol.* **41:**323–335.

31. Pickford, G. E., and J. W. Atz (1957). *The Physiology of the Pituitary Gland of Fishes.* New York Zoological Society, New York.

32. Ramaley, J. A. (1979). Development of gonadotropin regulation in the prepubertal animal. *Biol. Reprod.* **20:**1–31.

33. Schreibman, M. P. (1980). Adenohypophysis: structure and function. In *Evolution of Vertebrate Endocrine Systems* (P. K. T. Pang and A. Epple, eds.). Texas Tech Press, Lubbock, pp. 107–131.

34. Smyth, D. G., and S. Zakarian (1980). Selective processing of β-endorphin in regions of porcine pituitary. *Nature* **288:**613–615.

35. Stacey, N. E., A. F. Cook, and R. E. Peter (1979). Ovulatory surge of gonadotropin in the goldfish, *Carassius auratus. Gen. Comp. Endocrinol.* **37:**246–249.

36. Stetson, M. H., and E. G. Grau (1980). Hypothalamo-adenohypophysial relationships among vertebrates. In *Evolution of Vertebrate Endocrine Systems* (P. K. T. Pang and A. Epple, eds.). Texas Tech Press, Lubbock, pp. 59–84.

37. Sumpter, J. P., B. K. Follett, and J. M. Dodd (1978a). Studies on the purification and properties of gonadotrophin from ventral lobes of the pituitary gland of the dogfish (*Scyliorhinus canicula* L.). *Gen. Comp. Endocrinol.* **36:**264–274.

38. Sumpter, J. P., N. Jenkins, and J. M. Dodd (1978b). Gonadotrophic hormone in the pituitary gland of the dogfish (*Scyliorhinus canicula* L.): distribution and physiological significance. *Gen. Comp. Endocrinol.* **36:**275–285.

39. Tsuneki, K., and A. Gorbman (1975). Ultrastructure of the anterior neurohypophysis and the pars distalis of the lamprey *Lampetra tridentata. Gen. Comp. Endocrinol.* **25:**487–508.

40. Wallis, M. (1975). The molecular evolution of pituitary hormones. *Biol. Rev.* **50:**35–98.

41. Wallis, M. (1978). The chemistry of pituitary growth hormone, prolactin and related hormones and its relationship to biological activity. In *Chemistry and Biochemistry of Amino Acids, Peptides and Proteins* (B. Weinstein, ed.). Dekker, New York.

5

The Pars Intermedia and Pigmentary Control

In contrast to the higher vertebrates, a fairly constant morphological feature of the pituitary of poikilotherms is a prominent pars intermedia. A pars intermedia is totally lacking in birds and some adult mammals. The widespread occurrence of functional chromatophores (i.e., those capable of creating reversible color changes) in the skin of poikilotherms roughly parallels this phyletic distribution in pituitary morphology, and hormonal control of pigmentary function is a well-recognized role of the pars intermedia in lower vertebrates. This suggests that birds and mammals might have eliminated or reduced melanophore-stimulating hormone (MSH) formation, together with the loss of functional chromatophores. On the contrary, MSH is clearly present in the adenohypophysis of birds and mammals. As we shall discuss later, there is considerable current interest in the extrapigmentary effects of MSH in higher vertebrates. For now we will concentrate on the pigmentary effects of the hormone in poikilotherms.

Animal color changes, when we consider them as adjustments to the changing environment, are unique. The purpose of most adjustments to the environment is to achieve a more efficient physiological or reproductive state within the ranges of variation of temperature, light, water, or food encountered by the organism. The purpose of skin-color changes is almost always a ''social'' one: the concealment of an animal within his normal background from other animals, or the signaling to another individual of a state of sexual readiness. It is possible, as some authors have suggested, that coloration may be involved in body-temperature regulation, since dark surfaces absorb and light surfaces reflect heat. If so, this cannot be a common use of integumentary pigmentation, but analysis of this problem is too far from our aim in this chapter.

The controlling mechanisms for color changes may be genetic, involving mutation and selection over generations; they may be endocrine, involving periods of time from minutes to as long as part of a life cycle; they may be nervous or combinations of nervous and endocrine, involving the shortest time intervals. In some instances (e.g., with the tadpole's tail), it is clear that chromatophores are capable of responding directly to light stimuli, with no nervous or endocrine intervention.

The subject is clearly a large one, and it is limited here to consideration of the blood-borne factors, principally MSH, that regulate the color adaptations to the environment. The usual objects of action of MSH are chromatophores in the skin. Chromatophores are also found on blood vessels, on membranes of the nervous system, or in the peritoneum; however, these are usually unresponsive to MSH. MSH's action on chromatophores can be classified into two types of skin darkening: one type, known as the "morphological color change," occurs over a period of weeks and refers to an increase in the population of skin melanophores; it may be accompanied by an increase in the amount of pigment in skin cells. The other type is the rapid "physiological color change" due to the redistribution of pigment granules within the cell (Fig. 5.1).

A common and most extensively studied chromatophore is the melanophore that carries the black, melanin-containing pigment granules (melanosomes). In the absence of MSH, pigment granules become concentrated in the center of the cell. When blood levels of MSH are elevated, the melanophores respond by dispersing melanin granules throughout their periphery to impart a dark coloration to the skin. While MSH action on melanophores produces the most dramatic effect on overall skin coloration, other chromatophores, which contain red, yellow, orange, or reflecting pigments, may also be affected. Cells carrying yellow or red pigments are

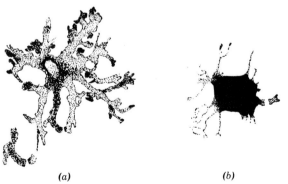

(a)   (b)

FIGURE 5.1. Two melanophores of the frog *Rana temporaria*: (*a*) with melanin granules dispersed throughout the cell; (*b*) with melanin granules concentrated in the center of the cell, the pigment-free cytoplasmic arms still barely visible. [After H. R. Hewer, *Proc. R. Soc. London*, **95**:31, 1923.]

xanthophores and erythrophores, respectively; since their pigments are fat-soluble compounds such as carotenoids, these cells are also known as "lipophores." Iridophores (also called guanophores or leucophores) contain purines such as guanine and hypoxanthine, which are organized into highly reflective crystals or platelets. These cells impart a white or glistening quality to the skin. The size and orientation of the reflecting plates within the cells determine, in part, the amount of light reflected by the skin.

PHYSIOLOGICAL COLOR CHANGE

Normally, when a cold-blooded vertebrate is placed on a dark or light background with overhead illumination, its skin color changes within a period of minutes to days, so that the organism better matches its background. In frogs and many other species the hormonal dependence of this rapid color change can be easily shown *in vitro*. When frog skin is removed from the animal and placed with its serosal (inside) surface in contact with a physiological salt solution, the melanin granules in melanophores are drawn toward the nucleus and form a small punctate mass (Fig. 5.2). When MSH or pituitary suspensions are added to the solution, the melanin granules are dispersed in the cytoplasm. Maximal dispersal of granules in *Rana pipiens* skin occurs after about one hour of exposure to MSH. The darkening of the skin associated with melanin dispersal can be measured by shining light through the skin or reflecting light off the skin and derermining the change in the amount of light absorbed (Fig. 5.3). When the salt solution containing MSH is exchanged for fresh solution with no hormone, the melanophores return to the punctate form, and light absorbance by the skin decreases within an hour or two. The kinetics of the melanophore response to MSH *in vitro* approximate those observed in the normal background adaptation of the animal.   Considering the morphological distribution and hormone responses of the pigment cells in various layers of anuran amphibian skin, Bagnara and colleagues have explained how color change is accomplished through the integrated function of dermal chromatophores. Frog skin chromatophores are organized into "dermal chromatophore units," which consist of xanthophores stacked on top of iridophores that lie above large melanophores (Fig. 5.4). The melanophores have dendritic processes that extend around and over the surface of the iridophores but below the xanthophores. In other words, in this configuration the melanophore is like an extensive basket that contains several iridophores; the xanthophores are sitting on top of the basket. When circulating levels of MSH are high, melanin granules are dispersed throughout the melanophore extensions, covering the surface of the iridophores (Fig. 5.4b). This blocks reflected light from the iridophores, and the skin appears dark. In the absence of MSH, melanin granules leave the dendritic extensions and become concentrated near the melanophore nucleus under the iridophore layer (Fig. 5.4a). Light coming

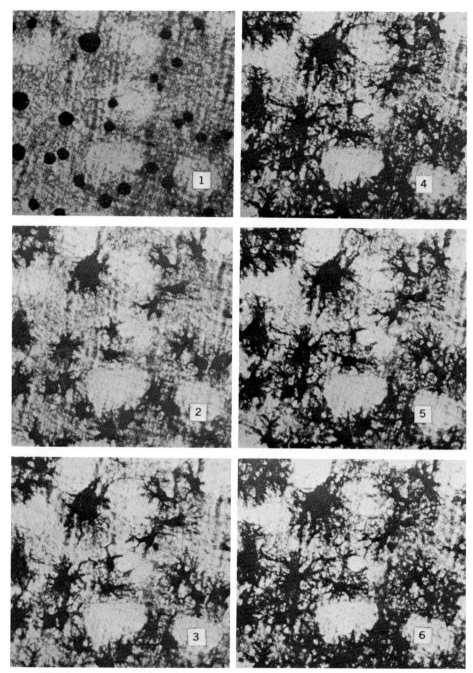

FIGURE 5.2. Successive photographs (at 15-minute intervals) of the same group of melan-ophores ($\times$ 210) in a piece of frog skin (*Rana pipiens*) in Ringer's solution. A suspension of homogenized frog pituitary (containing MSH) was added to the solution immediately after photograph 1 was taken. [From P. A. Wright, *J. Cell Comp. Physiol.*, **31**:111, 1948.]

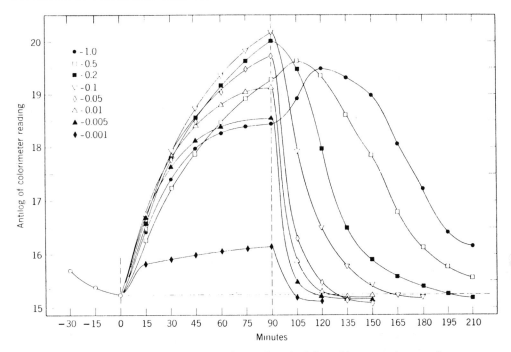

FIGURE 5.3. Plot of the color changes in pieces of excised frog skin exposed to varying concentrations of pituitary gland suspensions. Results of experiments in which pieces of excised frog skin mounted in Bakelite frames were exposed for 90 minutes to pituitary suspensions ranging in concentration from 1/1000 to 1 pituitary gland in 50 ml Ringer's solution. Dispersion and concentration of melanophore pigment were followed by the use of a photoelectric colorimeter, and the readings were converted to antilogarithms and averaged. The curve between −30 and 0 minutes represents average readings up to the time of exposure to pituitary suspensions. After 90 minutes of contact with pituitary suspensions, the skins were placed in Ringer's solution, which was changed every 30 minutes until the end of the experiment. Compare with photographs in Fig. 5.2. [From P. A. Wright, *J. Cell Comp. Physiol.*, **31**:111, 1948.]

through the upper surface of the skin is reflected off the iridophore platelets and through the xanthophores. Because light scatters as it passes through the epidermis, reflected light is blue as it leaves the iridophores, but it is filtered through the yellow pigment cells, so that only the green wavelengths emerge from the skin. In addition to dispersing pigments in melanophores, MSH induces a contraction of iridophores, although this effect on iridophores is better demonstrated by morphological color change in larval amphibians. It is interesting that the two different chromatophores in anuran skin react in opposite fashion to the same hormone to result in the coordinated darkening response.

It should be emphasized that this model of the dermal chromatophore unit is based on studies of several anuran amphibian species. Other poikilotherms have different chromatophore morphologies and hormone re-

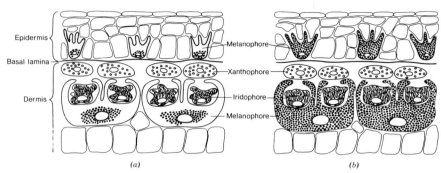

FIGURE 5.4. Diagrammatic representation of the organization of pigment cells into "dermal chromatophore units" in amphibian skin. Small melanophores are located in the epidermis while in the dermis there are large, basket-like melanophores with processes extending over iridophores. Xanthophores which contain yellow pigment granules are situated in the dermis just below the basal lamina. (*a*) In the absence of MSH, melanin granules are concentrated around the nucleus of the melanophores, and the iridophores are expanded. (*b*) In the presence of MSH, melanin granules are dispersed throughout the melanophore, and the iridophores are contracted. [After J. T. Bagnara, M. E. Hadley, and J. D. Taylor, *Gen. Comp. Endocrinol.*, Suppl. 2, 1969.]

sponses. Although in most anurans studied only the melanophores and iridophores respond to MSH, the hormone promotes expansion of xanthophores in the tree frog *Hyla arenicolor*. MSH has been shown to stimulate erythrophore dispersion in the minnow *Phoxinus phoxinus*. In some other bony fish species, the melanophores are unresponsive to MSH; color change is regulated by direct innervation of chromatophores rather than by a humoral mechanism. Direct neural control of pigmentation allows some fishes the advantage of rapid control of complex skin-color patterns. Control of color change has been studied in too few representative species to make any firm generalizations. However, based on what is known, we may conclude, tentatively, that MSH regulation of melanophore dispersion determines the physiological color change of most species of amphibians, reptiles, and elasmobranchs. The situation in teleosts shows a diversity of endocrine and direct neural control of chromatophores. Such diversity of pigmentary control in teleosts and some species of other classes illustrates an important point. The morphology of skin chromatophores and their particular responses to hormonal or neural factors are probably best adapted to fit the color change needs of the animal in its specific environment.

MORPHOLOGICAL COLOR CHANGE

The phenomenon of morphological color change differs from the physiological one in several aspects: (1) morphological change occurs over periods of weeks to months and is often associated with seasonal cycles; (2) physiological changes occur only in poikilotherms, whereas morphological changes have been observed in species from all vertebrate classes; and (3) morphological change involves primarily melanophores (or melanocytes) in the epidermal layer of skin rather than the dermal layer.

When some cold-blooded animals are maintained on illuminated black backgrounds for periods of a month or more, the melanin content of the skin is increased either because of greater melanin production or increased number of melanophores, or both. Much of the increased melanin production is due to heightened activity of some epidermal melanocytes, which may deposit melanosomes into extracellular spaces or, alternatively, donate their melanosomes to adjacent epidermal cells. Those epidermal cells that take up melanosomes do not have dendritic processes nor do they synthesize melanin as do melanophores. In some poikilotherms MSH stimulates the synthesis and, possibly, release of melanosomes by epidermal melanocytes. After the melanosomes are phagocytized by epidermal cells, they are retained dispersed throughout the cell cytoplasm and contribute to the permanent overall darkness of the skin. Thus melanosomes in epidermal cells cannot participate in rapid physiological color change. Although in some cases epidermal melanocytes may disperse their melanosomes throughout their cytoplasm in response to MSH, they have a minor effect on rapid color change, since epidermal melanocytes are generally smaller and thinner than dermal melanophores.

Homoiothermic vertebrates (birds and mammals) do not have functional dermal chromatophores; but they have epidermal melanocytes that are homologous to those of poikilotherms. In mammals there is a recognized "epidermal melanin unit" which consists of a melanocyte and several dozen adjacent epidermal cells (keratinocytes) that take up melanin granules (Fig. 5.5). Keratinocytes that take up melanosomes impart a dark coloration to the skin. Epidermal melanocytes produce larger melanosomes in the skin of Negroids and Australoids compared to Caucasoids and Mongoloids. Injection of MSH into humans produces a darkening response, which is due to dispersion of granules in melanocytes and increased production and transfer of melanin to keratinocytes. The physiological significance of this MSH effect in humans is doubtful, since skin pigmentation is predominantly controlled by genetic factors. However, this suggests that melanocytes have MSH receptors in humans. Melanization of skin after exposure to solar radiation (tanning) appears to be a direct effect of ultraviolet rays on the epidermal melanin unit. This occurs without MSH mediation. Epidermal melanocytes also contribute melanin granules to hair and feathers. MSH injections have been shown to promote melanization of growing hair in mice, guinea pigs, and the short-tailed weasel and of certain feathers in chickens. Again, the significance of these hormonal effects is tenuous in the face of genetic control of hair or feather color. One area that deserves further study is the possible hormonal control of seasonal morphological color change in some mammals, the short-tailed weasel in particular. In the winter this

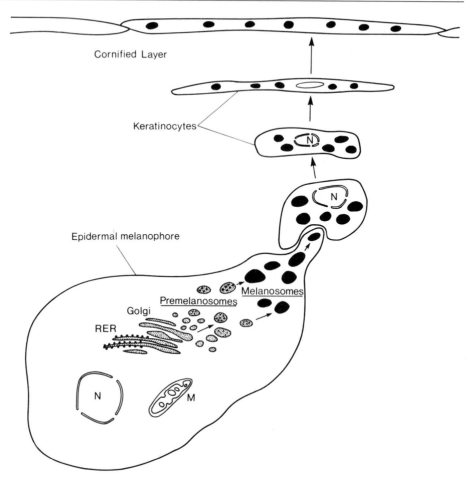

Cornified Layer

Keratinocytes

Epidermal melanophore

Melanosomes

Premelanosomes

Golgi

RER

N

M

FIGURE 5.5. Diagrammatic representation of an epidermal melanophore (melanocyte) and keratinocytes in the human epidermis. The melanocyte synthesizes melanin, which is packaged into premelanosomes. Premelanosomes become melanosomes after melanin synthesis is completed within the pigment vesicle. Melanosomes located in the processes of the melanocyte can be phagocytised by a keratinocyte. The keratinocyte is moved to the external, cornified layers of epidermis. Melanosomes in the keratinocyte impart a dark coloration to the skin. Epidermal melanocytes in other mammals or birds may donate their melanosomes to growing hair or feathers. [After W. C. Quevedo, *Am. Zool.*, **12**:35, 1972.]

weasel has a white coat, which conceals the animal against the background of snow. Accompanying the springtime melting of the snows, the weasel's coat turns brown to maintain a concealing coloration. Measurement of blood levels of MSH, and perhaps of MSH receptors on hair follicles, during the seasons might indicate the significance of the observed MSH effect. Seasonal changes in melanization of birds' feathers appear to be controlled variously by gonadal, thyroidal, and gonadotropic hormones.

HORMONAL CONTROL OF COLOR CHANGE

The first suggestion of an endocrine basis for control of vertebrate chromatophores appeared in the experiments of B. M. Allen and P. E. Smith (ca. 1914 to 1916), who found that hypophysectomized tadpoles developed with practically no melanophores but large silvery guanophores (Fig. 5.6).

Atwell, in 1919, showed that pituitary extracts darkened the hypophysectomized amphibian larva, and Swingle, in 1920, implanted different lobes of pituitary tissue into hypophysectomized tadpoles and observed that the pigmentary response was identifiable with the pars intermedia. In the 1920s, Hogben and his collaborators firmly established the pars intermedia as the source of MSH, developed the use of the frog for bioassay, and investigated in detail the reactions of chromatophores to MSH in various fishes, amphibians, and reptiles.

During the early studies on pituitary control of chromatophores, several investigators had claimed the existence of a hormone that acted in a fashion opposite to that of MSH and caused skin lightening. This factor (melanin-concentrating hormone, MCH) was originally postulated by Hogben and Slome in 1931. After many decades of attempts at isolating MCH and much

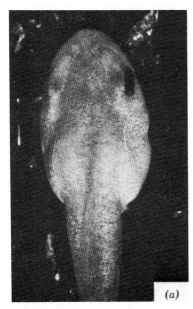 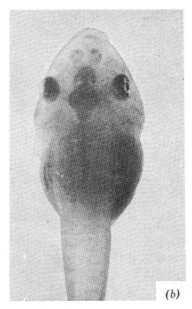

FIGURE 5.6. (*a*) Tadpole of *Rana sylvatica* hypophysectomized as an early tailbud embryo. The silvery sheen is due to the absence of melanophores and the multiplication of iridophores, which appear as a solid sheet. (*b*) The same tadpole 2 weeks after injection of 10 μg of bovine MSH. The principal change is the reduction of iridophores, revealing the brain case, eyes, olfactory organs, etc. There are still relatively few melanophores, barely visible in the tail. [From J. T. Bagnara, *J. Exp. Zool.*, **137**:265, 1958.]

discussion about its existence, it became generally accepted that such a hormonal factor is not present in the vertebrate pituitary. Since catecholamines, or serotonin and melatonin (in some species), are potent melanophore-concentrating agents, as is stimulation of adrenergic nerves, any skin-lightening activity of tissue extracts is usually suspected to be working through these agents rather than through true pituitary MCH. On the other hand, Novales and Novales have recently shown that pituitary endorphins may exert a pharmacological antagonism on MSH action. Moreover, Rance and Baker have recently isolated melanophore-concentrating activity from pituitaries of five species of bony fishes, while eliminating possible pharmacological action of several suspected agents. Westerfield, Pang, and Burns have shown that the teleost MCH activity of the pituitary appears to be due to a small peptide. Thus it is quite possible that MCH exists, at least in the teleost pituitary. The situation in teleosts is even more complicated considering the recent evidence of Ball and Batten. These investigators have shown in the sailfin molly that adaptation to a black background activates a cell type of the pars intermedia that is not an MSH cell. This suggests that dark background adaptation in some bony fishes is controlled by a pars intermedia hormone that is not MSH.

The morphological and biochemical changes in the pars intermedia of frogs during background adaptation have received much attention. The ultrastructure of MSH cells in frogs transferred from a light to a dark background shows an increase in the amount of rough endoplasmic reticulum (RER), a dilatation of RER cisternae, a greater development of Golgi elements, and a decrease in the number of secretory granules. Transfer of frogs back to a light background reverses these changes. Immunocytochemical studies have shown that the secretory granules react to αMSH and βMSH antisera. All of the morphological changes are indicative of activated synthesis and secretion of MSH in dark background adapted frogs. Wilson and Morgan have compared the pituitary and plasma concentrations of αMSH in the African clawed toad, *Xenopus laevis*, adapted to backgrounds of different color for one week (Table 5.1). The black background adapted animals had plasma αMSH concentrations 200 times greater and had about one-sixth as much αMSH in their pituitary compared with those adapted to a white background. In the dark background adapted animals the corresponding changes in αMSH levels indicate a greater rate of MSH secretion associated with depletion of the pars intermedia stores of hormone, which agrees with the observed decrease in the number of intracellular secretory granules. Furthermore, MSH is removed from the circulation of black background adapted frogs at a high rate (Table 5.1). Therefore, the pituitary must respond by greatly increasing its rate of synthesis of MSH to maintain a high concentration of hormone in its blood. It is not certain why the clearance of MSH is increased at a time when it should be maintained in the blood at a high level.

In the blinded animal the background adjustments of melanophores are

TABLE 5.1. The kinetics of αMSH in the adult African clawed toad (*Xenopus laevis*) adapted to illuminated backgrounds of different colors for one week[a]

	Background		
)	White	Gray	Black
Total pituitary αMSH content			
(ng)	73	68	11
Plasma concentration (pg/ml)	22	62	407
Clearance (ng/day)	1.6	4.5	29
Rate of turnover of pituitary			
content (days)	46	15	0.4

[a] From J. F. Wilson and M. A. Morgan, *Gen. Comp. Endocrinol.* **38:**172 (1979).

either greatly reduced or eliminated completely. Thus the lateral eyes appear to be important receptors of photic information for background adaptation. In animals that have hormonal control of chromatophores, photic information is passed along through neural pathways to the hypothalamus, which tonically inhibits MSH secretion. The exact mechanism by which the retina discriminates differences in background color is not known. However, a widely accepted theory is based on the differential illumination of the upper and lower portions of the retina. It is believed that when an animal is on a white background with overhead illumination, both the lower and upper parts of the retina are illuminated by direct and reflected light, respectively. This full illumination of the retina is translated into neural impulses, which are sent via the hypothalamus to block MSH secretion. In black background adapted animals the amount of light reflected from the background is diminished, so that the lower portion of the retina receives a proportionately greater amount of photic stimulation from direct overhead light. With the reduced stimulation of the upper part of the retina, neural impulses are sent to the hypothalamus, ultimately resulting in release of tonic inhibition of the pars intermedia and MSH secretion.

It might seem that this theory could easily be tested by recording from nerves in the pars intermedia of frogs on different backgrounds. However, both morphological and electrophysiological studies have shown that neural control of MSH cells is a complex matter. Electron microscopic studies show that, depending upon the species, there are at least two, and sometimes three, types of neuronal endings that may synapse with secretory cells in the pars intermedia. One type of nerve ending contains small, clear vesicles that are believed to be cholinergic. Another type, containing larger vesicles with electron-dense cores, is thought to be adrenergic. The third class of nerve ending contains the largest vesicles, which are characteristic of neurosecretory neurons. These neurosecretory endings are localized in the pars intermedia near its border with the pars nervosa, and they do not form synapses with MSH cells. Nonetheless, neurosecretions from these endings may reach the MSH cells by diffusion.

The varied relationships between nerve endings and MSH cells suggest that MSH release is controlled by several factors. This possibility has been supported by studies of the effects of neurotransmitters and peptides on MSH secretion. As we mentioned, the hypothalamus tonically inhibits MSH release. When the pars intermedia is transplanted into a frog at some site distant from the hypothalamus, the animal becomes dark. Also, if the pars intermedia is cultured *in vitro*, MSH will be secreted autonomously for weeks or months. The bulk of evidence shows that tonic inhibition of release is maintained by catecholamines—norepinephrine or dopamine in particular. Other neurotransmitters may stimulate MSH release. MSH secretion is induced by acetylcholine in frogs and mice, but not in rats. This cholinergic stimulation of MSH release may be due to direct action on the cells or indirectly through inhibition of catecholaminergic endings in the pars intermedia. It has also been shown that serotonin may stimulate MSH release in some species. Celis, Taleisnik, and colleagues have added to the list of factors controlling MSH with evidence that hypothalamic peptides are involved. The tripeptide Pro-Leu-Gly·NH$_2$ appears to be an inhibitor of MSH release in rats. Interestingly, this MSH-inhibiting factor (MIF) has a sequence identical to the terminal arm of oxytocin (see Chapter 3), and it is even more curious that the ring structure of oxytocin may have MSH-releasing activity (MRF). These workers claim that hypothalamic oxytocin may be the precursor to MIF and MRF and that the relative amount of enzymatic activity for degrading oxytocin in the hypothalamus plays a role in the control of MSH release. Most of the evidence for peptide MIF and MRF comes from studies of the rat. These peptides do not appear to influence MSH release in amphibians; however, possible peptidergic control of MSH release in amphibians has not been eliminated.

Electrophysiological studies of the nerves in the pars intermedia have provided some information on their source within the nervous system. However, additional work is needed to precisely define the neural pathways and the nature of their effects on MSH release. Hadley and Bagnara have proposed a hypothetical scheme for the control of MSH secretion in animals with an innervated pars intermedia (Fig. 5.7). In addition to the lateral eyes that may send photic information to the hypothalamus through higher brain centers, photoreceptors in the pineal gland may also receive information and regulate MSH release at several points. Electrophysiologic studies by Oshima and Gorbman show that there are at least two types of spontaneously active nerves in the pars intermedia. One type is indifferent to light while the other is inhibited by light. Opaque covering of the pineal gland blocks the inhibitory effect of light on the light-sensitive nerves. Removal of the lateral eyes has no effect on these neurons. These workers suggested that the light-indifferent neurons tonically inhibit MSH release while the light-

CONTROL OF MSH RELEASE

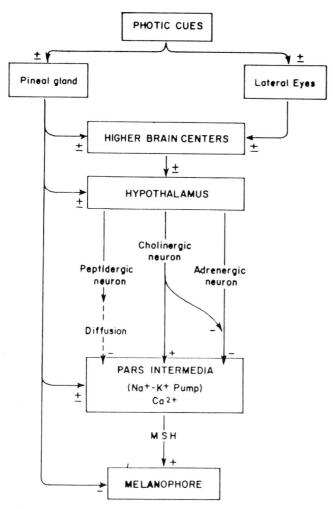

FIGURE 5.7. Scheme for the control of pars intermedia MSH secretion. Both stimulatory (+) and inhibitory (−) inputs to MSH release are indicated. [From M. E. Hadley and J. T. Bagnara, *Am. Zool.*, **15** (Suppl. 1):94, 1975.]

inhibited elements stimulate MSH secretion. Thus, the release of MSH would be determined by the balance of activity of the two neuronal types. The long latency (20 to 30 seconds) between light stimulation and the response of nerve endings in the pars intermedia suggests that the neurons do not go directly from the pineal gland to the pars intermedia, but instead may be interrupted by synapses or some humoral link in the hypothalamus or higher brain centers. Clearly, the control of MSH release involves the integration of many nervous and possibly humoral factors.

Ontogeny of Chromatophore Control in Anurans

Most tadpoles exhibit the curious phenomenon of taking on a light skin coloration when placed in the dark. This body-blanching response to darkness occurs irrespective of background coloration and does not occur in adults. A similar situation occurs in fishes; however, this phenomenon has received greatest attention in anuran amphibians. Apparently, these changes in response to overall photic stimulation during anuran development are a consequence of the maturation of the mechanism of color change regulation. A primary agent in the body-blanching response of tadpoles is the indole derivative of tryptophan, melatonin.

McCord and Allen reported in 1917 that feeding bovine pineal glands to tadpoles induced a dramatic skin blanching. The melanophore-concentrating substance of the pineal gland was isolated by Lerner and colleagues, who chemically identified it as melatonin. Melatonin is synthesized enzymatically from the amino acid tryptophan. Two important enzymes in this pathway are N-acetyl transferase (NAT), which adds an acetyl group to serotonin, and hydroxyindole-O-methyl transferase (HIOMT), which is the final enzyme in the melatonin pathway (see Chapter 14; Fig. 14.8). The melatonin-synthesizing activity of tissues can be determined by measuring the activities of either HIOMT or NAT, or both. Melatonin and its synthetic enzymes have been localized in the pineal gland, retina, and other brain areas. Melatonin is released into the general circulation by the pineal gland and possibly by the retina or other structures. The plasma concentration of melatonin shows a diurnal rhythm, with the highest levels occurring during the night. Pinealectomy of a wide variety of vertebrates eliminates the nighttime rise in circulating melatonin. In addition to its possible involvement in the regulation of color change, the pineal gland may participate in controlling seasonal cycles of reproduction (Chapter 14).

The melanophore-concentrating effect of melatonin in tadpoles is due to a direct action on dermal melanophores. Epidermal melanophores are not responsive to melatonin. In adult amphibians or fishes neither the epidermal or dermal melanophores contract in response to melatonin, except perhaps when given a high pharmacologic dose.

In order to put background adaptation and dark-induced blanching in perspective, three ontogenic stages of control of skin coloration in amphibians must be recognized: primary-stage tadpoles, secondary-stage tadpoles, and adults. Both classes of tadpoles show the blanching response to darkness, while adults do not. Primary-stage tadpoles cannot adapt to different backgrounds, apparently because they cannot inhibit MSH release. Background adaptation is possible only in secondary-stage tadpoles and adults.

When primary-stage tadpoles are placed in the dark, the dermal melanophores contract, while the epidermal melanophores remain expanded and the iridophores remain contracted. This response depends on an intact pineal gland, but occurs regardless of the presence of input from the lateral eye.

Although blood levels of melatonin have not been measured in tadpoles, these observations are consistent with the interpretation that in darkness the pineal gland releases melatonin into the circulation, where it induces body blanching by overcoming the MSH effect on dermal melanophores. When secondary-stage tadpoles are placed in the dark, the dermal melanophores contract, the epidermal melanophores contract partially, and iridophores are partly expanded. This effect on epidermal melanophores and iridophores suggests partial inhibition of MSH release and may be associated with increased melatonin in secondary-stage animals in the dark. Whether the pineal gland or lateral eyes are most elemental in the response of secondary-stage tadpoles is not clear. Slight inhibition of MSH release in adults maintained in darkness has been observed by Wilson and Morgan, who showed that plasma αMSH levels in *Xenopus* after seven days of light deprivation were similar to those of toads maintained on an illuminated gray background. Adult frogs have elevated levels of melatonin in circulation when placed in darkness. However, generally speaking, the skin of adults in the dark does not blanch, since melanophores have lost the ability to respond to these melatonin levels, and the plasma concentration of MSH, while lowered, is still sufficient to maintain melanophores in a partly expanded state. Thus in these three ontogenic stages there appears to be a developmental change in the mechanisms that control MSH release and chromatophore response. The dark-induced blanching response of tadpoles is lost in the adult, presumably due to loss of melatonin receptors on melanophores. The response of background adaptation develops during the transition between primary and secondary tadpole stages, apparently due to maturation of neuroendocrine control of MSH secretion.

Evidence against pineal involvement in background adaptation through release of melatonin into the blood peripheral circulation comes from studies of the adult rainbow trout *Salmo gairdneri*. Ralph, Owens, and Gern have measured circulating levels of melatonin in trout maintained on white, neutral, and black backgrounds. After several weeks, the fishes had color adapted, as indicated by measuring light reflectance from the skin. As expected, plasma levels of melatonin of all fishes were high at night and low during the day. However, there were no differences in melatonin levels among the groups on different backgrounds. The situation may be different in mammals. Rust and Meyer have shown that when melatonin is implanted into short-tailed weasels at the time they are normally growing a brown coat, the coat color changes to white, suggesting melatonin inhibition of MSH release. Melatonin treatment of weasels that have a pituitary implanted under the kidney capsule has no effect on coat color. This implies that melatonin has no direct effect on pituitary release of MSH but is acting through hypothalamic inhibition of MSH. The differences in the relationship between plasma melatonin and coloration in weasels and fishes may be due to species differences in control of MSH. Alternatively, the melatonin implants in weasels may have produced a pharmacologic effect. Additional work is needed to clearly define pineal gland involvement in vertebrate color adaptation.

Multiple Forms of MSH

Amino acid sequence studies reveal that the hormone MSH occurs in two fundamental forms: an α form, with 13 to 15 amino acid residues, and a β form, with 16 to 22 residues, depending on the species. A third form, called γMSH, has been detected in the sequence of pro-opiocortin. However, whether γMSH has any hormonal function or whether it is secreted *in vivo* has not been demonstrated. In general, αMSH is four to five times more potent in its melanotropic activity than are the β forms. As we have discussed in Chapter 4, the MSHs appear to be formed by enzymatic cleavage of the precursor molecule, β-lipotropin, which is derived from a still larger glycoprotein precursor, pro-opiocortin. The structures of MSHs have been determined for at least five mammalian species, two species of dogfish, and a salmon (Table 5.2). There is a fairly high degree of sequence homology among MSHs from different species and among α and β forms. Sequence comparisons of α and β forms from different species shows a higher degree of variability in the β form. The sequence of αMSH is identical in all mammalian species investigated. The αMSHs of both dogfishes are identical to each other but differ from those of mammals in having an amino acid substitution at residue 13 and lacking the acetyl group on the amino-terminal serine. One of the αMSHs of salmon is larger than most other αMSHs, while the βMSHs of salmon are shorter than other vertebrate MSHs. In contrast to this evolutionary conservatism of the α form, βMSHs of most species so far examined are different. In the chum salmon (*Oncorhynchus keta*) there appear to be two separate α and β forms. Kawauchi and Muramoto have suggested that there may be two separate genes coding for two separate pro-opiocortin precursor molecules in chum salmon. Two different camel βMSHs have been described; however, there seems to be only one camel αMSH. Considering all the structures of MSH that have been identified, there are only six amino acid positions that are the same in all forms. βMSH has not been found to occur naturally in human pituitaries. Lowry and co-workers have suggested that human βMSH is an artifact produced from degradation of lipotropin during prolonged extraction of pituitaries with acetic acid. Dogfish βMSHs differ from mammalian forms at additional amino acid positions. In fact, the βMSH sequences of the two dogfish species are as different from each other as they are from mammalian forms. This heterogeneity of the two dogfish βMSHs is not surprising, since these two dogfish are quite distant on the phylogenetic scale. There is no information on the amino acid sequences of MSHs from other vertebrate classes. However, studies using immunohistochemistry, radioimmunoassay, or biochemical separation techniques in conjunction with MSH bioassay have provided some clues to suggest that both α and β MSHs are present in pituitaries of

TABLE 5.2. Amino acid sequences of αMSH and βMSH from various vertebrates[a]

αMSH	Amino Acid Sequence 1	2	3	4	5	6	7	8	9	10	11	12	13	14	15
Mammalian	Ac·Ser·	Tyr·	Ser·	Met·	Glu·	His·	Phe·	Arg·	Trp·	Gly·	Lys·	Pro·	Val·	NH_2	
Dogfish	H·Ser·	Tyr·	Ser·	Met·	Glu·	His·	Phe·	Arg·	Trp·	Gly·	Lys·	Pro·	Met·	NH_2/OH	
Salmon I	H·Ser·	Tyr·	Ser·	Met·	Glu·	His·	Phe·	Arg·	Trp·	Gly·	Lys·	Pro·	Val·	NH_2	
Salmon II	Ac·Ser·	Tyr·	Ser·	Met·	Glu·	His·	Phe·	Arg·	Trp·	Gly·	Lys·	Pro·	Ile·	Gly·	His·OH

βMSH	Amino Acid Sequence 1	2	3	4	5	6	7	8	9	10	11	12	13	14	15	16	17	18
Ox, sheep	H·Asp·	Ser·	Gly·	Pro·	Tyr·	Lys·	Met·	Glu·	His·	Phe·	Arg·	Trp·	Gly·	Ser·	Pro·	Pro·	Lys·	Asp·OH
Pig	H·Asp·	Glu·	Gly·	Pro·	Tyr·	Lys·	Met·	Glu·	His·	Phe·	Arg·	Trp·	Gly·	Ser·	Pro·	Pro·	Lys·	Asp·OH
Horse	H·Asp·	Gly·	Gly·	Pro·	Tyr·	Lys·	Met·	Glu·	His·	Phe·	Arg·	Trp·	Gly·	Ser·	Pro·	Arg·	Lys·	Asp·OH
Camel I	H·Asp·	Gly·	Gly·	Pro·	Tyr·	Lys·	Met·	Glu·	His·	Phe·	Arg·	Trp·	Gly·	Ser·	Pro·	Pro·	Lys·	Asp·OH
Camel II	H·Asp·	Gly·	Gly·	Pro·	Tyr·	Lys·	Met·	Gln·	His·	Phe·	Arg·	Trp·	Gly·	Ser·	Pro·	Pro·	Lys·	Asp·OH
Monkey	H·Asp·	Glu·	Gly·	Pro·	Tyr·	Arg·	Met·	Glu·	His·	Phe·	Arg·	Trp·	Gly·	Ser·	Pro·	Pro·	Lys·	Asp·OH
Dogfish[b]	H·Asp·	Gly·	Ile·	Asp·	Tyr·	Lys·	Met·	Gly·	His·	Phe·	Arg·	Trp·	Gly·	Ala·	Pro·	Met·	Asp·	Lys·OH
Dogfish[c]	H·Asp·	Gly·	Asp·	Asp·	Tyr·	Lys·	Phe·	Gly·	His·	Phe·	Arg·	Trp·	Ser·	Val·	Pro·	Leu·OH		
Salmon I		H·Asp·	Gly·	Ser·	Tyr·	Lys·	Met·	Asn·	His·	Phe·	Arg·	Trp·	Ser·	Gly·	Pro·	Pro·	Ala·	Ser·OH
Salmon II		H·Asp·	Gly·	Ser·	Tyr·	Arg·	Met·	Gly·	His·	Phe·	Arg·	Trp·	Gly·	Ser·	Pro·	Thr·	Ala·	Ile·OH

[a] Rectangles enclose unvarying portions of the peptides.
[b] *Scyliorhinus canicula*
[c] *Squalus acanthius*

species representing all the major vertebrate classes except the cyclostomes. Researchers employing immunological techniques using antibodies to mammalian αMSH have detected αMSH in fishes, amphibians, mammals, and birds. In contrast, similar studies of divergent species using antibodies directed against mammalian βMSH have had only limited success. This lack of cross-reactivity with antibodies to mammalian hormone indicates novel structures of the β form of MSH in other species. Thus, the immunological studies agree with the finding of heterogeneity of βMSHs in those species in which amino acid sequences are known.

The smallest portion of MSH that still has melanotropic activity is the pentapeptide Met-Glu-His-Phe-Arg. This sequence is considered an essential part of the functional site of MSH, and it appears that most larger peptides that contain this sequence have intrinsic melanotropic activity. Thus ACTH, βLPH, and γLPH have some melanotropic effects, although they are much less potent than the MSHs. It is interesting that some amino acid substitutions are found in the region corresponding to this active site in the βMSHs of salmon and dogfishes. Despite this fact, dogfish and salmon βMSHs are potent melanotropic agents. It is of further interest that the sequence His-Phe-Arg-Trp, which forms a part of the functional site of MSH, is conserved in all the known structures of MSH (Table 5.2).

Mechanisms of MSH Action

The mode of action on melanosome dispersion and melanin synthesis has received much attention, partly because of the rapid response of melanophores and the ease of experimenting with frog, fish, or lizard skin *in vitro*. Certain parts of the intracellular chain of events initiated by MSH differ depending upon the animal species and on whether dermal or epidermal melanophores are studied. Therefore, a specific unified theory of MSH action on chromatophores cannot be offered. On the other hand, many of the cellular components involved have been identified.

As would be expected for a peptide hormone, MSH acts as a first messenger to stimulate the intracellular production of a second messenger, cyclic AMP (Chapter 1). Melanosome dispersion in melanophores (or contraction of iridophores) can be produced by treating skin with dibutyryl cyclic AMP, which penetrates the cell more easily than cyclic AMP. Addition of methyl xanthines such as caffeine or theophylline darkens skin by elevating intracellular cyclic AMP through inhibiting its degradation by cyclic AMP phosphodiesterase. It is not clear whether MSH elevates cyclic AMP by activating adenyl cyclase or inhibiting phosphodiesterase. In any event, high levels of cyclic AMP within the cell mimic all the actions of MSH, whether they be melanosome dispersion, melanin synthesis, or differentiation of stem cells into mature melanocytes. Receptors for MSH have not been isolated; however, they appear to be localized on the outer surface of the plasma membrane, since skin darkening is induced by MSH bound to sepharose beads and thereby prevented from entering the cell. Molecular details of MSH receptor elevation of cyclic AMP are not known, although Ca^{2+} or some equivalent divalent cation is required. Calcium does not appear to be required for melanosome dispersion once intracellular cyclic AMP is high. Prostaglandin (PGE) in particular has been implicated in melanophore response, since PGE increases adenyl cyclase and melanosome dispersion by a Ca^{2+}-independent mechanism.

Once cyclic AMP is elevated, it apparently activates protein kinases, which in turn regulate as yet ill-defined processes that are specific responses of the cell. For our discussion, these diverse MSH responses will be separated into melanosome dispersion, melanin synthesis, and melanocytogenesis.

In seeking a rational basis for analysis of MSH's action on melanosome dispersion, endocrinologists have in the past tried to find similar features in other biological phenomena. There are some similarities between the reversible movement of pigment granules and muscular contraction. There is also a resemblance between pigment movement and locomotion of chromosomes during mitosis. Accordingly, attention has been focused on the role of microtubules and microfilaments in chromatophores. Microtubules in the cytoplasm of melanophores are oriented in parallel with the extensions of the dendritic processes. It is thought that the tubules may form channels along which melanosomes move. In addition, these microtubules may in some fashion supply a motive force to granule dispersion. Treatment of melanophores with agents (colchicine, vinblastine, vincristine) that interfere with microtubule function prevents the normal dispersion or aggregation of melanosomes. Microfilaments may also play a role in melanosome movements, since these elements are also observed in the pigment cell cytoplasm. Cytochalasin B, a specific inhibitor of microfilament function, will interfere with melanosome movements in melanophores of a number of species. The challenging problem in elucidating the general functions of these elements concerns the varying roles of microtubules and microfilaments in melanosome dispersion or aggregation in dermal or epidermal melanophores of different species. For example, in the frog *Rana pipiens* MSH favors the formation of microtubules and reduces the number of microfilaments in epidermal melanophores. Thus, in this frog species microtubules favor melanosome dispersion, while microfilaments promote aggregation. However, in some fishes functional microtubules are necessary for both dispersion and aggregation of melanosomes. The situation is further confounded by the observations that neither microfilaments nor microtubules are prominent features of dermal melanophores of the toad *Xenopus laevis*. Overall, these observations suggest that the mechanism of MSH action on melanosome movement, aside from elevation of cyclic AMP, is an adaptive process that is determined by the particular structural and functional relationship of microtubules and microfilaments in a given animal species and chromatophore type.

A classical hypothesis of MSH action contends that the melanophore cytoplasm is alternately solated and gelated. Assembly and disassembly of microtubules may favor sol–gel changes, so that melanosomes become dispersed as the cytoplasm is solated. Formation of microtubules may then cause the cytoplasm to gelate in dendritic processes, excluding melanosomes and forcing their aggregation near the center of the cell.

Melanogenesis stimulated by MSH or cyclic AMP appears to occur through activation of tyrosinase, followed by *de novo* synthesis of the enzyme. Tyrosinase assembles the highly complex polymer structure of melanin by oxidation of many tyrosine molecules. In an unstimulated melanophore, tyrosinase is inhibited by binding with an inhibitory protein. Alternative theories of MSH action are based on metabolic changes within the cell. According to Wright (1955), an anaerobic source of energy is important in melanosome movement. Wright found that treating pieces of frog skin with metabolic poisons that block oxygen consumption had no effect on MSH-induced dispersion of melanosomes over a period of four hours. However, blocking glycolysis with iodoacetate inhibits the aggregation of melanosomes. Thus, in the absence of available energy from glycolysis, the melanophore remains expanded. MSH then may disperse melanosomes by blocking glycolysis. Horowitz proposed that MSH acts by oxidizing sulfhydryl (SH) groups, since agents that bind sulfhydryls darken lizard skin and compounds that donate sulfhydryls block MSH action. Although these ideas are interesting, they have not been pursued by other researchers. Additional work on integrating these theories with the second-messenger hypothesis and microtubule function may be promising.

Chromatophores are derived from stem cells that originally came from the embryonic neural crest region. Treatment of stem cells with MSH will initiate melanin synthesis and promote the development of the dendritic cytoplasmic processes that are characteristic of mature melanophores. Dibutyryl cyclic AMP will mimic these MSH effects on stem cell differentiation. Full development of mature melanocytes requires protein synthesis, since blockers of protein or RNA synthesis prevent development of the characteristic, large dendritic structures. Differentiation of stem cells into chromatophores may be regulated by synergistic actions of other hormones, since ACTH and corticosteroids influence some aspects of melanocytogenesis.

The actions of MSH exerted through elevation of cyclic AMP are quite varied and include movement of organelles, enzyme activation, and cell differentiation associated with protein synthesis. This illustrates a fundamental aspect of the second-messenger hypothesis. Specificity of hormone response is not determined by cyclic AMP; many peptide hormones act through elevation of intracellular cyclic AMP. Specificity is determined by the particular regulatory proteins (e.g., kinases) that respond to high levels of cyclic AMP. A better understanding of the mechanism of MSH action will be realized when the molecular details of protein kinase action are known.

Catecholamines in the Coordination of Color Change

As in most physiological processes under hormonal control, color changes in poikilotherms are regulated by several humoral factors. MSH-induced darkening may be modified by the synergistic or antagonistic action of circulating catecholamines. Epinephrine and norepinephrine, released into the circulation by stress to the animal, will cause the animal's skin to lighten (excitement pallor) or darken (excitement darkening) depending on the type of catecholamine receptor on its chromatophores. These responses are common in amphibians and reptiles. Excitement pallor is apparent to anyone who has picked up and handled a brown chameleon; the chameleon turns green within a few minutes. The direction of excitement-induced color change is probably adapted to the requirements of the species in its habitat. For example, if a brown chameleon basking on a tree trunk is chased by a predator, the chameleon may escape into the foliage and shortly become adapted to the green background of leaves as a result of catecholamine action.

The catecholamines' pigmentary effects are difficult to sort out *in vivo* since catecholamines may inhibit MSH secretion by the pars intermedia. Pharmacological studies of chromatophore responses *in vitro* have clarified the situation. Catecholamine receptors can be classified as either the alpha or the beta type. These types can be identified by using more or less specific alpha and beta agonists or antagonists. For example, the skin of *Xenopus* is darkened by the specific beta-receptor agonist isoproterenol. If *Xenopus* skin is exposed to a catecholamine along with an agent that blocks alpha receptors (phentolamine), the skin will still darken; however, if a beta blocker (phenoxybenzamine) is used, the skin remains pale. Thus the catecholamine-induced darkening in *Xenopus* is effected through beta receptors. Similar studies on skin from *Rana pipiens*, which lightens in response to catecholamines, show that this response is mediated by alpha receptors. Considering all the information, some generalizations emerge. Stimulation of alpha-adrenergic receptors causes paling, while stimulation of beta-adrenergic receptors induces darkening. The chromatophores of some species have only alpha- or only beta-adrenergic receptors. In other species chromatophores have both types of receptors, but one type predominates over the other. The predominant receptor type determines the direction of color change in response to catecholamines.

The coordinated control of color change depends on the interplay of several factors, which include circulating amounts of MSH and catecholamines and the type of adrenergic receptor present on the chromatophore plasma membrane. When catecholamine concentration in the plasma is high relative to MSH levels, the catecholamine effect on chromatophores will prevail. In those species whose chromatophores have beta receptors (darkening response), catecholamines and MSH will synergize to cause darkening. In species with alpha receptors (lightening responses), the hormones will antagonize each other's action. There is some evidence that catecholamine action on chromatophores involves the second messenger, cyclic AMP. Stimulation of beta receptors elevates cyclic AMP, while alpha stimulation brings about a decline in cyclic AMP. Thus the degree of expansion of the chromatophore will be determined by the summation of those factors that increase (MSH and beta stimulation) and decrease (alpha stimulation) the intracellular concentration of cyclic AMP.

EXTRAPIGMENTARY ACTIONS OF MSH

In general, there appears to be little involvement of MSH in the control of pigmentation in warm-blooded animals beyond the few examples we have mentioned. This has led some researchers to suggest that MSH may have no function in higher vertebrates and that it may be a vestigial hormone. However, several arguments can be brought against this view. Significant amounts of MSH are present in the pituitaries of mammals and birds. In addition, the structure of MSH (of the α form in particular) is remarkably constant in those species of higher vertebrates for which the amino acid sequence is known. Therefore, it could be argued that there must be some selective pressure, and hence some function of the hormone, that is responsible for the retention of MSH and its structural integrity during the evolution of higher vertebrates. This kind of reasoning has encouraged the search for extrapigmentary actions of MSH in mammals.

The observed effects of MSH in mammals are quite varied. Many of these studies are difficult to interpret, since they have not spurred additional research to evaluate the physiological significance of the observed actions of MSH. Furthermore, some MSH actions may result from its structural similarity to ACTH. Extrapigmentary effects of MSH have been reviewed by Novales (1974). The idea that MSH may have some role in reproduction is based on the evidence that MSH induces menstrual bleeding in amenorrheic women and may synergize with sex steroids to stimulate the preputial gland of the rat. On the other hand, injection of MSH causes a reduction in testis weight in rats and guinea pigs. Synthetic αMSH stimulates steroid production by rat adrenals; however, it is much less potent than ACTH. The steroidogenic action of αMSH may be a reflection of the fact that αMSH corresponds to amino acid residues 1 to 13 of ACTH. MSH has been implicated in many other seemingly unrelated physiological processes, which include accelerating heart rate, lowering blood calcium, stimulating sodium loss, mobilizing fat stores, stimulating erythropoiesis, and causing the aqueous flare response (apparently by increasing the protein content of the aqueous humor in the eye of the rabbit).

Most recently, interest in the extrapigmentary functions of MSH has focused on animal behavior and growth of the mammalian fetus. Earlier observations indicated that MSH acts on the nervous system. Injection of βMSH increases the amplitude of monosynaptic potentials in the spinal cord of cats. The hormone also increases high-amplitude waves in the electroencephalogram (EEG) of rats and frogs. In contrast, βMSH decreases amplitude variations in electrical discharges of the transparent knifefish. Clearly, MSH can modify neuronal function; these neuronal effects may be significant in the context of the behavioral changes that result from treatment of animals with peptides of the MSH–ACTH–LPH family. In many of the behavioral studies a peptide fragment consisting of the sequence Met-Glu-His-Phe-Arg-Trp-Gly was used. This sequence corresponds to residues 4 to 10 of αMSH and ACTH. Since this fragment has little effect on peripheral target organs, it is assumed that any observed behavioral changes are due to direct action on the nervous system. One interesting behavioral effect of this peptide fragment is enhancement of learning and memory processes. The pioneering work of de Wied, Bohus, and colleagues showed that hypophysectomized mice had slow acquisition and fast extinction in active avoidance tests. Active avoidance can be measured by the electric shock shuttle box technique. A rat is placed in a shuttle box in which one-half of the floor is electrified (Fig. 5.8). There is no electric current going through the floor before the test. With the rat in place, the buzzer is sounded (conditioned stimulus) and, after a few seconds, the electric current to the floor is turned on (unconditioned stimulus). The rat learns to avoid an electric shock by jumping over a barrier to the side of the box that is not electrified within the short interval between the conditioned and unconditioned stimuli. The time required for the rat to learn to jump fairly consistently over the barrier when the buzzer sounds is called the acquisition period. Other studies have examined how long the conditioned avoidance is retained. Once the rat acquires the behavior, the test protocol is changed so that sounding the buzzer is no longer followed by electrifying the floor. The rat will discover that staying on the floor will not result in an electric shock and will eventually lose the barrier-jumping behavior. This is known as the extinction phase, which may be interpreted as a function of behavior retention or memory. Treatment of hypophysectomized rats with the peptide fragment αMSH_{4-10} ($ACTH_{4-10}$) shortens the acquisition phase and prolongs the extinction phase. Thus MSH or ACTH from the pituitary may stimulate learning and facilitate memory. The physiological significance of these peptide-mediated behaviors is strengthened by the localization of bioassayable and immunoreactive αMSH and ACTH in many areas of the rat brain. Furthermore, hypophysectomized rats retain this brain MSH and ACTH, which suggests that these peptides may have a dual origin: pituitary and brain. However,

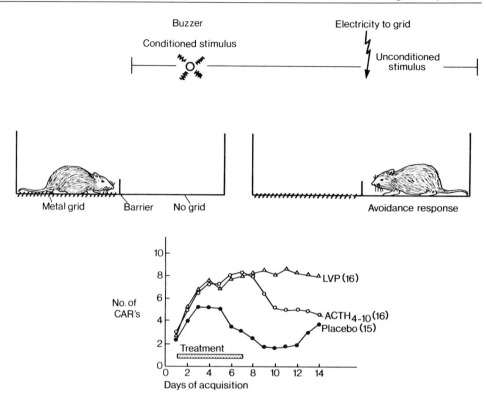

FIGURE 5.8. The effects of daily treatment of hypophysectomized rats with $ACTH_{4-10}$ (20 µg/day) and lysine vasopressin (LVP; 1 µg/day) for 7 days on avoidance acquisition in a shuttlebox. With the rat placed on the side of the box with a metal grid, the buzzer was sounded and the grid was electrified 5 seconds later. This test was repeated daily for 14 days. During the treatment period, the rats injected with the peptides learned to avoid the electric shock at a faster rate and more consistently than rats that were treated with a placebo (salt solution). After the treatment period, the rats treated with $ACTH_{4-10}$ lost their consistent performance in the test and behaved like the controls. The LVP-treated rats continued to perform well in the test. CAR = conditioned avoidance response. [From B. Bohus, W. H. Gispen, and D. deWied, *Neuroendocrinology,* **11**:137, 1973.]

the effect of hypophysectomy on avoidance behavior argues in favor of a role for the pituitary. Understanding MSH's or ACTH's action on learning and memory is complicated by observations that other peptides (β-endorphin, vasopressin) have similar effects on these processes. Future research on behavioral effects of peptides holds the promise of understanding brain function at the molecular level and possible hormonal treatment of mental disturbances.

Another area of recent interest concerns the role of MSH in the growth of the mammalian fetus. Removal of the brain and pituitary of a fetus slows fetal growth. Swaab and Visser have used replacement therapy on these fetuses to identify the growth-promoting factor that was eliminated by brain and pituitary removal. They found that αMSH stimulated intrauterine growth of these fetuses, whereas growth hormone, prolactin, $ACTH_{1-24}$, $ACTH_{4-10}$, TSH, LH, FSH, HCG, oxytocin, insulin, cyclic AMP, and extracts of the hypothalamus or placenta were ineffective. Furthermore, treatment of intact rat fetuses with purified αMSH antiserum slowed fetal growth. These researchers argue that αMSH may be important in human fetal growth. In the normal human fetus αMSH can be found in both the pars intermedia and pars distalis. In the congenital anomaly anencephaly, the brain fails to develop after about the third or fourth week of fetal development. In anencephalic humans the cerebral hemispheres are completely missing or very small; the hypothalamus, pars intermedia, and pars nervosa are usually absent. Although the pars distalis is present in anencephalics, it does not contain αMSH, and the intrauterine growth rate of anencephalics is lower than that of normal human fetuses. Thus it appears that the fetal brain and hypothalamus are required for the differentiation of the pars intermedia and production of pituitary MSH. The hypothesis of the control of human fetal growth by MSH of the pars intermedia is interesting, since the pars intermedia is not retained in the adult human.

ADDITIONAL READING

1. Bagnara, J. T., and J. D. Taylor (1972). Dermal chromatophores. *Am. Zool.* **12**:43–62.

2. Bagnara, J. T., and M. E. Hadley (1973). *Chromatophores and Color Change: The Comparative Physiology of Animal Pigmentation.* Prentice-Hall, Englewood Cliffs, New Jersey.

3. Ball, J. N., and T. F. C. Batten (1981). Pituitary and melanophore responses to background in *Poecilia latipinna* (Teleostei): role of the pars intermedia PAS cell. *Gen. Comp. Endocrinol.* **44**:233–248.

4. Bohus, B., W. H. Gispen, and D. de Wied (1973). Effect of lysine vasopressin and $ACTH_{4-10}$ on conditioned avoidance behavior of hypophysectomized rats. *Neuroendocrinology* **11**:137–143.

5. de Wied, D. (1965). The influence of the posterior and intermediate lobe of the pituitary and pituitary peptides on the maintenance of a conditioned avoidance response in rats. *Int. J. Neuropharmacol.* **4**:157–167.

6. Eberle, A. N. (1980). MSH receptors. In *Cellular Receptors for Hormones and Neurotransmitters* (D. Schulster and A. Levitzki, eds.). Wiley, New York.

7. Geschwind, I. I. (1966). Change in hair color in mice induced by injection of αMSH. *Endocrinology* **79**:1165–1167.

8. Hadley, M. E. (1972). Functional significance of vertebrate integumental pigmentation. *Am. Zool.* **12**:63–76.

9. Hadley, M. E., and J. T. Bagnara (1975). Regulation of release and mechanism of action of MSH. *Am. Zool.* **15** (Suppl. 1): 81–104.

10. Horowitz, S. B. (1958). The energy requirements of melanin granule aggregation and dispersion in the melanophores of *Anolis carolinensis. J. Cell. Comp. Physiol.* **51**:341–357.

11. Kawauchi, H., and K. Muramoto (1979). Isolation and primary structure of melanotropins from salmon pituitary glands. *Int. J. Peptide Protein Res.* **14**:373–374.

12. Nakanishi, S., A. Inoue, T. Kita, M. Nakamura, A. C. Y. Chang, S. N. Cohen, and S. Nama (1979). Nucleotide sequence of cloned cDNA for bovine corticotropin-β-lipotropin precursor. *Nature* **278**:423–427.

13. Novales, R. R. (1974). Actions of melanocyte-stimulating hormones. *Handbook of Physiology*, Sect. 7, Vol. 4, Part 2. Williams & Wilkins, Baltimore, pp. 347–366.

14. Owens, D. W., W. A. Gern, and C. L. Ralph (1978). Nonrelationship between plasma melatonin and background adaptation in the rainbow trout (*Salmo gairdneri*). *Gen. Comp. Endocrinol.* **34**:459–467.

15. Quevedo, W. C. (1972). Epidermal melanin units: melanocyte-keratinocyte interactions. *Am. Zool.* **12**:35–41.

16. Rance, T. A., and B. I. Baker (1979). The teleost melanin-concentrating hormone—a pituitary hormone of hypothalamic origin. *Gen. Comp. Endocrinol.* **37**:64–73.

17. Rust, C. C. (1965). Hormonal control of pelage cycles in the short-tailed weasel (*Mustela erminera bangsi*). *Gen. Comp. Endocrinol.* **5**:222–231.

18. Swaab, D. F., and M. Visser (1977). A function for α-MSH in fetal development and the presence of an α-MSH-like compound in nervous tissue. In *Frontiers of Hormone Research*, Vol. 4 (F. J. H. Tilders, D. F. Swaab, and T. J. B. van Winnersma Greidanus, eds.), Karger, Basel, p. 170.

19. Waring, H. (1963). *Color Change Mechanisms in Cold-blooded Vertebrates*. Academic, New York.

20. Westerfield, D. B., P. K. T. Pang, and J. M. Burns (1980). Some characteristics of melanophore-concentration hormone (MCH) from teleost pituitary glands. *Gen. Comp. Endocrinol.* **42**:494–499.

21. Wright, P. A. (1955). Physiological responses of frog melanophores *in vitro*. *Physiol. Zool.* **28**:204–218.

6

The Thyroid Gland

It is possible to define the thyroid gland in a fairly simple way as the vertebrate tissue that can accumulate iodide in great excess and can combine it chemically in the organic compound thyroxine. Defined in this way, the thyroid gland appears refreshingly simple. It may be contrasted with the pituitary and adrenal glands or the gastrointestinal tract, which produce numerous hormones, some of them complex proteins that, unlike thyroxine, usually vary from one species to the next. Unfortunately, much of the apparent simplicity of the thyroid gland disappears upon closer study, as we shall see, and some of the knottiest problems in comparative endocrinology involve this gland.

In recent years a tremendous surge of thyroidal research has been made possible by the fortunate availability of radioactive iodine. Since the thyroid hormone and its precursors are virtually the only iodine compounds in living organisms, the distribution of radioiodine can be interpreted as the distribution of these compounds. Thus a simple labeling device is available for thyroid function. For no other endocrine function is an element alone useful as a marker. The best that can be done in this way for other hormones is radiocarbon or radiohydrogen labeling of relatively complex hormone precursor compounds such as cholesterol.

COMPARATIVE GROSS ANATOMY

The basic histological unit of all vertebrate thyroid glands is the follicle, a hollow ball consisting of a single layer of epithelial cells enclosing a fluid-filled space (Fig. 6.1). The thyroid gland is a highly vascular (Fig. 6.2) assembly of follicles, and it may be variable in shape. However, in each vertebrate group, the shape of the gland is reasonably characteristic.

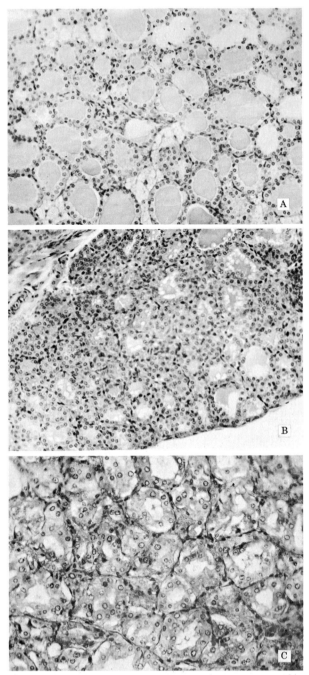

FIGURE 6.1. Thyroid follicles of the mouse in different states of stimulated activity (all at the same magnification). (*A*) Normal mouse thyroid. Cells are roughly cuboidal; stainable colloid with regular outer edge. (*B*) Thyroid after 7 days of feeding thiourea, a goitrogen that leads to TSH secretion by the pituitary. Cells are only slightly taller. Colloid in many follicles contains

In the cyclostomes and teleosts there is usually no organized thyroid gland. Instead, the follicles are scattered singly or in small groups in the loose connective tissue under the pharynx (Figs. 6.3 and 6.4). The pattern of distribution of these loose follicles usually follows the course of the ventral aorta and the roots of its branches into the gills. However, there are some exceptional teleosts (Bermuda parrot fish, swordfish, tuna) in which compact thyroid glands have been found; these may be bilobed, one lobe behind the other in the midline (Fig. 6.3). Although the thyroid area of teleosts is generally well supplied with blood, a most interesting lymphatic relationship has been described for the angler fish *Lophius*. In this species thyroid follicles are said to be grouped around a large lymphatic sinus, and this drains almost without interruption into the heart.

Perhaps the most unusual anatomic feature of the teleost thyroid is its tendency to undergo widespread dispersion out of the pharyngeal area. The most common nonpharyngeal site in which thyroid follicles may be found is the head kidney (Fig. 6.5). This was first discovered by Baker-Cohen (1959), who was investigating the cause of cysts in the kidneys of platyfish (*Platypoecilus*) with enlarged, goitrous thyroids. These cysts had the ability to store radioiodine. Further study revealed that the "misplaced" (hetero-topic) thyroid probably migrated from the pharyngeal position. Furthermore, smaller numbers of follicles were found in the brain, eye, esophagus, and spleen. Since Baker's discovery of the phenomenon, it has been reported in several other species of teleost fishes, so that it may be characteristic of the group. It has been said that this tendency for dispersion of thyroid follicles is due to the unencapsulated nature of the gland in teleosts.

In the cartilaginous fishes the thyroid is usually a unified gland, disk-shaped in the skates and rays and flask-shaped in the sharks. The narrowed part of the shark's thyroid is directed toward the pharyngeal floor, and in one of the primitive sharks, *Chlamydoselachus*, a rather wide duct extends from the narrowed end of the thyroid gland through the basihyoid cartilage to the pharynx. There is a tendency among the elasmobranchs for fusion of the venous and lymphatic channels on the thyroidal surface. In some elasmobranchs this produces a continuous venous sinus in which the gland becomes suspended (Fig. 6.6).

The amphibian thyroid is distinctly double, and the two, usually rounded lobes may be far apart, particularly in urodeles. Typically, they are associated with the hyoid cartilages and may be firmly attached (Figs. 6.3, 6.7, and 6.8). In *Amphiuma*, for example, the posterior ventral tips of the branchial cartilages are hollowed out and contain the two thyroid glands. Such glands, as can be imagined, are difficult to find by dissection. Among the more remarkable statements that have been made concerning the amphibian

many bubblelike "resorption vacuoles." (*C*) After 39 days of feeding thiourea. Cells are taller; in some places (near bottom of photograph) the thyroid epithelium is folded; the nuclei are enlarged and vesicular. The stainable colloid is almost completely absent.

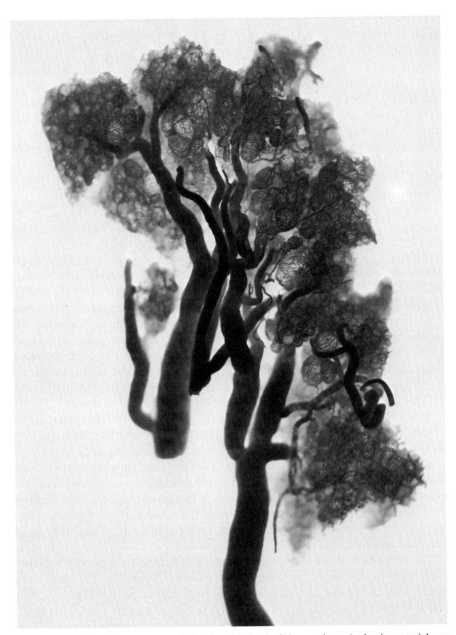

FIGURE 6.2. Circulatory pattern of the thyroid gland of the monkey. A plastic material was injected into the blood vessels; the tissues were then digested away, leaving only the plastic. The large vessels in the lower left are the principal arteries (narrower) and veins (broader). The globular structures represent the capillary basket around individual follicles. It is interesting to observe that, in general, the capillaries are parallel, running from an arteriole on one side of the follicle to a venule in the other side. [From T. W. Williams and C. C. Boyer, *Stereo-Atlas of Microanatomy*, 1960.]

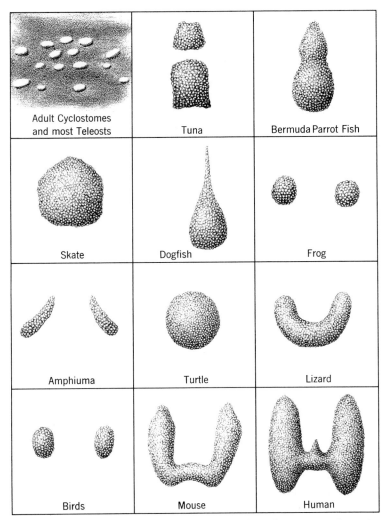

FIGURE 6.3. Outlines of the shapes of thyroid glands in various groups of vertebrates.

thyroid is that it may be absent from certain forms. This has been claimed as the reason underlying neoteny, or failure of metamorphosis, in the salamander *Typhlomolge rathbuni* and in the frog *Pelobates syriacus*. However, restudy of *Typhlomolge* has shown that it has small but typically follicular glands.

The reptilian thyroid gland, like the other reptiliam endocrine organs, has been studied relatively little, so that the full extent of its anatomic variation is not well known. However, the most common forms are those seen in the lizards and in the turtles (Fig. 6.3). In snakes and turtles the thyroid gland is a single discoid structure located in front of the heart at the branching of

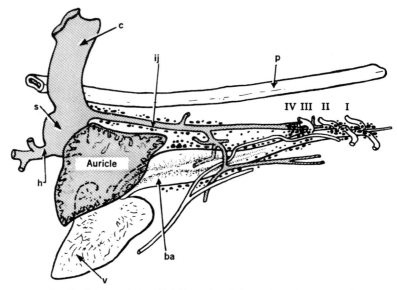

FIGURE 6.4. The distribution of thyroid follicles in relation to blood vessels and the pharynx in the normal adult platyfish. Thyroid follicles (in black) are shown in approximately natural size in proportion to the blood vessels. Veins are shaded, arteries are white. Individual afferent branchial arteries are numbered I through IV. *ba*, Bulbus arteriosus; *c*, cardinal vein; *h*, hepatic vein; *ij*, inferior juglar vein; *p*, pharynx; *s*, sinus venosus; *v*, ventricle. [After K. F. Baker-Cohen, *Comparative Endocrinology* (A. Gorbman, ed.), Wiley, New York, 1959.]

the systemic aortae. In lizards it lies straplike across the trachea or is bilaterally lobed, each lobe at the side of the trachea and connected to the other lobe by a broad bridge (isthmus) of thyroid tissue over the trachea. In a few lizards, there are two separated lobes (*Uromastyx, Monitor*).

In birds, the thyroid consists of two isolated, rounded lobes lying on either side of the trachea at the level of the clavicles (Figs. 6.3 and 6.9).

The mammalian thyroid (Fig. 6.3) typically resembles that of some lizards in being formed from two lobes connected by an isthmus that crosses the ventral side of the trachea. In the prototherian mammal *Echidna*, the kidney-shaped thyroid is unpaired and is situated within the thorax.

DEVELOPMENT OF THE THYROID GLAND

With the exception of the lampreys, the thyroid gland of all vertebrates has a relatively simple development from the floor of the pharynx. It appears early in development as a small pocket of tissue or a solid mass growing ventrad in the midline at the level of the first or second visceral pouches (Figs. 2.11, 6.10, and 6.11). This primary structure, whether solid or hollow, becomes flask shaped. The narrowed end of the anlage is known as the

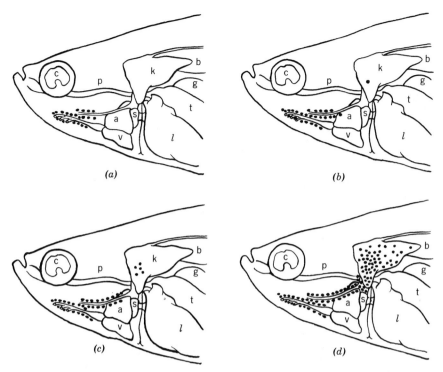

FIGURE 6.5. Increased posterior distribution of thyroid follicles (black dots) with advancing age in strain BH platyfish. In the kidneys the actual mean number of renal follicles per fish is shown for each age group. The other follicles are not shown in this same quantitative way, although an attempt at approximation was made. (*a*) 1 Month old; (*b*) 3 months old; (*c*) 6 months old; (*d*) 10 months old. *a*, auricle; *b*, air bladder; *c*, chorioid gland; *g*, gall bladder; *k*, kidney, *l*, liver; *p*, pharynx; *s*, sinus venosus; *t*, stomach; *v*, ventricle. [After K. F. Baker-Cohen, *Comparative Endocrinology* (A. Gorbman, ed.), Wiley, New York, 1959.]

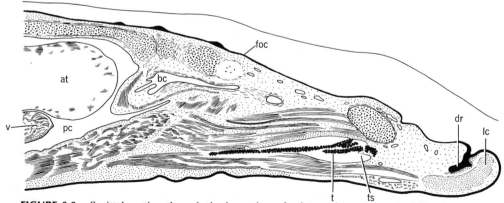

FIGURE 6.6. Sagittal section through the lower jaw of a late embryo (60 mm) of *Squalus acanthias*, the Atlantic dogfish. The thyroid tissue (*t*) is shown in black, formed by a long, chainlike mass of follicles embedded in a large venous sinus (*ts*). *at*, Atrium; *bc*, bulbus cordis, the base of the ventral aorta; *dr*, dental ridge; *foc*, floor of oral cavity; *lc*, cartilage in lip; *pc*, pericardial cavity; *v*, ventricle. [From E. H. Norris, *J. Morphol.*, **31**:187, 1918.]

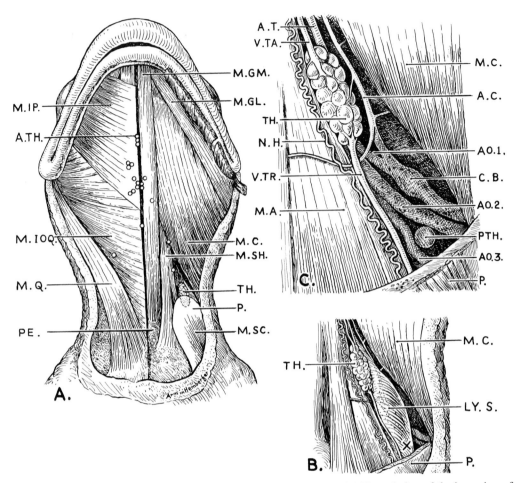

FIGURE 6.7. Thyroid structure of *Triturus viridescens*. (*A*) Ventral view of the lower jaw of the salamander with skin removed, revealing superficial muscles on the right side and, after dissection, deeper muscles and thyroid gland (*TH*) on left side. Sites of accessory thyroid follicles (*A.TH.*) from varying depths are projected as circles as though on the surface. (*B*) Site of left thyroid gland. Procoracoid cartilage (*P.*) is partly cut away to reveal entire thyroid lobe. The parathyroid (not visible) lies behind the point *x* but is obscured by the lateral lymph sac (*LY.S.*). (*C*) Higher magnification of *B*, with lymph sac removed to show the parathyroid and other details. *A.C.*, External carotid artery; *A.T.*, thyroid artery; *AO.1*, carotid artery; *AO.2*, systemic arch; *AO.3*, pulmocutaneous artery; *C.B.*, carotid body; *M.A.*, abdominohyoideus muscle; *M.C.*, ceratohyoid muscle; *M.GL.*, lateral geniohyoid muscle; *M.IOQ.*, interossa quadrata muscle; *M.IP.*, posterior intermandibular muscle; *M.Q.*, quadratopectoral muscle; *M.SC.*, supracoracoid muscle; *M.SH.*, sternohyoid muscle; *N.H.*, hypobranchial nerve; *P.*, procoracoid cartilage; *PE.*, pericardium; *PTH.*, parathyroid gland; *V.TA.*, thyroid advehens vein; *V.TR.*, thyroid revehens vein (external jugular vein). [From L. S. Stone and H. Steinitz, *J. Exp. Zool.*, **124**:469, 1953.]

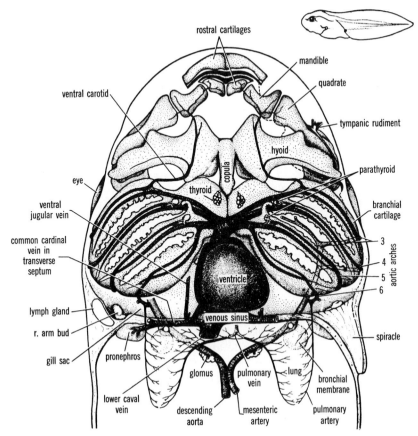

FIGURE 6.8. Ventral view of the skeletal, circulatory, and endocrine structures in the anterior part of a bullfrog tadpole (*Rana catesbeiana*, stage 26). The thyroid follicles are attached to the branchial cartilage anterior to the heart, near the midline. The parathyroids are lateral to the thyroids near the fourth and fifth aortic arches. (See also Figs. 6.7 and 6.16). [After E. Witschi, *Z. Naturforsch.*, **4**:230, 1949.]

thyroglossal duct, since it connects the thyroid to the tongue rudiment in the pharyngeal floor.

There seems to be considerable variability in the time of separation of the thyroglossal duct from the pharynx. Usually it breaks promptly. As the thyroid enlarges and moves away from the pharynx, if the duct is not yet broken, it becomes elongated at this time. A normally persisting thyroglossal duct has been described in the shark *Chlamydoselachus*; it may remain as an abnormal remnant in human adults.

The histological differentiation of the developing thyroid may proceed at highly variable rates in the different vertebrate groups. In the fishes and amphibians the thyroidal anlage separates from the pharyngeal endodermal floor so early that its cells, like other cells of the region, are still laden with

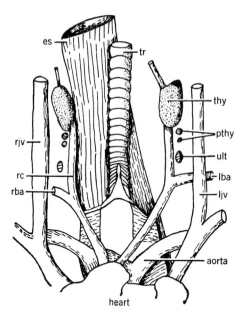

FIGURE 6.9. Thyroids, parathyroids, and ultimobranchial bodies of the domestic chicken in relation to the heart, trachea, and esophagus. *es,* Esophagus; *rjv,* right jugular vein; *rc,* right carotid; *rba,* right brachial artery; *ljv,* left jugular vein; *lba,* left brachial artery; *ult,* ultimobranchial body; *pthy,* parathyroids; *thy,* thyroid; *tr,* trachea. [After L. A. Adams and S. Eddy, *Comparative Anatomy,* Wiley, New York, 1949.]

yolk. Consequently, as the yolk is utilized, the early bilobed thyroid gland of the frog actually shrinks, despite an absolute increase in cell number.

Differentiation in amphibian embryos is rapid, so that *Rana pipiens* tadpoles with a body length of only 3 mm (10 mm total length) have a functioning thyroid gland. This corresponds to completion of about 10% of premetamorphic development in terms of time. In the chick embryo the thyroid gland is sufficiently differentiated to function on the seventh to ninth day of the 21 days of incubation. In mammalian embryos the thyroid begins to function when approximately 50% (man, pig, rabbit) to 80 or 90% (rat, mouse) of intrauterine development is completed.

Regardless of the rate of thyroidal differentiation, its pattern is similar in all vertebrates other than the cyclostomes. The pharyngeal rudiment increases in size while it is moving to its definitive location. A part of the "movement" of the thyroidal rudiment is only apparent. Actually, there is an extensive rearrangement of cervical tissues during this time, involving the heart and branchial structures; this sometimes creates the impression of extensive movement of the thyroid anlage, when in fact it moves relatively little. On the other hand, there is good evidence that when the thyroid anlage is not enclosed by a capsule (fishes), individual thyroid follicles may wander over a wide area (Fig. 6.5).

Cellular differentiation at this time goes through two stages. First, the originally solid primordium is penetrated by the surrounding mesenchymal tissues, forming the basic stroma and vascular supply. The cells of the primordium become separated into cords (Fig. 6.12). Second, the cords are separated into small cellular groups. In each group the cells become visibly

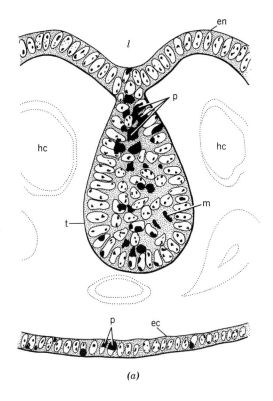

(a)

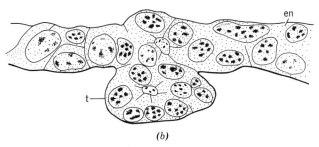

(b)

FIGURE 6.10. (*a*) Cross section through the thyroid gland and adjacent structures of a *Squalus acanthias* embryo, 5.8 mm long (× 5000). *ec*, Ectoderm; *en*, endoderm of pharyngeal floor; *hc*, head cavities (outline in stipple); *l*, lumen of pharynx; *m*, mitotic figure; *P*, pigment granules; *t*, thyroid primordium. [After E. H. Norris, *J. Morphol.*, **31**:211, 1918.] (*b*) Cross section through the thyroid primordium in the pharyngeal floor of a 22-mm embryo of the salamander *Ambystoma*. [After J. M. Sanders, *J. Morphol.*, **57**:597, 1935.]

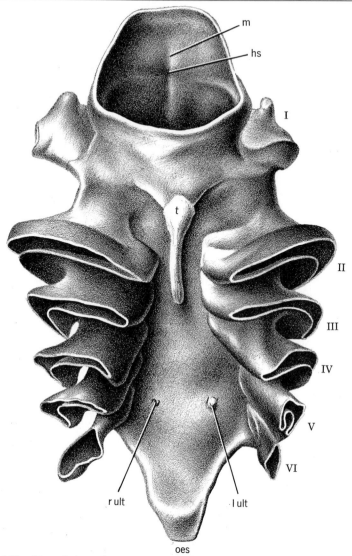

FIGURE 6.11. Ventral view of a wax reconstruction of the pharynx of a *Squalus* embryo 33.1 mm long. The gill pouches have been partly cut off. *m*, mouth; *hs*, base of hypophyseal stalk; *I* to *VI*, first to sixth gill pouches; *t*, thyroid; *r ult*, right ultimobranchial body; *l ult*, left ultimobranchial body; *oes*, esophagus. [After W. E. Camp, *J. Morphol.*, **28**:369, 1917.]

polarized, the nucleus in each moving to a basal position (Fig. 6.12). Intracellular droplets of colloidlike material may then be found. Finally, by release of these droplets, extracellular colloid and typical follicles are formed.

In the petromyzontid cyclostomes (lampreys) is found the most unusual pattern of thyroidal embryology. Here the thyroidal anlage forms from a long segment of the groove that lies in the midventral part of the pharynx.

Between the levels of the second to fifth branchial arches, this region is isolated and enclosed by horizontal shelflike growths from in front, from behind, and from both sides of the groove. In this way a tubular structure, the subpharyngeal gland, is formed, and a duct, which ultimately opens into the pharyngeal floor at the level of the fifth visceral arch, is differentiated.

The broad derivation of the thyroid anlage of lampreys contrasts with its restricted origin from the pharyngeal floor of all other vertebrates. By differential growth of the epithelial lining of the subpharyngeal gland, the originally simple cylinder is converted into a relatively complex structure (Fig. 6.13). The epithelium differentiates into a variety of types of cells, some of them ciliated and some not (Fig. 6.14). Most lampreys remain larvae for at least five or six years, and during this entire time the subpharyngeal gland differentiates no further. At the time of metamorphosis, some of the epithelial cellular types degenerate and others, to varying degrees, are rounded up into follicles to form the adult thyroid gland. Although there may be some variation in different species of lampreys, one ciliated type (*III* in Fig. 6.14) appears to be the principal cellular source of adult thyroid tissue. It is of interest that this type of subpharyngeal glandular cell is able to metabolize iodine all through the long period of larval life (Fig. 6.14), and it contains thyroglobulin, the characteristic protein of thyroid cells that is utilized in the synthesis of thyroid hormone (Fig. 6.15). Accordingly, it has a thyroidlike function even in the embryo. These thyroid-active cells are part of an exocrine gland in the larva. Not until metamorphosis is this primitive exocrine "thyroid" gland converted to an endocrine gland by closure of the duct. These facts are part of the basis for speculations concerning the evolution of the thyroid gland. The problem will be considered at a later point in this chapter.

Association of Thyroid and Branchiogenic Organs: An Embryological Problem

The thyroid gland is frequently associated intimately in adult mammals with structures of lateral pharyngeal origin in the embryo. These include the thymus, parathyroids, and ultimobranchial organs. In the fishes and amphibians there appears to be no tendency to such close association. In cyclostomes and higher fishes, for example, the thymic tissue remains close to the dorsal wings of the pharyngeal pouches, and there is no readily identifiable parathyroid tissue.

Ultimobranchial tissue, as the name implies, is derived in the embryo of fishes from the last pharyngeal pouches (Fig. 6.11), and it migrates backward to a position over the pericardium. Here it forms irregular follicular tissue whose function is to form the hormone calcitonin, a calcium-regulating factor. Functions of the parathyroid and ultimobranchial glands will be taken up in Chapter 7.

In amphibians, parathyroids form from the ventral wings of the third and

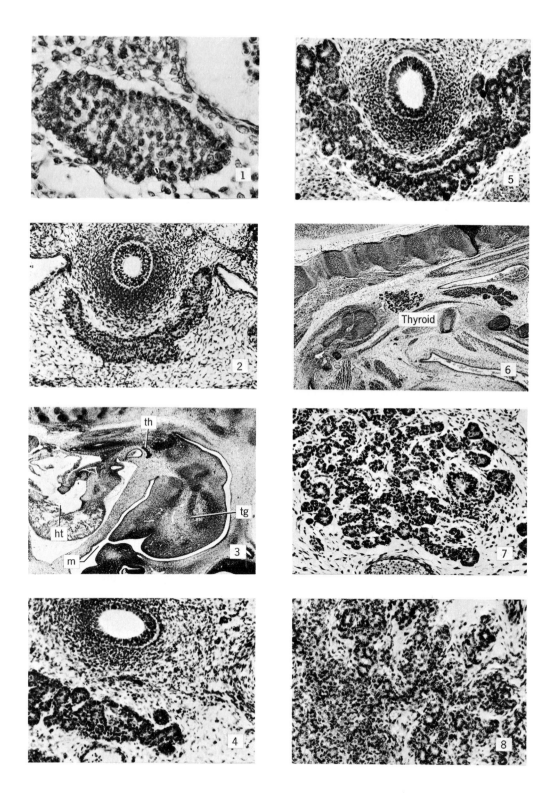

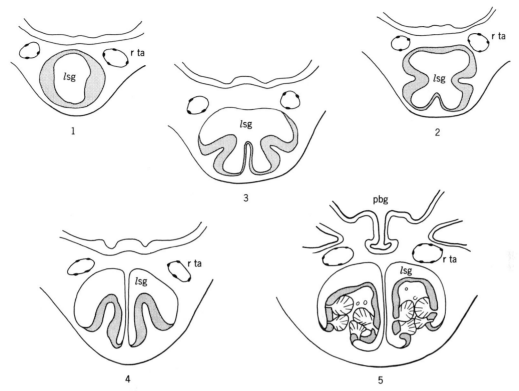

FIGURE 6.13. Cross sections through equivalent regions of the developing subpharyngeal gland of lamprey (*Lampetra planeri*) larvae (ammocoetes). (*1*) Subpharyngeal gland of a 5-mm embryo; (*2*) 6-mm embryo: two glandular lamellae arising from lateral walls and septum from ventral wall; (*3*) 6.3-mm embryo: further growth of septum and lamellae; (*4*) 7.2-mm embryo: completion of septum, dividing the single lumen longitudinally into two; (*5*) fully differentiated subpharyngeal gland: gland cylinders have formed within the lamellae, and the epithelium over the lamellae has differentiated into the cellular types illustrated in Fig. 6.14. *lsg*, Lumen of subpharyngeal gland; *pbg*, pseudobranchial groove; *rta*, right truncus arteriosus. [Adapted from G. Sterba, *Wiss. Ztschr. Friedr.-Schiller Univ.*, 1953.]

FIGURE 6.12. Typical states in the development of the rabbit's thyroid (gestation period, 35 days). (*1*) Gland at 12 days of gestation. The thyroglossal duct has disappeared. The only differentiation in the primordium is a first indication of its future bilobed shape. (*2*) Cross section of the thyroidal primordium at 14 days. Above it is the circular trachea in cross section. (*3*) Lower magnification of the thyroid at 14 days; sagittal view, region of the heart. *th*, Thyroid; *ht*, heart; *tg*, tongue; *m*, mouth. (*4*) Cross section of a portion of a 15-day thyroid. This is the earliest stage to show ^{131}I accumulation. Cells are arranged in cords and plates, but follicles are beginning to form. (*5*) Cross section of the thyroid of a 16-day fetus partly enveloping the trachea. Follicular differentiation is well started. (*6*) Low-power view of a parasagittal section of a 17-day thyroid. At this stage the thyroid produces radioautographs. (*7*) Higher magnification of a 17-day thyroid. (*8*) Portion of a 19-day fetal thyroid. [From A. J. Waterman in *Comparative Endocrinology* (A. Gorbman, ed.), Wiley, New York, 1959.]

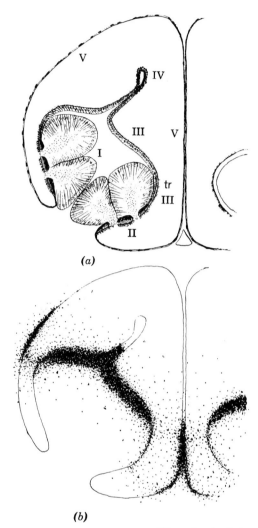

(a)

(b)

FIGURE 6.14. (a) Cross section of one-half of the differentiated subpharyngeal gland (endostyle) of an ammocoete of the brook lamprey. Over the glandular lamella is a ciliated epithelium; within it are four cylindrical glandular masses (type *I* cells) that secrete a mucoid substance. The covering epithelium is differentiated into morphologically different cell types (*II, III, tr III, IV*), and a squamous epithelium covers the remaining surface (type *V*). This animal was injected with radioiodine, and a piece of X-ray film was placed in contact with this section. When the film was developed, a black exposed area was found on it (a radioautograph). (b) Radioautograph made by *a* projected onto a tracing of the section. It appears, by such matching, that the cell types *III, tr III*, and *V* are able to accumulate ^{131}I in organic form in a "thyroidlike" manner. [From A. Gorbman and C. W. Creaser, *J. Exp. Zool.*, **89**:391, 1942.]

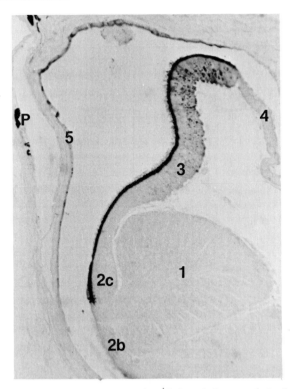

FIGURE 6.15.   Photograph of a part of a section of the subpharyngeal gland after "staining" by use of an antibody to mammalian thyroglobulin. The antibody-staining reaction is strongest in the type *3* cells and in the dorsal (labeled *2c*) type *2* cells (see also Fig. 6.14), and weak in the type *5* cells. These are also the cells that accumulate radioiodine and contribute to forming the adult thyroid follicles. In the type *3* cells there are large droplets of thyroglobulin within the cells, but in all three cell types most of the thyroglobulin is located near or at the apex (outer part) of the cell. *P* indicates a melanin pigment-containing cell, which should not be confused with the immunostained thyroglobulin. Magnification: 312 ×. [Photograph supplied by Dr. Glenda M. Wright from a doctoral thesis, University of Calgary.]

fourth pharyngeal pouches (Fig. 6.16). They do not migrate far and remain in the hyoid area near but separate from the thyroids. Ultimobranchial tissue, as in the fishes, becomes located near or on the pericardium (Fig. 6.17).

Reptilian ultimobranchial tissue behaves essentially as it does in fishes and amphibians; thymic tissue and the parathyroids, since they are derived from the dorsal and ventral parts of the lateral wings of the same visceral pouch, may remain attached for some time, and are thus closely associated in the posterior subpharyngeal region even in the adult. However, although it is exceptional, the thymus may be found embedded in the thyroid glands of certain species of reptiles.

In birds the thyroid remains free of direct contact with lateral pharyngeal structures (Figs. 6.9 and 7.6), but in mammals such an association is general.

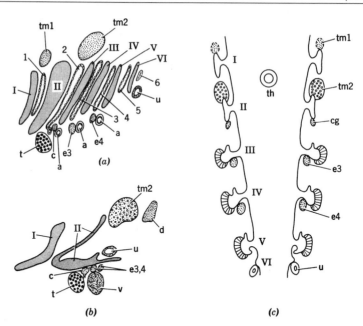

FIGURE 6.16. Diagrams summarizing the derivation of various glandular structures from the pharynx of the frog. (*a*) Lateral view, tadpole stage. Visceral arches (*I, II, III, IV, V, VI*) are shown as solid. Visceral pouches (*1, 2, 3, 4, 5, 6*) are shown as elongated spaces between the arches. Thymic lobes are dorsal to the pouches from which they take origin (*1* and *2*). Thyroid, parathyroids, carotid body, ultimobranchial body, and aortic arches are below the pharynx. (*b*) Lateral view, after metamorphosis. Dorsally, only *thymus 2* plus the ''dorsal gill remainder'' or dorsal *Kiemenrest* are left. Ventrally, the thyroid, parathyroids, carotid body, ultimobranchial body, and ventral gill remainder (ventral *Kiemenrest*) can be seen in the adult arrangement. Compare with Fig. 6.8. (*c*) Summary of the derivatives of the branchial pouches of the frog without indication of whether they are dorsal or ventral. *a*, Branchial arteries in cross section; *c*, carotid gland; *d*, dorsal *Kiemenrest*, or gill remainder; *e*, parathyroid glands; *t*, thyroid; *tm*, thymus; *u*, ultimobranchial body; *v*, ventral *Kiemenrest*, or gill remainder. [Based on Greil's modifications of Maurer's drawings, *Anat. Hefte*, 1905; taken from R. S. McEwen, *A Textbook of Vertebrate Embryology*, rev. ed., Holt, Rinehart & Winston, New York, 1931.]

Furthermore, it appears to be normal among mammals for the ultimobranchial tissue to become so closely integrated with the median thyroid anlage (Fig. 6.18) that there is difficulty in distinguishing one from the other. It has been claimed that the active thyroid tissue ''induces'' the ultimobranchial tissue to differentiate into a form like its own. Exceptional instances have been found in human pathology in which there was failure of contact between the median thyroid and the ultimobranchial tissue. In such cases the ultimobranchial tissue differentiates in an unusual morphological pattern. Furthermore, in rats or mice whose thyroid function is reduced experimentally or during normal aging, there is a ''dedifferentiation'' of the ultimobranchial zone of the thyroid.

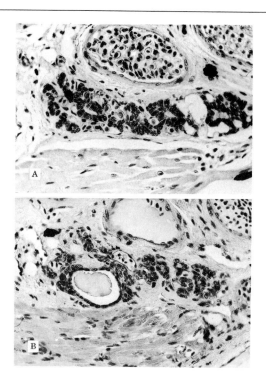

FIGURE 6.17. (*A*) Ultimobranchial tissue of the normal salamander *Triturus viridescens*. It is made up of follicular and cordlike groups of cells. (*B*) Ultimobranchial tissue of a salamander 21 days after hypophysectomy. Most of the organ is not very different from normal. In some thyroidlike follicles (one is shown), however, there is an accumulation of colloid and lowering of epithelial cell height. It is not known whether the effect on epithelial height is a direct response to the hypophysectomy or is merely due to stretching by the accumulating colloid. [From H. Steinitz and L. S. Stone, *Anat. Record,* **120:**435, 1954.]

Occasionally, the duct which originally joined the ultimobranchial body to the last pharyngeal pouch persists in mice (Fig. 6.19), so that in the adult there is a tubular connection from the thyroid to the *lateral* pharynx. Ultimobranchial follicles in adult thyroids often may be distinguished histologically from median thyroid tissues, since their epithelium may be stratified or, in some species, ciliated (Fig. 6.18). It is interesting that ultimobranchial follicles in adult mice, recognizable by their ciliated epithelium, do not metabolize iodine. Ultimobranchial tissue of the embryo, in addition to forming visibly differentiated follicular structures in mammalian thyroids, may also form nonfollicular and interfollicular structures. Such scattered or clumped cells are usually designated as "C cells." By use of immunocytochemical techniques, they have been shown to contain calcitonin, a hormone that will be treated in more detail in the following chapter.

It has been noted that, in mammals, intimate association between the ultimobranchial pouches and median thyroid is the rule. Other lateral pharyngeal derivatives show the same tendency to become entangled with thyroid tissue. The mammalian parathyroid glands typically remain upon the surface, or they may become deeply embedded within the thyroid. Thymic tissue is often, but much less typically, attached to the median thyroid. An interesting embryonic anomaly persisting in the adult is a cyst (often ciliated)

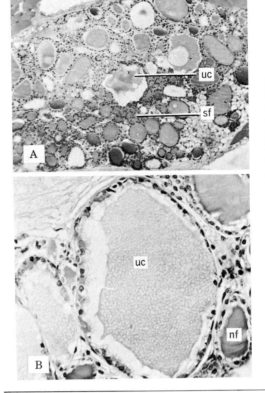

FIGURE 6.18. (*A*) Section through the thyroid gland of a C57-strain adult mouse. At the center and to the upper right of center are two irregularly shaped follicles, the primary ultimobranchial centers. Immediately below and to the right of the central one is a cluster of very small "satellite" follicles. Below the primary ultimobranchial follicles and their satellites are dark-staining follicles with heavily staining colloid. Above them are larger, lighter follicles. The upper light follicles metabolize radioiodine; the primary ultimobranchials and satellites do not. The small, dark follicles metabolize ^{131}I weakly. (*B*) A primary ultimobranchial follicle in the mouse showing the granular colloid and heteromorphic epithelium, partly composed of ciliated cells. *nf*, Normal follicle; *uc*, primary ultimobranchial follicle; *sf*, satellite follicle.

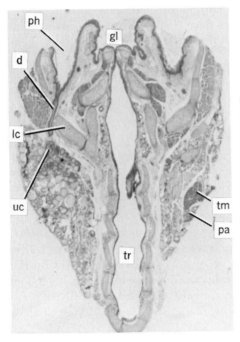

FIGURE 6.19. Frontal section of the trachea, posterior pharynx, and two thyroid glands of an I-strain mouse. Extending from the left posterior angle (piriform fossa) of the pharynx (*ph*) is a duct (*d*) that penetrates a laryngeal cartilage (*lc*) and ends in the thyroid in a series of primary ultimobranchial follicles (*uc*). (See Fig. 6.18.) These follicles blend in with the normal ones. In the right thyroid there are large ultimobranchial follicles, visible in the center, and a large mass of thymus (*tm*) and parathyroid (*pa*) tissue in the surface of the gland. *tr*, Trachea. The persisting duct is a rare developmental anomaly and represents the retention of the embryonic connection between the ultimobranchial body and the fourth pharyngeal pouch.

connecting the thymus to parathyroid and thyroid glands. This cyst, when found in the mouse, represents the lateral wing of the original pharyngeal pouch III.

THYROID HISTOLOGY AND CYTOLOGY

As has been mentioned before, the thyroid gland is the only vertebrate alveolar endocrine organ. Its follicles are lined by a simple epithelium, and each follicular lumen is filled with a coagulable fluid, called the "colloid." The colloid is the site of storage of a protein-bound form of the thyroid hormone, so that this gland is also unique in having the only extracellular storage of hormone within the gland. As will be discussed presently, the colloid may also be the site of at least part of the synthesis of thyroid hormone.

The epithelium is capable of extreme variation in shape within the same species and within the same thyroid gland in differing physiological states. A thyroid follicular epithelium composed of low squamous cells is associated with reduced function. A taller, columnar epithelium is most usually found in a very active gland (Fig. 6.1). Characteristic changes in the colloid may also be associated with different stages of function. A densely staining, uniformly eosinophilic colloid is found next to the squamous epithelium. The colloid of active glands is nonuniform, may be basophilic in part, and usually contains numerous nonstaining, vacuolelike spaces. It has been claimed that the "vacuoles" are artifacts arising from poor fixation. If this is so, then they are artifacts of such regular occurrence that their presence is as good a diagnostic feature as we have of glandular activation. The vacuoles, in fact, may indicate a high level of proteolytic release of thyroid hormone from the protein to which it is bound.

Cytological features, too, can be used as criteria of activity in the thyroid cell. The size of the Golgi apparatus and the number of mitochondria, in general, parallel functional activity. The number of secretion droplets in the cells also is a good index, and it has been suggested as the basis of a sensitive test for TSH.

By the use of electron microscopy, additional information has been made available. The thyroidal cytoplasm, in addition to the usual features such as endoplasmic reticulum and mitochondria, contains a larger than usual variety of granules of different sizes and densities (Figs. 6.20 and 6.21). Interpretation of the functions of these granules was at first difficult, but gradually, by combining electron micrographic information with that from timing of biochemical events and by timed autoradiography of radioiodine (Fig. 6.22), some understanding has resulted. Some of the granules are formed in the Golgi apparatus and contain newly synthesized thyroglobulin. Such granules move to the apical membrane (next to the follicle lumen) and discharge their content into the lumen by a process of exocytosis (i.e., by

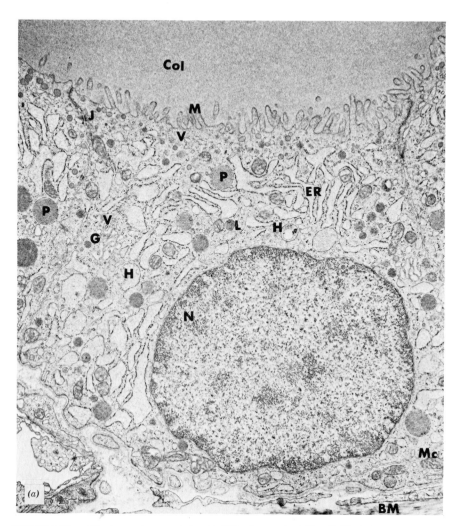

FIGURE 6.20a. Electron micrograph (× 11,000) of a rat thyroid cell. There is one complete cell in this field, from the apical surface above, bearing microvilli (*M*) and facing the colloid-filled lumen (*Col*) to the irregular basal surface at the basal membrane (*BM*). The cell-to-cell junctional apparatus (*J*) is labeled at the left, but is visible on the right edge as well. The nucleus (*N*) occupies a large fraction of the cell volume. Droplets (*V*) containing thyroglobulin (synthesized in the endoplasmic reticulum) are considered to be formed in the golgi apparatus (*G*) and released to the colloid by exocytosis at the apical cell membrane. Colloid taken in at the apical surface forms large droplets or phagosomes (*P*). These fuse with lysosomes (*L*) to form heterosomes (*H*), which leads to proteolysis and release of hormones. *ER*, Rough endoplasmic reticulum; *Mc*, mitochondrion. [Photograph provided by Dr. S. H. Wollman.]

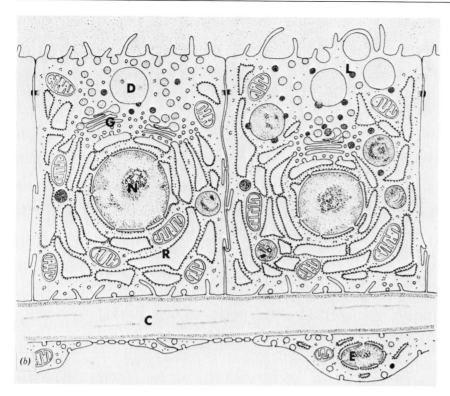

FIGURE 6.20b. Drawing of two mammalian thyroid follicular cells to further illustrate and clarify details in Fig. 6.20A. In the cell at the left emphasis is placed on the numerous, newly synthesized, small thyroglobulin-containing vacuoles that are moving from the Golgi region (G) toward the colloid surface of the cell above. Note the numerous small indentations of the apical cell surface between the microvilli, where exocytosis is taking place. In the cell at the right emphasis is placed on phagocytosis of colloid and events that follow. Note the large, phagocytosed vacuole that has just formed at the cell surface, and another below it and just to the right; a phagosome that has just fused with a lysosome (L) is shown in the left cell (labeled D). One just like it is shown unlabeled in the right cell in the same approximate location. In the right cell heterosomes with irregular structures, in various degrees of structural change, are shown deeper in the cell. Below the cells is the collagenous, fibrous basement membrane (C) and a blood capillary space lined by endothelium (E). [Drawing provided by Professor Hisao Fujita, Osaka University.]

fusion of their surrounding membranes with the plasma membrane). This process *adds* to the amount of plasma membrane. Other large granules, sometimes called "colloid droplets," are formed by endocytosis of colloid from the lumen. In this process apical cytoplasmic "pseudopods" extend into the lumen, surround a small bit of colloid and draw it into the cell in a manner resembling phagocytosis. This process *decreases* the total amount of plasma membrane. Pseudopod formation and endocytosis has been observed to be a rapid response by thyroid cells to injection of TSH. The

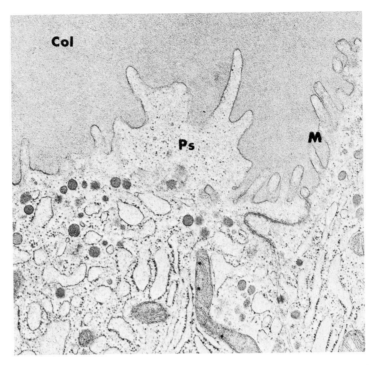

FIGURE 6.21. Electron micrograph ($\times$ 18,700) of the apical end of a rat thyroid cell showing a "pseudopod" presumably engulfing some colloid from the follicular lumen and in the process of forming a phagosome. The small, dark vacuoles—most numerous at the left, close to the cell membrane—are colloid vesicles that will be emptied into the colloid by exocytosis. *Col*, colloid in the follicular lumen; *M*, microvilli, *Ps*, pseudopodium. [Photograph provided by Dr. S. H. Wollman.]

cytoplasmic colloid droplets fuse with the so-called dense granules, which are believed to contain lysosomal proteolytic enzyme. After fusion with the lysosomes, the large granules develop an irregular heterogeneous appearance. It is presumed that proteolytic digestion of the iodinated thyroglobulin occurs at this point in the large droplets. This releases the hormone from protein bondage, and freed hormone can diffuse out of the cell. These details of the thyroid secretory cycle are illustrated, at least in part, in Figs. 6.20 through 6.23.

In the following part of this chapter the chemical events in the formation of thyroid hormone will be considered. It will be necessary to correlate them with the thyroidal cytological cycle just described. Among the interesting problems that must be taken up is the place in the cell where iodination of thyroglobulin takes place. Another morphofunctional question is where the digestion of thyroglobulin takes place. From the description above, it would appear to be intracellular, occurring within the large colloid droplets after

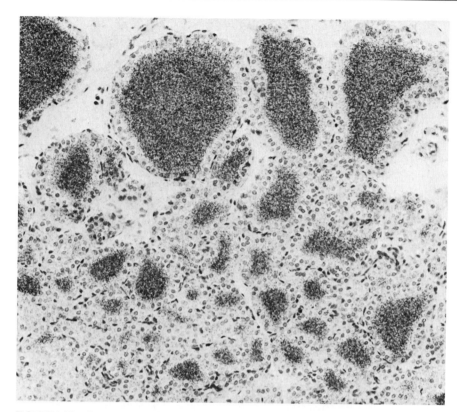

FIGURE 6.22. Rat thyroid follicles after 99 days of daily feeding of radioiodine [125]I. The larger dark granular areas (not to be confused with the stained, rounded small cell nuclei) show the distribution of organically bound radioiodine (by this time, the equilibrium of radioiodine and stable iodine may be assumed). Most of the bound radioiodine is in the follicular lumens. Some is in the cells (compare the granularity of the cytoplasm with that where no cells are located, as near the top of the photo). The luminal radioiodine may be taken to represent hormone stored in thyroglobulin. The much smaller amount of radioiodine in the cytoplasm may be taken to represent thyroglobulin in phagosomes taken from the colloid and on the way to secretion. Magnification 230 ×. [Photograph provided by Dr. S. H. Wollman.]

fusion with the lysosomes. However, there is some evidence that proteolytic enzyme can be secreted into the follicular lumen, and a certain amount of proteolysis can take place in the lumen itself.

The descriptive histology of most vertebrate thyroid glands falls within the limits defined so far in this discussion. However, certain unusual structures have been described and should be mentioned here. For example, Cowdry has observed that the thyroidal epithelium of certain elasmobranch fishes is flagellated. In the follicles of young adult lampreys, cytological remnants of subpharyngeal glandular ciliated structures have been found (Fig. 6.23). These include basal granules and the yellow- or orange-colored

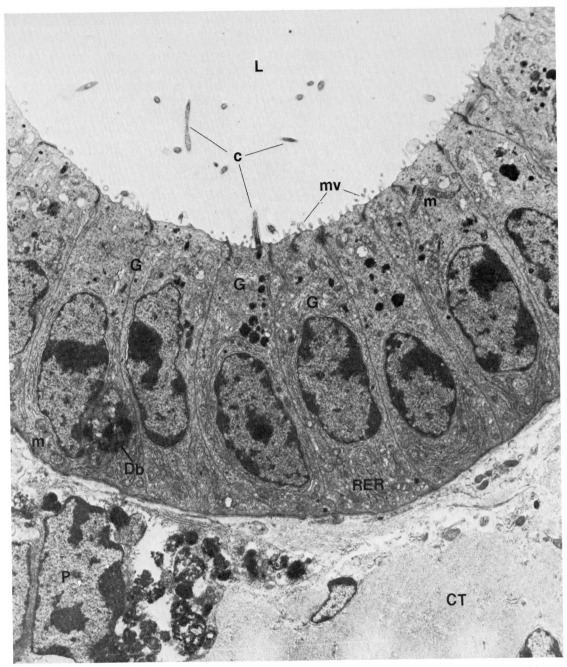

FIGURE 6.23. Part of a thyroid follicle of the adult lamprey *Petromyzon marinus*. This may be compared with the ultrastructure of the mammalian (Figs. 6.20 and 6.21) thyroid cells. A variety of granules do not show well at this magnification (5000 ×), but a large, dense-body heterosome (*Db*) is shown. *mv*, Microvilli; *G*, Golgi; *c*, cilia; *m*, mitochondria; *RER*, rough endoplasmic reticulum; *CT*, connective tissue. [Photograph provided by Dr. Glenda M. Wright from a doctoral thesis, University of Toronto.]

granules that are typical of the type III cells of the subpharyngeal gland. Earlier in this chapter it was mentioned that those parts of the adult mammalian thyroid that are derived from the ultimobranchial component in the embryo may differ histologically from the rest of the thyroid. Ultimobranchial-derived follicles may have a stratified squamous epithelium in some mammals and a ciliated epithelium in others. In the mouse (Fig. 6.18) there is usually a primary ultimobranchial follicle whose epithelium contains, alternately, ciliated and nonciliated cells. Around this is a group of satellite follicles lined with squamous cells. They are not otherwise distinguishable from normal thyroid follicles, yet they do not metabolize iodine as do normal follicles.

Nonfollicular ("parafollicular") thyroid C cells of mammals are now generally considered to be ultimobranchial-derived calcitonin-secreting cells. However, interfollicular thyroid cells have been described in many species of lower vertebrates. In such species there usually is a separate ultimobranchial gland that could not have contributed cells to the thyroid gland.

Cyclic Changes in Thyroid Morphology

Using the cytological and histological criteria of functional activity that have been mentioned (epithelial cell height, "vacuolization" of colloid, basophilia of colloid, number of secretion droplets or mitochondria, size of the Golgi apparatus, weight of the entire gland), many examples now have been found of regular cycles in the thyroid gland. However, in most cases these observations have only opened problems, not answered them. For example, in the life cycle of the salmon hypertrophy of the thyroid has been found at the time the young "parr" transforms into the "smolt," which is the migratory form that travels downstream to the ocean. It is tempting to assign to the thyroid hormone a causal role in precipitating the anatomic, physiological, and behavioral changes that result in successful migration, and many biologists have succumbed to the temptation. However, the fact remains that migration and thyroid hyperplasia are only two of many simultaneous events occurring in salmon at this phase of the life cycle. To assume that these two out of the many changes are directly related is not scientifically permissible without further experimental evidence. There is much left to learn of the relation of the thyroid to the phenomenon of migration in populations of fishes and of birds.

This correlation, incompletely understood though it may be, is perhaps better established than the relation of thyroidal hyperplasia to "metamorphosis" (eel, herring), and to gonadal activity (*Misgurnus, Rhodeus, Phoxinus*) found in other fishes. In some forms there is an apparently negative correlation between thyroidal and gonadal activity. This has been claimed in the pigeon, the frog, and certain lizards. Other functional correlations, positive or negative, that have been found include molting in a variety of vertebrates (amphibians, reptiles, and birds) and hibernation. Heightened thyroid activity is characteristic of periods of pregnancy and lactation in mammals and brooding activity in birds.

In general, the thyroid of poikilothermic vertebrates shows all the histological signs of low activity in the cold months and of maximum activity in the warmer months. It is interesting that hibernating mammals (hedgehog, marmot, ground squirrel) have a similar thyroidal cycle. Other warm-blooded vertebrates (squirrel, merino sheep, fox) have relatively active thyroids in the cold months. In domesticated homoiotherms such as the sheep, cat, and guinea pig—perhaps because they are protected from environmental extremes—these tendencies are less clear.

FUNCTION OF THE THYROID GLAND: THE METABOLISM OF IODINE

The special function of the thyroid gland, stated simply, is the accumulation of iodine and its union with tyrosine to form the thyroid hormone. This process appears to be, in at least several of its phases, under the control of the thyrotropic hormone of the pituitary (TSH). The various steps in the genesis of thyroid hormone are summarized diagrammatically in Fig. 6.24.

Iodide Accumulation

The first and perhaps the most important step is the accumulation of diffusible iodide. The degree of this accumulation can be measured as the ratio of the concentration of iodide in the thyroid to that in blood serum, i.e., the T/S ratio. A T/S ratio of about 25 is usual in rats. After stimulation by TSH, the ratio may increase to a value as high as 500 or more. The most reasonable interpretation of the mechanism of iodide accumulation is that it involves a transcellular active transport system ("iodide pump"). In fishes there is no clear evidence for a thyroid iodide pump, and relatively low T/S ratios have been found.

Consistent with the transport or "pump" hypothesis is the fact that the mechanism may be poisoned by certain anions, such as thiocyanate, perchlorate, nitrite, and periodate. In the presence of small concentrations of these inhibitors, the mammalian T/S ratio falls to a value of close to 1.0.

The thyroidal transport of iodide is an action of prime importance, making possible the efficient and rapid synthesis of thyroxine, but it is not limited to the thyroid gland. Marine plants, particularly red and brown algae, accumulate iodides, as well as other halides, and they manufacture a small amount of iodotyrosine. In the anterior digestive tract the chloride cells of the gills, the salivary glands, and the gastric glands also have this property. Furthermore, the mammary gland and the kidney are known to participate in halide (including iodide) transport. The notochord of lampreys has also been found able to accumulate high ratios of iodide in comparison with blood serum. Most of these halide-transporting tissues have been tested in the

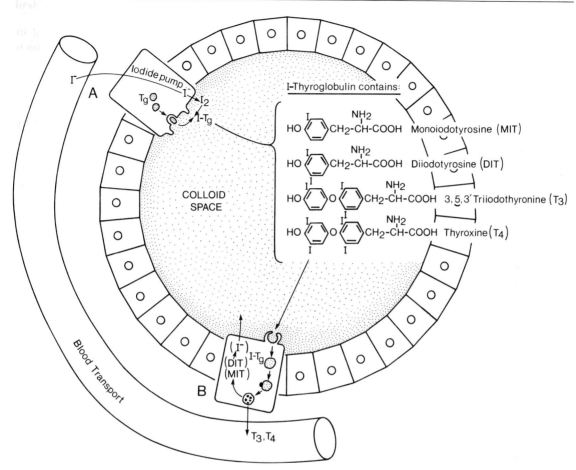

FIGURE 6.24. Diagrammatic summary of the biochemical events in the synthesis of thyroid hormone. A thyroid follicle is shown adjacent to a blood capillary. Two cells, *A* and *B*, are shown enlarged. Although the earlier events in thyroxinogenesis are shown in *A* and later events are shown in *B*, all events may occur simultaneously in each cell. In *A* the iodide pump and the synthesis and exocytosis of thyroglobulin are illustrated. The reentry of thyroglobulin (now iodinated) into the cell by endocytosis, the fusion of the resulting organelle with a lysosome, and the consequent liberation of iodotyrosines (MIT, DIT) and iodothyronines (T_3, T_4) from the iodothyroglobulin are illustrated in *B*.

presence of thiocyanate and are inhibited by it. In the only instance of nonthyroidal iodide accumulation, in the notochord, a thyroidlike discharge of accumulated iodide is produced by thiocyanate. Thus thyroidal iodide transport and retention is a property that is far from unique.

Because ^{131}I makes possible sensitive and precise studies of thyroxinogenesis, it has been used with interesting results in the study of embryonic thyroid function. Embryonic thyroxinogenesis will be discussed at greater length later, but it is significant at this point to mention that at least in some species thyroid function develops in steps or stages. It seems clear that in both chick and rabbit embryos there is an "iodide" stage during which mineral iodide is accumulated but no organic iodine is formed.

Organic Compounds of Iodine and Their Formation

Historical Background. Organically bound iodine was first described by Andrew Fife, in 1819, in gorgonian corals only eight years after the discovery of the element iodine by Courtois. In succeeding years much information was collected concerning the occurrence and concentration of iodine in plants, invertebrate animals, and in natural waters. Because the first separated iodoprotein came from gorgonians, it was called iodogorgonine. Hydrolysis of iodogorgonine by Drechsel in 1896 yielded diiodotyrosine, which was named at the time iodogorgoic acid (Table 6.1). In light of the relatively vast amount of information now available about thyroidal biochemistry, it seems remarkable that iodine was not discovered in the thyroid gland itself until 1896 by Baumann.

The beneficial effects of feeding burnt seaweed or sponge to humans afflicted with goiter, a thyroid deficiency disease, are said to have been known since the 12th century both in Oriental and European cultures. However, attribution of the beneficial effects to the iodine content of these prep-

TABLE 6.1. Organic Iodine Compounds in the Thyroid Gland

Iodogorgoic acid or diiodotyrosine, (DIT)

Monoiodotyrosine (MIT)

3, 5, 3', 5'-Tetraiodothyronine or thyroxine, (Tx or T_4)

3, 5, 3'-Triiodothyronine (T_3)

arations was not possible until more precise chemical information became available.

Separation of the thyroidal iodoprotein, thyroglobulin, by Oswald came in 1899. E. C. Kendall, 1915, reported the crystallization of thyroxine from hydrolyzed thyroglobulin. However, the final elucidation of the molecular structure of thyroxine and its synthesis were described in papers published in 1926 and 1927 by C. R. Harington, and by Harington and G. Barger. The later authors took note of the presence of diiodotyrosine in thyroid hydrolysates and suggested that thyroxine was formed by condensation of two molecules of diiodotyrosine, with the elimination of an alanine (CH_3CHNH_2COOH) residue (Fig. 6.25).

Iodination of Protein. The radioactive isotopes of iodine, principally ^{131}I, first became available for biochemical research in 1938 and 1939. The great mushrooming of research concerned with thyroidal iodine metabolism and hormonal synthesis in recent years was made possible by using these isotopes as "tracers" or "labels" to indicate with great precision the rates and qualitative and quantitative aspects of the reactions involved.

Within a period of less than one minute after injection of radioactive iodide into a rat, it can be found by autoradiographic techniques in a metabolized organic form in the thyroid colloid or near the apical plasma membrane of the thyroid cell. In thyroids of cold-blooded vertebrates this process is a little slower. The exact place where the iodination of thyroglobulin occurs has been impossible to decide because the precision of radioiodine localization is not quite sufficient to indicate whether it is just within the apical cellular membrane or just outside of it in the colloid space. The peroxidase enzyme, which is the probable agent for the oxidation of iodide

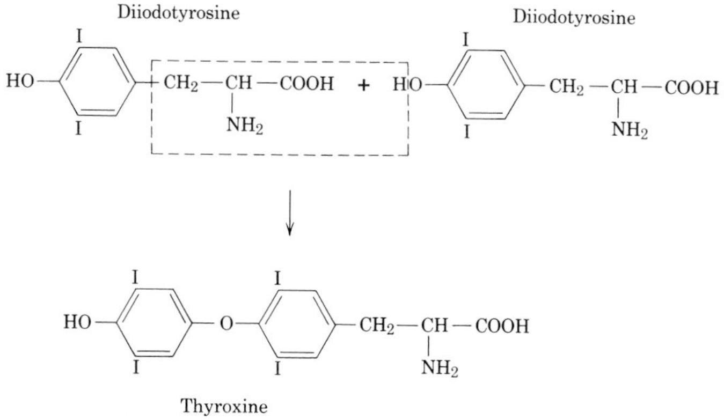

FIGURE 6.25. Formation of thyroxine by condensation of two diiodotyrosine molecules, according to the Harington hypothesis. However, it should be noted that within the thyroid gland the iodotyrosines are part of the thyroglobulin molecule, not free as shown here.

in order to make it reactive with thyroglobulin, is localized in the plasma membrane (Fig. 6.26), so that the iodination would seem to occur very close to the membrane, probably on the colloid side.

There are several other uncertainties concerning the process of thyroglobulin iodination, and among them is the chemical form of the iodine at the time when it is joined to the protein. Oxidation of iodide to molecular iodine through the action of the peroxidase is one possibility. However, if this were the process, there would most likely be more than one kind of iodoprotein in the thyroid, since molecular iodine will interact with tyrosine molecules of any protein. To provide more specificity to the thyroglobulin iodination process, it is proposed that iodide, oxidized to the iodinium (I^+) state, is

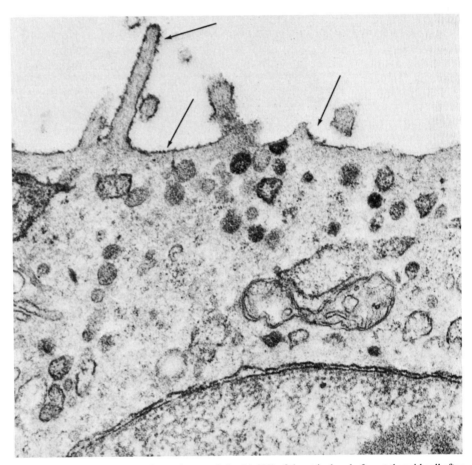

FIGURE 6.26. Electron photomicrograph ($\times$ 31,000) of the apical end of a rat thyroid cell after cytochemical staining for peroxidase activity. The enzyme reaction product is black. The heaviest deposition of peroxidase product is in the plasma membrane (arrows), the surface of microvilli (arrow), some apical vacuoles, and perhaps the nuclear membrane. [Photograph provided by S. H. Wollman.]

bound to the peroxide enzyme. In an extension of this mechanism, the oxidized iodine is carried on the enzyme as a radical, while another (specific) site on the enzyme interacts with tyrosine on the thyroglobulin, converting it to a radical. There would then follow an interaction between the two apposed radicals.

Whatever the precise mechanism may be, the result is a thyroglobulin molecule some of whose tyrosines bear one or two atoms of iodine (Fig. 6.4). Apparently not all the tyrosines of the thyroglobulin molecule are equally susceptible to iodination, and there is evidence that some tyrosines, which at first are not available for iodination, become available, or "exposed," as the molecule changes shape during the iodination process. As shown in Fig. 6.27 (an artificial situation in which casein is being iodinated), the relative amounts of monoiodotyrosine and diiodotyrosine in the protein change as the supply of iodine is increased. At lower iodine levels, monoiodotyrosine predominates; at higher levels, diiodotyrosine predominates. A similar relationship is found in the intact (in vivo) thyroid. At very high concentrations of iodine, the process of thyroglobulin iodination is actually inhibited (Wolff-Chaikoff effect), possibly through a direct action on the peroxidase system.

The coupling of iodotyrosine molecules in the manner shown in Fig. 6.25 yields iodothyronine compounds. Coupling apparently can occur between iodotyrosines on the same thyroglobulin molecules or on different molecules.

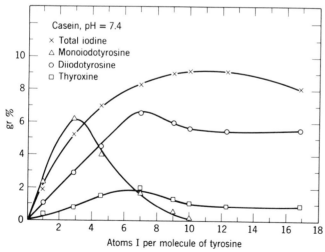

FIGURE 6.27. The relative yields of iodinated compounds when casein is incubated at 37°C with different molecular proportions of iodine. Total iodinated protein increases until a proportion of nine atoms of iodine per molecule of tyrosine (in the protein) is achieved. Increasing the proportion of iodine in the reacting mixture beyond this does not increase the iodination of protein. Other conclusions offered by these data are discussed in the text. [Adapted from R. Michel, Thesis, University of Paris, 1950.]

It is clear that some coupling, and thus hormone formation, will occur *in vitro* when a variety of proteins are subjected to iodination (Fig. 6.27). However, there is evidence that iodotyrosine coupling is much more efficient in the presence of enzymes extractable from thyroid tissue, especially peroxidase.

Iodine supply affects the relative proportions of tetraiodo- and triiodothyronine (T_4 and T_3), formed by coupling of iodotyrosines. As pointed out earlier, a lower availability of iodine leads to a greater proportion of monoiodotyrosine. Coupling of mono- and diiodotyrosine would be expected to be the mechanism for the formation of T_3. However, at still lower levels of iodine, thyroglobulin is increasingly poor in iodine. Under such circumstances, efficiency of coupling is greatly reduced and there is a greater-than-expected decrease in iodothyronine formation. Among other things, this would indicate that uniodinated tyrosines in thyroglobulin do not couple.

Iodination of Nonthyroidal Proteins. Studies of the *in vitro* iodination of proteins other than thyroglobulin were first carried out in 1939 by Ludwig and von Mutzenbecher. This work and experiments that followed have provided a very useful perspective on thyroidal iodination and the type of iodination of proteins that occurs in the invertebrates. It has been found that a maximum yield of thyroxine from casein is obtained when the protein is placed in an iodine solution containing six atoms of iodine for each molecule of tyrosine in the protein (Fig. 6.27). While the formation of mono- and diiodotyrosine is about equal at lower concentrations of iodine, at concentrations of more than three atoms of iodine per molecule of tyrosine diiodotyrosine is formed almost exclusively. This important fact will be referred to again. Furthermore, there is never a time in the reactions *in vivo* when only monoiodotyrosine is produced, as there is during incubation of cell-free thyroid fractions or in early chick embryo thyroids. Although there is a rough parallelism between the amount of tyrosine in a protein and its thyroxine-forming potency, there is by no means a strict relation between these two parameters (Table 6.2). In fact, thyroglobulin *in vitro* does not appear to be a particularly good thyroxine-forming protein. Its content of tyrosine is low when compared to casein, silk fibroin, and insulin. The fraction of its tyrosines that will form thyroxine when iodinated is lower than in casein (protein of milk) and zein (protein of corn) (Table 6.2). It is interesting that the tyrosines of silk fibroin, apparently because of the rigidity and fibrous shape of the protein molecule, are converted inefficiently to thyroxine.

Factors Affecting the Organic Phase of Iodine Metabolism

It is a fact that thyroid glands stimulated by hypophyseal TSH manufacture an increased amount of thyroxine. However, it is unclear whether this is merely one consequence of the more active accumulation of iodide or

TABLE 6.2. The yield of thyroxine obtained by iodination[a] of proteins and peptones.

Product Studied	Initial Tyrosine Content (%) A	Yield of Thyroxine After Iodination (%) B	Ratio $\dfrac{B \times 100}{A}$
Casein	7.20	1.65	22.3
Fibroin	12.00	0.40	3.3
Insulin	12.20	1.35	12.7
Thyroglobulin	3.30	0.68	20.6
Zein	5.84	1.61	27.5
Peptone of casein I	1.07	0.04	3.7
Peptone of casein II	2.70	0.14	5.2

[a] Six atoms of iodine were added for each calculated molecule of tyrosine. Method of Reineke and Turner, after Roche and Michel, *Recent Progr. Horm. Res.*, **12**:1 (1956).

whether TSH may affect also other rate-determining steps in the process of thyroxinogenesis.

Inhibition of the organic phase by a series of chemicals, on the other hand, is well established. These chemical inhibitors include excess iodide, *p*-aminobenzoic acid, sulfonamides, thioureas, thiouracils, and aminothiazoles (see Table 6.3). These antithyroid drugs differ from thiocyanate in that their inhibition of thyroxine synthesis is not overcome by additional iodide. Thus they interfere at a different level of iodine metabolism. Since they prevent the formation of iodotyrosines but permit iodide accumulation by the thyroid, they must block the formation of oxidized iodine. They produce this inhibition not only *in vivo*, but also in thyroid slices incubated *in vitro*.

TABLE 6.3. Antithyroid or goitrogenic substances

Thiourea   2-Mercapto-imidazole   *p*-Aminobenzoic acid

2-Thiouracil   2-Aminothiazole   Sulfonamides

In thyroid slices the inhibition of iodotyrosine formation occurs at antithyroid drug concentrations that have no effect on respiration of the slices. Most current evidence indicates that the antithyroid chemicals interfere with the peroxidase-catalyzed step in which iodine, in a form that is reactive with tyrosine, is produced.

THYROGLOBULIN

Thyroglobulin is the most abundant protein in the thyroid gland, and it is relatively easily purified. Its properties have been analyzed from numerous standpoints. It is a relatively large molecule with a molecular weight variously determined from 600,000 to 750,000; its isoelectric point is about 4.6. The amino acid content of thyroglobulin is unusual only in its rather high arginine content (12.7%). A carbohydrate is normally contained in thyroglobulin, and histochemical reagents that reveal glycoproteins (e.g., the periodic acid–Schiff or PAS reaction) strongly color the thyroid colloid. When thyroglobulin in hydrolyzed, the carbohydrate hexosamine is found among the products.

When mammalian thyroglobulin is processed in an ultracentrifuge, it separates into several fractions of different molecular size. These fractions are generally designated by their sedimentation rate constants as 5S (smallest), 12S, 19S, and 27S (largest). The most abundant fraction is the 19S form, which is the one whose molecular weight is generally given as 600,000. The 27S form appears to be a dimer (double molecule) of the 19S form. The smaller forms may be constituents of the 19S thyroglobulin, but they are not exact-multiple subunits of the 19S form. Furthermore, they are often less well iodinated than the 19S form. The predominant thyroprotein in all vertebrates is the 19S form, with the exception of the cyclostomes. In hagfishes the prevailing thyroprotein has a sedimentation constant of 3 to 8S. In younger larval lampreys the 3 to 8S iodoprotein is the most abundant. However, as the larva approaches metamorphosis, the proportion of 19S thyroglobulin increases, and in the adult lamprey, after metamorphosis, only 19S thyroglobulin is found.

Despite wide variations in thyroid function or in age, the physical properties of thyroglobulin are not much altered. Even the iodine and thyroxine contents of thyroglobulin may vary greatly without materially influencing the physical properties of the protein.

The iodine content of thyroglobulin has been found to range from less than 0.1% (goitrous states, low iodine diets) to 1.2% (in the fetal calf). The thyroxine content varies in a manner paralleling the total iodine content (Table 6.4) of the thyroglobulin. It is of interest that in all vertebrate thyroids suitably tested thyroxine contains 25 to 30% of the thyroidal iodine regardless of the total iodine level. An interesting and paradoxical fact illustrated in Table 6.4 is the lack of correspondence between iodine content in the thyroid

TABLE 6.4. The proportion of total iodine present as thyroxine in the thyroids of various vertebrates

Species	Mean Thyroid Weight (Mg)	Mean Total Iodine (Mg %)	Mean Thyroxine Iodine (Mg %)	Thyroxine as % of Total Iodine
Shark (*Squalus suckleyi*)	84	29	8	27.9 ± 0.5
Turtle (*Pseudemys scripta*)	173	126	41	31.8 ± 1.3
Chicken (white leghorn)	56	105	27	25.0 ± 0.7
Turkey	108	143	36	24.7 ± 0.7
Guinea pig	57	42	12	28.3 ± 1.2
Rabbit	133	50	15	28.9 ± 1.1
Dog	833	230	74	32.0 ± 0.6
Rat	26	41	12	29.3 ± 0.6
Horse	11200	75	23	29.6 ± 1.2
Cattle		128	41	31.6 ± 1.0
Sheep	977	133	40	29.7 ± 0.7

and its concentration in the environment in which an animal lives. The shark *Squalus*, for example, living in an iodine-rich environment, has only 29 mg% iodine in its thyroid; the freshwater turtle (*Pseudemys scripta troosti*) has 126 mg% iodine in its thyroid, even though it resides in an iodine-poor environment.

Thyroglobulin, because of its molecular size, cannot normally enter the blood from the lumen of the follicle. Furthermore, if it is injected into an animal, it is always antigenic, even in the homologous animal species. Certain chronic inflammatory diseases of the thyroid (Hashimoto's disease) have been supposed to be due to escape of small amounts of thyroglobulin from the thyroid and the development of circulating antibodies. Such auto-antibodies against thyroglobulin have been demonstrated in the blood sera of patients with chronic thyroid inflammations. The initial leakage of thyroglobulin past the follicular cell boundary could be caused by disease or by mechanical injury. Injury to thyroid tissue by large doses of radioiodine leads to the appearance of thyroglobulin in the blood.

PROTEOLYSIS AND DEHALOGENATION

Since the protein-bound thyroid hormone is imprisoned in the follicular colloid, it is necessary to split it from the thyroglobulin to make it diffusible. This is accomplished by proteolytic digestion. Cytologically this process is visible on electron micrographs in the fusion of iodothyroglobulin vacuoles within the thyroid cell with lysosomes. Presumably it is the proteolytic enzymes within the lysosomes that catalyze the complete hydrolysis of the thyroglobulin. Although several proteases now have been found in the thyroid, the principal enzyme is one that has maximum activity at pH 4.0. Proteases with such an acid optimum fall into the general class of tissue enzymes known as cathepsins. Thyroidal catheptic activity is increased by TSH treatment and decreased by hypophysectomy. Almost all studies of this protease have been made in mammals. However, even the subpharyngeal gland of the ammocoetes contains a protease with an optimal pH near 4.0. The actual digestion of the iodoproteins of the ammocoete, as suggested before, occurs in the intestine, and any released thyroid hormone must be absorbed there. It is interesting, therefore, that the thyroprotease whose presence is obligatory after the duct of the subpharyngeal gland closes is present long before it is needed.

It appears, then, that the hydrolysis of thyroglobulin must proceed at a given rate, largely under the control of the pituitary, which regulates the concentration of the digestive enzyme. If this is so, a small proportion of iodinated amino acids free of protein should be found in the thyroid gland. Analysis of butanol extracts of fresh thyroid shows that this is true, though usually less than 5% of the total thyroidal iodine is in the protein-free form (mono- and diiodotyrosine and thyroxine).

Of these three amino acids, only thyroxine is found in the peripheral blood in significant amounts. Until recently, the reason for the virtual absence of mono- and diiodotyrosine in the circulating blood of mammals was unknown. The discovery of an enzyme that specifically deiodinates mono- and diiodotyrosine but spares the iodothyronine compounds (thyroxine and triiodothyronine) provided an answer to the puzzle.

Thus, it would appear that protease releases all iodinated amino acids from thyroglobulin, but those that represent immature forms of the thyroid hormone are destroyed by the desiodase (known also as dehalogenase and deiodinase). The liberated iodide apparently returns to the pool and is reused in the thyroidal iodine cycle. The concentration of desiodase, like that of the thyroprotease, is under the control of TSH. The desiodase titer rises after TSH injection.

COMPARATIVE ASPECTS OF THYROXINOGENESIS

In a qualitative sense it seems quite clear that all vertebrates form and secrete comparable hormones from their thyroid glands, namely thyroxine and perhaps triiodothyronine (T_4 and T_3). Quantitatively also, most vertebrates are quite comparable in having approximately 1 to 5 μg of T_4 per 100 ml of blood. However, there are broad excursions from these norms representing fluctuations in environmental iodine supply as well as cyclic and seasonal events in the life patterns of particular species (e.g., hibernation, variation in abundance and kind of food, reproductive periods, temperature extremes, etc.). In fact, it is remarkable that blood plasma levels of thyroxine are as uniform as they are if we consider that there is enormous variation in the amount of iodine in the environment. For example, seawater fishes are exposed to about 60 μg/liter of iodine (as iodate and iodide), while freshwater fishes live in concentrations one-tenth to one-thousandth as high. In addition, we must remember that the level of T_4 in the blood is the resultant of several processes that add (glandular secretion) or remove (metabolism, urinary excretion, fecal elimination, tissue penetration) thyroxine from the blood (Fig. 6.28). Beyond this, species vary in the number of thyroxine-binding proteins that occur in the blood (from practically none to three or four). Such proteins, in theory, increase the capacity of the blood to hold thyroid hormones. Furthermore, species vary in the degree to which they convert T_4 to T_3 by removal of one atom of iodine in the peripheral tissues.

Finally, it must be clear that a continuously variable hypothalamic (TRH) and thyrotropic (TSH) set of controls is superimposed over all these factors. These factors have been best studied among the laboratory mammals and

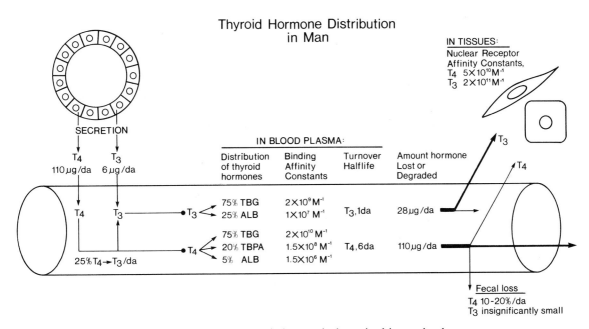

FIGURE 6.28. The distribution of thyroid hormones in humans is determined in part by the relative affinities of hormone-binding proteins in the plasma and tissues. Thyroxine-binding globulin (TBG) has a 10-fold higher affinity for T_4 than for T_3. Thyroxine-binding prealbumin (TBPA) binds T_4 but does not bind T_3. Serum albumin (ALB) binds T_3 more strongly than T_4, but the affinities of ALB are low for both hormones. The overall effect of thyroid hormone binding in blood plasma is a tendency for T_4 to remain in plasma, while T_3 is relatively free to penetrate the peripheral tissues. Thus the turnover of T_4 in blood plasma is six times slower than that of T_3. The binding affinity of T_3 for the nuclear receptor in tissues is 100 times that for TBG. This favors the movement of T_3 out of the plasma and into peripheral cells.

in humans. However, some interesting comparative data have been obtained from lower vertebrates, and these can be discussed at least briefly.

Iodine Turnover Rate

The simplest approach to the problem of the rate of hormonal production is to observe the speed with which a dose of ^{131}I, given as the iodide, enters the thyroid, accumulates to a peak value, and then leaves the gland in hormonal form. This may be accomplished by placing a radioactivity-counting device over the thyroid gland of an animal at specific intervals after injecting radioiodide; alternatively, this may be done by injecting a large number of animals with radioiodide, killing groups of them at intervals thereafter, and averaging the radioactivities found in individual thyroids at any time interval (Fig. 6.29).

In theory, any radioiodide injected into an animal at a certain time be-

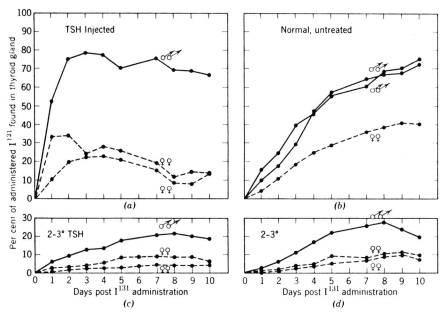

FIGURE 6.29A. Thyroidal accumulation of radioiodine in the terrapin turtle *Terrapene carolina* under different conditions. Each curve represents the record of the same turtle over a period of 10 days. Thyroidal radioactivity was measured *in vivo* by an external counting detector. In all instances it is clear that females are less active in this respect than males. The normal pattern (*b*) is a gradual thyroidal accumulation of the radioisotope for the full 10 days. This must mean that the iodine has not left the body (has not been excreted) during this time. TSH greatly accelerated thyroidal ^{131}I uptake, so that the same maximum was reached in 2 days. Low temperatures (2 to 3°C) greatly reduced ^{131}I uptake, and even TSH (*c*) could not stimulate it at this temperature. [From C. J. Shellabarger, A. Gorbman, F. Schatzlein, and D. McGill. *Endocrinology,* **59:**331, 1956.]

comes distributed within a short time to form a labeled part of all the iodine in the organism. The ^{131}I goes through all of the metabolic experiences of the total iodine, but it is always recognizable as the iodine that was introduced at a certain point in time. Therefore, radioiodinated tyrosine and thyroxine are dated in the sense that they can be distinguished from the unlabeled compounds that were present before.

Time curves, such as those in Figs. 6.29, 6.30, and 6.31, provide an estimation of the turnover rate in thyroidal iodine metabolism. The interpretation of these curves is complicated, since the labeled iodine enters the thyroid over a period of time but at a decreasing rate (much of the iodide is excreted). Furthermore, some of the hormone that leaves the gland is deiodinated, and its label returns to the thyroid. Finally, if the radioiodine is held in some tissue or organ other than the thyroid for a length of time, this further changes the picture.

Though they appear at first as annoying complexities, these are the actual factors in the iodine metabolism of the animal, and they will vary with the organism and its physiological and environmental conditions. For example, curve *b* in Fig. 6.29*B* (for the white-throated sparrow) is typical for many vertebrates, including mammals with active thyroids. There is a rapid period

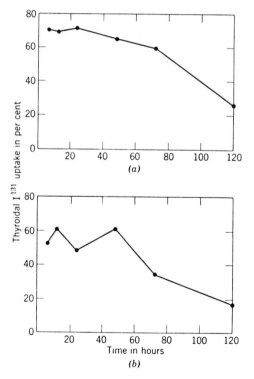

FIGURE 6.29*B*. Radioiodine accumulation in the thyroids of two species of birds, the weaver finch (*a*) and the white-throated sparrow (*b*), kept under similar circumstances in the laboratory. These records are unusual for vertebrates, because these two birds concentrate circulating ^{131}I very rapidly in their thyroids (60 to 70% within 6 hours) and then release it relatively slowly. The *apparently* slow release could be the result of the continuing return of ^{131}I to the thyroid from the tissues after hormone deiodination. [From O. Berg, A. Gorbman, and H. Kobayashi, *Comparative Endocrinology* (A. Gorbman, ed.), Wiley, New York, 1959.]

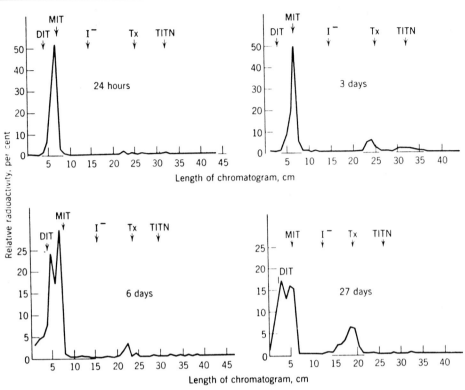

FIGURE 6.30. The chemical forms of ^{131}I in the thyroid gland of the turtle (*Pseudemys floridanus*) at various intervals after intraperitoneal injection of radioiodine. The graphs represent the relative radioactivity of spots on filter paper chromatograms that correspond to the various known iodine compounds: *DIT*, diiodotyrosine; *MIT*, monoidotyrosine; *I*⁻, iodide; *Tx*, thyroxine; *TITN*, triiodothyronine. It is clear that it requires a long time for radioiodine-labeled hormone to appear in significant quantity. [From C. J. Shellabarger, A. Gorbman, F. Schatzlein, and D. McGill, *Endocrinology* **59**, 1956.]

of uptake,* which reaches a peak value (in this instance 60% of the original dose) in about six hours. The radioiodine level then decreases, presumably because of the gradual loss of ^{131}I in organic form; most of it is gone by 100 hours after injection. A small residue remains, but this could be explained by the gradual arrival of ^{131}I from some temporary storage depot (e.g., muscle tissue) or from deiodination of previously secreted hormone in the tissues.

The circulating iodine of marine teleosts is high because seawater contains

* The word *uptake* is perhaps a poor one, but it is in such general use that we shall employ it here. In general, in connection with a radioisotope, it refers to accumulation of the isotope by a particular organ (e.g., thyroidal uptake). The term *percent uptake* is often used to indicate the fraction of the total dose of isotope given that is accumulated by an organ at a stated time after administering of the isotope.

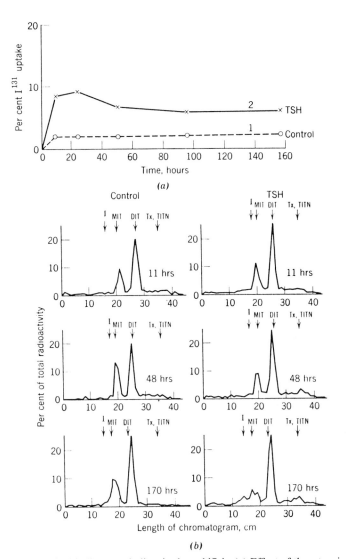

FIGURE 6.31. Thyroidal iodine metabolism in the goldfish. (*a*) Effect of thyrotropic hormone on peak accumulation and turnover of ^{131}I. *Curve 1:* untreated goldfish; the peak value, 3% of the injected ^{131}I dose, is reached after 12 hours. *Curve 2:* goldfish pretreated 4 or 5 days with mammalian TSH. Note that TSH-treated fishes release about one-third of their peak accumulation of radioiodine after 48 hours, while the untreated fishes hold 100% of their peak accumulation for the length of the experiment (156 hours). (*b*) Radiochromatograms of trypsin and papain hydrolysates of thyroid tissue of control and TSH-treated goldfishes sacrificed at intervals after injection of a tracer does of radioactive iodine. Figures show distribution of radioactivity along the length of chromatograms developed with butanol-acetic acid. Arrows indicate the position of known iodinated compounds chromatogrammed in parallel with the thyroid hydrolysates: *I*, iodide; *MIT*, monoiodotyrosine; *DIT*, diiodotyrosine; *TITN*, triiodothyronine; *Tx*, thyroxine. Note the absence of thyroxine from control series and its presence after TSH treatment. [From O. Berg and A. Gorbman, *Proc. Soc. Exp. Biol. Med.*, **86:**156, 1954.]

about 45 to 60 μg of iodine per liter. In general, the blood iodine level in fishes reflects the supply in the water. Since only a small part of the relatively high level of circulating iodine needs to be taken up by the thyroid of marine fishes to satisfy its needs, the apparent uptake of *tracer* iodine will be low. In freshwater fishes a much larger part of the circulating stable iodine must be taken up by the thyroid to form an equivalent amount of hormone, so that the apparent percent uptake of ^{131}I will be high. The iodine content of the environmental water obviously influences the thyroidal uptake of tracer iodine. The same effects on tracer iodine uptake can be produced in mammals by restricting or adding to the normal dietary iodine, and the increases or decreases in ^{131}I uptake are due to the same factors. For these reasons it is sometimes difficult to draw conclusions concerning the absolute value of radioiodine uptake information, although qualified conclusions may be justified.

In general, the amphibians and reptiles (Fig. 6.29A) have slow iodine cycles that resemble those of teleosts. This is true even though the terrestrial or freshwater habitats of amphibians and reptiles constitute iodine-poor environments. Birds and mammals, on the other hand, have more rapid thyroidal iodine turnover cycles. It may be more than coincidental that the most active thyroids are in the homoiothermic forms. One of the most active thyroids reported, for example, is that of the white-throated sparrow *Zonotrichia*, whose thyroidal uptake reaches a maximum of as much as 70% of the injected dose of ^{131}I within three to six hours after injection (Fig. 6.29B). The loss of thyroidal radioiodine is also relatively rapid.

When turtles are kept in dry environments, unusually high thyroidal radioiodine uptakes are known to appear, although the thyroid is comparatively inactive. In these reptiles a maximum of about 80% of the originally injected radioiodine is found in the thyroid, but it accumulates gradually over a period of eight days. The important question here is where and in what form has the radioiodine been stored druing the long interval? The reservoir proves to be the extremely voluminous urinary bladder, which during periods of desiccation is not emptied but is used as a source of reabsorbed fluid. The radioiodine is thus saved by the same mechanism as that used for conservation of water. The same species of turtles, when kept in ample water, has a normal teleostlike cycle of thyroidal radioiodine usage.

QUALITATIVE ASPECTS OF THE THYROIDAL CYCLE

The value of the quantitative turnover studies of thyroidal iodine metabolism is greatly increased if a qualitative analysis is made at the same time. In such an analysis the chemical compounds into which the iodine evolves at progressive time intervals are determined. As might be expected, iodotyrosines appear in detectable quantities first (Figs. 6.30 and 6.31), and, as a rule, monoidotyrosine (MIT) appears in greater quantities than diiodoty-

TABLE 6.5. The MIT/DIT ratio
in the chick

Time after Injection of ^{131}Iodine (hrs)	MIT/DIT
$\frac{1}{4}$	2.9
1	1.7
5	1.4
12	1.1
22	0.9
48	0.8

rosine (DIT) (Table 6.5). As the relative amount of DIT increases and that of MIT decreases, the iodothyronines appear.

In mammals labeled iodothyronines appear in detectable amounts during the first 24 hours after giving tracer iodine—often much more quickly. Relatively few birds have been tested (chick, white-throated sparrow), but they too appear to form iodothyronines quickly. Thyroxine (T_4) is the predominant iodothyronine in all vertebrates, and about one-third of the total iodine in the thyroid gland is in this form. A variable and smaller proportion of thyroidal iodine—usually less than 10%—is in the form of triiodothyronine (T_3) (Table 6.6).

An attractive possibility is that the production of more T_3 is favored when the iodine supply is lowered. According to Lachiver and Leloup, this actually happens in experiments in which iodine-deficient diets are fed to rats; first, a larger-than-usual proportion of MIT to DIT is formed, then the proportion of T_3 increases. Since T_3 is in many respects more active physiologically than T_4, this could be a useful mechanism to protect the organism against restriction of the environmental supply of iodine. That is, as the iodine supply is lowered, a smaller amount of hormone is produced, but it is more potent. The mud minnow *Umbra limi* has been found to manufacture mostly T_3 at one time of year and T_4 at other times. It is not known whether this is related to environmental iodine supply.

TABLE 6.6. The distribution[a] of radioiodine in thyroidal fractions at 24 to 72 hours after injection of ^{131}I

	MIT	DIT	T_4	T_3	Iodide
Rat (Roche et al.)	33	33	22	6	6
Man (Braasch et al.)	19	27	38	9	7
Chick (Vlijm)	28	40	20	3	7

[a] Expressed as percent of the total radioactivity of the thyroid.

Various cold-blooded vertebrates have been found to make little or no detectable T_4 (in tests with radioiodine) or to synthesize it very slowly. This is true of certain fishes (Fig. 6.31) (goldfish and the sunfish *Lepomis gibbosus*, both freshwater forms), amphibians (*Necturus, Amphiuma*), and reptiles (turtles) (Fig. 6.30.). The amount of thyroid hormone provided by this kind of thyroid metabolism—if, indeed, it provides any—makes it questionable whether the hormone has any normal physiological role in these animals. In the goldfish, at least, thyrotropic hormone stimulates an increased quantitative level of thyroidal function and a production of some T_4. In the untreated goldfish no new thyroxine appears for as long as a week after injecting ^{131}I.

SECRETION AND TRANSPORT OF THYROID HORMONES

As is summarized in Fig. 6.24, the visible cytological events that represent the secretion of the thyroid hormones T_3 and T_4 are clear. Units of iodothyroglobulin from the follicular lumen are taken back into the surrounding cells by the process of phagocytosis (endocytosis) to form large droplets. These colloid droplets fuse with lysosomes to form phagolysosomes. At this time the proteolytic enzymes from the lysosomes promote hydrolysis of the iodothyroglobulin. The T_3 and T_4, thus freed, can now diffuse into the surrounding capillaries. It is of interest that MIT and DIT are found in normal human blood only in extremely small amounts. Apparently, they are deiodinated by a specific enzyme that has no action on T_3 and T_4 and whose activity is stimulated by TSH. Some calculations show that in this way as much iodine is freed for thyroidal reuse as is secreted as T_3 and T_4. Thus iodotyrosine deiodination is an important source of reused iodine for hormonal metabolism.

In the blood of many vertebrate species the thyroid hormones T_3 and T_4 are quickly bound to one or more proteins. Only 0.05% of human circulating T_4 and 0.3% of circulating T_3 are free to diffuse, and are in equilibrium with the hormone bound to protein. Not many species have been studied in this respect, but in fishes, for example, there are some species that have no thyroid hormone-binding proteins; a larger number of fish species, however, have at least one such protein. The blood plasma thyroid hormone-binding proteins have been best studied in man, where three major proteins have been identified: thyroxine-binding globulin (TBG), thyroxine-binding prealbumin (TBPA), and serum albumin (ALB). The least abundant of these, TBG, carries about 75% of all plasma thyroxine because its affinity for the hormone is 100-fold stronger than that of the more abundant TBPA and 10,000-fold stronger than that of ALB (Fig. 6.28). TBG also carries about 75% of all plasma T_3, but its binding affinity for T_3 is only one-tenth of its affinity for T_4. For this reason, although the total amount of T_3 in the blood plasma is somewhat less than that of T_4 (one-fiftieth), it is able to leave the blood more easily to penetrate the peripheral tissues. Furthermore, Fig. 6.28 indicates that the intracellular (nuclear) receptor for T_4 has about the same binding affinity for T_4 as does TBG, its major plasma carrier. Thus, we may reason that the movement of T_4 from the blood toward its target tissues will be relatively slow and primarily motivated by the difference in thyroxine-binding affinity between TBPA and ALB on the one hand, and the tissue receptor for T_4 on the other. T_3, in contrast, is bound more strongly to its tissue receptor than to any carrier protein in the blood plasma. Accordingly, its movement between blood plasma and peripheral cells is motivated by this difference. While this interpretation in humans seems quite rational and partially explains the greater biological activity of T_3 over T_4, examination of other species clouds the picture somewhat.

Some mammalian species (e.g., rat, dog) lack TBG, and in these most of the plasma thyroid hormone is carried by albumin. Similarly, in the few reptiles and birds that have been appropriately studied, ALB is the most important or principal thyroid hormone carrier. In most such instances the T_3 and T_4 receptors in tissue have not yet been studied, but it would seem that their affinities for hormone would be greater than that of ALB. This would assure a more rapid clearance of T_3 and T_4 from the blood. In the chicken and duck, T_3 and T_4 are bound equally by plasma protein.

As mentioned before, some fishes seem to lack plasma T_3- and T_4-binding proteins altogether. Thus it becomes appropriate to ask what is the function of the plasma hormone-binding proteins. Obviously, it is not an essential function. However, at the least, if T_3 and T_4 are carried on protein, they would avoid glomerular filtration in the kidney and possible significant loss in the urine. Furthermore, in terrestrial animals, whose dietary sources of iodine may be irregular, a store of thyroid hormones in the blood should help to even out the fluctuations in hormone availability to the tissues. At any rate, it is clear that the strength of the binding of thyroid hormones to carrier proteins in blood will have an influence on the availability of these hormones to the tissues. Since there are two principal thyroid hormones, T_3 and T_4, the differences in their binding to plasma proteins will account, at least partly, for their apparent biological activities relative to each other.

Kinetic studies of thyroid hormone secretion rates and of thyroid hormone transport show that there is much more T_3 in the blood and tissues than is normally secreted by the thyroid gland. Furthermore, injection of radioactive-labeled T_4 is followed soon by the appearance of labeled T_3 in the blood and tissues. Thus a considerable fraction of the secreted T_4 is converted to T_3 by removal of an atom of iodine from the phenolic ring. In several species of fishes it is estimated that from 40 to 70% of all T_4 is thus deiodinated. In fact, in some fishes (e.g., brook trout), although there is little T_3 made by the thyroid gland, 50% of the hormone in the blood is T_3. The anatomic site of this deiodination in vertebrates remains unknown.

Movement into hormonal target tissues is not the only possible fate for thyroid hormones in the blood. Figure 6.32 summarizes the various alter-

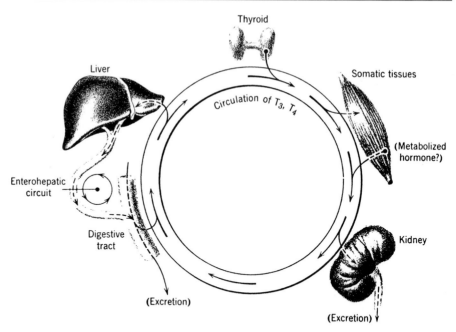

FIGURE 6.32. Pattern of release, circulation, metabolism, and excretion of thyroid hormone.

natives. Some hormones will be lost in the urine. Some are selectively removed by the liver and secreted into the bile. That this route can be important is shown by an experiment in which the bile duct is tied. Under these circumstances in a fish, up to 60% of circulating labeled thyroxine is found in the bile within several days. Normally, thyroid hormones secreted into the bile are moved to the intestine, where a certain fraction (depending on the species) is reabsorbed into the blood and the rest is lost in the egesta. The route blood → intestine → blood is known as the enterohepatic circuit.

BEGINNING OF FUNCTION IN THE DEVELOPING THYROID GLAND

Because thyroid hormones have remarkable morphogenic abilities in the adult animal, their possible participation in developmental events has been studied frequently. However, in order to evaluate this question properly, it must be shown first that these hormones actually are made during embryonic life and ascertained at what time during development they appear. Technically, this is a difficult job, since it calls for measurement of the smallest quantities of hormones secreted by the most minute organs.

For the thyroid gland the question of the beginning of its functioning is particularly significant, since many of the actions of its hormones may be considered maturational. Thus a role for the thyroid hormone during embryonic development might be expected. The well-known stimulation of amphibian metamorphosis is an illustration of this.

Several kinds of criteria have been used to judge the time of the beginning of thyroidal function. Perhaps the least satisfactory of these is morphology. The formation of the first follicles, intracellular colloid, extracellular colloid, and so on, are no doubt valuable clues, but, unfortunately, their exact relation to hormone formation is not clear. Extraction of the embryonic glands or their implantation into test animals will reveal the presence of hormone, but a negative result might mean only that an insufficient amount of material was tested. For the thyroid, the most sensitive method available has been the use of radioactive iodine. In providing a simple answer to the question of when does thyroid function begin the radioautographic technique has been valuable. This technique can show iodine accumulation in the gland in amounts only slightly exceeding those of neighboring tissues (Fig. 6.33). As more and more sensitive techniques have been employed, the first detectable differentiation of thyroidlike function has been found at increasingly earlier stages. Hilfer has been able to find biochemical evidence of thyroid function in the rudiment of the thyroid gland of the chick embryo as it first buds from the floor of the pharynx. However, this level of thyroid function probably is of little significance with respect to influencing differentiation of other parts of the embryo.

Because different investigators have used different methods and criteria, perfect agreement does not exist. However, in general, an approximation can be made concerning the time of functional onset in the thyroids of various species. In the endostyle of larval lampreys, iodine metabolism is demonstrable early (in the first of the five years of larval life). In frogs (*Hyla regilla* and *Rana pipiens*) thyroid function can be demonstrated in the small larva before hatching. The ammocoetes and tadpole larvae serve as examples of organisms in which thyroid function begins relatively early. In the chick and in various mammals (man, sheep, rabbit, pig), significant levels of thyroid function begin when one-third to one-half of the incubation or gestation period is completed. In the rat and mouse, on the other hand, about 90% of gestation is completed before a significantly increased level of thyroid function begins.

What is the reason for this great difference in the relative time of onset of function in different animals? The only reason that has been suggested is a teleological one, namely that the thyroid secretion differentiates earlier in free-living embryos (ammocoete, tadpole) because it may be essential for certain activities in the free-living process. The same argument appears to hold for interrenal function.

The simplicity of the biosynthesis of thyroid hormone has made possible the study of an interesting problem: does the ability to synthesize T_4 appear suddenly, or does it develop one step at a time? It has been claimed that in the chick embryo the earliest functional stage (seven to eight days) is one in which iodide can be accumulated but no organic iodine compounds can

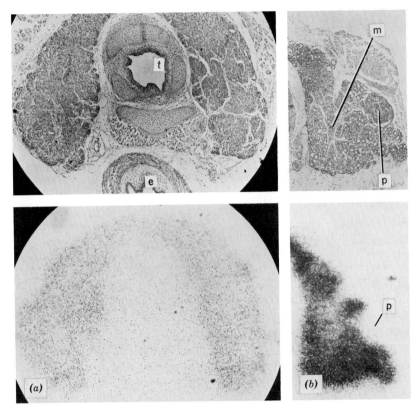

FIGURE 6.33. Sections through the thyroids of (*a*) 19-day and (*b*) 21-day rat embryos. The mothers of these embryos were injected with a tracer dose of radioiodine to determine when the embryonic thyroid could first concentrate this element. Below each photograph is the radioautograph made by putting a piece of X-ray film in contract with the tissue section for a few hours. Since the tissue was processed through aqueous and alcoholic solvents before sectioning, only protein-bound ^{131}I remains in the section. The 19-day thyroid contains barely enough ^{131}I to show a difference from the background (the nonthyroid tissue). The thyroid consists of cords of cells and a few follicles at the periphery. The 21-day thyroid has many differentiated follicles, except in the central (medullary) region. Its radioautograph is very strong, clearly different from the background. However, the radioactivity is least in the central region, where follicular differentiation is slowest. See also Fig. 6.12. *e*, Esophagus; *m*, medulla of thyroid; *p*, parathyroid; *t*, trachea. [From Gorbman and Evans, *Endocrinology*, **32**:113, 1943.]

be formed. Following this, there is a brief MIT stage (ninth day) when this amino acid, but not DIT, can be demonstrated. The abilities to form DIT and T_4 follow, apparently simultaneously. This type of biochemical maturation by steps has not yet been found in other forms, though there appears to be an "iodide stage" in the rabbit embryo.

In mammals the exchange of thyroid hormones and precursors across the placenta is an interesting phenomenon. Iodide is readily transmitted to the fetus when injected into the mother. The same is true of labeled T_4. The

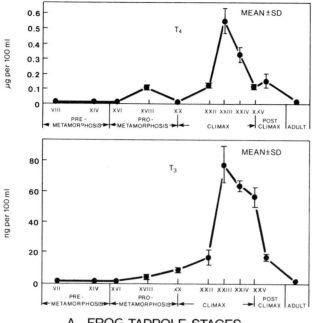

A. FROG TADPOLE STAGES

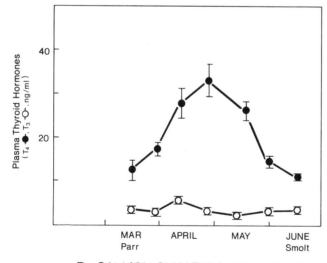

B. SALMON SMOLTIFICATION STAGES

FIGURE 6.34. Changes in blood concentrations of thyroid hormones (*A*) during the metamorphosis of the bullfrog and (*B*) during the parr–smolt transformation of yearling coho salmon. A sharp increase in both T_4 and T_3 is observed during the metamorphic climax of the bullfrog tadpole. During smoltification of the salmon, circulating T_4 levels increase gradually, while the level of T_3 changes only slightly. [(*A*) From E. Regard, A. Taurog, and T. Nakashima, *Endocrinology*, **102:**674, 1978; (*B*) from an unpublished experiment by W. W. Dickhoff, University of Washington.]

reverse probably also takes place, since thyroidectomized pregnant dogs show no signs of hypothyroidism until their puppies are born. Such pups are born with enlarged thyroids, apparently having supplied their mother with thyroid hormone during the latter part of pregnancy.

At or near the normal term of pregnancy, the thyroids of rabbit and pig fetuses have about the same ^{131}I-concentrating ability as their mothers. The full-term bovine fetal thyroid, however, has a sevenfold greater ^{131}I-concentrating ability than the mother's thyroid. The thyroglobulin isolated from such fetal bovine thyroids is more than 30 times as radioactive as the maternal thyroglobulin. These and more recent experiments indicate that the mammalian fetal thyroid is sensitive to TSH and that the fetus and the mother have separate and different TSH concentrations in their blood sera. Indeed, it seems clear from several kinds of experiments that the placenta is impermeable to TSH.

In viviparous sharks, snakes, and teleosts, transmission of radioiodine from mother to embryo has been found, and if the embryonic thyroid is sufficiently differentiated, the radioiodine is deposited in it in protein-bound form. Thus even in the absence of a placenta, this type of metabolic exchange takes place.

An interesting phenomenon has been found in some older developing organisms, namely a surge in thyroid hormone secretion at a particular phase of development. In frog tadpoles, for example, such a surge has been found at the time of the "climax" of metamorphic changes when the aquatic larva is transforming into an amphibious adult (Fig. 6.34). Both T_3 and T_4 increase suddenly in the plasma at this time. In salmon a similar, temporary increase in plasma T_4 occurs during the springtime transformation of the freshwater parr stage to the seawater smolt stage. In this case (Fig. 6.34), T_3 levels are not affected. Equivalent studies in other species have not been made, but there is a similar surge in plasma T_3 and T_4 in rats during the first few weeks after birth. The mechanisms for producing such thyroid hormone surges are not understood, nor is their precise role in development well evaluated, except, perhaps, in the case of the tadpole.

NONTHYROIDAL METABOLISM OF IODINE AND HORMONE FORMATION: EVOLUTION OF THYROID FUNCTION

It has been mentioned earlier in this chapter that the basic property of thyroid tissue, the transport of iodide, is found in other organs and tissues. These include the notochord, chloride cells of the gills, gastric glands, salivary glands, mammary glands, and kidney. A similar phenomenon occurs in certain marine algae.

If iodide transport is so general a phenomenon, can thyroid hormone also be formed outside the thyroid gland? The evidence for this in experimental animals is not good, but on the basis of indirect information it has been claimed that extrathyroidal T_4 synthesis does occur. The stomach and mammary gland may form MIT, but it is doubtful whether they can form any more advanced organic iodine compounds. Similarly, in the iodoproteins separated from various marine invertebrates, most of the iodine is in the form of MIT. Some invertebrates, on the other hand, form significant proportions of DIT (iodogorgoic acid), which is only a step from T_4.

Using radioactive iodine, endocrinologists have been able to explore many groups of invertebrates for their ability to form iodoproteins. Except for the echinoderms and protozoans, it may be said that members of virtually all of the larger phyla of invertebrates synthesize iodoproteins to some extent (Figs. 6.35 and 6.36). More careful radiochromatographic studies have been

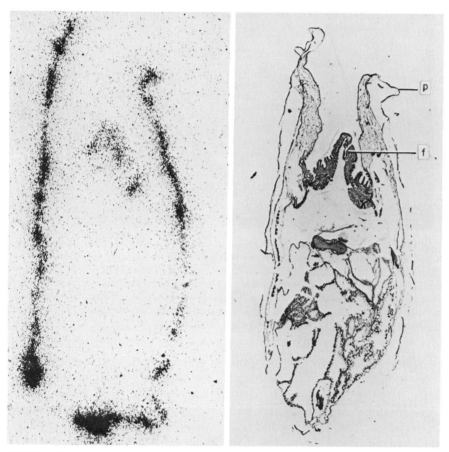

FIGURE 6.35. Section through a small, bivalve mollusc *Musculium partumeium* (right), which had been kept in ^{131}I-containing water. On the left is the radioautograph of the same section. Because the animal was fixed in an acetic acid–containing fluid, the mineral shell is dissolved. The radioautograph shows that organically bound (protein-bound) ^{131}I is localized in the periostracum (p), a fibrous protein (scleroprotein) covering the shell, and, to a smaller extent, in the base of the foot (f).

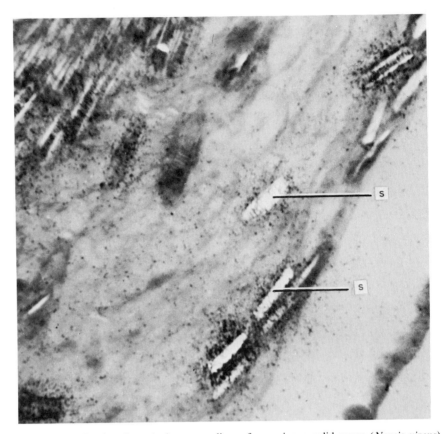

FIGURE 6.36. Section through the parapodium of a marine annelid worm (*Nereis virens*). Superimposed upon the section is the radioautograph made by localized ^{131}I in the tissue. Because of the magnification, the radioautograph appears as black dots. The black dots are localized around the setae (*s*), hairlike structures of scleroprotein and chitin in the parapodium, indicating that radioiodine in protein-bound form has become localized there. The iodoprotein of *Nereis* parapodia has been studied by chemical (chromatographic) analysis, and the iodine is present principally as monoiodotyrosine and diiodotyrosine.

performed in annelids and mollusks; in certain species of the latter group it seems clear that T_4 is synthesized, sometimes in surprisingly high quantities.

Accordingly, we must accept the idea that T_4 preceded the thyroid gland in evolution. The thyroid gland is a relatively efficient and rapid producer (and storage organ) for T_4, but it would appear that invertebrates living in a high-iodine environment (seawater contains 40 to 60 μg/liter) can slowly form this compound. Whether T_4 has any normal physiological role in most invertebrates is, however, highly questionable.

Does the wide phyletic distribution of the ability to form thyroid hormone and its precursors offer any suggestions with regard to evolution of thyroid function? Figure 6.37 summarizes such a theory. This theory is based on the fact that at some point in time T_4 began to be utilized in metabolic processes of animals to their benefit. The added survival value, or adaptive value, of larger and more dependable sources of iodoprotein created the need for an organ like the thyroid, which can carry an animal through periods of iodine "famine" and release hormone as it is needed.

The first sources of iodoprotein must have been more or less accidental and located in or near the anterior digestive tract (Fig. 6.37). In annelids and mollusks it is known that the pharyngeal teeth and the radula (rasping tongue) can form radioiodoprotein. In *Amphioxus* and other protochordates, Barrington has found that the midventral pharynx (endostyle) contains ra-

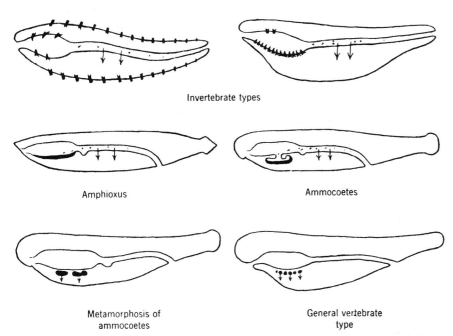

Invertebrate types

Amphioxus

Ammocoetes

Metamorphosis of
ammocoetes

General vertebrate
type

FIGURE 6.37. Summary of the distribution of iodoproteins (shown as solid black), iodotyrosine, and iodothyronine compounds in the animal kingdom, suggesting a pattern of evolution of thyroid function. Iodoproteins in most invertebrate phyla are generally found in fibrous, tough, exoskeletal structures (setae, byssus threads, periostracum, etc.) and in pharyngeal teeth. It is supposed that when this readily available material first became of metabolic value to animals, its source was pharyngeal, and it was hydrolyzed in the digestive tract to release its hormone. Once there was adaptive value in having larger, more dependable sources of iodoprotein, the pharyngeal source of iodoprotein became of major importance (second "invertebrate type"). Amphioxus and ammocoetes both exhibit this type, except that the iodoprotein is no longer a scleroprotein, but is associated with exocrine pharyngeal glandular activity. The advance of ammocoetes over amphioxus is in the separation of the iodoprotein-forming gland from the rest of the pharynx. At metamorphosis, the ammocoete thyroid forms by closure of the duct and becomes dependent upon its own, locally active protease for hydrolysis of the iodoprotein. It is at this point that an internally secreting thyroid, typical of all vertebrates, is differentiated.

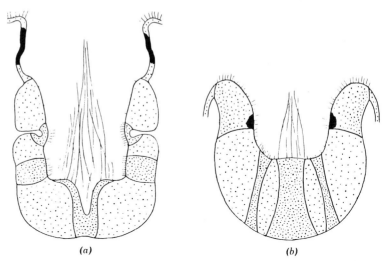

(a)   *(b)*

FIGURE 6.38.   Diagrams of cross sections of the endostyles of (*a*) *Ciona* and (*b*) *Amphioxus* showing the relationships of the iodination centers to the other regions of the organs. In both animals these centers (black) lie near the lip of the endostyle and immediately above the glandular tracts (light stippling; three pairs in *Ciona* and two pairs in *Amphioxus*). The iodination centers have the ability to accumulate radioactive iodine, and they extend the full length of the endostyle. [After E. J. W. Barrington, *Comparative Endocrinology* (A.Gorbman, ed.), Wiley, New York, 1959.]

dioiodoprotein-forming tissue in a large part of its length (Fig. 6.38). In larval lampreys the radioiodoprotein-forming part of the pharynx is almost completely separated from the pharynx, but still releases its iodoprotein into the pharynx through a duct. At metamorphosis, this structure becomes a true follicular thyroid gland.

THE FUNCTIONS OF THE THYROID HORMONES

General

The list of organs, organ systems, and metabolic processes affected by thyroid hormones is longer by far than that for any other hormone. If one seeks to find some unifying pattern or principle among these diverse functions of T_4, in the present state of our knowledge this proves impossible. What common factors could there be between (1) guanine deposition in fish scales, (2) melanin deposition in bird feathers, (3) threshold stimulus sensitivity in nerve receptors, (4) closure of epiphyses in bones, (5) schooling behavior in fishes, (6) creatine–creatinine conversion, and (7) water diuresis?

It has been argued, because of this variety of actions, that thyroid hormone must influence cellular metabolism at some elementary level from which all special metabolic effects would branch out. Yet, if thyroid hormone influenced general cellular metabolism at such an elementary level, why are not its effects even more widespread? How can we explain what specificity of action does T_4 have? These are some of the questions that should be borne in mind in considering the numerous phenomena that can be classified as morphological, physiological, and general metabolic effects of thyroid hormone.

To gain perspective into these details, various suggestions have been made in the past. For example, Gudernatsch has characterized most of the actions of T_4 as maturational. It is true that many of the morphological actions of T_4 fall into this class, but many of the functional effects do not. Others have tried to interpret all actions of thyroid hormone as due to a general, relatively unspecific, increase in metabolic rate. This view also requires so many exceptions that it is of little orienting value.

Morphological Effects of Thyroid Hormones

Metamorphosis.   One of the most spectacular actions of T_4 is the stimulation of metamorphosis in amphibian larvae. This was discovered in 1912 by Gudernatsch when he fed bits of horse thyroid to frog tadpoles. When so treated, the tadpoles quickly lost their horny teeth (used for eating plant material), grew hindlimbs and then forelimbs, shortened their intestines in anticipation of carnivorous feeding, resorbed their swimming tails, modified their skin structure for terrestrial life, and emerged from the aquatic to the terrestrial environment (Fig. 6.39).

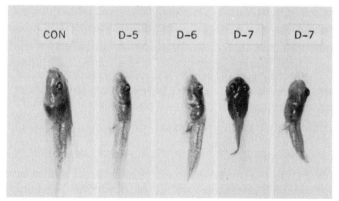

FIGURE 6.39. *Rana pipiens* tadpoles kept in spring water (*CON*) or in $5 \times 10^{-8} M$ DL-thyroxine (*D-5* through *D-7*) for periods of up to one week. The *CON* tadpole increased 10% in length during the week-long period (from 38 to 42 mm). The *D-5* tadpole was killed after 5 days in thyroxine solution. The *D-6* tadpole was killed after 6 days in thyroxine solution; forelimbs had emerged in this specimen. The *D-7* tadpoles, killed after 7 days in thyroxine solution, had *decreased* 42% in length; an erupted forelimb is visible on one of them. After 7 days of treatment, the eyes bulged, the hind limbs grew, and the tail fins were greatly reduced. [From an unpublished experiment by Jane C. Kaltenbach, Mount Holyoke College.]

These changes can be precipitated long before they would normally occur, resulting in a subnormally sized frog, since differentiation is induced before full tadpole growth is expressed. Thyroidectomized tadpoles do not metamorphose but instead grow to a giant size. All tissues and systems are involved, and virtually all seem to be directly responsive to the thyroid hormone. One way in which this has been investigated is by the implanting of a small pellet of T_4-containing agar or cholesterol in various places in the tadpole.

In such experiments, locally restricted metamorphic changes are produced (Fig. 6.40). Since the metamorphic event occurs only in the neighborhood of the T_4 pellet (where the hormone concentration is highest), this may be taken to mean that the responding tissue is directly sensitive to T_4 and does not depend on some prior reaction in another part of the embryo. Adrenal cortical steroids accentuate the metamorphic response to T_4, whether general or local, particularly the destructive phases (tail shortening, piercing of the operculum by the forelimb).

The tadpole-metamorphosis response is extremely sensitive, concentrations under 1 μg/liter (less than one part T_4 per billion parts of water) being minimally effective for leopard frog tadpoles at 25°C. This concentration is approximately 10^{-9} M. As a standard for comparison, total T_4 (protein-bound and free) is approximately 10^{-8} M in human blood, and most *in vitro* biochemical tests for T_4 action use concentrations 10^{-5} to $10^{-4} M$. T_3 usually is more effective than T_4. Triiodothyropropionic acid (the deaminated form of T_3) has been found to be about 300 times more active than T_4, but Frieden states that this is because this substance is absorbed much more rapidly by the tadpole than is T_4.

Detailed analysis of the responses of individual tadpole tissues to thyroid hormones shows that different tissues become sensitive to the hormones at different times and that their rates of response are widely variable. Furthermore, there are different orders of relative sensitivity of tadpole tissues to the various thyroid hormones and hormone analogues that have been tested, so that one is a better stimulant of leg growth, another is a more efficient stimulant of tail fin resorption, and so on.

Available information about the normal concentration of thyroid hormone in blood and tissues of tadpoles shows that it is low at the start of metamorphosis, reaches a maximum, and then falls again before completion of metamorphosis (Fig. 6.34). Accordingly, placing a tadpole in a relatively high concentration of T_4 produces a rapid, uncoordinated, and atypical metamorphosis, which usually terminates in death. Conversely, if a tadpole is hypophysectomized (so that it produces little thyroxine of its own) and is placed in a low concentration of T_4 (less than 1 μg/liter), then only partial metamorphosis ensues. Only those metamorphic events with a low T_4 requirement occur. Such partly metamorphosed tadpoles (Fig. 6.41) may be kept for a year in a static condition and will develop to a further stage only if the T_4 concentration is raised.

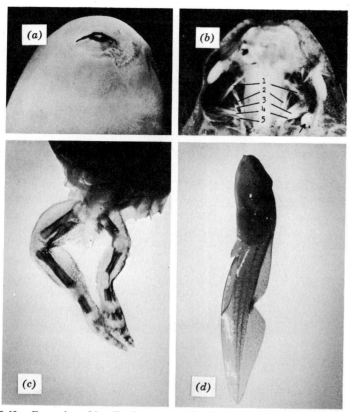

FIGURE 6.40. Examples of localized metamorphic changes in *Rana pipiens* tadpoles in response to implanted pellets containing thyroxine. (*a*) Pellet containing 20% thyroxine and 80% cholesterol placed to one side of the mouth; labial teeth and fringed lip are lost on that side (right side). (*b*) Pellet containing 20% thyroxine (shown by small arrow at lower right) implanted into the right orbit of the eye; the principal local effect was a hypertrophy of ocular muscles (*1*, inferior oblique; *2*, rectus medialis; *3*, retractor bulbi; *4*, rectus inferior; *5*, rectus lateralis). (*c*) Pellet containing 5% thyroxine implanted into the left limb at stage X (Taylor and Kollros stage). Tadpole killed 22 days later at stage XIV, and cleared to show skeleton. All bones, as well as the leg as a whole, grew in length and width. Ossification was more complete in the leg bones adjacent to the thyroxine pellet. (*d*) Pellet containing 40% thyroxine implanted into the dorsal tail fin at a stage IV; after 10 days (stage VIII), the tadpole was killed. Resorption (notchlike area) of the fin and darkening occurred at the site of implantation. [From unpublished experiments of Jane C. Kaltenbach, Mount Holyoke College.]

As might be expected, thyroid hormone action upon tadpoles can be blocked by inhibitors of DNA transcription and of protein synthesis (e.g., actinomycin, puromycin). Appropriate analysis has shown that thyroid hormones stimulate both DNA and RNA synthesis. Even resorption of the tadpole's tail depends upon RNA synthesis. One might expect that if thyroid hormone stimulates the development of so many different kinds of tissues, transcription of many qualitatively different kinds of RNA should be de-

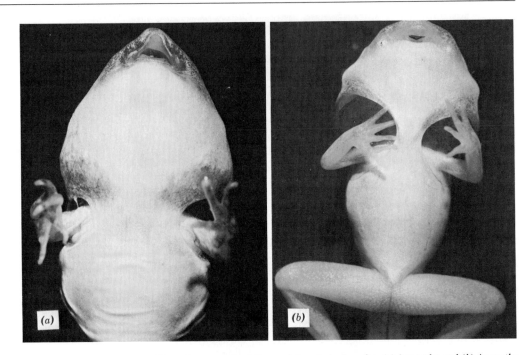

FIGURE 6.41. Hypophysectomized *Rana pipiens* tadpoles after (*a*) 3 months and (*b*) 4 months in thyroxine solution (0.6 μg/liter) at 25°C. In *a* the upper jaw has fully transformed to the adult type, but the lower jaw retains a fragment of larval beak. The skin window on the animal's right has two separate openings with a thin strand of skin between them. In *b* the specimen retains more larval mouth parts (horny beaks, frill-edged lips, teeth) than does the specimen in *a*. However, leg development is far advanced. Skin windows enlarged to several times the usual maximum. The gills remain large and functional. [From J. J. Kollros, *Comparative Endocrinology* (A. Gorbman, ed.), Wiley, New York, 1959.]

tectable in a T_4-treated tadpole. It has not yet been possible to show that stimulated RNAs in T_4-treated tadpoles are qualitatively different from those in untreated tadpoles.

Neoteny.   Different amphibian species exhibit a wide range in the rate and degree of completion of metamorphosis. In those instances that have been investigated, accompanying variations in production of thyroid hormone have been found. Species that have a prolonged larval stage are said to be neotenous, and some of them can even breed while they retain larval somatic structure. Thus, neoteny might be considered, at least in the latter instance, a form of development in which somatic and reproductive development no longer bear the same relation to each other that they have in "normal" species.

Milder expressions of neoteny are found in certain frogs (races of *Rana esculenta* and all bullfrogs, *Rana catesbeiana*), which spend several years as tadpoles. These species are readily induced to complete metamorphosis by T_4 treatment. In some salamanders (*Triton alpestris, Triton taeniatus, Ambystoma tigrinum*), races or populations are found that differ from the normal races of same species in remaining larvae for prolonged periods, or even permanently. These too respond readily to T_4 by completion of metamorphosis.

Some genera of salamanders contain neotenous species that differ from other species of the same genus in remaining larvae permanently and breeding in this state, (e.g., the Mexican axolotl *Ambystoma mexicanum, Eurycea tynerensis, Eurycea neotenes*). Such species are responsive to T_4, but to different degrees. For example, even in 10^{-5} to 10^{-6} M T_4 *Eurycea tynerensis* will only partially metamorphose. It seems clear that in such species there is a relative insensitivity of certain tissues to T_4.

Finally, there is a group of "perennibranchiate" salamanders that are permanently larval, breeding in this state, and that appear almost completely unresponsive to high doses of T_4. This group—exemplified by *Necturus, Siren, Pseudobranchus,* and *Cryptobranchus*—has been well investigated for its sensitivity to T_4, and only scattered reports of slight responses, particularly of the skin, exist. Thus within the class Amphibia, a complete and wide range of tissue responsiveness to T_4 has been found. It would seem that here is a good study material for the biochemist interested in the cellular mechanism of T_4 action.

It is tempting to equate the presence or absence of sensitivity to thyroid hormones with presence or absence of thyroid hormone receptor proteins in the various tissues. Although some initial data exist showing that T_3 and T_4 receptors exist in hormone-sensitive amphibians, no study has yet been made of T_3 and T_4 receptor activity in tissues of neotenous amphibians or in perennibranchiates.

Metamorphosis in Nonamphibian Vertebrates.   If metamorphosis is defined as a period of rapid development following a period of relatively slow development, then it may be said to occur in vertebrates other than amphibians. The transformation of the larval lamprey (ammocoete) to the adult has been considered as a metamorphosis, as has the change of the leptocephalus to the elver to the adult eel. In neither of these instances in the cyclostome and teleost does T_4 accelerate development. As mentioned earlier, despite its unresponsiveness to T_4, the ammocoete larva is known to manufacture thyroid hormone in its subpharyngeal gland, the precursor of the adult thyroid.

The developing salmon is undoubtedly the teleost whose "metamorphosis" has received the most attention. The young fishes develop in fresh water to an intermediate stage, the parr. At the end of this stage there is a surge of plasma T_4 (Fig. 6.34) and a lesser one of T_3. This surge is correlated with various morphological changes, none as striking as those in the tadpole but including a deposition of guanine in the skin that gives a silvery color to it. At the same time, there are behavioral changes, resulting in a downstream migration to seawater and the development of an ability for osmoregulation in seawater. The transformed downstream migrant is called a smolt. T_4 injection in the parr results in accelerated silvering of the skin, but tolerance to seawater does not necessarily follow. It is concluded that thyroid hormone is involved in the smoltification of salmon, but it may not be the only hormone involved in this development.

In the tropical mudskipper *Periophthalmus*, an amphibious fish, it was claimed by Harms more than 40 years ago that T_4 hastens those structural changes in eyes, skin, and fins that are adaptations to terrestrial life. Harms enthusiastically backed the idea that T_4 is a hormone of general phylogenetic significance as the stimulant of "Landtierwerdung," primarily responsible for the emergence of vertebrates from the aquatic environment. Most remarkable was his claim that by thyroid treatment he caused blennies, truly aquatic fish, to remain out of water. Unfortunately, it has been impossible for later workers to confirm this claim.

In summary, it would appear that metamorphosis in fishes is probably only partially dependent on the thyroid and that T_4-induced complete metamorphosis is peculiar to the Amphibia. Among the Amphibia, those species that undergo metamorphosis require thyroid hormone for its completion; those species that are neotenous either fail to produce sufficient thyroid hormone or have a metamorphic mechanism that has lost (or failed to acquire) a sensitivity to T_4. Insensitivity to thyroid hormones is most likely due to the absence of specific receptor proteins in cells. Synthesis of such specific proteins must be assumed to be a genetic feature. Thus differences in tissue sensitivity to thyroid hormones in related species probably are phenotypic expressions of evolved genetic differences between such species These are intriguing problems for further study by embryologists and endocrinologists.

Maturational Effects of Thyroid Hormones

Although it is clear that thyroid-controlled metamorphosis is a phenomenon that is largely restricted to amphibians, many of the less spectacular morphological effects of thyroxine may be considered maturational. Included under this heading would be the action of thyroid hormones on the central nervous system, integument, skeleton, and gonads, as well as on growth and regeneration. A word of caution should be introduced at this point concerning the use of the word *maturational* to describe the structural changes stimulated by T_4. Although it is true that this adjective accurately describes these changes, it should be remembered that almost all morphological actions of hormones (pituitary hormones, sex hormones) represent a change from a relatively undeveloped to a developed state, and so are "maturational."

Thyroxine and Growth.   It has been observed frequently (but not universally) that thyroidectomized young animals do not grow well. Much confusion and disagreement now exists in the interpretation of the specific role of thyroid hormones in somatic growth. This confusion has resulted from several factors:

1. If it does have such a role, T_4 is not the only hormone that affects growth.

2. Thyroidectomy and T_4 treatment have been applied in different species, and in different experiments, at different phases of the life cycle.

3. Vastly different dosages of hormone have been used in different experiments, so that different levels of action may have been tested, some of them toxic and some normal or "physiological."

4. Many of the consequences of thyroidectomy are obvious metabolic disturbances. Accordingly, the role of thyroid hormones may be merely to create the "climate" in which true growth factors are expressed ("permissive action").

In young fishes such as guppies (*Lebistes*), platys (*Platypoecilus*), or swordtails (*Xiphophorus*), treatment with antithyroid drugs or the destruction of thyroid tissue with radioactive iodine results in growth retardation according to many investigators, but has little or no effect according to others. The reasons for these discrepancies are obscure. Radiothyroidectomized salmon grow at an approximately normal rate. Giving thyroid hormone to young fishes usually has no growth-promoting effect and may, in fact, curb normal growth in the dosages usually used. In more critical tests, Pickford has found that hypophysectomized killifish (*Fundulus*) do not grow when their thyroids are stimulated by TSH, but they do respond to hypophyseal growth hormone.

In amphibians, as has been brought out earlier in this chapter, thyroidectomy results in *increased* growth of tadpoles, beyond their normal limits, and T_4 clearly arrests growth. Actually, T_4 treatment of tadpoles, by promoting a rapid loss of water from the tissues, causes a sharp drop in body weight. Little or no information exists concerning the control of growth in young postlarval amphibians or reptiles.

In young birds and mammals, thyroidectomy either arrests or slows the growth rate, and T_4 feeding corrects the fault (Fig. 6.42). In newborn thyroidectomized rats, the skull is broad and round, the ears thickened, the long bones are delayed in ossification, and the DNA content of liver and muscle is reduced. Thyroid hormone treatment begun before 15 days of age corrects these abnormalities and deficiencies. After this age, hormone treatment is relatively ineffective in correcting the effects of neonatal hypothyroidism. H. M. Evans and co-workers have made a careful analysis of the relative roles of growth hormone and T_4 in the growth of rats from the time

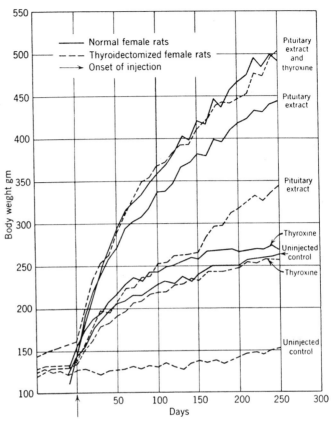

FIGURE 6.42. Growth of normal and thyroidectomized rats given thyroid and pituitary hormones. [From H. M. Evans, M. E. Simpson, and R. Pencharz, *Endocrinology*, **25**:175, 1939.]

of birth. They found that while growth hormone can strongly stimulate growth in thyroidectomized infantile animals, T_4 is ineffective in hypophysectomized specimens (Figs. 6.42 and 6.43). The dose of T_4 used, 5 µg/day, is sufficient to restore a normal growth rate and basal metabolic rate in thyroidectomized baby rats. Furthermore, in either intact or thyroidectomized animals growth hormone can stimulate the rate and extent of growth to a supernormal level; T_4 treatment of intact baby rats at best will only equal the normal growth rate, or may, depending upon dosage, actually depress body weight below the norm. However, T_4 plus growth hormone, given together, can produce a level of growth in rats not achieved by any other experimental means (Fig. 6.42).

Thus T_4 may act as a synergist of growth hormone, but it does not in itself have the ability to stimulate growth. The basis for this synergism is unknown. Two possibilities that have been suggested, but not yet experimentally tested, are the following: (1) T_4 may increase the sensitivity of the

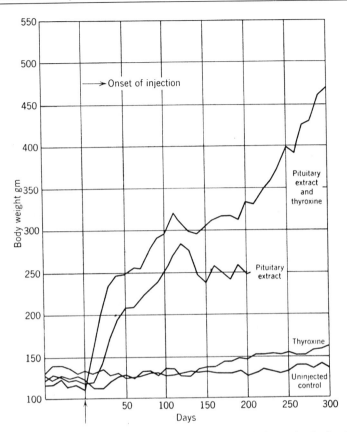

FIGURE 6.43. Growth of rats lacking both the thyroid and pituitary glands that have been injected with either thyroxine or pituitary hormones, or both. [From H. M. Evans, M. E. Simpson, and R. Pencharz, *Endocrinology*, **25**:175, 1939.]

tissues to growth hormone; (2) T_4 may influence the amount of growth hormone synthesized and released by the adenohypophysis (in intact or thyroidectomized animals). There are numerous other possibilities.

Thyroxine and Postembryonic Differentiation. It is clear that in thyroidectomized young vertebrates growth and differentiation are separable phenomena. Tadpoles may become "giant" in the absence of thyroid hormone, but they fail to progress in development. Although thyroid hormones may play an ancillary role in growth, they appear to have a primary role in differentiation.

The *endoskeleton* is a target of T_4 that shows the separation of the phenomena of growth and differentiation. In thyroidectomized rats bone growth, like body weight, is arrested and the histological structure of the bones remains of the youthful type. In this state hypophyseal growth hormone will induce growth, largely by stimulation of proliferation at the epiphyseal cartilages; however, little if any differentiation occurs. On the other hand, when T_4 is given to a hypophysectomized immature rat, it induces rapid differentiation (an increase in "bone age") and ossification of the epiphyses of long bones without appreciably affecting length.

The particular effects of T_4 upon differentiation of bone depend upon the dosage level, and various patterns of bone growth can be observed when the hormone is given to thyroidectomized animals or to cretinous children. In hyperthyroidism there appears to be a partial decalcification of bones. Studies in young T_4-treated mammals injected with radioactive sulfur and calcium show that there is an increased deposition of sulfur, presumably in the organic part of the skeleton, and an increased turnover, or exchange, of calcium in the mineral part of bones. There is disagreement concerning the effect of T_4 upon serum and urinary calcium.

The growth and eruption of teeth are clearly under thyroid control in various mammalian species. The eruption of the incisors of young rats is so dependable an expression of thyroid function that it has been suggested as the basis for a bioassay of thyroid hormones. In hypothyroid children (cretins), the eruption of both deciduous and permanent teeth is greatly delayed. For example, it has been reported that a cretin almost 12 years old had a "dental age" of 5 years. A 34-year-old cretin who still retained both deciduous and unerupted permanent teeth in her jaw also has been described (Fig. 6.44).

Another interesting skeletal response to thyroid state is that of the horns of sheep and the antlers of deer. In deer (Fig. 6.45) the growth of horns can be greatly accelerated by T_4 injections; other hormonal factors are also normally involved.

In young fishes, T_4 treatment affects the growth of fin rays, so that fins of large and unusual shapes are produced. However, not all fins are equally affected. T_4 treatment stimulates abnormal growth of the head of fishes (Fig. 6.46). A part of the effect is due to osteogenic distortion of the cranial bones (as in experiments with *Gambusia*, the mosquito fish). However, a large part of the observed response in salmon, trout, and guppies is due to proliferation of orbital connective tissue and the resultant protrusion of the eyes

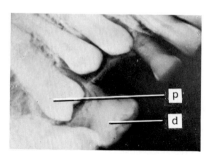

FIGURE 6.44. An X-ray photograph of part of the jaw of a cretin, a woman 34 years old. The deciduous teeth are still in place (*d*). The permanent teeth (*p*) have not erupted and remain deep in the bone of the jaw behind the deciduous teeth. [Photograph supplied by E. Zegareli, Columbia University.]

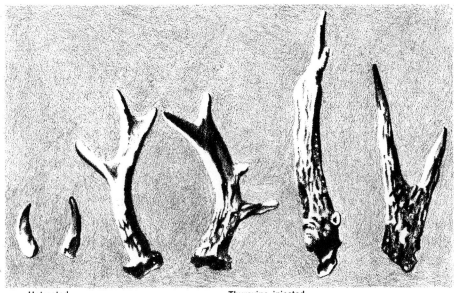

Untreated   Thyroxine-injected

FIGURE 6.45. Effect of thyroxine on the growth of antlers in young deer (*Capreolus capreolus*). All antlers are from animals of the same age. The small pair on the left belonged to an untreated animal. The remaining specimens show various patterns of response in thickness of bone and degree of branching. [After W. V. Buddenbrock, *Vergleichende Physiologie*, Verlag Birkhauser, Basel, 1950.]

(exophthalmos). Since the heads of radiothyroidectomized trout grow normally in size and proportion, it would appear that the disproportionate growth just described must represent a special response to a hyperthyroid state.

The question of whether osteogenic tissue is directly sensitive to T_4 appears answered by work such as that of Fell and Mellanby, who found that this hormone induces maturational changes in the cartilage of chick embryo limb buds in organ culture.

The *integument* and its derivatives respond in many ways, structurally and physiologically, to the thyroid hormones. Changes in mitotic rate, epidermal molting, feather and hair and scale growth, pigmentation, glandular activity, fluid content, and vascularity have been described in extremely extensive literature. It will be impossible to do more than pass over some of the salient features here.

T_4 treatment in all classes of vertebrates is accompanied by an increased epidermal mitotic rate. The proliferative effect of T_4 is not uniform; T_4 causes a decreased mitotic rate in the cornea. Its specificity has been questioned by Leblond, who found that hypophysectomy blocks the mitotic response in intestinal epithelium. However, growth hormone overcame this

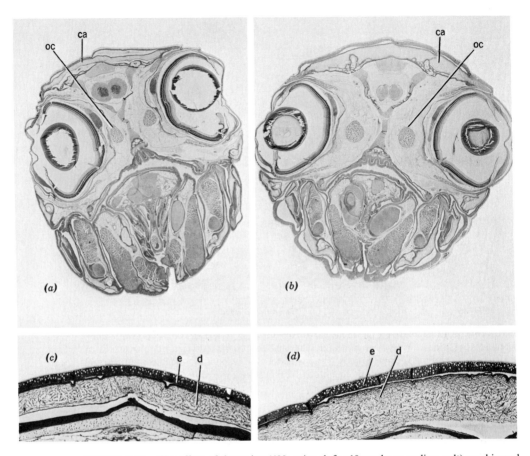

FIGURE 6.46. The effect of thyroxine (400 μg/week for 10 weeks as sodium salt) on skin and head structures in young, parr-stage salmon (*Salmo salar*). (*a*) Section through the head of a control specimen, injected with saline solution; (*b*) section through head of a thyroxine-injected parr; (*c*) section through the skin of the control specimen; (*d*) section through the skin of the thyroxine-treated parr. Distortion in the shape of the head is apparent in the thyroxine-treated fish. In the control, the longest dimension is vertical (dorsoventral). In the thyroxine-injected fish the longest dimension is the width. A large part of this increase in width is due to an increase in loose connective tissue behind the eye (*oc*). However, changes in the thickness and shape of skeletal cartilage (*ca*) are also seen. In the skin the large dose of thyroxine has a small effect on the epidermis (*e*), but results in a considerably thickened dermis (*d*). [Previously unpublished photographs supplied by Gilles LaRoche, University of California, illustrating experiments published in 1952 by LaRoche and Leblond.]

block. This objection cannot apply universally, if it applies at all, to epidermis, since the skins of hypophysectomized tadpoles (as well as other tissues) respond well to T_4.

The epidermal effects of T_4 are variously expressed in different vertebrate groups. In amphibians, reptiles, and birds, molting (ecdysis) of cornified cells or feathers is promoted by T_4 and inhibited by thyroidectomy. The epidermis of cold-blooded forms is thickened after thyroidectomy and because of its relative opacity it is changed in color. Vascularity of amphibian skin and of the teleost *Periophthalmus* is increased after T_4 treatment because of partial penetration of the epidermis by blood capillaries. This obviously increases the usefulness of the skin as a respiratory organ.

Various kinds of integumentary pigmentary effects have been noted in different vertebrates. Fishes, as mentioned earlier, commonly deposit guanine in the skin after thyroid treatment and become silvery. Silvering can be induced in teleostean species that do not normally exhibit it.

In birds there has been much work done on the effects of thyroid hormones upon melanin pigmentation of the newly forming feather. Endocrine control over differentiation, pigmentation, and molting of feathers is the subject of a voluminous literature. The developing feather germ is a complex structure in which shape, size, barbulation (development of filaments with interlocking hooks, giving the feather a stiff, flat shape), amount of pigment, pattern of pigmentation, and the nature of the pigment are separately influenced by the sex steroids, adrenal steroids, and thyroid and pituitary hormones. The analysis of the interaction of genetic, endocrine, and other factors in the growing feather is a fascinating topic, too complex to treat here adequately.

Insofar as the thyroid enters this picture, several things may be said. Thyroidectomy generally inhibits molting, and T_4 enhances it. There is great species variation in the sensitivity of the molting mechanism to changes in the thyroid state. Domestic fowl, pigeons, pheasants, and partridges are examples of sensitive forms; crows and jackdaws are relatively insensitive. In at least some species in which the analysis has been sufficiently detailed, it is clear that T_4 is acting in synergism with sex steroids in the induction of molting.

In the regeneration of feathers after molting or after plucking, T_4 is stimulatory, again in synergism with certain of the steroid hormones. It is not yet clear whether this is a true synergism or whether the thyroid or sex hormones merely cause the feather germ to be receptive to the action of the other hormone. The threshold sensitivity to the molt-inducing action of T_4 varies in feathers in different parts of the body, some being resistant even to high doses (flight and tail feathers). Furthermore, only feathers past a certain critical phase of their growth cycle will be induced to molt by T_4.

In the regenerating feather the two features most apparently susceptible to thyroid action are barbulation and pigmentation. Thyroidectomy of domestic fowl results in a feather that grows very few barbules and hence does not form a flat "vane" by interlocking of the barbs. Furthermore, in both cocks and hens the "cocky" (neutral) feather pattern is produced. Castration produces no further changes in feathering. Injected estrogens likewise do not alter the "cocky" feather pattern. To return to the "henny" type of feathering requires both T_4 and estrogen. This, again, illustrates a situation in the morphogenesis of the feather in which synergistic hormones—or a "sensitizing" or "priming" hormone plus a morphogenetic hormone—are required.

In respect to melanin pigmentation of the feather, thyroidectomy produces characteristic changes. In leghorn fowl feathers that should normally regenerate as black, instead are brownish, reddish, or nonpigmented. T_4 injection, on the other hand, favors the black phase (Fig. 6.47). Since the yellow, orange, red, brown, or black phases represent different oxidation phases of melanin, this effect has been related to the metabolic effects of T_4 in these birds. However, the pigmentary response in other species of birds may be opposite, T_4 favoring lighter colors and thyroidectomy darker. Feathers contain other pigments aside from melanin, particularly the lipochromes, and these respond to T_4 treatment in different ways.

Again, it must be repeated that T_4 is only one of a group of hormones affecting pigmentation. The sex hormones also are involved, not only with regard to hue, but also to the pattern of color deposition. As Witschi has shown in the weaver finch, melanin pigmentation of the feather germ may respond even to pituitary hormone (LH), so that the role of T_4 in this phenomenon remains to be further clarified. An example of the metabolic effects that must be the basis of T_4 action has been supplied by Kobayashi, who has found that T_4 induces a rapid increase in alkaline phosphatase activity in the skin and feather germs of pigeons.

In thyroidectomized roosters there are regressive changes in the comb and the spurs. The comb is known to be primarily under endocrine control by androgenic steroids. However, since androgens cannot repair the thyroidectomy effect, it must be presumed, as in previous instances, that T_4 serves a synergistic or potentiating role in comb growth, acting together with the androgen. The spurs, on the other hand, do not respond to the presence or absence of androgens, so that their growth must be considered to be either under the sole regulatory influence of T_4 or, as has been suggested, of T_4 plus hypophyseal growth hormone.

In mammals, particularly in humans, the effect of hypothyroidism on the skin is so characteristic that the condition has been given the name *myxedema*. In thyroidectomized domestic mammals (cattle, sheep), the hair coat is thinner and the individual hairs are more coarse and brittle than normal. In humans there is a tendency toward loss of hair. The rate of hair growth has been measured in thyroidectomized and T_4-injected rats and guinea pigs; It is faster in hyperthyroidism and slower in hypothyroidism.

The skin of hyperthyroid (thyrotoxic) humans characteristically is thin, warm (due to vascularity), and moist (due to glandular activity). The skin in myxedema is thickened, dry, and cool. Histologically, the chief change in myxedematous skin is in the dermis. This is thickened by infiltration of

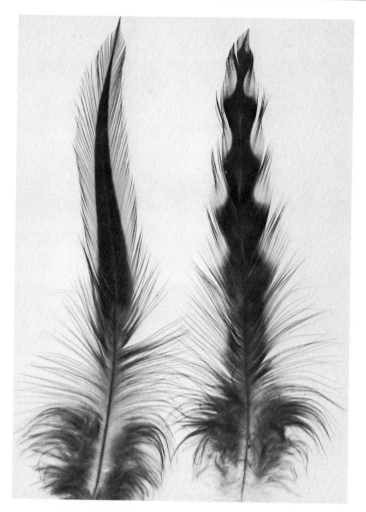

FIGURE 6.47.   Dorsal neck hackle feathers of caponized brown leghorn fowl. The feather on the left, from a bird that received no endocrine treatment, illustrates the normal pigmentary pattern. The feather on the right is from a bird treated with thyroxine (10 mg every seventh day during the growth period). Thyroxine increases the width of the melanin-pigmented central band. The effect of thyroxine wears off after the second weekly injection, since the melanin-pigmented band varies in width. The widest part of the band corresponds to the time just after injection of thyroxine. [Photograph made from feathers supplied by Mary Juhn, University of Maryland.]

fluid, and the collagenous fibers appear swollen. The ground substance in the infiltrating fluid appears to be of a mucinous nature and stains characteristically. The chief chemical components have been identified as the mucopolysaccharides hyaluronic acid and chondroitin sulfuric acid.

The *reproductive system* has been reported in almost all vertebrate groups to be delayed in differentiation or to regress to various degrees after thyroidectomy of immature or mature animals. Treatment of swordtails (*Xiph-ophorus*) with antithyroid drugs has been reported as markedly delaying sexual maturation. Destroying the thyroid glands of these fishes with radioactive iodine delays but does not prevent sexual maturation. In other fish species the thyroid appears to have an influential but not primary control over reproductive function.

In Amphibia a similarly unclear relationship exists between the thyroid glands and the gonads, though the testis appears to be less dependent upon thyroid function than the ovary. In reptiles, birds, and mammals it appears that at least some thyroid hormone is necessary for reproductive function, since thyroidectomy arrests or decreases gametogenesis and, apparently, also sex hormone secretion. T_4 remedies the abnormalities induced by thyroidectomy, but in higher doses it may be actually inhibitory to gonadal development.

In several species of birds there is a distinct and curious antagonism between thyroid and gonadal function. In an Indian bird, the spotted munia, the gonads remain in a permanent breeding state after thyroidectomy. In juvenile males the testis matures more rapidly than normal after thyroidectomy. Similarly, it has been found in a European quail that the annual cycles of thyroid and gonad activity alternate with each other. T_4 injected during the long-day period of the year, when testicular development is highest, causes a depression of plasma testosterone. Similarly, castration of male quail during the long-day period, when plasma T_4 is low, provokes a rise in plasma T_4. The mechanism for such an antagonism between thyroid and gonad function probably involves the hypothalamic controllers, and it deserves further study.

In mammals phases of reproduction specifically disturbed by thyroidectomy or hypothyroidism are the estrous cycle, fertility, pregnancy, and lactation in females; and testicular growth, spermatogenesis, accessory sex glands, and fertility in males. T_4 has been found to increase (at least temporarily) the milk yield from cows and the productivity of eggs by hens.

Regeneration is another phenomenon in which the influence of T_4 has been explored. Regeneration of limbs is found only in some fishes and amphibians, and it is more successful in younger than in older members of a species. Hypophysectomy in fishes abolishes the capacity to regenerate amputated fins, but, although opinion is divided in this regard, it appears that treatment with antithyroid drugs ("chemical thyroidectomy") does not necessarily prevent such regeneration. On the other hand, treatment of some species (the catfish *Ameiurus*; the mosquito fish *Gambusia*) with thyroid hormone or TSH will initiate fin regeneration under conditions that normally prevent it, such as lowered temperatures.

In urodele amphibians, in which such work has been conducted extensively, thyroid hormone usually inhibits limb regeneration. The source or growing point from which undifferentiated tissues appear to contribute toward the reconstruction of skeletal, muscular, and other structures is the "cap" or blastema covering the amputation surface and the tissue immediately behind the blastema. T_4 treatment may prevent the formation of the blastema if it is started early during regeneration. If given after blastema formation, it may briefly stimulate regeneration, but in the usual dosages employed it causes maturation of the undifferentiated tissues and halts the regenerative process.

Since the pituitary gland also appears involved in limb regeneration, it is possible that, as in other instances already cited, endocrine influences over this process may involve the thyroid only in a synergistic or permissive role.

The *adult nervous system* is highly responsive to changes in thyroid function; in the developing organism it also exhibits fundamental structural changes. Both the size and mitotic rate of the brain can be augmented by treating growing amphibians and mammals with thyroid hormones. Implantation of an agar or cholesterol pellet containing T_4 into the brains of frog tadpoles produces specific local morphogenetic changes, such as involution of Mauthner's cells. Accordingly, it seems probable that nerve tissue is directly responsive to thyroid hormone and that the role of T_4 in these changes is not indirect or synergistic with other hormones, as in some previously cited examples of T_4-affected structural phenomena. Thyroidectomy of young rats or treatment with antithyroid drugs results in smaller-than-normal brains, delayed neuronal maturation and smaller size, a reduction in the number of axons in the cerebral cortex, and reduced myelin deposition in fiber tracts.

If thyroidectomy is performed early enough in young rats, succinic dehydrogenase activity in the cerebrum is reduced, and it may be restored only if T_4 replacement is begun before the 20th day. In shark embryos T_4 induces an early differentiation of stainable neurosecretory material in the hypothalamus.

The *digestive tract* in certain species and under certain circumstances may be profoundly altered by changes in thyroid function. When the herbivorous tadpole metamorphoses into the carnivorous frog, the intestine loses 80% of its total length. These changes, successively involving complex degenerative and differentiation phases, are precipitated by thyroid treatment, but the specificity of their response to T_4 is yet unknown. In embryos of teleost and elasmobranch fishes, it has been claimed that T_4 accelerates the absorption of yolk from the large yolk sac and the final differentiation of the body wall near the yolk stalk.

In young rats T_4 increases the mitotic rate of the liver and the intestinal mucosa. This increase is not produced in hypophysectomized rats and is thus interpreted to be an effect of a pituitary hormone (STH?) potentiated by T_4.

Physiological and Metabolic Functions of Thyroid Hormones

General. In the preceding paragraphs a series of morphological actions of thyroid hormones has been presented. The thyroidal effects that now follow may be considered as functional or metabolic. To reiterate, the separation of the complex list of thyroid hormonal actions into such categories has been made only for convenience, so that there would be at least some organization and order in this chapter.

In the preceding section it has been impossible to discuss structural changes without frequent reference to function; the converse will be true in the following section. It must be remembered that at the basis of any thyroid hormone action is a series of chemical events that occur after the entry of the hormone into the cell. It is known that thyroid hormone can accumulate in certain tissues and within the cell in certain cytoplasmic units, primarily the mitochondria. Since mitochondrial accumulation of T_4 may be a general phenomenon, perhaps at least the first chemical events leading to the great variety of effects in the many responding tissues are the same in all responding cells.

In the following paragraphs the physiological responses will be given first. These are characteristic functional changes in certain organs or organ systems. Following this the so-called metabolic effects, alterations in body chemistry that are not limited to a single system, will be given. Finally, a brief discussion of the current theories of thyroid hormone action at the cellular level will conclude this chapter. When the riddle of how the thyroid hormone acts is solved, the logical order will be the reverse of this one. However, as will emerge later, we are still far from this "logical" presentation of the subject.

Nervous System and Neuromuscular Phenomena. Aside from the morphological manifestations already mentioned, there is a surprisingly long list of changes in the nervous system that are functional consequences of changes in thyroid state. Nervous function at all levels is influenced by the thyroid: exchange of water and salts between cell and body fluids, spontaneous electrical activity, sensitivity threshold to a variety of stimuli, reflex time, motor behavior, and mental acuity. Furthermore, thyroid regulation of neural activity is found in all major vertebrate groups. This may be contrasted, for example, with control over oxygen consumption, which seems best established in warm-blooded vertebrates.

One of the early theories formulated to explain the rise in metabolic rate in animals fed thyroid material was based on the possibility that the hormone stimulated the central nervous system. According to this theory, increased spontaneous nervous stimulation of muscle maintains a higher than normal state of tonus; this, in turn, requires an increased oxidation rate in the organism. Against this theory are the following facts: (1) slices of tissues taken from thyroxine-injected animals have a higher oxygen consumption rate *in vitro* than tissues from noninjected animals; (2) animals treated with curare (a muscle-paralyzing drug), or whose muscles are paralyzed by spinal cord section, still have an increased oxygen consumption after T_4 treatment.

However, it is true that muscles of thyroxine-injected animals are in a relatively higher than normal state of tonus and may even exhibit (in humans) spontaneous tremors. In hypothyroid animals, including humans, muscles are relaxed and flaccid, and respond slowly and without vigor. Accordingly, this maintenance of muscle tone, though it may account only for a fraction of the total oxygen consumption of hyperthyroid animals, must be regarded as contributing to the oxygen consumption of the *intact* warm-blooded animal after thyroid treatment.

Blood flow through the brain and vascular resistance have been measured both in humans and in dogs in different thyroid states. T_4 injection accelerates, and thyroidectomy slows the cerebral blood circulation, the range between the extremes being about 30 to 40%. This alone might account for some of the functional manifestations listed above.

The rate of contraction of the heart and the volume of blood pumped per unit of time are phenomena that readily respond to thyroid treatment in warm-blooded organisms. High doses of T_4 may induce an extremely rapid but inefficient heart rate, a condition known as tachycardia.

Digestive Tract. Although there is disagreement concerning the relationship between thyroid state and glandular secretion in the digestive tract, it seems well established that T_4 stimulates motor activity in the stomach and intestine, thus accelerating the movement of food through the gut. The secretion of hydrochloric acid by gastric glands in humans is frequently reduced by *either* hyper- or hypothyroidism.

T_4 markedly increases the rate of absorption of glucose, galactose, oleic acid, and vitamin A from the intestine. This function in the rat is not affected by hypophysectomy, and so is independent of any of the pituitary hormones and, presumably, of the adrenal gland. It has been proposed that this is a basic effect upon the intestinal epithelial metabolic transport mechanism, presumably through an influence on cellular phosphorylation.

The principal effect of hyperthyroidism upon the liver is a depletion of glycogen.

Kidney, Gills, Water Distribution, and Water Excretion. A mechanism that is consistently responsive to changes in the thyroid state of mammals is water transfer in the kidneys. T_4 or hyperthyroidism cause an increased loss of water in the urine (diuresis, diabetes insipidus); thyroidectomy or hypothyroidism result in a decreased urine volume. This effect might be considered as a consequence of increased metabolic rate, but it does not follow the increase in metabolic rate produced by the drug dinitrophenol. A rather spectacular experiment by Brull, in 1940 (apparently not repeated by later workers), indicates that the action of T_4 upon the kidney may be direct. He transplanted two kidneys—one from a normal dog and the other from a thyroxine-injected dog—into a third dog, connecting each to a renal artery of the host. Urine from their respective ureters was collected. The kidney from the thyroxine-treated dog produced more urine.

In myxedema in humans and in hypothyroidism in rats, there is an increase in interstitial fluid. T_4, in addition to prompt diuresis, causes a loss of interstitial fluid from the skin and muscle but an increase in water in the liver and blood.

There have been numerous studies of the possible role that thyroid hormones play in salt and water metabolism in fishes exposed to variations in external salinity. Most of the evidence for such a role is indirect and open to question, and much of it is contradictory. For example, in tests in which T_4, radiothyroidectomy, or antithyroid drugs were used, the following conclusions have been drawn: thyroid hormone antagonizes acclimatization to a change in environmental salinity in the stickleback and carp; has no effect on acclimatization in trout, killifish, and salmon; and facilitates such acclimatization (or osmoregulation) in marine teleosts (*Serranus*, *Cantharus*, and *Coricus*; also salmon parr and trout).

Oxygen Consumption and Body-Temperature Regulation. The first function associated with the thyroid gland, recorded during the infancy of endocrinology by Magnus-Levy in 1895, was the control of oxygen consumption in man. Since Magnus-Levy's time, this function has been repeatedly confirmed in virtually all birds and mammals properly tested. Various adjectives and phrases have been used to describe the part played by the thyroid in the body. It is a "governor" of metabolism, or a "thermostat," or it serves to "fan the fires of life" or to "regulate the rate of living."

Accordingly, it has come as a surprise that in the cold-blooded vertebrates this function has been difficult—usually impossible—to demonstrate. In fact, the experiments in which it has been shown that thyroid hormone treatment of adult fishes, amphibians, or reptiles was followed by a rise in oxygen consumption are so few that they are well known for their exceptional nature.

In the amphibians, Taylor, by implanting thyroid glands in salamanders, and Warren, by feeding leopard frogs desiccated thyroid, produced increases in oxygen consumption. There are two well-known and often-quoted papers describing a similar response in fishes: in parrotfishes given fish thyroid extract and in goldfishes given T_4 or TSH. Both of these papers are countered by negative results in the same species as well as in many other species of fish.

Since T_4 is known to increase spontaneous motor activity in fishes (Table 6.7), it is possible that some of the exceptional claims may be based on increased oxygen consumed in response to muscular movements during the tests. Shark embryos treated with thyroid hormones have been found to respond by increasing oxygen consumption. However, the pattern of response is peculiar, since oxygen consumption may return to normal despite continued treatment (Fig. 6.48). The oxygen consumption of lizards (*Anolis*) has been found to be relatively unresponsive to T_4 at usual room temperatures, but clearly responsive at 30°C. (Fig. 6.49). This finding, by Maher and Levedahl, of a temperature-dependent respiratory oxygen consumption response to thyroid hormones has been confirmed in other species of reptiles and in amphibians.

When oxygen consumption is measured at successive time intervals after thyroid hormone is given to a responsive species, it is found that no effect is detectable for a period from several hours to several days. This delay in the metabolic effect of the hormone is known as its latent period. The reason for the delay is as yet unknown, but two possible explanations have been suggested: (1) thyroxine must first be altered to a chemically active form; (2) the hormone stimulates the buildup or release of certain enzymes that are active in the metabolic processes eventually measured. In support of the first alternative it has been claimed that certain forms of the thyroid hormone (T_3, triiodothyroacetic acid) have no latent period. or a reduced one, and may be the "tissue hormones." However, this is not yet clearly established for more than a few species. Support for the second possibility is found in the general intracellular actions of thyroid hormones (discussed below) upon the genome and upon transcription and translation of genes coding for certain enzymes.

If separate organs or tissue slices are removed from T_4-injected mammals, their oxygen consumption, as measured by Warburg manometry, is above normal. Conversely, tissues of thyroidectomized animals have a decreased respiratory rate compared to controls. Not all tissues are equally responsive; the brain, spleen, and gonads are little or not at all affected by such changes in thyroid state. Furthermore, tissues of T_4-treated cold-blooded vertebrates do not, as a rule, show a respiratory response.

If *in vitro* tests of tissue respiration are made by adding T_4 to the fluid medium *after* the tissue is taken from the body, it is generally agreed that no respiratory increase results. This can mean that T_4 (and those of its analogues similarly tested) is not the "tissue hormone," or that its action on respiratory metabolism is indirect, or that it requires a cofactor.

The increased rate of oxidative metabolism in thyroid-stimulated animals results in the release of a certain amount of heat, the exact caloric quantity of which is related to the dose of T_4. The value of this to a warm-blooded animal is that it provides the means for raising body temperature. Thus the secretion of T_4 in homoiotherms is considered part of a complex thermoregulatory mechanism. Thyroidectomized mammals are unable to survive colder-than-normal temperatures: their body temperature, like that of poikilotherms (cold-blooded animals), tends to parallel that of the environment.

Regulated calorigenesis (heat production) in warm-blooded vertebrates is a complex function and the result of several kinds of metabolic activity (to be discussed in more detail below). One source of heat (variously estimated to account for 25 to 50% of total calorigenesis) is the continuous active transport of sodium ions to maintain the unequal concentration of these ions between intra- and extracellular fluids. It is believed that this "sodium pump" is regulated, at least in part, by thyroid hormones. Adrenergic innervation and catecholamine (adrenaline, noradrenaline) adminis-

TABLE 6.7. Thyroid hormones and nervous function

Animal Species or Group	Nature of Experiment	Observations	References
Elasmobranch fishes *Squalus suckleyi*	Injection of embryos with thyroxine or triiodothyronine	Advance in time of differentiation of neurosecretion in the hypothalamus	Gorbman and Ishii (1960)
Teleost fishes *Periophthalmus* (mudskippers) *Blennius pavo* (blenny)	Addition of thyroid hormone to aquarium water	Behavioral changes, principally a tendency to remain out of water	Harms (1929, 1935)
Blennius pavo (blenny)		No increased tendency to remain out of water—contradiction of previous result	Caglar (1950)
Anguilla anguilla (eel)	Addition of thiourea to aquarium water	Decreased rheotaxis (inferred promotion of rheotaxis by thyroid hormones)	Vilter (1944) Fontaine (1948)
Oncorhynchus kisutch (salmon) *Salmo gairdnerii* (trout)	Addition of thyroxine to water or injection of thyroxine	Increased rate and amount of swimming, decreased schooling	Hoar, Keenleyside and Goodall (1955)
Carassius auratus (goldfish)		Changes in electrial EEG of the brain	Oshima, 1965
Amphibians *Rana pipiens* *Rana temporaria* (frogs)	Brain implants of thyroxine-containing pellets, feeding thyroid powder.	Premature maturation of certain discrete reflexes (eyelid closure) or of certain cells or cell groups (Mauthner's cell, mesencephalic V nucleus). Stimulation of mitosis in brain	Kollros (1942, 1943) Kollros and Pepernik (1952) Pesetsky and Kollros (1956) May and Mugard (1955)

Organism	Method	Effect	Reference
Rana temporaria (frog)	Rheobase and chronaxic determination in nerve-muscle preparations of thyroidectomized frogs.	Rheobase and chronaxie increased threefold. (Sensitivity to electrical stimulation decreased)	LeGrand and Ajoulat (1931)
Birds	Thyroxine or thyrotropic hormone injection	Induction of premigratory unrest or "Zugunruhe"	Merkel (1938)
Reptiles *Anolis carolinensis* (lizard)	Thyroxine injections	Behavioral effects: increase in general activity and pugnacity (territoriality)	Evans (1959) Evans and Clapp (1939)
Pseudemys floridanus (turtle)			
Mammals Man	Thyroid feeding of cretins	Increase in mental acuity and alertness. Increase in number of "alpha waves" in electroencephalogram	Brown, Bronstein, and Kraines (1939) Brody (1941)
Cat, rabbit, dog, guinea pig, and particularly rat	Thyroidectomy, thyroxine injection	Thyroid treatment causes increased spontaneous bioelectric activity of brain, increased excitability of brain (decrease of reaction time), increased respiration and mineral metabolism in brain, lowered threshold of excitability of certain reflexes (ear twitch, audiogenic seizures, electroshock seizures).	Asimoff (1928) Muller (1936) Timiras and Woodbury (1956) Brody and Kunde (1926) Kunde and Neville (1926) Horsten and Boeles (1949)

TABLE 6.7. (*Continued*)

Animal Species or Group	Nature of Experiment	Observations	References
Rat	Thyroidectomy	Reduced spontaneous motor activity and maze-learning ability	Richter (1933)
Infantile rat	Radiothyroidectomy, goitrogen treatment	Depresses growth and cellular differentiation of central nervous system and delays development of reflexes. Depresses concentration of succinic dehydrogenase in cerebrum. Normal level restored if thyroxine given early in life.	Eayrs and Taylor (1951) Eayrs and Horn (1955) Barnett (1948) Hamburg and Flexner (1957)
Infantile rat	Triiodothyronine	Advances differentiation of audiogenic seizure and swimming reflexes by 1 to 4 days.	Hamburg and Vicari (1955)

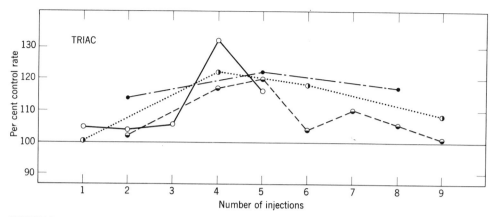

FIGURE 6.48. The effect of triiodothyroacetic acid (10 μg every other day) on oxygen consumption in late embryos of the shark *Squalus suckleyi*. The control oxygen consumption (saline-injected sharks) is taken as 100%. The four lines above the control represent the responses of four different groups of animals, each group containing four specimens and identically treated. [From A. W. Pritchard and A. Gorbman, *Biol. Bull.*, **119**:109, 1960.]

tration have a basic role in thermogenesis, which can be blocked by drugs such as propranolol (beta-adrenergic blockers). In the thermogenic actions of adrenergic substances, thyroid hormones have a potentiating or synergistic action.

When the temperature surrounding an intact mammal is suddenly lowered, TSH is secreted, the thyroid is stimulated, and body thermoregulation is eventually achieved. Thermoregulation is a neuroendocrine reflex, since it can be blocked by surgical lesions of the hypothalamus. Activation of the thyroid by lowered environmental temperatures is revealed by physiological tests of thyroid function (e.g., radioiodine uptake), by increased thyroid hormone concentration in the blood, and by histological changes in the thyroid gland. Conversely, raising the external temperatures tends to produce the opposite changes.

In many homoiotherms cycles of changes in thyroid histology parallel the seasons. The gland appears histologically active in winter, inactive in summer. Domestic animals (perhaps because of partial protection) and humans (because of more complete protection from environmental extremes) show these changes to a lesser degree. In cold-blooded vertebrates the opposite cycle is seen: active thyroids in warm seasons and inactive thyroids in cold seasons.

Since hibernation, or winter sleep, of certain wild mammals (dormouse, hedgehog, marmot) is associated with a lowered body temperature (hypothermia), it is of interest to know if the thyroid is involved. Experiments in which these animals are suddenly cooled show that their thyroids are not activated as in other mammals. This has been interpreted as a failure in the neuroendocrine mechanism, so that mammalian hibernators become poi-

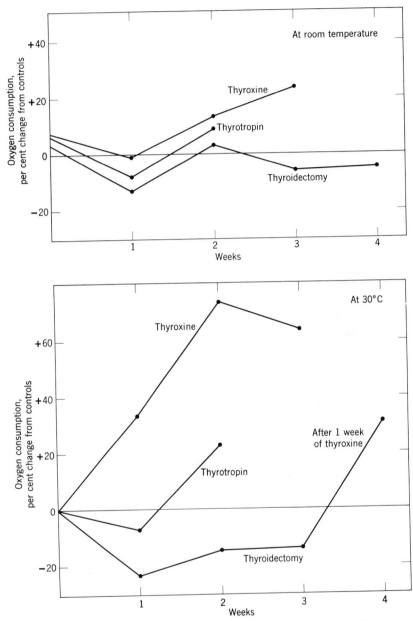

FIGURE 6.49. Effect of *l*-thyroxine (10 μg per day), thyrotropin, and thyroidectomy on oxygen consumption by the lizard *Anolis carolensis* at two different temperatures. These data show that the small respiratory responses obtained at room temperature (22 to 25°C) are greatly magnified at 30°C. [From M. J. Maher and B. Levedahl, *J. Exp. Zool.*, **140**:169, 1959.]

kilothermic under certain circumstances. Furthermore, their thyroids become inactive in the cold season, which is the opposite of normal thermoregulatory mammals. However, this may be an effect rather than a cause, since rats whose body temperature is forcibly lowered by rectal cooling also show involutional changes in the thyroid.

In marmots hormonal iodine in the blood is at a minimum during hibernation, and so is the T_4 content of the thyroid. T_4 treatment will prevent ground squirrels from beginning normal hibernation. In one species of ground squirrel, *Spermophilus richardsoni* there is a clear increase in plasma T_4 and T_3 during hibernation. All these facts point to no clear role for the thyroid in hibernation. In hedgehogs thyroidectomy does not precipitate hibernation or prevent it. Furthermore, it is known that hormones of other glands may be involved, so that no simple mechanism can be stated at the present time. It is likely that the primary regulator of hibernation is the hypothalamus and that multiple endocrine and nonendocrine factors are influential in the phenomenon.

Nitrogen Metabolism.   The particular effects of thyroid hormones upon nitrogen metabolism—an extremely wide and diverse subject—vary with dosage and with the physiological state of the organism. It has been mentioned earlier that suitable dosages of T_4 in young animals, especially in concert with growth hormone, can stimulate growth and thus the deposition of new protein. Under these circumstances, a *positive* nitrogen balance is elicited (i.e., more nitrogen enters the body than leaves it). The deposition of guanine in the skin of fishes can considered another example of an anabolic action of T_4.

On the other hand, it is easily demonstrated that higher dosages of T_4 cause body wastage, particularly of muscle tissues, and a negative nitrogen balance. Hoar (1957) described an increase in nitrogen excretion (mostly as ammonium compounds) in T_4-treated goldfishes with no accompanying increase in oxidative metabolic rate. In mammals and humans in whom many metabolic studies have been made, T_4 causes an increase in nitrogen excretion, mostly in the form of urea and some creatinine.

In salmonid fishes thyroid hormone treatment can stimulate amino acid incorporation (i.e., *new* protein formation) into hemoglobin and other plasma proteins, and into liver proteins. A low dose of T_4 in such fishes reduces nitrogen loss from the urine in the form of urea and ammonium ion.

Creatinine is normally a relatively minor urinary constituent. Its continued loss through the urine in hyperthyroid humans is contemporary with a loss of creatine and creatine phosphate from the muscles. Creatine and phosphocreatine are important in the energy exchange cycle in muscle function. This explains the wastage, weakness, and easy fatigue of muscles in thyrotoxic people. The point at which T_4 exerts its action in the synthesis of creatine or in its metabolic conversion into creatinine is not known.

Several researchers have reported that T_3 and T_4, given to the intact rat or to liver cell preparations *in vitro*, stimulate amino acid incorporation into mitochondrial proteins. For example, it has been found that T_3 added to cultures of rat mitochondria will induce labeled amino acid incorporation within two to three minutes. Concentrations and dosages of T_3 in these experiments are high (about $1 \times 10^{-5} M$). Furthermore, the media in which the mitochondria are incubated often contain little protein, so that the effective concentration of T_3 may be much higher than *in vivo*, where protein binding reduces the free T_3 and T_4 levels by a large factor. Thus it is easy to consider such rapid mitochondrial responses to T_3 as abnormal or unphysiological manifestations. Nevertheless, it is interesting that only mitochondria of normally responsive tissues (liver and muscle, but not spleen or testes) show such T_3-stimulated protein synthesis. Thus it is a tissue-specific phenomenon.

Lipid Metabolism   There are characteristic alterations in metabolism of the lipids associated with changes in thyroid state. Most characteristic are the drop in serum cholesterol in hyperthyroidism and its rise in hypothyroidism. This is not due merely to increased breakdown and utilization for energy, since dinitrophenol, which increases the metabolic rate in mammals, does not materially affect the serum cholesterol level.

Plasma concentrations of lipids other than cholesterol are often affected by changes in thyroid state, but in a direction opposite to that of cholesterol. Thyroid hormone treatment of fishes or mammals favors lipolysis (a release of stored fat from adipose cells), raising the free fatty acid content of blood plasma. T_4, even *in vitro*, has a lipolytic effect, particularly when acting together with adrenaline. Epididymal fat pads of thyroidectomized rats require three times as much adrenaline as do fat pads from normal rats for stimulation of cyclic AMP levels and subsequent lipolysis.

Carbohydrate Metabolism.   Generally, hypothyroidism is associated with hypoglycemia; hyperthyroidism or administration of T_4 often produce hyperglycemia. Under extreme circumstances, the hyperthyroid condition has been characterized as "thyroid diabetes." However, the effects of the thyroid state upon carbohydrate metabolism in lower vertebrates are inconsistent and unpredictable.

Other relationships of thyroid function to carbohydrate metabolism will be amplified below, particularly with respect to glycolysis and production of lactate.

MECHANISM OF ACTION OF THYROID HORMONES

When the actions of a hormone are as widespread in the organism as those of T_3 and T_4, we should be prepared to find a large variety of specialized or adaptive actions in different vertebrate species. This must be so even when we do not yet understand the adaptive values of the differences that are found. For example, certain mammalian thyroid researchers, when they found no effect of T_3 upon respiratory oxygen consumption in frogs, concluded that T_3 has *no* action or function in adult Amphibia. To draw such a conclusion, they had to ignore all of the proven actions of thyroid hormones upon adult amphibian central nervous functions, upon phases of intermediary metabolism, and on skin structure. Similarly, even within the mammalian group, some tissues (liver, muscle, etc.) are listed as responsive to thyroid hormone, and some (brain, gonad, and spleen) as unresponsive. Here, again, the criterion of responsiveness has been increased oxygen consumption. Yet, there are many kinds of bioelectric and other functional changes in the brain that are related to thyroid state. It remains possible, furthermore, that there are as yet unrecognized functional responses in mammalian spleen and gonads, even though there is no increase in oxygen consumption of these tissues after treatment with thyroid hormone.

If it is true that not all species and not all tissues respond in the same way to thyroid hormones, then we must be prepared to find that different cellular mechanisms may be utilized by these hormones in various types of tissues. An immediate opportunity for expression of such differences in mechanism is offered by two types of intracellular binding receptor proteins, one in the mitochondria and one in nuclei. Both of these thyroid hormone receptors have similar binding affinities—about 1×10^{-10} M. The mitochondrial receptor was characterized in rat liver by Sterling and Milch, who showed that it is limited to mitochondria. Unlike the cytoplasmic receptors for steroid hormones, which move with their bound hormone into the nucleus, the mitochondrial T_3 and T_4 receptors remain extranuclear. It would appear, therefore, that mitochondrial and nuclear receptors must compete for binding of T_3 and T_4 in a tissue like rat liver, in which both receptors occur. Since the mitochondria are loci for certain important cellular metabolic activities (cytochrome oxidation, oxidative phosphorylation) that can be measured by respiratory oxygen consumption that supports them, it is tempting to relate this phase of thyroid hormone action to the mitochondrial receptor. However, there remain reasons for questioning whether the mitochondria are indeed primary intracellular targets for thyroid hormone action, though it can hardly be doubted that they are in some way involved.

1. When T_3 or T_4 are injected into a mammal, no effect upon oxygen consumption is seen for 12 to 24 or more hours. *In vitro* responses of isolated mitochondria to T_3 or T_4 (amino acid uptake and incorporation into protein, increase in oxidative phosphorylation) are almost immediate.

2. The effect of thyroid hormones on oxygen consumption of the whole animal can be blocked by actinomycin or puromycin, suggesting that the action depends upon nuclear transcription and/or cytoplasmic translation of DNA and RNA.

3. Mitochondrial responses can be evoked readily by the D isomers of T_3 or T_4, which are relatively inactive in the whole organism. Similarly, the deaminated forms of T_3 or T_4 are quite active in isolated mitochondria, but much less so *in vivo*.

4. Generally, the concentrations of T_3 and T_4 used in *in vitro* tests with isolated mitochondria are several orders of magnitude higher than those seen in the blood plasma of intact vertebrate organisms.

Cellular Actions of Thyroid Hormones Resulting in Increased Oxygen Consumption

As cellular biochemists have developed a better understanding of intermediary metabolism and energy exchange, it has become increasingly clear that thyroid hormones influence this complex of reactions at different points and in different ways, as well as in different parts of the cell. Probably the most important type of action that thyroid hormones have is in regulating the synthesis—and therefore the total concentration—of certain key enzymes involved in intermediary metabolism. In addition, it has been reported that thyroid hormones can affect certain intracellular metabolic processes even without new protein synthesis (e.g., in the presence of inhibitors of genomic transcription and translation). The latter effect on the *activity* of an enzyme or substrate is more difficult to understand, unless the hormone is utilized as a coenzyme or in some still more different way.

It is probably inappropriate, or useless at this point, to instruct the student who has not studied cellular biochemistry in the interlocking details of intermediary metabolism. However, Figs. 15.1 and 15.2 contain a superficial summary, or overview, of some of the processes and reactions in question, with many steps omitted. One of the principal metabolic pathways for carbohydrate metabolism is that of glycolysis, or reduction of larger molecules to the three-carbon compounds pyruvate and lactate. During this multistep, enzyme-catalyzed process, oxidation occurs by donation of hydrogen atoms to NAD. Ultimately, these hydrogen atoms are oxidized by an aerobic process (see Fig. 15.1) utilizing the cytochrome electron transfer system (in mitochondria), and at the same time ATP is generated from ADP with part of the additional energy so produced. This particular function is referred to as oxidative phosphorylation. Characteristically, there is a "normal" relationship, or ratio, between the amount of phosphate incorporated into ATP and the amount of respiratory oxygen consumed. This is the P:O ratio.

If the fate of pyruvate is followed, it may be seen that this metabolic substrate can enter the citric acid cycle (Krebs cycle) by either of two routes. It can be oxidatively decarboxylated, converting it to a two-carbon acetate, which, in combination with coenzyme A, reacts with oxaloacetate to form citrate. Alternatively, by reaction with CO_2, it can be converted to oxaloacetate. The citric acid cycle is essentially a chemical method for oxidation of two-carbon units derived, as shown in Fig. 15.1, from glycolysis or lipolysis. As mentioned above, such oxidations utilize hydrogen acceptors (NAD, NADP, FAD), which shuttle hydrogens into the mitochondrial cytochrome electron transport system for aerobic oxidative phosphorylation and ATP formation. Thus, from a number of steps in the metabolism of carbohydrates and fat (as well as of amino acids), where there are oxidations that utilize hydrogen acceptors, it is possible to involve the mitochondrial cytochrome oxidative system and to influence the requirement by the organism for respired oxygen.

At what points in this scheme are the thyroid hormones involved? Actually, there is a long list of enzymatically regulated metabolic steps that have been found to be stimulated by appropriate levels of T_3 and T_4, including, as examples, the following: hexokinase-mediated phosphorylation of glucose, yielding glucose-6-phosphate; oxidation of succinate in the Krebs cycle; action of glycerophosphate dehydrogenase in the reduction of dihydroxyacetone phosphate (an intermediate product of glycolysis) to α-glycerophosphate. Glycerophosphate enters the mitochondrion, where it is oxidized back to dihydroxyacetone phosphate (which can return to the cytoplasm), yielding its hydrogen to NAD for transport to the oxidative phosphorylation chain. This is one of the mechanisms whereby electrons are carried into the cytochrome oxidase system to increase the need for oxygen.

Rather than list at length the enzymatic steps in intermediary metabolism that *may* be regulated by thyroid hormones, we can use Table 6.8 as an example of a specific study in the rat by Bargoni (1968). Here the activities of enzymes involved in a variety of steps in glycolysis are compared in normal rats, rats fed a goitrogenic drug (propylthiouracil) to make them hypothyroid, and rats fed thyroid powder to make them hyperthyroid. Furthermore, the enzyme activities are contrasted in three tissues: liver, kidney and skeletal muscle. It is clear from the table that changes in thyroid state affect virtually every step in the glycolytic pathway, but not to the same extent in each tissue. Generally, hypothyroidism decreases, and hyperthyroidism increases the activities of the individual enzymes in this series, but there are exceptions. For example, aldolase activity is increased in kidneys of hypothyroid rats, and liver phosphoglucomutase activity is decreased in hyperthyroid rats. The least overall action of thyroid hormone on glycolysis was found in the kidney.

Similar tables could be made to illustrate T_3 and T_4 responsiveness of enzyme activities in the Krebs cycle, or in fat or protein metabolism, with somewhat similar results. Generally, the stimulation of oxygen consumption in the organism or tissue by thyroid hormones parallels the responsiveness of its intermediary metabolism to these hormones.

Exploration of the actions of thyroid hormones on the intermediary metabolism of cold-blooded vertebrates has been relatively neglected, but there is ample evidence that some such actions are exerted in the liver and muscle

TABLE 6.8. Variation in the activity[a] of enzymes in the metabolic pathway of anaerobic glycolysis. Comparisons between tissues of rats fed thyroid powder and rats fed a goitrogen, propylthiouracil[b]

	Liver		Kidney		Muscle	
	Propylthiouracil	Thyroid	Propylthiouracil	Thyroid	Propylthiouracil	Thyroid
Total synthesis of lactate from glycogen	−34	+27	0	0	0	+30
Total synthesis of lactate from glucose	−40	+90	0	+25	−50	+160
Phosphorylase	−40	−80	0	0	0	0
Phosphoglucomutase	0	−41	0	0	0	0
Hexokinase	−76	0	0	0	0	+225
Phosphoglucose isomerase	−16	0	0	0	−23	+30
Phosphofructokinase	0	+58	0	+72	0	0
Aldolase	−13	0	+18	+29	0	0
Phosphotriose isomerase	−22	+57	0	0	−49	0
Phosphoglyceraldehyde dehydrogenase	−30	+23	0	0	−20	0
Phosphoglycerate kinase	−32	+26	0	0	−31	+49
Phosphoglycerate mutase	0	+58	0	+49	0	0
Enolase	−46	+97	−35	+72	0	0
Pyruvate kinase	−21	0	0	0	−33	0
Lactic dehydrogenase	0	+76	0	0	0	+15

[a] Values given are percentage change from values in normal rats.
[b] From N. Bargoni, *Bull. Soc. Chim. Biol.*, **50**:2427–2449 (1968).

of amphibians and fishes. However, in these forms there is usually no stimulation of oxygen consumption by thyroid hormones. In amphibians and reptiles Maher and Levedahl first made the interesting observation that thyroid hormones do not stimulate oxygen consumption if the animal is kept at a low temperature, but there is a stimulation of oxygen consumption at higher temperatures in the normal range (e.g., 20 to 25°C). If the thyroid hormones stimulate intermediary metabolism in poikilothermic animals below 20°C and in mammalian brain, why is there no increase in respiratory oxygen consumption? This question remains to be answered.

Thyroid Hormones and Membrane Transport of Ions

Several hormones are implicated in phenomena occurring at the plasma membrane of the cell; these involve electrolyte transport by active mechanisms (requiring energy) against a concentration gradient of the electrolyte. The most prominent of these hormones are adrenal corticosteroids, insulin, prolactin, and thyroid hormones. Matty and Green found that within a few minutes after applying T_4 or T_3 to amphibian skin or to the urinary bladder, there was an increased transport of sodium ion (Na^+), and this was accompanied by increased oxygen consumption by the tissue. The hormone concentrations used were high: 1×10^{-6} or 1×10^{-7} M.

More recently, Edelman and Ismail-Beigi have proposed that a major part of the increase in oxygen consumption caused by raised levels of T_3 in mammals is due to the action of the hormone on outward transport of Na^+ from cells. It is proposed that this action ("sodium pump") to maintain the unequal distribution of Na^+ between mammalian cells and the surrounding body fluids requires a major expenditure of ATP energy. This energy is made available by activation of a plasma membrane–bound ATPase. Ultimately, the ATP energy is provided by respiratory oxygen, as discussed above. The drug ouabain, which blocks Na^+ movement, abolishes the stimulation of oxygen consumption by T_3 in rat liver and kidney preparations.

Thyroid Hormone Potentiation of Catecholamines

There is considerable evidence that thyroid hormones and adrenal medullary hormones such as noradrenaline increase oxygen consumption in a test tissue (the epididymal fat pad of the rat). Both hormones increase the rate of lipolysis, and it has been claimed that thyroid hormone treatment increases the number of cell membrane receptors for noradrenaline. Thus one possibility is that thyroid hormone potentiates the lipolytic action of catecholamines, in addition to directly increasing the activity of certain enzymes that take part in lipolysis and β-oxidation of fat. A suggestive datum is the fact that blockage of adrenergic receptors—by use of the beta blocker propranolol—considerably relieves the symptoms of hyperthyroidism in human patients.

Actions of Thyroid Hormones on the Nucleus: Protein Synthesis and Tissue Differentiation

It has been pointed out above that one rapid intracellular action of thyroid hormones is upon amino acid uptake and protein synthesis within the mitochondria. This phenomenon occurs in experiments with rat liver and kidney cell preparations, but it is difficult to evaluate because it generally requires unphysiologically high concentrations of hormone. At any rate, it appears to be a different phenomenon from the T_3- and T_4-stimulated protein synthesis seen in the whole organism. Such synthesis requires hours to days for its expression, and it can be prevented by actinomycin and chloramphenicol, which block genomic transcription and RNA translation.

It should be realized that many of the phenomena mentioned above (growth, differentiation of new structures, changes in the activity of certain enzymes) involve new synthesis of protein. Hence their ultimate explanation involves the way in which they interact with the nuclear genetic apparatus. J. R. Tata has pointed out that there is a regular time sequence for the cellular biochemical phenomena triggered by thyroid hormones in frog and rat tissues: an increase in nuclear RNA within three to four hours, an increase in RNA polymerase, formation of new ribosomes that incorporate some of the new RNAs that leave the nucleus at this point, synthesis of new enzymes and structural proteins. These phenomena extend over a period of several days after a single exposure to T_3 or T_4.

The value of synthesis of enzymes that participate in intermediary metabolism is clear, though the reasons for emphasizing different enzymes in a chain of reactions in different tissues remain obscure. In some tissues the T_3-regulated synthesis of a single enzyme or protein may have important adaptive meaning. For example, E. Frieden has shown that T_4 stimulates the new synthesis of carbamyl phosphate synthetase, a rate-limiting enzyme in the formation of urea. In aquatic animals nitrogenous waste is excreted in ammoniacal form, since it can readily be diluted in the abundant water available to the organism. Thus it has been interpreted by Frieden that the T_4-evoked synthesis of carbamyl phosphate synthetase is part of the conversion of the aquatic tadpole into a terrestrial frog. During metamorphosis there are accompanying changes from a larval to an adult form of hemoglobin with appropriate differences in oxygen carrying capacity that are adaptive for terrestrial life.

Many properties of the thyroid hormone–evoked genomic response system are inferred from indirect information, since more direct information is lacking. For example, it would appear that the responsiveness of certain parts of the genome to T_3 or T_4 is limited to certain stages of development. Brain respiratory oxygen consumption is stimulated in the newborn rat, but not in the adult rat. Dendritic differentiation of Purkinje cells in the rat cerebellum is influenced by T_4 at birth, but not three weeks later. Similarly, there are many differences between responses to T_4 in tadpole tissues and in the corresponding tissues of the adult frog. Furthermore, even in tissues in the same developing animal there are qualitative differences in responses to thyroid hormones. For example, skin and connective tissues of the tadpole tail are programmed to degenerate and be absorbed, while similar tissues on the trunk of the same tadpole respond by further differentiation and growth. Involution of the tadpole tail is a positive response to T_3 and T_4, since it can be blocked by actinomycin. We have already noted that the particular metabolic enzymes responsive to T_3 in the adult rat differ in different tissues, implying that different parts of the genome are being transcribed in these tissues.

Responsiveness or lack of responsiveness to thyroid hormones in developing neotenous or adult tissues depends in part on whether nuclear receptors for the hormones exist in these tissues. The presence or absence of such receptors must be a genetically programmed phenomenon; it has not yet been adequately investigated, though methods for such study already exist. When qualitatively different enzymes or other proteins are synthesized at different times in the same tissue, or in different tissues at the same time (in response to T_3 and T_4), we are dealing with the problem of developmental differentiation. Such problems are being studied by developmental biologists, but no clear picture has yet emerged.

We must not lose sight of the fact that these efforts are among the first, perhaps fumbling, attempts to decipher the exact metabolic role of a hormone. Eventually we may be able to inscribe the hormones into the metabolic charts and show where they affect specific chemical changes leading to biosynthesis and morphogenesis.

ADDITIONAL READING

1. Allen, B. M. (1938). The endocrine control of amphibian metamorphosis. *Biol. Rev.* **13**:1.

2. Baker-Cohen, K. F. (1959). Renal and other heterotopic thyroid tissue in fishes. In *Comparative Endocrinology* (A. Gorbman, Ed.). Wiley, New York, pp. 283–301.

3. Barrington, E. J. W. (1959). Some endocrinological aspects of the Protochordata. In *Comparative Endocrinology* (A. Gorbman, Ed.). Wiley, New York, pp. 250–265.

4. Berg, O., A. Gorbman, and H. Kobayashi (1959). The thyroid hormones in invertebrates and lower vertebrates. In *Comparative Endocrinology* (A. Gorbman, ed.). Wiley, New York, pp. 302–319.

5. Brookhaven Symposia in Biology, No. 7 (1955). *The Thyroid.* Brookhaven National Laboratory, Upton, New York.

6. Gorbman, A. (1955).Some aspects of the comparative biochemistry of iodine utilization and the evolution of thyroidal function. *Physiol. Rev.* **35**:336–346.

7. Gorbman, A. (1959). Problems in the comparative morphology and physiology of the vertebrate thyroid gland. In *Comparative Endocrinology* (A. Gorbman, ed.). Wiley, New York, pp. 266–282.

8.   Gross, J. (1957). The thyroid in relation to energy metabolism. In *Hormonal Regulation of Energy Metabolism* (L. W. Kinsell, ed.). Thomas, Springfield, Ill, pp. 133–159.

9.   Gudernatsch, J. F. (1912). Feeding experiments on tadpoles. I. The influence of specific organs with internal secretion. *Arch. Entwicklungsmech. Organ.* **35:**457.

10. . Harington, C. R. (1933). *The Thyroid Gland, Its Chemistry and Physiology*. Oxford University Press, Oxford.

11.   Harris, G. W. (1959). Neuroendocrine control of TSH regulation. In *Comparative Endocrinology* (A. Gorbman, ed.). Wiley, New York, pp. 202–222.

12.   Hoar, W. S. (1957). Endocrine organs. In *The Physiology of Fishes* Vol. 1 (M. E. Brown, ed.). Academic, New York, p. 245.

13.   Kendall, E. C. (1915). The isolation in crystalline form of the compound containing iodine, which occurs in the thyroid. Its chemical nature and physiologic activity. *JAMA* **64:**2042–2043.

14.   Kollros, J. J. (1959). Thyroid gland function in developing cold-blooded vertebrates. In *Comparative Endocrinology* (A. Gorbman, ed.). Wiley, New York, pp. 340–350.

15.   Lehninger, A. L. (1958). Oxidative phosphorylation. *Science* **128:**450–456.

16.   Lehninger, A. L. (1959). Respiratory-energy transformation. *Rev. Mod. Phys.* **31:**136.

17.   Lehninger, A. L. (1960). Energy transformation in the cell. *Scientific American,* **202:**102–114. (These three interesting reviews by Lehninger provide a useful background for further understanding of cellular phosphorylation mechanisms and the possible role of thyroxine in them.)

18.   Lehninger, A. L., B. L. Ray, and M. Schneider (1959). The swelling of rat liver mitochondria by thyroxine and its reversal. *J. Biophys. Biochem. Cytol.* **5:**97.

19.   Lynn, W. G., and H. E. Wachowski (1951). The thyroid gland and its functions in cold-blooded vertebrates. *Quart. Rev. Biol.* **26:**123–168.

20.   Miner, R. W., ed. (1949). Thyroid function as disclosed by newer methods of study. *Ann. New York Acad. Sci.* **50:**279–507.

21.   Pitt-rivers, R., and J. R. Tata (1959). *The Thyroid Hormones*. Pergamon, New York.

22.   Rawson, R. W. (1955). The chemistry and physiology of the thyroid. In *The Hormones*, Vol. III (G. Pincus and K. V. Thimann, eds.). Academic, New York, p. 433.

23.   Roche, J., and R. Michel (1956). Nature and metabolism of thyroid hormones. *Recent Progr. Horm. Res.* **12:**1.

24.   Salter, W. T. (1940). *The Endocrine Function of Iodine*. Harvard University. Press, Cambridge.

25.   Salter, W. T. (1950). The chemistry and physiology of the thyroid hormone. In *The Hormones*, Vol. 2 (G. Pincus and K. V. Thimann, eds.). Academic, New York, p. 181.

26.   van Dyke, J. H. (1959). The ultimobranchial body. In *Comparative Endocrinology* (A. Gorbman, ed.). Wiley, New York, pp. 320–339.

27.   Waterman, A. J. (1959). Development of the thyroid-pituitary system in warm-blooded amniotes. In *Comparative Endocrinology* (A. Gorbman, ed.). Wiley, New York, pp. 351–367.

28.   Werner, S. C., and S. H. Ingbar, eds. (1982). *The Thyroid*. Hoeber-Harper, New York. (This volume is particularly valuable for its summaries of recent clinical information.).

7

Calcium Homeostasis

GENERAL

The regulation of plasma calcium and phosphate involves the action of several hormones upon several target organs, and the topic is best discussed as an integrated whole. The major organs involved in this regulation include bone, kidney, and the intestine. A diagrammatic interpretation of the functions of these organs in the control of plasma calcium is presented in Fig. 7.1. The major hormones thought to be involved in calcium regulation in higher vertebrates include parathyroid hormone, vitamin D metabolites, and possibly calcitonin. The interactions of these hormones with their targets will be considered in turn and a summary of their relative importance in calcium homeostasis will be presented at least for certain vertebrates. Brief reviews of the structure and function of the major target organs involved in calcium homeostasis are also included.

Perhaps it is useful to begin by mentioning the importance of calcium and phosphate, and why they need to be regulated. Calcium in the extracellular fluids exists in a number of forms, which total about 10 mg/dl (10 mg/100 ml) or 2.5 mM. The biologically active form, calcium ion, makes up about half of this total, but since the ionic form is rather difficult to measure with accuracy, total calcium values are usually presented. If calcium levels fall below about 7 mg/dl, or 1.75 mM, as they may after surgical parathyroidectomy, in many species parathyroid tetany occurs. This consists of uncontrollable muscle contractions resulting from hyperexcitability of nerve and muscle membranes, resulting in turn from decreased calcium supply to the cells. Parathyroid tetany can result in death from suffocation if paralysis of the respiratory muscles occurs. In "lower" vertebrates tetany appears to be more of an intermittent phenomenon, lasting several minutes and then disappearing until the animal engages in exertion or active movement.

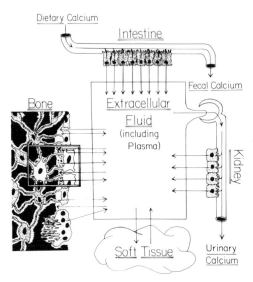

FIGURE 7.1. Regulation of plasma calcium concentrations by bone, kidney, and intestine. Concentrations of calcium in the extracellular fluids result from exchanges of this substance between the body fluids and the digestive tract, kidney, and soft and hard tissues. The two principal avenues of loss of calcium are via urinary and fecal routes. The input of calcium in terrestrial vertebrates is via ingestion. [From R. V. Talmage and R. A. Meyer, Jr., *Handbook of Physiology,* Vol 7 (R. O. Greep et al., eds.), American Physiological Society, Washington, D.C., 1976.]

Calcium has many other important functions as well. It is a key regulator in the activation of intracellular enzymes, and is needed for excitation–contraction coupling in all forms of muscle and in excitation–secretion coupling in exocrine and endocrine glands. It is a factor necessary for blood clotting, normal cell permeability, fertilization, for the actions of many hormones, and for cell adhesion. While one accepts as dogma that calcium values in the blood are precisely regulated in vertebrates, this is not really true. With the exception of the rat and human, in which plasma calcium concentrations are indeed very stable, most mammals and other vertebrates can shift their normal plasma calcium values by 10% or more within a short period of time and still maintain normal physiological functions.

Phosphate also exists in many forms. The form that is most studied is inorganic phosphate, which includes mainly free monobasic and dibasic ions, sodium biphosphate, and protein-bound phosphate. These substances constitute the major buffers in urine and minor buffers in the extracellular fluids. Phosphate is needed for the production of essential phosphorus-containing compounds such as nucleic acids, phosphoproteins, and phospholipids. Phosphorylation or dephosphorylation of key metabolic enzymes causes their activation or inactivation in biochemical pathways. Both calcium and phosphate are major components of bones and teeth. An average value for inorganic phosphate in vertebrate plasma is about 1 mM (about 3 to 4 mg/dl), but the values can vary rather widely. Variations in inorganic phosphate concentrations do not lead to the severe symptoms seen during calcium disturbances; however, a number of disease states are characterized by abnormal plasma phosphate values.

BONE STRUCTURE AND PHYSIOLOGY

Bone is a living tissue that serves as a supporting skeleton and a calcium storehouse. It consists of hydroxyapatite crystals (double salt of calcium carbonate and calcium phosphate) deposited on an organic matrix. The matrix consists mainly of collagen fibrils, which serve as a template for hydroxyapatite deposition. Bone cells consist of three major types: osteoblasts (or surface osteocytes), which function in collagen synthesis and thus in bone building; (deep) osteocytes, which may play roles in both bone deposition and bone resorption; and osteoclasts, which function in bone resorption. Bone as a tissue is formed into organs known as bones. The long bones of the limbs of larger vertebrates generally are taken as typical. Bones consist of a cylindrical shaft—the diaphysis—and caplike structures—the epiphyses. The diaphysis and sometimes the epiphyses are hollow, the central or marrow cavity being filled with various soft tissues (fat or blood-forming cells). The outer surface of a bone is its periosteal surface. The inner surface, facing the marrow cavity, is the endosteal surface.

The bone cells function in bone growth and in bone remodeling. Bone remodeling can be defined as an ongoing process of exchange of calcium and other components of surface apatite crystals with components of the bathing fluid. This can result from direct effects of bone cell activity or by simple exchange mechanisms, as explained below. Typically, osteoblasts and osteoclasts are located side by side along endosteal or periosteal surfaces and act simultaneously or sequentially in bone remodeling. Bone remodeling continues throughout the life of organisms even if bone growth ceases in the adult.

As the osteoblasts secrete collagen matrix around themselves, and as this matrix becomes mineralized, these cells gradually come to be located away from the bone surface and are termed (deep) osteocytes. They are located in lacunae (holes) surrounded by mineralized bone, and there appears to be little or no space between the osteocyte and the hard bone (Fig. 7.2a). The lacunae are interconnected by a network of tiny canaliculi that run throughout the bone. While it was once thought that the osteocytes were inactive physiologically, this is no longer a valid conclusion. The osteocytes send out cytoplasmic projections into the canaliculi that have been found to form tight junctions with the cytoplasmic processes of other osteocytes and osteoblasts (Fig. 7.2d). Thus there may be a kind of transport system linking the surface and deep bone cells. Osteocytes have been suggested by Bélanger et al. (1967) to participate in bone resorption (dissolution). This phenomenon, termed *osteocytic osteolysis*, is based upon histological evidence of partial demineralization of the perilacunar bone in response to large doses of parathyroid hormone. These changes are independent of changes in osteoclast number and are not related to bone remodeling.

Both osteoblasts and osteocytes have a similar ultrastructural appearance

(Fig. 7.2*a*,*b*). They are uninucleate and have typical cell inclusions. Both have been shown to contain microtubules and microfilaments, which may function in intracellular calcium movement, Osteoclasts are recognized easily by their large size and multinucleate nature (Fig. 7.2*c*). They have a very extensive brush border, the ''ruffled border,'' located on the side of the cell that lies against the bone surface (Fig. 7.2*c*,*e*). The cells are rich in lysosomes containing hydrolytic enzymes, which would aid in the breakdown of organic constituents of bone. Osteoclasts develop mainly from undifferentiated precursor cells that originate from tissues other than bone, although there are also reports that osteoblasts can be transformed into osteoclasts. Since they are multinucleate, several progenitor cells may have fused to form each osteoclast.

Stimulation of osteoclast production or activity can result from increased activity of existing osteoclasts, transformation of inactive (resting) to active osteoclasts, or increased production of new osteoclasts from osteoprogenitor cells. All three events would increase the breakdown of bone and liberation of calcium and phosphate, but are phenomena of relatively long duration. Osteoclasts are thought to function in regulation of bone remodeling rather than in the minute-to-minute maintenance of plasma calcium values.

There is, in addition, a large flux of calcium in and out of bone by exchange mechanisms that do not involve altered cellular activities. One of these is a simple exchange of ions at the surface of the ''exchangeable'' bone at the bone crystal surface. Calcium in the crystal lattice can exchange with calcium ions in the bathing solution or with ions such as sodium, potassium, or magnesium. This then could allow the liberation of calcium from bone without significant simultaneous net loss of bone mineral.

Since the extracellular fluid is supersaturated with calcium and phosphate, increased bone deposition can occur spontaneously at any time in places where bone or collagen already exists. Conversely, dissolution of bone could occur if the calcium level in the extracellular fluid is decreased, thus encouraging the movement of calcium from bone to extracellular fluids. These simple physicochemical relationships allow the addition or removal of bone mineral without the loss of the collagen matrix. In order for these fluxes to occur, there must be a lack of equilibrium between bone and blood calcium levels (if they were identical, then there would be no higher flux overall in one direction than in the other). There must, therefore, be some sort of barrier that normally separates bone from the extracellular fluid. Such a barrier has been suggested since the 1950s. The bone–blood interrelationship involves three compartments: the bone mineral, the bone fluid, and the extracellular fluid. If the extracellular fluids and bone fluid have similar calcium and phosphate values, then the barrier must be at the bone surface between the bone mineral and bone fluid phases. It has been suggested that such substances as pyrophosphate, hydrogen ions, or other substances at the bone surface could act to maintain a functional barrier and thus the ''disequilibrium'' between bone and bone fluid calcium concentrations.

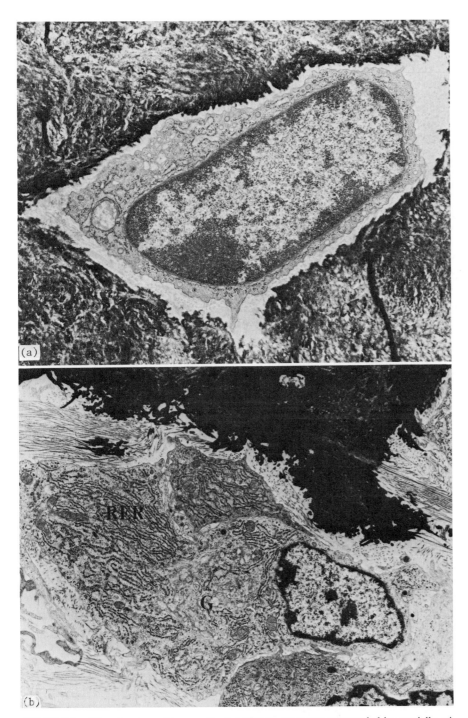

FIGURE 7.2. Ultrastructure of bone cells. (*a*) Mature osteocyte surrounded by partially mineralized bone matrix (× 14,500). Cell organelles in osteocytes are sparse. [From M. E. Holtrop, *Ann. Clin. Lab. Sci.*, **5:**264, 1975.] (*b*) Osteoblasts lying on the bone surface (black)

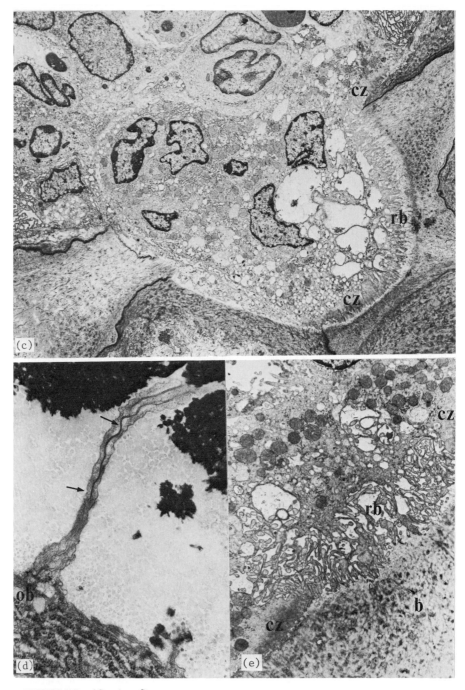

FIGURE 7.2. (*Continued*)

($\times$ 8200). These cells are characterized by an abundance of rough endoplasmic reticulum (*RER*) and a large Golgi region (*G*). [From M. E. Holtrop, *Ann. Clin. Lab. Sci.*, **5**:264, 1975.] (*c*) An osteoclast ($\times$ 4000). These cells are multinucleated and contain many mitochondria, vacuoles

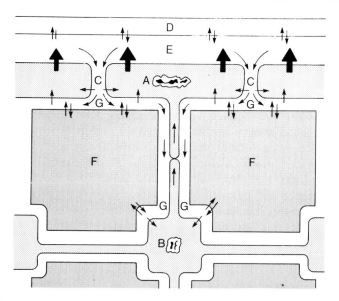

FIGURE 7.3. The Talmage model of exchange of calcium between skeletal bone and body fluids. According to this concept calcium is continually entering the "bone-fluid" (*G*) compartment through channels (*C*) between periosteal osteoblasts (*A*). The deeper osteocytes (*B*) take up calcium from the bone fluid, but they lose it via cell-to-cell transfer toward the periphery, finally reaching the osteoblasts. Here an outward-directed pump (heavy black arrows) moves calcium into the extracellular-fluid compartment (*E*), which is in equilibrium with blood (*D*). The circuit is repeated by entry of more calcium from the extracellular compartment to the bone-fluid compartment via the interosteoblastic channels. Calcium may enter or leave the bone-fluid compartment from the surface of the bone mineral (*F*). [From A. M. Parfitt, *Metabolism*, **25**:909, 1976.]

However, more recently the suggestion has been made that the functional barrier lies between the extracellular fluid and bone fluid compartments and that these do not have similar concentrations of calcium and phosphate. It is now thought that bone fluid calcium values are about one-third those of the extracellular fluid (as the calcium entering bone fluid quickly moves into bone). The barrier could then be a membrane consisting of osteoblast cells.

(including lysosomes) and free ribosomes. Part of the cell surface, the ruffled border (*rb*), is highly folded and provides a great increase in cell surface area, which is important in cell secretion and absorption. On each side of the ruffled border are clear zones (*cz*), generally devoid of cell organelles and containing actinlike filaments. These areas may enable the osteoclast to adhere to the bone surface. [From M. E. Holtrop and G. J. King, *Clin. Orthopaed.*, **123**:177, 1977.] (*d*) Cell process from an osteoblast (*ob*) making side-to-side contact with another cell process, forming a tight junction (arrow) (× 21,250). These processes contain microfilaments and provide a means of transport and communication among osteocytes and between osteocytes and osteoblasts. [From M. E. Holtrop and J. M. Weinger, *Calcium, Parathyroid Hormone and the Calcitonins*, Excerpta Medica, 1971, p. 365.] (*e*) Detailed view of ruffled border (*rb*) and clear zone (*cz*) areas of an osteoclast (× 5700). The bone (*b*) is demineralized. [From Holtrop and King, *Clin. Orthopaed.*, **123**:177, 1977.]

This model has been developed by Talmage (Fig. 7.3) to explain how plasma calcium can be regulated quickly without involvement of osteoclastic bone resorption. This model makes the assumptions (1) that the bone fluid (G) is kept separate from the extracellular fluids (E), (2) that extracellular-fluid calcium tends to continually enter the bone fluid along its concentration gradient by flowing in channels (C) between the osteoblasts, (3) that the bone fluid is closely associated with the calcified bone (F) and (4) that there is a calcium pump (heavy arrows) located on the distal surface of the osteoblast cells to move calcium quickly back into the extracellular fluid. Thus, under normal conditions calcium would move continually from the extracellular fluids into bone fluid and then into the bone or surrounding osteoblasts, and be actively pumped out into the extracellular fluids. Parfitt has emphasized that this mechanism is the major one by which plasma calcium levels are maintained and that it is independent of changes in activity or number of osteoclasts.

KIDNEY STRUCTURE AND PHYSIOLOGY

The kidney performs three major functions: filtration, tubular reabsorption, and tubular secretion. Filtration of substances occurs from capillaries supplying Bowman's capsule (the glomerulus) across the intervening membranes into the lumen of the capsule (see Fig. 12.4). This fluid is essentially an ultrafiltrate of blood plasma, containing the same concentrations of plasma constituents, with the exception of the plasma proteins. The glomerular filtration rate (GFR) is determined mainly by intravascular pressure causing the blood fluid constituents to leave the glomerular capillaries. One can easily estimate the GFR by measuring the excretion rate of a substance dissolved in blood plasma that is freely filterable in the glomeruli, but which thereafter is neither reabsorbed nor secreted by the renal tubules. One such substance is the polysaccharide inulin; the clearance of inulin provides a good approximation of the GFR. The clearance of a substance by the kidney is defined as the concentration of the substance per ml of urine (U) divided by the concentration of the substance per ml of plasma (P) times the volume (V) of urine (in ml) excreted per minute, or $U/P \times V$. This simply defines the amount of substance that is being "cleared" or "cleaned" from the body in a given time.

The renal clearance of a substance can be divided by the simultaneous clearance of inulin to correct for any changes that might have occurred in the GFR during the time of a test. This is referred to as the *relative clearance*, or *fractional excretion* of the substance, i.e., the clearance of the substance relative to that of inulin. For example, if the relative clearance of potassium (C_K/C_{In}) is 1.0, this means that there was no net change in the concentration of potassium along the tubule and that the same amount of potassium that was filtered was excreted. However, if the relative clearance of potassium

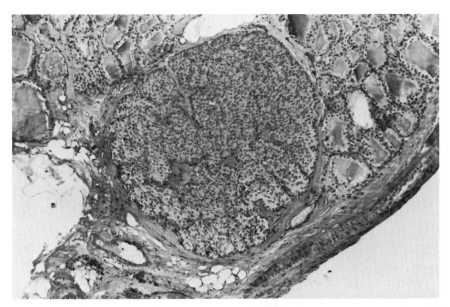

FIGURE 7.4. Histological structure of the rat parathyroid gland (× 115). The parathyroid is the round structure in the center, embedded just beneath the fibrous capsule (*lower right*) of the thyroid gland. Note that the parathyroid is composed of solid cords of cells, while the surrounding thyroid tissue is follicular. [Photo provided by Dr. Yuichi Sasayama, University of Toyama.]

is 0.5, this indicates that 50% of the potassium filtered by the glomeruli was reabsorbed into the body fluids across the tubules. Alternatively, the relative clearance of potassium might exceed 1.0, indicating that more potassium is being excreted than was filtered, and therefore tubular secretion of potassium occurred along the tubule. Thus, we can define tubular reabsorption as a process by which substances filtered by the glomeruli are partially or completely reabsorbed into the blood before they are excreted. Glucose, for example, at normal blood concentrations, is completely reabsorbed from the renal tubules following filtration, and sodium and calcium are also highly conserved. Tubular secretion is a process by which substances present in the peritubular capillaries can be added to the filtrate along the renal tubule, so that more of the substance than was filtered can be excreted. Examples of substances that leave the body mainly via this method are hydrogen ions, and many drugs and other substances foreign to the body, such as penicillin. Tubular reabsorption and secretion can occur anywhere along the nephron. To pinpoint the exact locations of transport, micropuncture or microperfusion studies are required.

The vertebrate kidney is an excellent example of the generalization that organ function is dependent upon organ structure. The structure of the kidney tubule varies markedly from one class of vertebrates to another. In fishes, amphibians, and reptiles, the tubules are short, only moderately convoluted, and lack the loop of Henle that is needed to concentrate urine by reabsorption of water along the tubule. Birds have a mixed population of nephrons, with some nonlooped, "reptilian-type" nephrons, as well as both short-looped and long-looped "mammalian-type" nephrons. Because avian and mammalian renal tubules have a loop of Henle, they can produce a urine that is more concentrated than their extracellular fluids.

Almost all of our information regarding how calcium and phosphate are handled by the kidney tubules is derived from studies of a few species of mammals. Studies with drugs and micropuncture indicate that both phosphate and calcium are normally reabsorbed in both the proximal and distal convoluted tubules. In a large number of lower vertebrate species, net (in excess of the glomerular filtrate) phosphate secretion occurs, though this does not occur in mammals. In all vertebrate classes calcium is highly conserved by the kidney.

THE PARATHYROID GLAND

The parathyroid glands of mammals, as the name suggests, are closely associated with the thyroid glands and often are embedded within the thyroid tissue. The glands consist of one or two pairs and measure 1 to 2 mm in diameter. Accessory, or additional, parathyroid tissue is a common finding in mammals. Although the glands had been described by anatomists in the 1800s, it was not until 1909 that MacCallum and Voegtlin recognized the parathyroids as important factors in calcium regulation. They realized that the tetanic convulsions that followed thyroidectomy in mammals were caused by decreased plasma calcium values resulting from the loss of the parathyroid glands. It is only in mammals that the thyroid and parathyroid glands are so closely associated anatomically, although there appears to be no physiological reason for this relationship. In nonmammalian vertebrates the parathyroid glands are more discrete, but are also found in the neck or thorax region in close association with the thyroid, thymus, and ultimobranchial glands. That the parathyroids are endocrine glands was determined by Collip and Clark who were able, in 1925, to reverse the hypocalcemia of parathyroidectomized animals with acid extracts of parathyroid glands.

The parathyroid glands of mammals are composed mainly of so-called chief cells, the source of parathyroid hormone. These cells are arranged in characteristic cell cords between which run blood vessels, nerves, and connective tissue (Fig. 7.4). The chief cell has a fairly uniform structure. The nucleus is large, and the cytoplasm contains a conspicuous endoplasmic reticulum and Golgi apparatus, typical of protein-secreting cells. However, generally very few large secretory granules are seen in the cytoplasm, indicating that parathyroid hormone is not stored to any extent. Both light and dark forms of chief cells are seen with the electron microscope. While they have been suggested to represent different stages in the activity of the glands, it is more likely that they are artifacts of fixation. The water-clear cell described by some histologists is probably a variant of the chief cell.

In addition, in some species of mammals an infrequent second cell type, the oxyphil, has been described. The cytoplasm of these cells is characteristically packed with mitochondria. The function of these cells is unknown, but since they have been most typically found in older animals, it has been suggested that they are correlated with aging or may represent degenerating chief cells. These cells have also been described in chicken and turtle parathyroid glands.

The parathyroids of birds, consisting of a single pair or two closely associated pairs of glands separated from the thyroids, are structurally very similar to those of mammals (Fig. 7.5). Usually, they are located along the carotid arteries, anterior to the heart, between the larger thyroid gland and the ultimobranchial body region (Fig. 7.6). The parathyroids are very small and measure less than 1.0 mm in diameter in most avian species. Their yellowish color and small size distinguish them from the larger, reddish thyroid glands. In chickens the two pairs of glands may be very closely associated and contained within the same capsule, and thus resemble a single

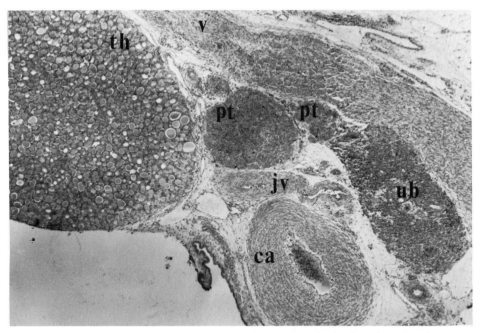

FIGURE 7.5. Histological aspects of several glandular structures in the thoracic region of an 18-day chick embryo. Areas of two closely associated parathyroid glands (*pt*) lie posterior to the thyroid (*th*). Below the parathyroids are the collapsed jugular vein (*jv*) and thick-walled carotid artery (*ca*). Further posterior is the ultimobranchial body (*ub*). The vagus nerve (*v*) is above (median to) the glandular structures. [From N. B. Clark and L. L. S. Mok, University of Connecticut, unpublished data.]

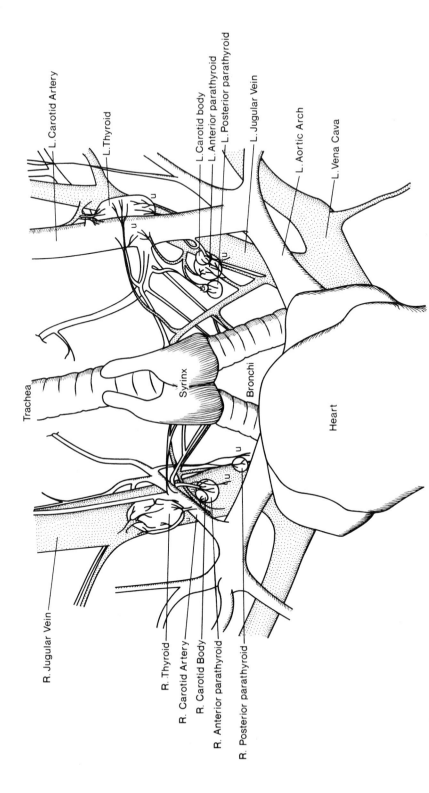

FIGURE 7.6. Thoracic area of the starling (*Sturnus vulgaris*) showing location of the two pairs of parathyroid glands, scattered ultimobranchial follicles (*u*), and carotid bodies. The latter are enclosed within the anterior parathyroid glands in most passerine birds. [Figure provided by Dr. R. F. Wideman, Jr, Pennsylvania State University.]

pair of glands. Accessory parathyroid tissue is found commonly within the thyroid or ultimobranchial glands. In many avian species the parathyroid glands may completely envelop the carotid bodies; the functional significance of this close anatomical relationship is unknown.

There are one or two pairs of parathyroids in reptiles. (There are reports in the older literature that some species possess three or more pairs of parathyroid glands, but this is probably incorrect.) Reptilian parathyroids are about the same in size, color, and histological appearance as those of birds (Fig. 7.7a). In turtles and lizards the glands possess many follicles, often filled with stainable material, which may represent stored parathyroid hormone. The location of the parathyroid glands in reptiles is somewhat variable. In snakes, the anterior pair is near the common carotid bifurcation in the region of the jaw, while the posterior pair is widely separated, in the region of the heart, embedded in the thymus tissue (Fig. 7.8a). In other reptilian groups the parathyroid glands are more closely associated with each other. In turtles, the anterior pair is embedded in the thymus, while the posterior pair lies in a concavity formed by the aortic arch. In lizards (one or two pairs) and crocodiles (one pair), the glands are located near the heart in close association with the thyroids and ultimobranchial bodies (Fig. 7.8b). While few studies of ultrastructure of reptilian parathyroids have been made, it is generally considered that the glands are composed of a single cell type. However, two cell types—chief cells and stellate cells—have been described in the iguana parathyroid gland. The latter are more electron dense and may function in support.

Amphibians probably represent the most diverse group as far as parathyroid structure (and function) are concerned. The structure and location of the parathyroids of urodele amphibians (salamanders) appear to be similar to those of birds and reptiles, although the glands are considerably smaller (generally about 0.25 mm in diameter). The glands—one or two pairs located near the carotid and systemic arches—are composed of richly vascularized cell cords (Figs. 7.7c, 7.8c). They are reported to appear at the time of metamorphosis, and therefore are not present in neotenous forms at all. There are no reports of seasonal variations in parathyroid structure in urodeles; however, few studies have been made.

In anuran amphibians (frogs, toads) the parathyroids do not consist of the typical cell cord structure. Instead, the cells are arranged in whorls and appear quite different histologically from those of urodeles or other vertebrate groups. The cells in the center of the glands are spindle shaped, smaller than the peripheral cells, and contain little cytoplasm. Capillaries penetrate into the glands to the cells of the central zone (Fig. 7.7e). The central zone in some species has been reported to become very small or to disappear altogether in the summer. Increased mitotic activity in the parathyroid glands of toads has been seen during the spring.

Anurans generally have two pairs of parathyroid glands. They are yellowish in color and are located anterior to the heart near or embedded in

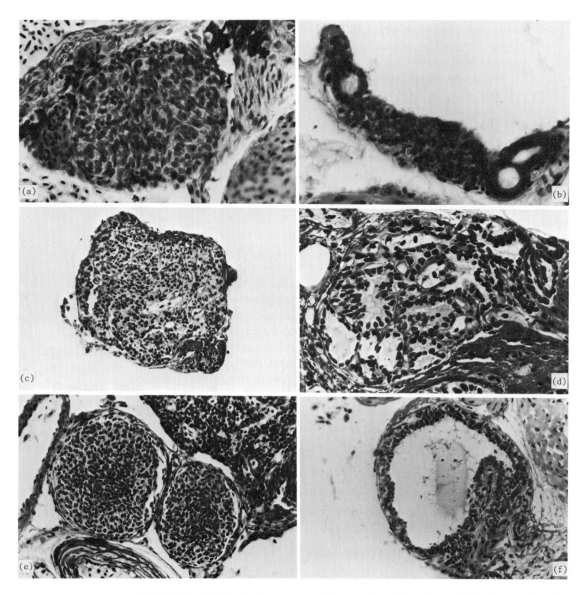

FIGURE 7.7. Histological appearance of the parathyroid glands and ultimobranchial bodies in various vertebrate species. (*a*) Parathyroid gland of the lizard *Takydromus tachydromoides* (× 470); (*b*) ultimobranchial gland of the lizard *Takydromus tachydromoides* (× 470); (*c*) parathyroid gland of the newt *Cynops pyrrhogaster* (× 115); (*d*) ultimobranchial gland of the newt *Cynops pyrrhogaster,* showing follicular structure (× 230); (*e*) pair of parathyroid glands of the frog *Rana nigromaculata* (× 230); the cells are arranged in compact whorls rather than cell cords; (*f*) ultimobranchial gland of the frog *Rana nigromaculata,* consisting of a single, large follicle. [Figures provided by Dr. Y. Sasayama, University of Toyama, Japan.]

the jugular bodies (Fig. 7.8*d*). They measure about 0.25 to 0.5 mm in diameter. Accessory parathyroid tissue has been described in some species. Electron micrographs of anuran parathyroid gland cells indicate that there is a single type of cell that can exist in either a dark or a light form. The parathyroid glands of anurans are present during larval stages from about the time of development of the internal gills.

Parathyroid glands are not found at all in freshwater or marine teleosts, and fishes do not respond to the administration of parathyroid hormone. Obviously, it is important that fishes, like other vertebrates, be able to regulate their extracellular-fluid calcium levels. Investigations in this area have established several hormones that might be acting as equivalents to parathyroid hormone to raise blood calcium values. These include two pituitary hormones, prolactin and ACTH, and will be discussed later.

It is of interest that the parathyroid glands in several vertebrate groups are known to undergo seasonal structural variation. The reasons for these changes are not known but may be the result of alterations in environmental temperature or of other environmental factors. Seasonal cycles in parathyroid structure have been reported in starlings, several species of lizards and frogs, and hibernating bats, and may be a rather common feature in vertebrates. More such systematic studies should be done.

Another rather common anatomical feature of parathyroid tissue is its frequent occurrence as accessory parathyroid "rests." This seems to be especially prevalent in birds, as parathyroidectomies in chickens are ineffective or have only a short-term effect unless extensive amounts of accessory parathyroid tissue are removed from the ultimobranchial glands. It is possible that the short-term effect of parathyroidectomy in amphibians (both anurans and urodeles) can be explained by the presence of accessory parathyroid glands. Alternatively, there may be additional hypercalcemic factors in these groups.

Until recently, there has been no question that the hormone-secreting cells of the parathyroid gland originate from endodermal tissue from the third and fourth pharyngeal pouches during embryonic development. However, this long-standing assumption has been challenged by Pearse, who believes that these cells are originally derived from neural crest cells that migrate to the region of the pharyngeal pouches during early development. He has presented evidence for neural crest origin of the parathyroid glands in frogs and feels that this may be a characteristic pattern in other vertebrate groups as well. Pearse's hypothesis will require further substantiation before it receives general acceptance.

Parathyroid Hormone Structure and Biosynthesis

The complete amino acid sequence is known for bovine, porcine, and human parathyroid hormone, while partial sequences of the hormone are known for the chicken (Fig. 7.9). In mammals the hormone is a straight-chain

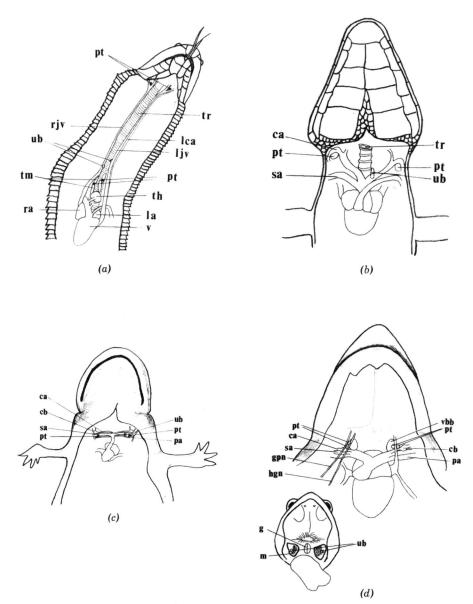

FIGURE 7.8. Location of the parathyroid glands and ultimobranchial bodies in various groups of amphibians and reptiles. (*a*) Location of two widely spaced pairs of parathyroid glands (*pt*) and a pair of ultimobranchial glands (*ub*) in the snake *Elaphe quadrivirgata*. *rjv*, right jugular vein; *tm*, thymus; *ra*, right atrium; *tr*, trachea; *lca*, left carotid artery; *ljv*, left jugular vein; *th*, thyroid; *la*, left atrium; *v*, ventricle. (*b*) Location of a single pair of parathyroid glands (*pt*) and a single left ultimobranchial body (*ub*) in the lizard *Takydromus tachydromoides*. *ca*, carotid arch; *sa*, systemic arch. (*c*) Location of a single pair of parathyroid glands (*pt*) and left ultimobranchial body (*ub*) in the newt *Cynops pyrrhogaster*. *cb*, carotid body; *pa*, pulmocutaneous arch. (*d*) Location of two closely adjacent pairs of parathyroid glands (*pt*) and bilateral ultimobranchial bodies (*ub*) in the frog *Rana nigromaculata*. *gpn*, glossopharyngeal nerve; *hgn*, hypoglossal nerve; *vbb*, ventral branchial body; *g*, glottis; *m*, muscle. [Figures provided by Dr. Y. Sasayama, University of Toyama, Japan.]

polypeptide consisting of 84 amino acids and a molecular weight of 8400 daltons. In studies of the biological activity of portions of the molecule, it has been determined that amino acids 1 to 34 contain the complete biological activity. Thus synthesized parathyroid hormone can be purchased and consists of only the N-terminal amino acids 1 to 34.

During chromatographic purification procedures for parathyroid hormone, it was found that hypercalcemic activity was present in more than one fraction. Additionally, in radioimmunoassay tests synthetic parathyroid hormone and plasma parathyroid hormone behaved as though there were differences between them. This led to further tests that identified a 90–amino acid prohormone consisting of amino acids 1 to 84 of parathyroid hormone plus six additional amino acids attached at the N-terminus (molecular weight 9000). Further analysis revealed a still larger precursor which exists free for only a few seconds before cleavage to the prohormone. This has been called "preproparathyroid hormone." Preproparathyroid hormone has 23 additional amino acids attached to the amino terminus of the molecule (preceding the amino terminus of proparathyroid hormone) and thus has 115 amino acids and a molecular weight of about 14,000 daltons. The structures of these precursors to bovine parathyroid hormone (PTH) are shown in Fig. 7.10. Preproparathyroid hormone is believed to be the initial synthetic product of the parathyroid chief cell and, therefore, contains all of the structural information coded in the parathyroid hormone gene.

Habener has described in detail the following steps of parathyroid hormone biosynthesis in the bovine parathyroid cell (Fig. 7.11):

1.   Preproparathyroid hormone is synthesized on the ribosome in the cytoplasm.

2.   As the polypeptide chain grows (from the N-terminus) it emerges from the ribosome and associates with the membrane of the endoplasmic reticulum. This "pre" portion of the molecule apparently functions as a signal protein to allow the molecule to enter the cisternae of the endoplasmic reticulum.

3.   The "pre" portion of the molecule (amino acids -7 to -29) is cleaved, and proparathyroid hormone moves to the Golgi region. (The fate of the 23–amino acid "pre" sequence is not known; it may be rapidly degraded.)

4.   The proparathyroid hormone molecule exists for about 20 minutes and is cleaved to parathyroid hormone in the Golgi region. This involves the loss of amino acids -6 to -1 and is an energy-requiring process. Microtubules are thought to be involved in some way in the cleavage.

5.   Parathyroid hormone is packaged into secretory granules at the Golgi apparatus or may be released from the cells without being packaged into granules ("bypass"). PTH is the major form of parathyroid hormone extractable from the parathyroid gland. Electron microscopic studies of parathyroid glands generally show few stored secretory granules, indicating

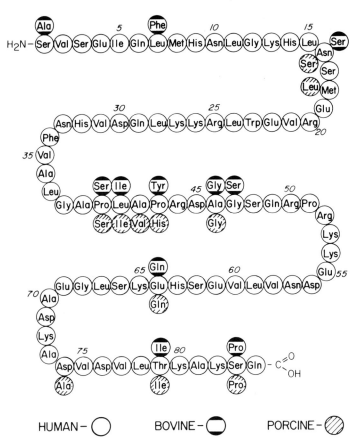

FIGURE 7.9. Amino acid sequences of human, bovine, and porcine parathyroid hormones. Sequences are quite similar. Where differences exist from human parathyroid hormone, the bovine amino acid substitutions at any position are shown black; porcine amino acid substitutions are shown cross-hatched. For a key to the abbreviations of amino acids see Appendix. [Based on H. T. Keutmann, M. M. Sauer, and G. N. Hendy, *Biochemistry*, **17:**5723–5729, 1978.]

that parathyroid hormone is either degraded or released rapidly, and not stored to any extent. The hormone is either transported to the plasma membrane for release or degraded within the cell. According to Cohn and colleagues, production of parathyroid hormone appears to proceed at a constant rate; the amount of hormone released depends upon the rate of degradation. This process appears to be regulated by the calcium levels of the extracellular fluids, so that high calcium levels will stimulate intracellular degradation of the hormone and low calcium concentrations will inhibit it.

6.   Upon release from the parathyroid chief cell, parathyroid hormone

(amino acids 1 to 84) cleaves at about amino acid 34. This may occur immediately after release or at the receptor. In any event, parathyroid hormone has a half-life of only 2 to 4 minutes and disappears from the circulation rapidly. The rest of the molecule (the C-terminal two-thirds of the molecule) persists in the extracellular fluids about 10 times longer than the N terminus. The C-terminal fragment has no biological activity, but it can be measured by radioimmunoassays for parathyroid hormone and thus results in estimates of circulating parathyroid hormone levels that are erroneously high.

Regulation of Parathyroid Hormone Secretion

Secretion of parathyroid hormone is a self-regulating system. The cells are sensitive to blood calcium levels, so that low concentrations of extracellular-fluid calcium stimulate parathyroid hormone secretion and high levels of calcium inhibit it (Fig. 7.12). However, parathyroid hormone release is not a simple linear response. Rather, parathyroid hormone output changes little in the normal range of extracellular-fluid calcium (9 to 11 mg/dl; C in Fig.

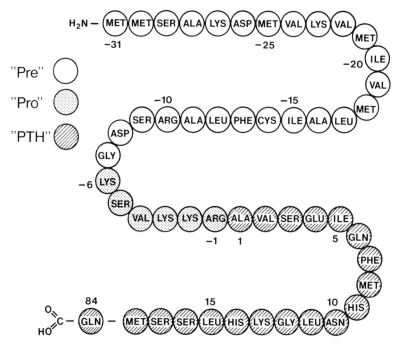

FIGURE 7.10.   Amino acid sequence of bovine preproparathyroid hormone. The PTH portion of the molecule is numbered 1 to 84, but the portion from amino acid 19 to amino acid 83 is omitted to avoid repetition (see Fig. 7.9). Proparathyroid hormone includes six additional amino acids, here numbered −1 to −6. Preproparathyroid hormone includes 25 residues in addition, here numbered −7 to −31. [From J. F. Habener and H. M. Kronenberg, *Fed. Proc.*, **37**:2561, 1978.]

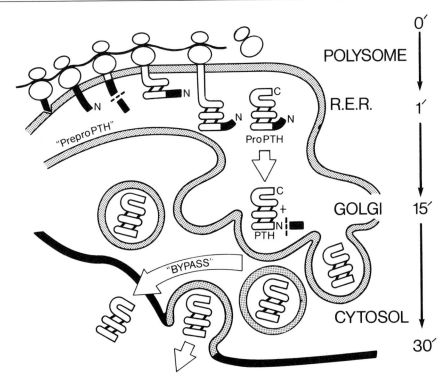

FIGURE 7.11. Scheme representing the intracellular synthesis of parathyroid hormone. Pre-proparathyroid hormone is synthesized between the polysome and the endoplasmic reticulum (*R.E.R.*). It moves along the matrix of the *R.E.R.*, during which time it is partially cleaved to proparathyroid hormone. In the Golgi lamellae proparathyroid hormone is cleaved to yield parathyroid hormone, which is packaged into secretory granules. These granules in the cytoplasm may be secreted by exocytosis (shown by short white arrow). Alternatively, parathyroid hormone may not be packaged but be released directly into the cytosol ("bypass"). [From D. V. Cohn, J. J. Morrissey, R. P. MacGregor, and J. W. Hamilton, *Comparative Endocrinology* (P. Gaillard and H. Boer, Eds.), Elsevier/North-Holland, Amsterdam, 1978, p. 273.]

7.12), but does increase markedly as the plasma calcium falls below 9 mg/dl (*B* in Fig. 7.12). Parathyroid hormone secretion rate becomes maximal at 6 to 7 mg/dl. Furthermore, there is always a low level of parathyroid hormone secretion. Figure 7.12 depicts data derived from human studies, but similar relationships could be expected in most other mammalian and submammalian groups.

How is it that the parathyroid cells respond to small changes in extracellular-fluid calcium concentration, whereas other cells apparently do not? It has been suggested that since parathyroid cells contain few mitochondria (compared with other cells), they cannot sequester much calcium and must respond immediately to increased calcium entrance into the cells. Thus, according to Cohn's hypothesis, hypercalcemia would stimulate intracellular degradation of hormone and decrease parathyroid hormone output. Since more proparathyroid hormone is synthesized than is required, hypocalcemia would decrease the degradation of proparathyroid hormone and thus would result in increased output of hormone, leading to hypercalcemia and homeostatic control of plasma calcium values.

Physiological Effects of Parathyroid Hormone

Parathyroid hormone has been reported to affect calcium transport in three targets: bone, kidney, and gut. The hypercalcemic activity of the hormone could result from a variety of different actions on these targets. In early studies investigators tried to ascertain which of the many effects of the hormone was the primary one and which were secondary (indirect) effects.

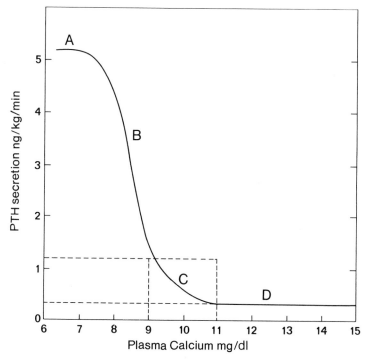

FIGURE 7.12. Parathyroid hormone secretion at different total blood calcium concentrations. *A* is the maximum secretory rate regardless of how low the blood calcium concentration may be. *B* is a rapidly changing secretory rate, proportional to the changes in blood calcium concentration over a range of approximately 7–9 mg/dl. Parathyroid hormone is mobilized rapidly in response to calcium levels falling below 9 mg/dl. *C* represents the small changes that occur in parathyroid hormone secretion in the normal range of blood calcium concentrations (9–11 mg/dl). *D* is the minimal parathyroid hormone secretory rate regardless of how high the blood calcium level may rise. [From J. F. Habener, *Polypeptide Hormones: Molecular and Cellular Aspects*, Elsevier/Excerpta Medica, Amsterdam, 1976, p. 197.]

It is now clear that there are several primary effects of parathyroid hormone and that many events occur simultaneously following the release or administration of the hormone. Most of the generalizations outlined below are based upon studies of a few species of laboratory mammals, such as the rat and dog.

Bone. Parathyroid hormone action results in an almost bewilderingly large number of changes in bone. The hormone stimulates bone adenyl cyclase activity and cyclic AMP production; however, it is still not certain whether cAMP is a necessary first step in the mechanism of action of the hormone in any of these events. Parfitt, in an excellent essay (1976), has described many of the effects of parathyroid hormone on bone, and put these into a rational order. There are both long-term and short-term effects, and these may occur independently of each other. The major effects are as follows:

1. Parathyroid hormone stimulates the conversion of connective tissue precursor cells into osteoclasts. This is a long-term effect (18 to 36 hours) that increases the rate of bone turnover and the mobilization of both calcium and phosphate. There is no evidence that cAMP is involved directly in this process.

2. Parathyroid hormone stimulates existing "resting" osteoclasts to enter into an active state. This effect requires about 6 to 18 hours and results in transient mobilization of calcium and phosphate. No cAMP involvement is necessary.

3. Parathyroid hormone increases the metabolic production by bone cells, especially osteoclasts, of various organic acids and enzymes that are almost certainly concerned with bone resorption. These include citric acid, lysosomal enzymes, collagenase, hyaluronic acid, and others. The time required for increased production of these substances varies widely, but generally is about 24 hours.

4. Parathyroid hormone stimulates (deep) osteocytes to move calcium from partially mineralized bone around the lacunae first into the bone fluid and thence into the extracellular fluid. This effect, which has been estimated histologically as decreased density of perilacunar bone, has been noted as early as two hours following parathyroid hormone administration, but is more marked after longer time intervals. This process requires cAMP formation and would function to correct decreases in plasma calcium and phosphate values.

5. Parathyroid hormone action leads to an increased permeability of the osteoblast membranes to calcium and thus increases the influx of calcium into these cells. Since cells contain a powerful outwardly-directed calcium pump, the calcium is quickly moved to the extracellular fluid (see the Talmage model, Fig. 7.3). This mechanism is thought to regulate the minute-to-minute values of plasma calcium and to be the first of the short-term

effects of parathyroid hormone on bone cells. Careful studies of changes in plasma calcium concentrations have revealed a small but consistent dip in plasma calcium within several minutes following parathyroid hormone administration that occurs before the characteristic hypercalcemic response, lending further evidence for this mechanism.

Thus all three populations of bone cells appear to be sensitive to parathyroid hormone and to be involved in the regulation of different aspects of calcium homeostasis: (1) the osteoblasts and osteocytes that line the bone surface (surface osteocytes) regulate the quick flux of calcium out of bone and thus determine the steady-state level of plasma calcium; (2) the (deep) osteocytes mobilize calcium from bone surrounding the lacunae without a breakdown of bone matrix and can provide increased amounts of calcium and phosphate rapidly; and (3) the osteoclasts increase in number and activity and resorb bone, freeing both bone mineral and matrix and thus regulating remodeling.

On the other hand, there are many researchers who feel that the minute-to-minute regulation of plasma calcium by parathyroid hormone does not involve bone at all and can be explained by the direct effect of the hormone on calcium reabsorption by the kidney or the indirect effects of parathyroid hormone on vitamin D stimulated calcium absorption from the gut.

Kidney. The renal actions of parathyroid hormone have been studied intensively in mammals. Parathyroid hormone enhances calcium reabsorption and phosphate excretion and produces a moderate water diuresis. These effects appear to be mediated by increased cAMP production in the renal tubular cells. Thus the hormone causes calcium conservation and increased excretion of phosphate by the kidney. Since bone resorption results in increased mobilization of *both* calcium and phosphate, this mechanism may rid the body of the extra phosphate freed during bone breakdown without the simultaneous loss of calcium.

In mammals renal calcium reabsorption appears to be linked with sodium reabsorption and occurs in both proximal and distal parts of the nephrons. Parathyroid hormone enhances the reabsorption of calcium by the distal parts of the tubules only. The hormone also enhances calcium reabsorption by the renal tubules of birds. In contrast, the renal reabsorption of calcium is not sensitive to the presence or absence of parathyroid hormone in normal snakes and turtles. This suggests that nephrons of the mammalian type are a necessary target for parathyroid hormone–mediated renal calcium reabsorption, but this is only speculation. Studies of renal clearance of calcium and of hormonal effects on this process have not yet been reported in amphibians.

The mechanisms by which the kidneys handle phosphate probably involve simultaneous reabsorption and secretion fluxes along the nephrons. The net (overall) effect of parathyroid hormone in mammals is to inhibit phosphate reabsorption, while in most of the nonmammalian species examined the net effect of the hormone is to stimulate tubular phosphate secretion. Both processes result in phosphaturia; however, only in the nonmammalian vertebrates is the amount of phosphate in the urine in excess of that which was filtered in the glomeruli. In fact, in many parathyroid-intact nonmammals, phosphate secretion occurs normally. There is at present no adequate model to explain how parathyroid hormone can affect both reabsorption and secretion of phosphate in the renal tubules.

Intestine.   Parathyroid hormone has been reported to enhance calcium absorption from the gut of experimental mammals, but since the required dose is high (about 100 international units), this effect may not be physiological. Also, this effect of the hormone varies greatly depending upon the amount of calcium in the diet. For example, if dietary calcium levels are high, then parathyroidectomy or parathyroid hormone administration have little effect on intestinal calcium absorption. In any case, the presence of vitamin D is an absolute requirement for intestinal calcium absorption.

It is presently thought that the effects of parathyroid hormone on gut calcium absorption are indirect. That is, parathyroid hormone stimulates the production of 1,25-dihydroxyvitamin D_3 (1,25-(OH)$_2D_3$), the physiologically active form of this vitamin. It has been shown, for example, that parathyroidectomy decreases the production of 1,25-(OH)$_2D_3$ in hypocalcemic rats, while parathyroid hormone restores the production of the metabolite to normal.

Comparative Studies of Parathyroid Hormone Function

Interest in the function of the parathyroids in nonmammalian vertebrates has intensified over the last decade, so that it is now becoming easier to make accurate generalizations concerning adaptive features in particular groups. Although large gaps remain in the literature, Dacke's recent (1979) book dealing with the comparative aspects of calcium has helped bring much of the pertinent literature together.

Birds.   Studies of parathyroid function in birds have been almost entirely confined to domestic chickens, although a few studies have been devoted to the function of these glands in Japanese quail and starlings. In general, the parathyroids of birds appear to function in the same manner as those of mammals. Untreated parathyroidectomy results in hypocalcemia, tetany, and death within only a few hours (if no accessory tissue is present), while parathyroid hormone administration can reverse these effects.

Parathyroidectomy in birds significantly increases the loss of renal calcium and decreases urinary phosphate excretion, while parathyroid hormone returns the levels toward normal. When parathyroid hormone is infused into the renal portal vein of one kidney of a hen while the phosphate excretion from both kidneys is measured separately, a unilateral increase in phosphate excretion is induced. This appears to show that the chicken kidney tubules are directly responsive to parathyroid hormone with respect to phosphate secretion and excretion.

The process of producing calcified eggshells also involves the movement of large amounts of calcium from one site to another. Elevated sex hormone concentrations induce the production by the liver of a yolk protein, phosvitin (see Chapter 13), that has a high affinity for calcium and phosphate. Accordingly, plasma calcium and phosphate levels increase sharply during the process of egg laying. High plasma levels of estrogens, in conjunction with testosterone or progesterone, also stimulate the production of a loosely structured bone within the marrow cavities in birds. This "medullary" bone is especially noticeable in the long bones. Medullary bone is very labile and appears to function as a storage place for calcium, rather than for support. Calcium from the medullary bone is subsequently transferred to the oviduct "shell gland," where it is used in the formation of the eggshell.

Cyclic eggshell formation thus results in the movement of large stores of calcium from gut or bone first to the marrow cavities and then to the shell gland. Parathyroid hormone is thought to be involved in this process because phosphate excretion is increased during this time, at least in chickens. It has been postulated that this mechanism facilitates the excretory loss of the phosphate that is liberated from medullary bone during eggshell formation.

Reptiles.   Parathyroidectomy of reptiles generally results in severe hypocalcemia, tetany, and death. In some species plasma calcium concentrations fall as low as 70% below normal. Serum phosphate levels rise sharply following parathyroidectomy in most reptiles. Administration of parathyroid hormone to either normal or parathyroidectomized reptiles generally results in significant hypercalcemia and hypophosphatemia.

There have been only a handful of studies of the effects of parathyroid hormone on renal excretion of calcium, phosphate, or other ions in reptiles. The changes that occur in plasma phosphate values following parathyroidectomy or parathyroid hormone administration in lizards, turtles, and snakes are thought to reflect shifts in renal phosphate excretion patterns. This has been found to be the case in the water snake *Natrix*. While the renal tubules of this species of snake normally secrete phosphate, this is abolished by parathyroidectomy. Within 30 minutes of parathyroid hormone administration to parathyroidectomized snakes, net phosphate secretion is again reestablished. On the other hand, calcium excretion patterns of the reptilian kidney appear not to be affected by parathyroid hormone.

Another interesting aspect of the effect of parathyroid hormone in reptiles is the long latency period before its presence or absence is reflected by changes in extracellular-fluid calcium or phosphate values. For example, in turtles it takes several days, or even a week or more, for the effects of parathyroidectomy or parathyroid hormone administration to be seen.

Amphibians. In general, parathyroidectomy of amphibians results in hypocalcemia and hyperphosphatemia, but these effects may last only for a short time before the plasma levels of calcium and phosphate return to normal. The reasons for the apparent recovery from the operation are not clear, but it is possible that amphibians possess more than one hypercalcemic hormone (see below). In addition, the time of year that the operation is performed has a large influence on the severity of symptoms. For example, parathyroidectomy of a frog in summer, when the gland has a normal histological appearance, has a much greater effect than if the operation were done in winter (when the glands are vacuolated and appear degenerated). It has been found in a few species of anurans that there is a natural seasonal fluctuation in plasma calcium values. However, this fluctuation does not correlate well with the histological appearance of the parathyroid gland.

Parathyroid hormone administration to anurans will reverse the effects of acute parathyroidectomy, or cause hypercalcemia and hypophosphatemia in intact frogs. These changes occur quite rapidly, usually within two hours.

There are only a few studies of effects of parathyroidectomy or parathyroid hormone administration on renal excretion patterns of amphibians, and in most of these renal clearance studies were not performed. Needless to say, it is very difficult to perform renal clearance experiments in such small animals; thus the best we can do is interpret studies in which intermittent samples of bladder urine were collected from the test animals. In these, there are reports that parathyroidectomy results in increased excretion of calcium, phosphate, sodium, and water—all indicating decreased reabsorption by the renal tubules.

It is of interest that the parathyroid glands of urodeles are reported not to develop until the time of metamorphosis and that neotenous and some aquatic salamanders have no parathyroids at all. Recently it has been shown that there is a diversity of response of different species of urodele amphibians to parathyroidectomy. While some salamanders respond to parathyroidectomy with lowered blood calcium values and tetany, more primitive ones show no changes in blood calcium after parathyroidectomy. Of course, neotenous salamanders must have some alternative system for regulating their extracellular-fluid calcium values. Those species of salamanders that are insensitive to parathyroidectomy do show a drop in serum calcium in response to hypophysectomy. Pang and Oguro have suggested that the pituitary hormone responsible for raising serum calcium values in these urodeles is prolactin. These findings in urodeles may relate to the short-term effects of parathyroidectomy in anurans as well.

Fishes. As stated earlier, parathyroid glands are absent in fishes. However, it is essential that fishes be able to regulate their extracellular-fluid calcium levels. Marine fishes need to be able to excrete the excess calcium ions that they obtain from seawater, while freshwater fishes, in order to maintain their plasma calcium ions, must not lose them to the environment.

It has been known for some time that hypophysectomized fishes maintained in water low in calcium content do not survive well and, among other changes, show decreased plasma calcium values. This suggests that there may be a factor, or factors, from the pituitary responsible for elevating blood calcium concentrations in fishes. Doses of cortisol, ACTH, or prolactin are all effective in hypophysectomized killifish in reversing hypocalcemia. In addition, extracts of the anterior portion of the killifish pituitary and middle portion of the carp pituitary, which are rich in prolactin cells, induce hypercalcemia in killifish. Since prolactin is effective at lower doses than the other hormones, prolactin has been suggested to be the hypercalcemic hormone in fishes. The hormone appears to act by enhancing calcium uptake from environmental water by the gills.

Some researchers feel that prolactin, while hypercalcemic, takes too long to act (two days) to be the physiological factor responsible for these changes. Parsons has pointed out structural similarities between the sequence of several amino acids in the 1-to-11 fragment of the ACTH molecule and amino acids 15 to 25 of bovine parathyroid hormone (part of the biologically active region) (Fig. 7.13).

Immunological studies also have lent support to the existence of a pituitary hypercalcemic factor in fishes. If antibodies are raised against bovine PTH_{1-34}, eel pituitary extract (but not human pituitary extract or porcine ACTH) will cause complete displacement of the bovine PTH from the antibody. This would indicate that the antibody "sees" a sequence in the eel pituitary extract that is similar to parathyroid hormone. In physiological experiments, pituitary extracts of guinea pig, rat, eel, and cod caused significant hypercalcemia in intact trout within two hours, whereas mammalian parathyroid hormone was without effect. Parsons has suggested the name *hypercalcin* for the piscine hypercalcemic pituitary factor. The hypothesis that hypercalcin is ACTH is attractive, since it would suggest evolution of the structure and function of a hypercalcemic hormone throughout the vertebrates, rather than a shift from use of one hormone to another in different vertebrate classes.

Similarity of Amino Acid Sequence in
ACTH and Parathyroid Hormone

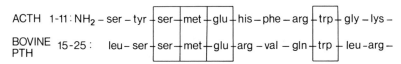

FIGURE 7.13. Similarities in portions of the ACTH and PTH molecules. Identical portions are enclosed in rectangles.

CALCITONIN

Calcitonin is among the most recently discovered hormones, described by Copp and colleagues in 1962. They perfused a high calcium medium (13 mg/dl) directly into a blood vessel of the thyroparathyroid apparatus (thyroid glands and the enclosed parathyroid glands) of the dog. Despite the infusion of calcium locally, systemic blood calcium *decreased* by about 10% within an hour and returned to normal in about two hours. Plasma phosphate values changed in a similar manner in response to the high calcium perfusate. Copp hypothesized that the decrease in blood calcium was caused by the release of a hormone from the thyroid or parathyroid glands and termed the proposed hormone *calcitonin*. Since parathyroid hormone was known to regulate calcium values, it was guessed at first that this new hypocalcemic hormone also was a product of the parathyroid glands. At about the same time, Hirsch and his co-workers noted a similar drop in systemic blood calcium values in rats that were thyroidectomized by electrocautery. Oddly, this response did not occur in animals that were surgically thyroidectomized. They suggested that this change was caused by a hormone released from cells in the thyroid gland itself and, cognizant of Copp's work, named it *thyrocalcitonin*. The site of origin of the hormone was soon solved, as it was possible to repeat the experiments and obtain hypocalcemia in parathyroidectomized animals. Thus the mammalian thyroid gland was determined to be the source of this new hormone.

The excitement generated by the discovery of calcitonin was intense, since it had long been felt that the minute-to-minute regulation of the calcium levels in the extracellular fluids could not be controlled adequately by parathyroid hormone alone. Thus many, if not most, workers in the parathyroid field embarked upon studies of this new hormone, with a resulting explosion of research and publications in this field.

Calcitonin Structure

The first task was to determine which thyroidal cell type secretes calcitonin. Pearse had previously defined the thyroid follicular cells as *type A*, the endothelial cells of the thyroid capillaries as *type B*, and the interfollicular or parafollicular cells as *type C* cells. It was these latter cells that were determined eventually to be the source of calcitonin. The C cells are not easy to distinguish from thyroid follicular cells by histochemical methods, but are strikingly clear if an immunocytochemical method is used (Fig. 7.14).

Once the cellular source of calcitonin was identified, it took only 18 months for the hormone to be isolated in pure form, the amino acid sequence determined, and the entire molecule synthesized. Porcine calcitonin was characterized by Potts and co-workers in 1968, and now the complete amino acid sequences for eight more calcitonins are known, including those of humans, sheep (ovine), cows (bovine), salmon, and eel. The general structure of all of these molecules is essentially the same, each consisting of 32 amino acids with a 1–7 disulfide bridge and proline amide as the C-terminal residue. The molecules are fairly stable and have a molecular weight of about 3600 (Fig. 7.15). Salmon calcitonin has both a higher affinity for receptors and a lower susceptibility to degradation, and thus has the highest biological activity.

However, there are oddities about the calcitonin molecules. For example, even in mammals there is a wide variation in the amino acid sequence from species to species (Fig. 7.15). In the first five calcitonin molecules characterized, only 9 of the 32 amino acids were homologous. Human calcitonin is more like salmon calcitonin in primary structure than it is like pig calcitonin. Also, there does not appear to be any "active core" or fragment that contains most of the biological activity; instead, the entire hormone is needed for an adequate biological response. On the other hand, the changes in the amino acid structures of the known calcitonin molecules are generally conservative and can be caused by single-base mutations in the genetic code. The disparity in the structures of calcitonins has led to difficulties in assaying for hormone in various vertebrate classes. The criterion used as the basis for the standard bioassay of calcitonin is its hypocalcemic activity in young rats. Acid extracts of mammalian thyroid tissue injected subcutaneously decrease blood calcium values by as much as 10 to 15% one hour later. Small amounts of hormone, such as those circulating in the plasma, cannot be measured accurately by this method. Radioimmunoassays for calcitonin are much more sensitive and can detect amounts of the hormone as small as 1 pg/ml. However, the differences in hormonal structure from species to species sometimes result in a lack of immunological cross-reactivity. Fortunately, it appears that salmon calcitonin will cross-react with calcitonins from other nonmammalian vertebrates.

At the same time that the more biochemically oriented endocrinologists were characterizing calcitonin in mammals, comparative endocrinologists were searching for the hormone in nonmammalian vertebrates. Acid extracts or homogenates of thyroid glands of the lower forms, however, did not induce hypocalcemia when tested in the rat. This was puzzling until it was rediscovered that the "parafollicular" C cells in the embryo are derived from the last pharyngeal pouch, from whence the ultimobranchial body develops. In nonmammalian vertebrate embryos the ultimobranchial pouches, after breaking away from the pharynx, remain as separate organs near the heart. They do not become incorporated into the developing thyroid, as they do in mammals. Ultimobranchial body extracts do indeed induce hypocalcemia in rats in the test assay for calcitonin activity.

The ultimobranchial bodies generally consist of scattered, isolated cells and follicles and are located in the region of the parathyroids and thyroid glands (Figs. 7.5, 7.6, and 7.8). They are often difficult to detect because of their diffuse nature, small size, and lack of a delimiting connective tissue capsule. In reptiles, the ultimobranchial body on the left side may be well

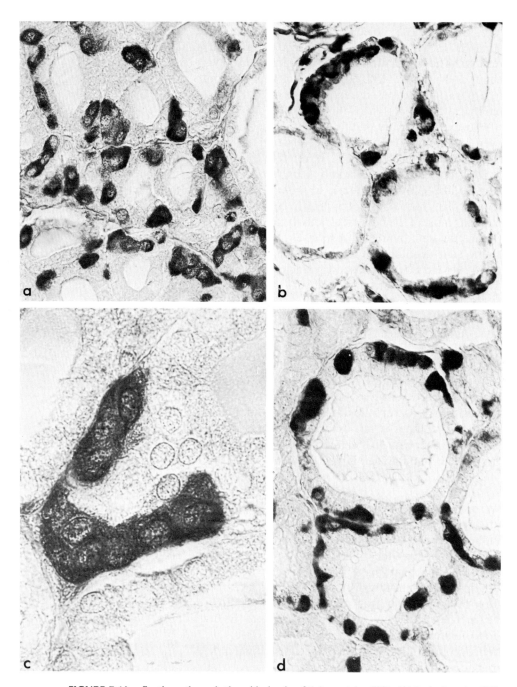

FIGURE 7.14. Sections through thyroid glands of (*a*) a rat (× 592), (*b*) hedgehog (× 592), (*c*) rat (× 1480), and (*d*) horse (× 592). The sections were not stained with any of the histological coloring agents, but were exposed to an antibody to synthetic human calcitonin linked to a peroxidase enzyme. After reaction of the calcitonin-containing cells with the antibody, the sections were exposed to a chemical substrate, which, after oxidation by the enzyme, resulted

developed, while the one on the right side may be reduced to a few cells or follicles or be absent altogether. In fishes the ultimobranchial body tissue is located along the pericardial membrane and esophagus anterior to the heart (Fig. 7.16).

Control of Calcitonin Secretion

The mammalian parafollicular cells appear to be stimulated to release calcitonin by high levels of calcium in the extracellular fluid. In addition, the release of calcitonin can be induced by infusions of the gastrointestinal hormones gastrin and cholecystokinin. Whether this is an adaptive physiological response, in "anticipation" of absorption of calcium from foods digested in the stomach and intestine, is uncertain since food rich in other substances (such as fats) will also stimulate cholecystokinin release.

Physiological Effects of Calcitonin

Besides causing decreased plasma concentrations of calcium and phosphate, calcitonin has been reported to increase the urinary excretion of calcium, phosphate, sodium, potassium, and magnesium. It also enhances urine flow (diuresis). The mechanism by which calcitonin affects renal excretory patterns is not certain. It is possible that many of these effects may be due to the pharmacological doses of the hormone used in experiments. It is also possible that some of the reported renal effects of calcitonin actually may be secondary responses to increased release of parathyroid hormone in response to a primary decrease in plasma calcium caused by calcitonin. However, in some studies using low doses of calcitonin in parathyroidectomized animals, the increased water and electrolyte excretion persists. Calcitonin is known to increase cyclic AMP production in renal proximal tubular cells, and thus the hormone may be acting at this site to reduce renal tubular reabsorption of water and electrolytes.

It is of interest that calcitonin will cause hypocalcemia in nephrectomized animals; thus the drop in extracellular-fluid calcium cannot be due solely to changes in calcium excretion by the kidney. Attention has therefore been focused on the effects of the hormone upon bone. *In vitro* studies have shown that calcitonin can reduce the effect of parathyroid hormone on the release of calcium and phosphate from bone (Fig. 7.17). This assay must be done indirectly, as addition of calcitonin alone to the bone culture causes no significant change. It is thought that calcitonin acts to inhibit bone resorption. For example, persons suffering from medullary carcinoma of the

---

in deposition of a black reaction product in the labeled cells. Most of the calcitonin-containing C cells appear to be between thyroid follicles, though they may intrude between thyroid epithelial cells to various degrees. In the hedgehog (*b*), entire follicles, or large parts of them, appear to be made up of calcitonin-containing cells. [Photographs provided by Dr. Sabine Blähser of the Justus-Liebig University, Giessen.]

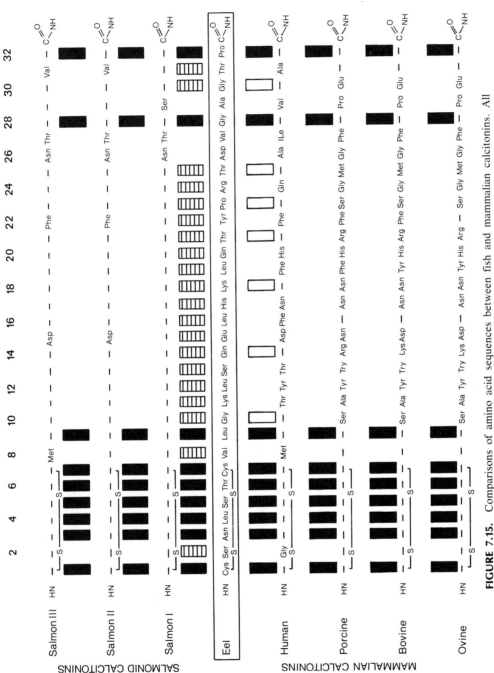

FIGURE 7.15. Comparisons of amino acid sequences between fish and mammalian calcitonins. All comparisons are against the sequence in eel calcitonin, shown in the center. Dashes indicate exact homologies with eel calcitonin, while the absence of a bar at any position in the molecule indicates that the amino acid at this position is different from eel calcitonin. A black bar indicates that same amino acid is in that position in *all* vertebrates examined. A cross-hatched bar indicates amino acids homologous in eel and salmon I calcitonin, the most similar of the fish calcitonins. A white bar indicates homologies between eel and human calcitonin, which thus far is the mammalian calcitonin most similar to that of the eel. [After M. Otani et al., *Calcium Regulating Hormones* (R. V. Talmage et al., eds.), Excerpta Medica, Amsterdam, 1975, p. 111.]

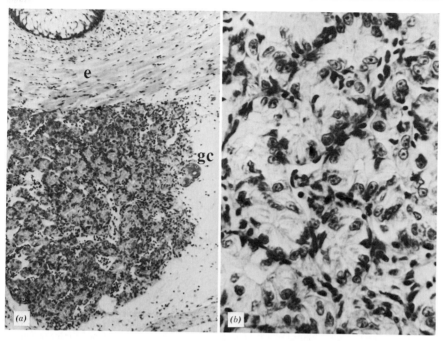

FIGURE 7.16. Histology of the ultimobranchial gland of the goldfish (*Carassius auratus*). (*a*) Low-power photomicrograph (× 140), showing the location of the ultimobranchial body adjacent to the esophagus (e). On the right side of the gland, ganglion cells (gc) can be seen. (*b*) Higher-power photomicrograph (× 620) of the ultimobranchial gland, showing its follicular appearance. [Figures provided by Dr. M. Oguri, Nagoya University, Japan.]

thyroid ("C cell" cancer) show greatly reduced bone remodeling. The mechanism by which calcitonin acts to decrease bone resorption is not certain, but since this effect persists in the presence of protein synthesis inhibitors, calcitonin may be acting to inhibit the intracellular calcium pump in bone (see Fig. 7.3).

The effects of calcitonin on the gut are controversial. There are conflicting data as to whether calcitonin affects either calcium absorption from the gut or the production of 1,25-dihydroxyvitamin D_3. At present it appears that calcitonin has no important effect on the absorption of calcium from the gut and that the intestine is not involved in the hypocalcemic action of calcitonin.

Comparative Studies

Attempts to show that calcitonin affects blood calcium and phosphate levels in nonmammalian vertebrates have met with little success. Injection of either mammalian or salmon calcitonin or ultimobranchial extracts into lower vertebrates generally has been without effect on plasma calcium or phosphate values. However, extracts of ultimobranchial bodies of lower vertebrates

A	B	C	D	E	F
Cont.	.5uPTE /ml.	.5uPTE +13uCT /ml.	13uCT /ml.	Buffer	.5uPTE/ ml.+ Buffer

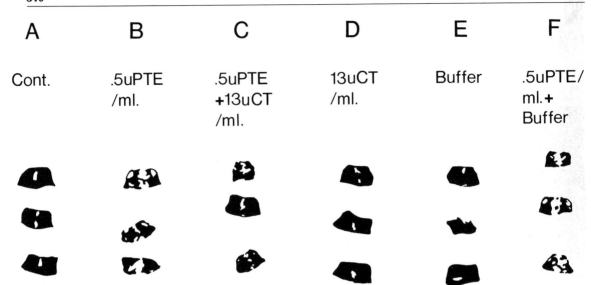

FIGURE 7.17. The results of an experiment in which small squares of flat bone from the cranium (calvaria) of young rats were cultured with parathyroid gland extract (PTE), calcitonin (CT), neither hormone (control or buffer), or both hormones. Bone is stained black, and areas from which bone tissue is resorbed are white (unstained). Parathyroid gland extract promoted extensive resorption of calcified bone (*B* and *F*). Calcitonin inhibited the action of parathyroid hormone (*C*), but by itself had no effect on bone resorption (*D*). [From M. A. Aliapoulios, P. Goldhaber, and P. Munson, *Science*, **151**:330, 1966.]

do cause significant hypocalcemia in the assay using the young rat. This implies that calcitonin is indeed present in the ultimobranchial bodies of lower vertebrates. The lack of a hypocalcemic effect in the lower vertebrates could be due to many factors, such as improper dosage or timing of sampling, or differences in hormone structure from species to species. Moreover, the effects of calcitonin may be reversed or masked if calcitonin stimulates endogenous parathyroid hormone secretion. It is possible that calcitonin may be acting on something other than calcium regulation in the nonmammalian vertebrate. Indeed, there is some evidence that the major effects of calcitonin might be on water and electrolyte excretion, and thus the hormone may play a role in plasma volume regulation or osmoregulation.

Physiological Significance of Calcitonin

Despite the great research interest generated by the discovery of calcitonin, its significance in normal calcium regulation is still uncertain. In mammals there is some evidence that calcitonin decreases bone resorption and increases renal excretion of calcium, both of which result in hypocalcemia. However, the effects are small. In lower forms there is even less experimental evidence for a role of the ultimobranchial body or of calcitonin in calcium regulation. It has been suggested that calcitonin protects the skeleton at times when it is important to decrease bone resorption, such as during lactation, pregnancy, starvation, limb immobilization, or hibernation. Another suggestion is that calcitonin may suppress calcium release from bone at times of hypercalcemia following meals. This might then allow maximal uptake of dietary calcium and maximal deposition of calcium in bone. Since the effect of calcitonin on blood calcium is so small, even its role as an agent for "fine tuning" of the mechanism of calcium homeostasis is debatable.

However, calcitonin almost certainly has some function and is not, as some have suggested, an evolutionary relic. Since the ultimobranchial gland and thyroid C cells are well innervated and well vascularized, and since there is evidence of cellular activity of the gland, as well as of seasonal changes in activity associated with hibernation (bat, hedgehog, marmot, hamster, dormouse), one might argue teleologically that calcitonin must have a physiological role.

VITAMIN D

While vitamin D has been known for a long time as a vitamin essential for the absorption of calcium from the gut and for bone calcium mobilization, only recently has it become to be considered as a calcium-regulating hormone. In fact, vitamin D itself (vitamin D_3 is cholecalciferol) can be considered a prohormone that gives rise to the active metabolite 1,25-dihydroxycholecalciferol (1,25-$(OH)_2D_3$) (Fig. 7.18). It has also been recognized that vitamin D has important effects on the regulation of phosphate as well as calcium and that it has physiological effects not only on bone and gut, but probably on the kidney as well.

The biosynthesis of vitamin D metabolites is outlined in Fig. 7.18. Vitamin D_3 is a steroidlike compound that can be synthesized in the skin from 7-dehydroxycholesterol under the influence of ultraviolet light or may be obtained from the diet. It is hydroxylated in the liver to 25-OHD$_3$, which represents the major metabolite in the blood. This metabolite, in turn, can undergo hydroxylation in the kidney to 1,25-$(OH)_2D_3$, the major physiologically active form. This step is stimulated by low extracellular-fluid phosphate concentrations, by parathyroid hormone, or by estrogen. Alternatively, 25-OHD$_3$ can be transformed to 24,25-$(OH)_2D_3$, which has about 10% of the activity of the 1,25-$(OH)_2D_3$ form, as measured by the ability to stimulate calcium absorption from the gut. The conversion of 25-$(OH)_2D_3$ to 24,25-$(OH)_2D_3$ is stimulated by high phosphate concentrations and inhibited by parathyroid hormone and estrogen.

Researchers are still discovering new metabolites of vitamin D and assaying their biological activity. The physiologically active metabolite 1,25-$(OH)_2D_3$ is known to undergo several conversions. For example, it can be

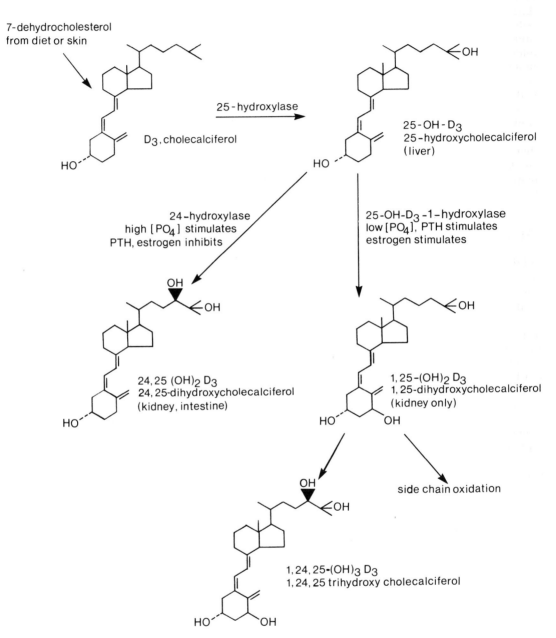

FIGURE 7.18. Pathways in the metabolism of vitamin D, indicating the enzymes and the conditions that promote or inhibit the various steps, as well as the places where the various steps occur.

hydroxylated to $1,24,25\text{-}(OH)_3D_3$. This metabolite is about as active as $1,25\text{-}(OH)_2D_3$ in stimulating calcium and phosphate absorption from the intestine, but it is considered to be a step in the inactivation of the hormone rather than a further activation product. In addition, several metabolites have been described in which there is side-chain oxidation of $1,25\text{-}(OH)_2D_3$. These have not yet been isolated and their biological importance is uncertain.

Effects of Vitamin D on the Intestine

Vitamin D accelerates the transport of calcium and phosphate across the gastrointestinal tract against a concentration gradient. Thus both calcium and phosphate are actively transported across the mucosal cells. The duodenum shows the most marked stimulation of transport in the presence of vitamin D. The mechanism by which this occurs is an object of much study. It is known that the transport does not require parathyroid hormone and that increased calcium transport begins about three hours after vitamin D administration. Actinomycin D blocks this response, indicating that protein synthesis must occur before the increased transport. The mechanism by which vitamin D affects the intestinal cells is believed to be very similar to that by which steroid hormones act upon their target cells. However, not all of the steps have been proven. Figure 7.19 outlines the probable mechanism of action of vitamin D on calcium transport across the intestinal mucosa. 1,25-dihydroxyvitamin D_3 enters the cell across the basal surface of the mucosal cell, binds to a cytosol receptor, and is transported to the nucleus, where it triggers the transcriptive and translational processes needed for the synthesis of transport proteins. These proteins carry calcium from the gut lumen across the brush border into the intestinal cell. All evidence at present suggests that the transport proteins function at the epithelial cell brush border. Whether they act also at the basal and lateral membranes is uncertain. Sodium is required for the movement of calcium across the basolateral membranes. Phosphate transport is also stimulated by $1,25\text{-}(OH)_2D_3$, but little is known about the mechanism.

The identification of the transport protein(s) for calcium (and phosphate) is still unresolved. Intestinal calcium-binding protein has been isolated from the chick and several mammals; it was thought to be the carrier protein made in response to vitamin D stimulation. However, questions have been raised because, at least in mammals, the calcium-binding protein does not appear until after increased calcium transport has begun, and the protein still remains at a high level after calcium transport returns to normal.

Effects of Vitamin D on Bone

It is well known that vitamin D deficiency in young animals leads to rickets; in the adult the condition is termed *osteomalacia*. Both diseases are characterized by undermineralized bones, decreased plasma calcium, and de-

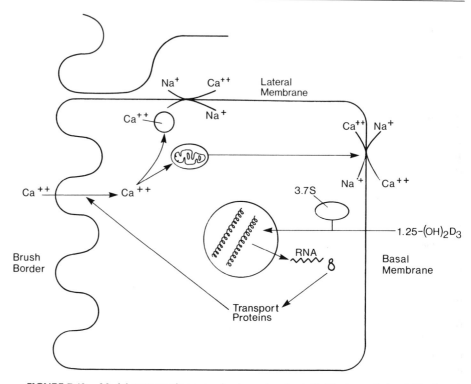

FIGURE 7.19. Model representing a mechanism whereby 1,25-dihydroxycholecalciferol may initiate calcium transport across the mucosal cells of the intestine. It is thought that 1,25-$(OH)_2D_3$ interacts with a 3.7S cytosol receptor, which enters the nucleus and stimulates DNA transcription and protein synthesis. These proteins presumably act at the exposed brush border of the intestinal cells, permitting the entry of Ca^{2+} from the digestive lumen. In the cytoplasm the Ca^{2+} is either packaged in vesicles or taken up by mitochondria. Calcium is expelled from either of these organelles at the lateral or basal cell surfaces by a sodium-dependent process. [From H. F. DeLuca, *Vitamin D Metabolism and Function,* Springer-Verlag, Berlin, 1979.]

creased movement of calcium from bone to medium *in vitro.* The treatment of such animals with vitamin D metabolites results in increased bone calcification, increased mobilization of calcium from bone, and return of plasma calcium to normal.

Because of these results, it has long been thought that vitamin D metabolites cause bone mineralization directly. However, there is little evidence for this. Instead, it is the elevation of plasma calcium and phosphate in response to 1,25-$(OH)_2D_3$ (by increased transport across the gut) that allows calcification to proceed normally.

The major effect of vitamin D upon bone appears to be on bone calcium mobilization. *In vitro* bone culture studies have shown that vitamin D_3 itself is ineffective in causing bone resorption, unless massive doses are given.

However, physiological doses of 25-OHD$_3$ or 1,25-(OH)$_2$D$_3$ are powerful stimulators of bone resorption *in vitro*; (1,25-(OH)$_2$D$_3$ is about 100 times more potent than 25-OHD$_3$). These effects on bone can be measured histologically or by release of ^{45}Ca from bones previously exposed to the isotope. Both 1,25-(OH)$_2$D$_3$ and parathyroid hormone are necessary for bone calcium mobilization to occur. There is some controversy at present regarding the relative importance of each hormone in bone remodeling. Some consider 1,25-(OH)$_2$D$_3$ to be a permissive factor for parathyroid hormone action upon bone. Conversely, since vitamin D metabolites act in such small doses compared to parathyroid hormone, bone remodeling may be mainly under the control of 1,25-(OH)$_2$D$_3$. It is important to remember that the effects of these hormones on bone are not believed to be important in maintaining plasma calcium values.

Effects of Vitamin D on the Kidney

Few renal clearance studies have been done to ascertain if vitamin D metabolites directly affect the renal resorption of calcium and phosphate. There are some mammalian studies that suggest that 1,25(OH)$_2$D$_3$ increases renal reabsorption of calcium by the renal tubules; however, other studies have shown no effect of the hormone on such transport.

Comparative Studies

Recent research has shown that the kidneys of species from all vertebrate classes contain the enzyme systems necessary for converting vitamin D$_3$ to 1,25-(OH)$_2$D$_3$. There have been few studies of the function of 1,25-(OH)$_2$D$_3$ in nonmammalian vertebrates, partly because of the unavailability, until recently, of commercial supplies of the metabolite. Large doses of vitamin D$_3$ in sharks, cyclostomes, or lungfishes have no significant effect on plasma calcium values, although hyperphosphatemia and increased bone resorption have been reported in eels. It has been suggested that since fishes take up calcium actively through the gills, a mechanism to take up calcium from the gut is of little importance.

Vitamin D$_3$-enhanced calcium uptake has been demonstrated in the frog duodenum; this process is facilitated by the presence of the parathyroid gland and by high plasma calcium levels. Other studies of this system in amphibians or reptiles are lacking.

The role of 1,25-(OH)$_2$D$_3$ in birds has received more attention; these studies are confined almost completely to domestic chickens and quail because of their economic importance. The hormone has been shown to be important in stimulation of bone resorption and intestinal calcium absorption. Intestinal calcium-binding protein has been found to be induced by 1,25-(OH)$_2$D$_3$ in chicks, the time of the vitamin D stimulus and the appearance of the calcium-binding protein being well correlated. Furthermore, the

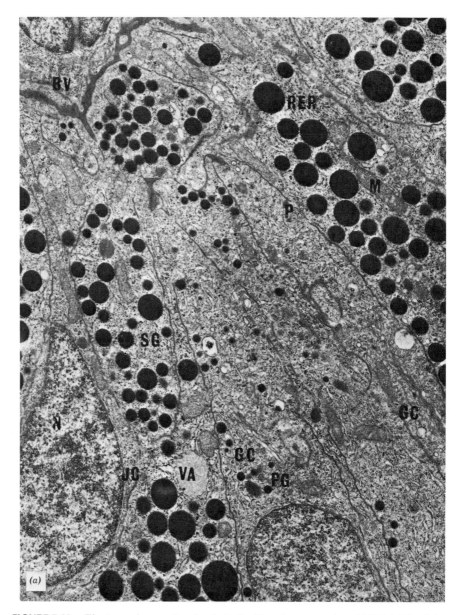

FIGURE 7.20. Electron micrographs of cells in the Stannius corpuscles of killifish (*Fundulus heteroclitus*) kept either in fresh water (*a*) or in seawater (*b*). In calcium-poor fresh water the cells appear quiescent. Secretory granules (*SG*) accumulate, rough endoplasmic reticulum (*RER*) is reduced in amount, mitochondria (*M*) are few and filamentous. In calcium-rich seawater, on the other hand, almost all secretory granules are discharged; rough endoplasmic

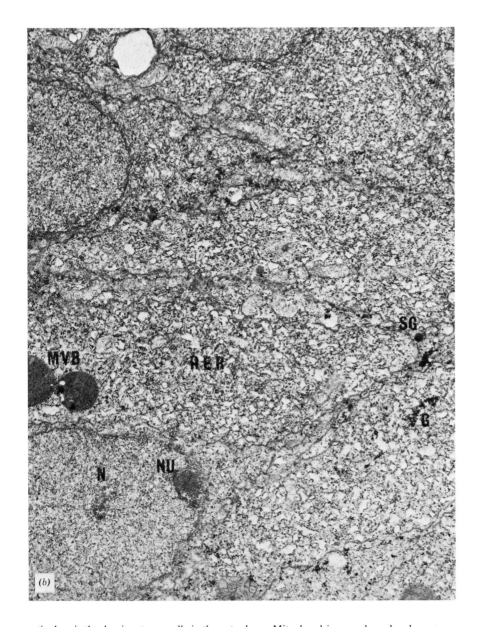

(b)

reticulum is the dominant organelle in the cytoplasm. Mitochondria are enlarged and numerous; nucleoli (*NU*) are prominent. *BV*, blood vessel; *G*, glycogen; *GC*, Golgi complex; *JC*, intercellular junctional complex; *MVB*, multivesicular body; *N*, nucleus; *P*, space between plasma membranes of adjacent cells; *PG*, prosecretory granules; *VA*, vacuole. [From R. S. Cohen, P. K. T. Pang, and N. B. Clark, *Gen. Comp. Endocrinol.*, **27**:41e, 1975.]

binding protein is absent in vitamin D-deficient chicks. Thus the chick calcium-binding protein may well be the transport protein that is induced by 1,25-$(OH)_2D_3$.

Studies of egg-laying birds have shown that there is a cyclic production of vitamin D metabolites. Highest plasma levels of 1,25-$(OH)_2D_3$ coincide with times of estrogen secretion; this can be inhibited by ovariectomy or other treatments to reduce estrogen levels. This process is undoubtedly important in supplying calcium during egg laying. The mechanism by which estrogen stimulates the production of 1,25-$(OH)_2D_3$ is not yet clear.

STANNIUS CORPUSCLES AND HYPOCALCIN

In addition to calcitonin, holostean and teleostean fishes possess a unique substance that may be important in lowering their blood calcium concentrations. This substance, named *hypocalcin* by Pang, is obtained from extracts of the Stannius corpuscles, small organs lying on the surface or embedded in the kidney of many fish species. Hypocalcin can be separated from a pressor substance also present in the corpuscles by extraction with hydrochloric acid. Removal of the Stannius corpuscles (in eels, goldfish, or killifish) results in increased plasma calcium values. Extracts of the glands will return the calcium values to normal in "stanniectomized" fishes. The Stannius corpuscles appear to be sensitive to circulating levels of calcium. The glands of killifish maintained in seawater show evidence of active protein synthesis, e.g., active Golgi regions and dilation of the cisternae of the endoplasmic reticulum. In contrast, killifish glands maintained in calcium-deficient seawater or in fresh water are filled with secretory granules and appear inactive (Fig. 7.20).

Hypocalcin is a protein with a molecular weight of about 4000 daltons. While "stanniectomized" fishes show bone changes such as increased calcium content and decreased numbers of osteoclasts, recent evidence shows that "stanniectomy" results in increased calcium uptake by the gills from environmental water. Injection of corpuscle extract rapidly reverses this effect both *in vivo* and *in vitro* preparations. The *in vitro* studies suggest a direct effect of hypocalcin upon calcium uptake by the gill. Ma and Copp have developed a sensitive assay for hypocalcin based upon its ability to inhibit Ca^{2+}-ATPase in the gill membrane of trout.

It is uncertain at present whether there is a functional relationship between hypocalcin and calcitonin. However, Chan has reported hypertrophy of the ultimobranchial body in "stanniectomized" eels.

SUMMARY

The regulation of extracellular-fluid calcium and phosphate at normal concentrations is dependent upon the presence of at least three major hormones acting on one or more of three major target organs. One might ask which of the three targets appears to be the most crucial in the regulation of calcium homeostasis. Alternatively, one might examine which hormone seems most essential in this regulation.

For example, it has been argued by Nordin and co-workers that the kidney is the most important and principal regulator of calcium homeostasis, since plasma calcium levels must be largely determined by the fraction of filtered calcium reabsorbed by the kidney tubules. Renal calcium reabsorption is directly affected by parathyroid hormone. The differences in plasma calcium concentrations in hypoparathyroid, normal, and hyperparathyroid patients, or between normal and parathyroidectomized animals, can be largely accounted for by changes in tubular reabsorption of calcium.

Nordin argues further that the gut is less important in determining plasma calcium levels. Ingestion of a large amount of calcium (100 mg/kg) normally will increase plasma calcium values in humans by only about 1 mg/dl, while overnight starvation has no effect on plasma calcium concentrations. Similarly, Nordin suggests that the role of bone in calcium homeostasis has been overemphasized and that bone functions only as the ultimate source of calcium when insufficient amounts are present in the diet. Of the many actions of parathyroid hormone on bone, only the effect on the osteoblast membrane would result in rapid adjustments in plasma calcium values.

It is important to remember that the actions of parathyroid hormone and vitamin D on calcium metabolism follow rather different time courses. Parathyroid hormone secretion is a rapid response to a hypocalcemic stimulus. The hormone has rapid effects and a half-life of only several minutes in mammals and birds. In contrast, the responses of targets to vitamin D take several hours, and the half-life of the hormone may be several days. Thus the response to hypocalcemia may be summarized in a simplified manner, as in Fig. 7.21. The absorption of calcium from the gut is a long-term effect believed to protect the skeleton from continuous calcium loss by introducing more calcium into the system from the environment.

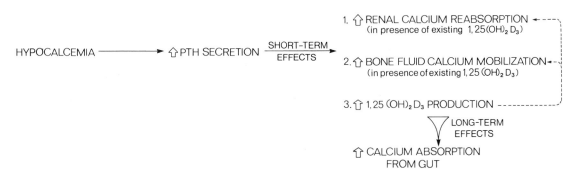

SHORT-TERM AND LONG-TERM RESPONSES TO HYPOCALCEMIA

FIGURE 7.21. Summary of the immediate and long-term effects of hypocalcemia. Further explanation is given in the text.

From these arguments one may conclude that the reabsorption of calcium by the kidney tubules and the pumping of calcium across the bone membrane are the major actions responsible for the minute-to-minute regulation of plasma calcium. In both cases, parathyroid hormone (along with permissive levels of 1,25-$(OH)_2D_3$) acts quickly to raise the calcium values of the extracellular fluid. Long-term regulation of plasma calcium values brings into play increased absorption of calcium from the gut and, possibly, actual bone resorption.

The role of calcitonin may be to reverse the effects if hypercalcemia resulted from increased calcium mobilization. Thus it might act to suppress bone calcium resorption and to increase the renal excretion of calcium and phosphate. However, high blood calcium in itself would decrease parathyroid hormone secretion, and the entire system could therefore be self-regulating.

ADDITIONAL READING

1. Anderson, M. P., and C. C. Capen (1976). Ultrastructural evaluation of parathyroid and ultimobranchial glands of iguanas with experimental nutritional osteodystrophy. *Gen. Comp. Endocrinol.* **30:**209–222.

2. Baksi, S. N., and A. D. Kenny (1977). Vitamin D_3 metabolism in immature Japanese quail: effects of ovarian hormones. *Endocrinology* **101:**1216–1220.

3. Bélanger, L. F., C. Bélanger, and T. Semba (1967). Technical approaches leading to the concept of osteocytic osteolysis. *Clin. Ortho. Rel. Res.* **54:**187–196.

4. Blähser, S. (1978). Immunocytochemical demonstration of calcitonin-containing C-cells in the thyroid glands of different mammals. *Cell Tissue Res.* **186:**551–558.

5. Bonjour, J-P., and H. Fleisch (1977). The effect of vitamin D and its metabolites on the renal handling of phosphate. In *Vitamin D: Biochemical, Chemical and Clinical Aspects Related to Calcium Metabolism* (A. W. Norman, K. Schaefer, J. W. Coburn, H. F. DeLuca, D. Fraser, H. G. Grigoleit, and D. von Herrath, eds.). de Gruyter, Berlin, pp. 419–431.

6. Brehm, H. V. (1964). Experimentelle Studien zur Frage der jahreszyklischen Veränderungen. Morphologische Untersuchungen an Epithelkörperchen (Glandulae parathyroideae) von Anuren. *Z. Zellforsch. Mikros. Anat.* **61:**725–741.

7. Bussolati, G., and A. G. E. Pearse (1967). Immunofluorescent localization of calcitonin in the 'C' cells of pig and dog thyroid. *J. Endocrinol.* **37:**205–209.

8. Chan, D. K. O. (1972). Hormonal regulation of calcium balance in teleost fish. *Gen. Comp. Endocrinol.*, Suppl. **3:**411–420.

9. Clark, N. B. (1965). Experimental and histological studies of the parathyroid glands of fresh-water turtles. *Gen. Comp. Endocrinol.* **5:**297–312.

10. Clark, N. B. and W. H. Dantzler (1972). Renal tubular transport of calcium and phosphate in snakes: role of parathyroid hormone. *Am. J. Physiol.* **223:**1455–1464.

11. Clark, N. B., and R. F. Wideman, Jr. (1977). Renal excretion of phosphate and calcium in parathyroidectomized starlings. *Am. J. Physiol.* **233:**F138–F144.

12. Cohen, R. S., P. K. T. Pang, and N. B. Clark (1975). Ultrastructure of the Stannius corpuscles of the killifish, *Fundulus heteroclitus*, and its relation to calcium regulation. *Gen. Comp. Endocrinol.* **27:**413–423.

13. Cohn, D. V., J. J. Morissey, R. R. MacGregor, and J. W. Hamilton (1978). The role of calcium in the biosynthesis and secretion of parathormone. In *Comparative Endocrinology* (P. J. Gaillard and H. H. Boer, eds.). Elsevier/North-Holland, Amsterdam, pp. 273–278.

14. Collip, J. B., and E. P. Clark (1925). Further studies on the physiological action of a parathyroid hormone. *J. Biol. Chem.* **64**:485–507.

15. Copp, D. H., E. C. Cameron, B. A. Cheney, A. G. F. Davison, and K. G. Henze (1962). Evidence for calcitonin—a new hormone from the parathyroid that lowers blood calcium. *Endocrinology* **70**:638–649.

16. Cortelyou, J. R. (1967). The effect of commercially prepared parathyroid extract on plasma and urine calcium levels in *Rana pipiens*. *Gen. Comp. Endocrinol.* **9**:234–240.

17. Cortelyou, J. R., A. Hibner-Owerko, and J. Mulroy (1960). Blood and urine calcium changes in totally parathyroidectomized *Rana pipiens*. *Endocrinology* **70**:441–450.

18. Dacke, C. G. (1979). *Calcium Regulation in Sub-Mammalian Vertebrates*. Academic, London.

19. DeLuca, H. F. (1979). Vitamin D. Metabolism and function. In *Monographs on Endocrinology*, Vol. 13 (F. Goss, A. Labhart, T. Mann, and J. Zander, eds.). Springer-Verlag, Berlin.

20. Habener, J. F., and H. M. Kronenberg (1978). Parathyroid hormone biosynthesis: structure and function of biosynthetic precursors. *Fed Proc.* **37**:2561–2566.

21. Henry, H., and A. W. Norman (1975). Presence of renal 25-hydroxyvitamin-D-1-hydroxylase in species of all vertebrate classes. *Comp. Biochem. Physiol.* **50B**:431–434.

22. Hirsch, P. F., G. F. Gauthier, and P. L. Munson (1973). Thyroid hypocalcemic principle and recurrent nerve injury as factors affecting the response to parathyroidectomy. *Endocrinology* **73**:244–252.

23. Hugi, K., J-P. Bonjour, and H. Fleisch (1979). Renal handling of calcium: influence of parathyroid hormone and 1,25-dihydroxyvitamin D_3. *Am. J. Physiol.* **236**:F349–F356.

24. Laverty, G., and N. B. Clark (1981). Renal clearance of phosphate and calcium in the fresh-water turtle: effects of parathyroid hormone. *J. Comp. Physiol.* **B141**:463–470.

25. Levinsky, N. G., and D. G. Davidson (1957). Renal action of parathyroid extract in the chicken. *Am. J. Physiol.* **191**:530–536.

26. Ma, S. W. Y., and D. H. Copp (1978). Purification, properties and action of a glycopeptide from the corpuscles of Stannius which affects calcium metabolism in the teleost. In *Comparative Endocrinology* (P. J. Gaillard and H. H. Boer, eds.). Elsevier/North-Holland, Amsterdam, pp. 283–386.

27. MacCallum, W. G., and C. Voegtlin (1909). On the relationship of tetany to the parathyroid glands and to calcium metabolism. *J. Exp. Med.* **11**:118–151.

28. McWhinnie, D. J., and J. R. Cortelyou (1967). Parathyroid glands of amphibians. II. Structural and biochemical changes in amphibian tissues elicited by parathyroid hormone under varying conditions of season and temperature. *Am. Zool.* **7**:857–868.

29. McWhinnie, D. J., and L. Lehrer (1972). Seasonal variation in amphibian phosphate metabolism and its relation to parathyroid structure and function. *Comp. Biochem. Physiol.* **43A**:911–925.

30. Martindale, L. (1973). Phosphate excretion in the laying hen (*Gallus domesticus*). *J. Physiol.* **231**:439–453.

31. Maurer, F. (1899). Die Schilddrüse, Thymus und andere Schlundspalten-derivate bei der Eidechse. *Morphol. Jahrb.* **27**:119–172.

32. Morrissey, R. L., and R. H. Wasserman (1971). Calcium absorption and calcium-binding protein in chicks on differing calcium and phosphorus intake. *Am. J. Physiol.* **220**:1509–1515.

33. Munson, P. (1976). Physiology and pharmacology of thyrocalcitonin. In *Handbook of*

Physiology, Vol. 7 (R. O. Greep and E. B. Astwood, eds.). American Physiological Society, Washington, D. C., pp. 443–464.

34. Narbaitz, R. (1979). Response of shell-less cultured chick embryos to exogenous parathyroid hormone and 1,25-dihydroxycholecalciferol. *Gen. Comp. Endocrinol.* **37:**440–442.

35. Nordin, B. E. C., M. Peacock, and R. Wilkinson (1972). The relative importance of gut, bone and kidney in the regulation of serum calcium. In *Calcium, Parathyroid Hormone and the Calcitonins* (R. V. Talmage and P. L. Munson, eds.). Excerpta Medica, Amsterdam, pp. 263–272.

36. Oguro, C., and A. Tomisawa (1972). Effects of parathyroidectomy on the serum calcium concentration of the turtle, *Goeclemys reevsii. Gen. Comp. Endocrinol.* **19:**587–588.

37. Oguro, C., M. Uchiyama, P. K. T. Pang, and Y. Sasayama (1978). Serum calcium homeostasis in urodele amphibians. In *Comparative Endocrinology* (P. J. Gaillard and H. H. Boer, eds.). Elsevier/North Holland, Amsterdam, pp. 269–272.

38. Pang, P. K. T., M. P. Schreibman, and R. W. Griffith (1973). Pituitary regulation of serum calcium levels in the killifish, *Fundulus heteroclitus* L. *Gen. Comp. Endocrinol.* **21:**536–542.

39. Pang, P. K. T., R. K. Pang, and W. H. Sawyer (1974). Environmental calcium and the sensitivity of killifish (*Fundulus heteroclitus*) in bioassay for the hypocalcemic response to Stannius corpuscles from killifish and cod (*Gadus morhua*). *Endocrinology* **94:**548–555.

40. Pang, P. K. T., A. D. Kenny, and C. Oguro (1980). Evolution of the endocrine control of calcium metabolism. In *Evolution of Vertebrate Endocrine Systems* (P. K. T. Pang and A. Epple, eds.). Texas Tech Press, Lubbock, pp. 323–356.

41. Pang, P. K. T., M. P. Schreibman, F. Balbontin, and R. K. Pang (1978). Prolactin and pituitary control of calcium regulation in the killifish, *Fundulus heteroclitus. Gen. Comp. Endocrinol.* **36:**306–316.

42. Parfitt, A. M. (1976). The action of parathyroid hormone on bone: relation of bone remodeling and turnover, calcium homeostasis, and metabolic bone diseases. II. PTH and bone cells: bone turnover and plasma calcium regulation. *Metabolism* **25:**909–955.

43. Parsons, J. A., D. Gray, B. Rafferty, and J. Zanelli (1978). Evidence for a hypercalcemic factor in the fish pituitary related to mammalian parathyroid hormone. In *Endocrinology of Calcium Metabolism*, Proceedings of the 6th Parathyroid Conference, Vancouver, 1977 (D. H. Copp and R. V. Talmage, eds.). Excerpta Medica, Amsterdam, pp. 111–114.

44. Pearse, A. G. E., and T. Takor Takor (1976). Neuroendocrine embryology and the APUD concept. *Clin. Endocrinol.* **5:**(Suppl.) 229S–244S.

45. Potts, J. T., Jr., and G. D. Aurbach (1976). Chemistry of the Calcitonins. In *Handbook of Physiology*, Vol. 7 (R. O. Greep and E. B. Astwood, eds.). American Physiological Society, Washington, D. C., pp. 423–430.

46. Potts, J. T., Jr., H. D. Niall, H. T. Keutmann, H. B. Brewer, Jr., and L. J. Deftos (1968). The amino acid sequence of porcine thyrocalcitonin. *Proc. Natl. Acad. Sci. USA* **59:**1321–1328.

47. Prashad, D. N., and N. A. Edwards (1973). Phosphate excretion in the laying fowl. *Comp. Biochem. Physiol.* **46A:**131–137.

48. Prashad, D. N., M. E. C. Robbins, and J. A. Parsons (1979). Urinary excretion of cyclic AMP in the laying fowl. *Comp. Biochem. Physiol.* **64A:**133–135.

49. Ranly, D. M., and P. R. Runnels (1969). The effect of parathyroid extract on phosphorus excretion in the chick embryo. *Texas Rep. Biol. Med.* **27:**795–801.

50. Reynolds, J. J. (1974). The role of 1,25-dihydroxycholecalciferol in bone metabolism. *Biochem. Soc. Spec. Pub.* **3:**91–102.

51. Robertson, D. R. (1974). Effects of the ultimobranchial and parathyroid glands on sodium and water excretion in the frog. *Endocrinology* **94:**940–946.

52. Robertson, D. R. (1975). Effects of the ultimobranchial and parathyroid glands and vi-

tamins D_2, D_3 and dihydrotachysterol$_2$ on blood calcium and intestinal calcium transport in the frog. *Endocrinology* **96**:934–940.

53. Robertson, D. R. (1978). The annual pattern of plasma calcium in the frog and the seasonal effect of ultimobranchialectomy and parathyroidectomy. *Gen. Comp. Endocrinol.* **33**:336–343.

54. Rosen, V., G. Laverty, and N. B. Clark (1980). Stimulation of calcium release from cultured embryonic chick bones by parathyroid glands of the freshwater turtle. *Gen. Comp. Endocrinol.* **41**:150–155.

55. Roth, S. I., and A. L. Schiller (1976). Comparative anatomy of the parathyroids. In *Handbook of Physiology*, Vol. 7 (R. O. Greep and E. B. Astwood, eds.). American Physiological Society, Washington, D. C., pp. 281–311.

56. Simkiss, K (1967). *Calcium in Reproductive Physiology*, Chapman & Hill, London.

57. So, Y. P., and J. C. Fenwick (1979). *In vivo* and *in vitro* effects of Stannius corpuscle extract on the branchial uptake of ^{45}Ca in stanniectomized North American eels (*Anguilla rostrata*). *Gen. Comp. Endocrinol.* **37**:143–149.

58. Sutton, R. A. L., C. A. Harris, N. L. M. Wong, and J. Dirks (1977). Effects of vitamin D on renal calcium transport. In *Vitamin D: Biochemical, Chemical and Clinical Aspects Related to Calcium Metabolism* (A. W. Norman, K. Schaefer, J. W. Coburn, H. F. DeLuca, D. Fraser, H. G. Grigoleit, and D. von Herrath, eds.). de Gruyter, Berlin, pp. 451–453.

59. Talmage, R. V. (1970). Morphological and physiological considerations in a new concept of calcium transport in bone. *Am. J. Anat.* **129**:467–476.

60. Waggener, R. A. (1930). An experimental study of the parathyroids in the Anura. *J. Exp. Zool.* **57**:13–55.

61. Wasserman, R. H., and A. N. Taylor (1966). Vitamin D_3-induced calcium-binding protein in chick intestinal mucosa. *Science* **152**:791–793.

62. Wittle, L. W., and J. N. Dent (1979). Effects of parathyroidectomy and of parathyroid extract on levels of calcium and phosphate in the blood and urine of the red-spotted newt. *Gen. Comp. Endocrinol.* **37**:428–439.

8

Gastrointestinal Hormones

The efficient digestion of a meal requires the coordination of an amazing number of physiological events. The digestive process is initiated by the meal itself and is integrated locally by the successive segments of the digestive tube. Coordination of digestion is achieved through neural and hormonal responses to the physical and chemical properties of the food within the lumen of the gut. In this chapter we propose to consider mainly the endocrine mode of integration of the digestive process.

The alimentary canal of vertebrates is basically a tube whose lumen is topographically continuous with the outside of the body. This tube is unusually complex in that it may be coiled to various degrees and in vertebrates, at least, it has certain localized structural outgrowths. The anatomy of the alimentary canal varies considerably among vertebrates and clearly is adaptable to changing selection pressures in evolution. Whether this potential for adaptation is related in part to the hormones of the gastrointestinal tract is a question that awaits investigation.

In mammals the chemical digestion of food begins with the action of saliva, followed by muscular transfer to the stomach via the esophagus (Fig. 8.1). The secretion of pepsinogen and hydrochloric acid in the stomach initiates proteolytic digestion. The stomach passes the partly digested mass of food to the small intestine, where most of digestion occurs. The first part of the small intestine (the duodenum) is the site of delivery of the secretions of such glands as the liver, pancreas, Brunner's glands, and crypts of Lieberkühn. These localized glandular outgrowths of the small intestine secrete particular substances necessary for the complete extracellular reduction of foodstuffs to forms that can be absorbed into the body in the lower parts of the small intestine (the jejunum and the ileum). The large intestine is specialized for the absorption of water.

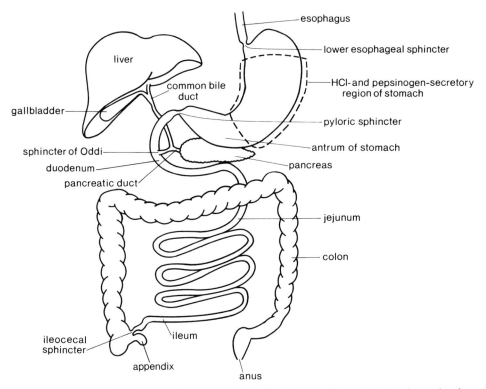

FIGURE 8.1. A diagrammatic representation of the human digestive tract and associated organs.

The regulation of this complex of processes occurs in a coordinated way, so that movement down the digestive tube and delivery of digestive secretions to the food bolus always occur at the right time, in the right sequence, and with the right velocity. The gastrointestinal hormones play a major role in ensuring the efficiency of these processes in mammals and, probably, in all other vertebrates as well.

GASTROINTESTINAL ENDOCRINE CELLS

Gastrointestinal endocrine cells are distributed diffusely in the epithelial lining of the alimentary tract (Fig. 8.2). They are not collected into compact glands as are the cells of most endocrine organs. This may be a primitive feature of the gastrointestinal endocrine system, but it also has physiological significance in that the diffuse cells produce an integrated signal in response to a diffuse stimulus, such as variable amounts of food entering the stomach over variable intervals. Thus the integrated response must occur to a degree that is correct or equivalent for the total quantity of food ingested. Because the gastrointestinal endocrine cells are widely scattered in a great mass of nonendocrine tissue, removal of a single cell type in order to study the endocrine consequences is impossible. Coupled with the fact that whole gastrointestinal tissue extracts contain several different hormones with different biological activities, this helps explain why progress in understanding the diffuse gastrointestinal endocrine system historically has lagged behind other fields of endocrine research. More recently, however, the development of improved chemical purification and hormone assay methods has led to rapid advances in our understanding of the hormones of the gut.

Gastrointestinal endocrine cells usually have microvilli that project into the lumen of the gut, enabling them to interact with luminal contents (Fig. 8.2). In fact, gut endocrine cells have been considered to be comparable in this way to the taste cells of the tongue. This chemoreceptive ability enables them to transduce the specific chemical information available in particular foods into a chemical code, namely the hormonal signal. Thus, gastrointes-

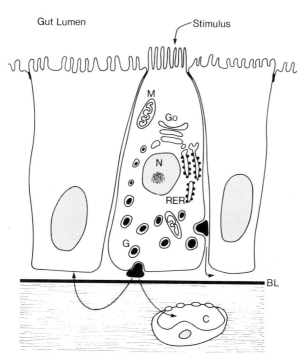

FIGURE 8.2. A generalized gastrointestinal endocrine cell. Chemicals in the lumen of the gut are "sensed" by the microvilli at the cell apex; this information results in exocytosis of the secretory product at the base of the cell. The secretory product may enter a capillary to exert an endocrine effect on target cells at some distance, or in some cases it may diffuse to neighboring cells in the gastrointestinal mucosa to exert a paracrine effect locally. *BL*, basal lamina; *C*, capillary lumen; *G*, secretory granule; *Go*, golgi region; *M*, mitochondria; *N*, nucleus; *RER*, rough endoplasmic reticulum.

tinal endocrine cells are the only endocrine cells in vertebrates that are directly influenced by perturbations of the environment external to the body.

The dual distribution of peptide-secreting cells in the gut and pancreas has convinced some workers that they should be considered together functionally as the gastroenteropancreatic hormone system. A total of 15 cell types are widely recognized in the gastroenteropancreatic endocrine system of mammals (Table 8.1). Of these, 14 are present in the gastrointestinal epithelium and four are found also in the pancreas. Only insulin-containing B cells are found exclusively in the vertebrate pancreas. Gastroenteropancreatic endocrine cells store their secretory products in cytoplasmic granules. The granules in each type of cell have distinct diameters and densities when examined in the electron microscope. The availability of specific antisera raised against gut peptides has allowed the matching of the particular cell types recognized in the electron microscope with specific secretory products by use of immunocytochemical techniques (Table 8.1).

Gastroenteropancreatic endocrine cells share the ability to take up 5-hydroxytryptophan (5-HTP) and to decarboxylate it to 5-hydroxytryptamine (5-HT) intracellularly. They have been categorized by the acronym *APUD* (Amine Precursor Uptake and Decarboxylation) because of this amine-handling property. The significance of the cytoplasmic association of amines and peptides in peptide-secreting cells is unclear. It has been suggested by Pearse that all peptide hormone-secreting cells are APUD cells. Pearse has proposed further that all APUD cells are derived embryologically from the

TABLE 8.1. Tissue distribution and cell classification of gastroenteropancreatic peptides

Peptide	Designation of Cell	Principal Location
Gastrin	G	Stomach, duodenum
Secretin	S	Upper small intestine
Cholecystokinin	I	Upper small intestine
Gastric inhibitory peptide	K	Upper small intestine
Vasoactive intestinal peptide	D_1	Entire gut
Substance P	EC; EC_1	Entire gut, stomach, duodenum
Motilin	EC_2	Small intestine
Glucagonlike	L	Entire intestine
Bombesin	P	Stomach, duodenum
Neurotensin	N	Lower small intestine
Somatostatin	D	Stomach, pancreas (islet)
Pancreatic polypeptide	PP	Pancreas (islet and acinar), Small intestine
Glucagon	A	Pancreas (islet), stomach (some species)
Insulin	B	Pancreas (islet)

neuroectoderm, but this generalization has proven controversial and remains in doubt. It may be, however, that peptide-secreting endocrine cells are evolutionary derivatives of amine-secreting neurons.

HORMONAL STATUS OF GASTROINTESTINAL PEPTIDES

The complexity of gastrointestinal physiology in terms of the number of active—presumably hormonal—peptides the gut contains and the extensive interactions between individual peptides on target tissues makes it difficult to unravel the precise physiological role of each gut peptide. For several of these peptides there is substantial information available about chemical structure, cell type of origin, control of release, and major biological effects following administration by injection or infusion. However, the many interactions between endogenous hormones and between the hormones and nervous reflexes has made it very difficult to identify with certainty the specific physiological function of a single hormone. It appears that unphysiologically large (pharmacologic) doses of all of the gastrointestinal peptides can influence all gastrointestinal processes. Therefore, distinguishing between physiological and pharmacologic actions is an especially difficult task in the case of the gastrointestinal hormones. Nevertheless, it is expected that most of the active peptides of the gut will eventually be shown to be normal physiological regulators of specific digestive processes.

It is not yet possible to give precise estimates of the physiological roles of some of the gastrointestinal hormones. In this chapter the gastrointestinal peptides that have been isolated in pure form from the gastrointestinal mucosa or pancreas, and for which the amino acid sequence has been determined, are emphasized. Discussion of insulin, glucagon, somatostatin, and pancreatic polypeptide (PP) is reserved for the following chapter.

Gastrin

Gastrin is the best studied of the gastrointestinal peptides, and it is widely accepted as a true hormone. Even in the case of gastrin, however, the full extent of its repertory of physiologically significant actions is not yet agreed upon by all workers.

Experiments suggesting the existence of gastrin were first described by Edkins in 1905, but it was not until 1964 that the chemical structure of gastrin was determined by Gregory and Tracy. Since then the amino acid sequences of several mammalian gastrins have been determined (Table 8.2). Mammalian gastrin has been shown to exist in several molecular forms (Table 8.3). Gastrin peptides of 34, 17, 14, and 4 amino acid residues in length (designated as gastrin-34, gastrin-17, etc.) have been described. Furthermore, each of these size variants, except the tetrapeptide, exists in both unsulfated (gastrin I) and sulfated (gastrin II) forms. The major gastrin com-

TABLE 8.2.   Amino acid sequences of gastrin-17 in some mammals[a,b]

		Man	Hog	Dog	Cow and Sheep	Cat
17.	Glp[c]					
16.	Gly					
15.	Pro					
14.	Trp					
13.	Leu	Met	Met	Val		
12.	Glu					
11.	Glu					
10.	Glu		Ala			
9.	Glu					
8.	Glu				Ala	Ala
7.	Ala					
6.	Tyr-R[d]					
5.	Gly					
4.	Trp					
3.	Met					
2.	Asp					
1.	Phe-NH$_2$					

[a] Except as noted, the amino acid sequences are identical to human gastrin.
[b] The numbering of amino acid residues is unconventional: from the carboxyl to the amino terminus. Note that the C-terminal amino acid may bear an amido (NH_2) group, not to be confused with a free amino group.
[c] Glp = pyroglutamyl.
[d] R = H (gastrin I); R = SO_3H (gastrin II).

ponents present in extracts of the antrum of the stomach are gastrin-17 I and II. However, the most prominent components in blood are gastrin-34 I and II. Gastrin-14 and gastrin-4 are minor components in mammals, and there are species differences in the relative proportions of the various components. It is apparent from Table 8.3 that all of the proposed forms of gastrin are fragments of gastrin-34, and this raises the possibility that all gastrins may be synthesized in the G cell as gastrin-34 and subsequently converted to the shorter molecules. Forms of gastrin larger than gastrin-34 have been identified by molecular fractionation techniques, but their amino acid sequences are unknown. The significance of the sulfate groups in the gastrin-II forms is unclear because few differences have been observed between the actions of sulfated and unsulfated forms.

The C-terminal region of gastrin is the center of biological activity of the whole molecule. It is not surprising, then, that the species differences in amino acid sequences of gastrins (Table 8.2) are confined to the less biologically important N-terminal ends of the gastrin-17 molecule. The tetrapeptide amide (Trp-Met-Asp-Phe-NH$_2$) has the full range of actions of gastrin, but is lower in potency than the other molecular forms when tested by

TABLE 8.3. Amino acid sequences of various forms of gastrin in man

	Gastrin-34	Gastrin-17	Gastrin-14	Gastrin-4
34.	Glp[a,b]			
33.	Leu			
32.	Gly			
31.	Pro			
30.	Gln			
29.	Gly			
28.	His			
27.	Pro			
26.	Ser			
25.	Leu			
24.	Val			
23.	Ala			
22.	Asp			
21.	Pro			
20.	Ser			
19.	Lys			
18.	Lys			
17.	Gln	Glp[b]		
16.	Gly	Gly		
15.	Pro	Pro		
14.	Trp	Trp	Trp	
13.	Leu	Leu	Leu	
12.	Glu	Glu	Glu	
11.	Glu	Glu	Glu	
10.	Glu	Glu	Glu	
9.	Glu	Glu	Glu	
8.	Glu	Glu	Glu	
7.	Ala	Ala	Ala	
6.	Tyr-R[c]	Tyr-R[c]	Tyr-R[c]	
5.	Gly	Gly	Gly	
4.	Trp	Trp	Trp	Trp
3.	Met	Met	Met	Met
2.	Asp	Asp	Asp	Asp
1.	Phe-NH$_2$	Phe-NH$_2$	Phe-NH$_2$	Phe-NH$_2$

[a] The numbering of amino acid residues is unconventional: from the carboxyl to the amino terminus. Note that the C-terminal amino acid may bear an amido (NH$_2$) group; not to be confused with a free amino group.
[b] Glp = pyroglutamyl.
[c] R = H (gastrin I); R = SO$_3$H (gastrin II).

injection. The hormonal significance of the gastrin-4 identified in tissue extracts, then, is questionable. Possibly, gastrin-4 may act as a neurotransmitter in the gut.

The identifying or characteristic biological action of gastrin is stimulation of gastric hydrochloric acid secretion. Gastrin also stimulates pepsinogen secretion, but this may be an indirect action dependent upon prior acid secretion. Another major biological action of gastrin in mammals is stimulation of contraction of the powerful smooth muscle of the gastric antrum, resulting in the mixing and disruption of ingested food. Recently, the important role of gastrin in stimulation of growth of the acid- and pepsinogen-secreting mucosa of the stomach has been appreciated. Digested proteins and amino acids are the most potent stimulants for the release of gastrin from the gastric antral mucosa in mammals. Tryptophan and phenylalanine are the most potent of the amino acids in releasing gastrin. Other specific chemical components of food play only a minor role in gastrin release. The importance of nervous reflexes, both vagal and local reflexes of the stomach wall, as releasers of gastrin is unclear.

Most gastrointestinal hormones seem to act independently of other hormones of the endocrine system, but the relationship between gastrin, calcium, and calcium-regulating hormones is a conspicuous exception. Food entering the stomach stimulates the release of gastrin, which in turn has been shown to stimulate the release of calcitonin in some species. It seems clear that gastrin-stimulated calcitonin release is adaptive in that it anticipates the calcium load the body faces after a meal and aids in minimizing hypercalcemia during intestinal calcium absorption. Parathyroid hormone or high levels of blood calcium can also stimulate the release of gastrin, and calcitonin can reduce or even prevent such gastrin release. This negative feedback system helps promote blood calcium homeostasis during intermittent periods of calcium ingestion. This may be of special importance to suckling mammals facing the unusually high calcium stress of frequent and large ingestions of milk.

Bombesin, a peptide isolated from the skin of certain frogs and subsequently identified by immunological techniques in gastrointestinal tissues, is also a potent stimulant of gastrin release in mammals. It is not known whether bombesin or a bombesinlike peptide is a physiologically significant releaser of gastrin.

Accumulated acid in the lumen of the stomach appears to be the major physiological inhibitor of gastrin release. This provides a physiologically useful negative feedback system whereby increasing stomach acid concentrations, stimulated by gastrin, inhibit further gastrin secretion. Several peptides have been identified that can inhibit gastrin release. Most of these peptides also directly inhibit the action of gastrin on gastric acid secretion. Peptides that have these dual effects when applied either *in vivo* or *in vitro* include somatostatin, gastric inhibitory peptide, vasoactive intestinal peptide, secretin, glucagon, and calcitonin. It is unknown whether any of these substances has a physiological role as an endogenous inhibitor of gastrin release.

Sensitive and precise radioimmunoassays for mammalian gastrins have been developed. It has been shown that the fasting blood gastrin concentration in humans is about 20 fmoles/ml (1 fmole/liter equals 10^{-15} M; 20 fmoles/ml is equivalent to about 40 pg/ml when related to a standard of gastrin-17), which rises to a peak response of about 40 fmoles/ml after eating a meal.

Cholecystokinin

In 1928, Ivy and Oldberg showed that a humoral substance originating from the small intestine stimulated gallbladder contraction. Harper and Raper, in 1943, showed that similar extracts also stimulated pancreatic enzyme secretion. Logically enough, the earlier workers named the factor that was active on the gallbladder *cholecystokinin*, and the later workers named the factor that was active on the pancreas *pancreozymin*. It remained for Jorpes and Mutt, in 1964, to demonstrate that both biological activities were properties of a single peptide. This hormone is now called cholecystokinin (CCK) because of the historical priority of the discovery of its action on the gallbladder.

Jorpes and Mutt determined the amino acid sequences of two molecular forms of porcine CCK of 33 and 39 residues in length (Table 8.4). Their structural analysis revealed that CCK-33 is a C-terminal fragment of CCK-39 and that the C-terminal pentapeptide sequence of CCK is identical to that of gastrin. Recently, the predominant molecular form of CCK in hog and human intestinal extracts was shown to be CCK-8, the C-terminal octapeptide fragment of the larger forms. Minor components corresponding to peptides larger than CCK-39 and similar in size to CCK-4 were also identified. CCK-4, of course, is identical to gastrin-4. The molecular form or forms of CCK that may circulate in the blood are unknown.

As was found for gastrin, the C-terminal region of CCK is the center of biological activity of the whole molecule. That is, CCK/gastrin-4 has all of the biological actions of both CCK and gastrin. Distinction between CCK and gastrin receptors is apparently achieved by the requirement for a sulfate substitution on the tyrosine side chain in position 7 of CCK. The sulfated tyrosine residue in CCK is only one position removed from the corresponding tyrosine in gastrin, but this slight change in position confers great target organ specificity.

Cholecystokinin has a wide variety of effects on the gastrointestinal tract and its outgrowths. The actions that are thought to be physiologically significant include (1) stimulation of pancreatic enzyme secretion, (2) augmentation of secretin-stimulated pancreatic bicarbonate secretion, (3) stimulation of gallbladder muscle contraction and relaxation of the sphincter of Oddi, (4) stimulation of intestinal motility, (5) inhibition of gastric emptying,

TABLE 8.4. Amino acid sequences of various forms of cholecystokinin[a,b]

	CCK-39	CCK-33	CCK-8	Caerulein	CCK-4
39.	Tyr				
38.	Ile				
37.	Gln				
36.	Gln				
35.	Ala				
34.	Arg				
33.	Lys	Lys			
32.	Ala	Ala			
31.	Pro	Pro			
30.	Ser	Ser			
29.	Gly	Gly			
28.	Arg	Arg			
27.	Val	Val			
26.	Ser	Ser			
25.	Met	Met			
24.	Ile	Ile			
23.	Lys	Lys			
22.	Asn	Asn			
21.	Leu	Leu			
20.	Gln	Gln			
19.	Ser	Ser			
18.	Leu	Leu			
17.	Asp	Asp			
16.	Pro	Pro			
15.	Ser	Ser			
14.	His	His			
13.	Arg	Arg			
12.	Ile	Ile			
11.	Ser	Ser			
10.	Asp	Asp		Glp[c]	
9.	Arg	Arg		Gln	
8.	Asp	Asp	Asp	Asp	
7.	Tyr-SO$_3$H	Tyr-SO$_3$H	Tyr-SO$_3$H	Tyr-SO$_3$H	
6.	Met	Met	Met	Thr	
5.	Gly	Gly	Gly	Gly	
4.	Trp	Trp	Trp	Trp	Trp
3.	Met	Met	Met	Met	Met
2.	Asp	Asp	Asp	Asp	Asp
1.	Phe-NH$_2$	Phe-NH$_2$	Phe-NH$_2$	Phe-NH$_2$	Phe-NH$_2$

[a] The numbering of amino acid residues is unconventional: from the carboxyl to the amino terminus.

[b] The CCK structures are the porcine molecules; caerulein is a frog skin molecule.

[c] Glp = pyroglutamyl.

and (6) stimulation of growth of the exocrine pancreas. Cholecystokinin can also elicit satiety, but definitive evidence for the physiological significance of this action is lacking, although it is attractive to hypothesize that satiation is a normal behavioral action of this hormone.

The original observation that indicated that CCK may elicit behavioral satiety was that rats which were surgically prepared with a gastric fistula (to prevent ingested food from entering the small intestine) did not limit their meal size as they would normally and that injected CCK caused them to stop eating prematurely under these conditions. A working hypothesis was then advanced that as food chyme enters the small intestine, it stimulates CCK release into the blood, and the CCK then interacts with the ventro-medial hypothalamus of the brain to induce satiety. This is an attractive hypothesis because it provides a quantitative relationship between the amount of food eaten and the intensity and duration of the resulting behavioral satiety. The CCK-secreting cell transduces intraluminal chemical information into a blood-borne signal to the brain indicating the nutritional status of the food in the small intestine even before it is absorbed into the body. The validity of the CCK satiety hypothesis is still open to debate. A particularly interesting question that awaits experimental clarification is the role, if any, that the brain's own CCK (see below) may play in eliciting satiety. Other evidence suggests strongly that CCK is not the only satiety cue. It is probable that the control of feeding behavior is complex and that CCK is only one of several potential satiety signals available to the animal.

Cholecystokinin is released from epithelial cells lining the upper small intestine by intraluminal fat, peptides and amino acids, and by calcium and magnesium ions. The stimuli for the release of CCK are adaptively related to the actions of the hormone in that CCK stimulates the expulsion of bile from the gallbladder and the secretion of the enzyme lipase from the pancreas. In the small intestine bile and lipase aid in fat digestion. Similarly, the amount of proteolytic enzymes secreted from the pancreas is regulated by CCK, which is released into the bloodstream in direct relationship to the load of peptides and amino acids entering the small intestine from the stomach. However, CCK also stimulates pancreatic amylase secretion, even though carbohydrates do not seem to stimulate CCK release. CCK seems to stimulate the "parallel" secretion of pancreatic enzymes (equal amounts of all of the many types of pancreatic enzymes), although some evidence for nonparallel (selective) secretion of enzymes has been reported.

Release of CCK has been estimated by measurement of target organ responses such as pancreatic enzyme secretion or gallbladder contraction. Measurement of circulating blood levels of CCK by radioimmunoassay has not yet yielded results that are widely accepted by workers in this field. This is because of several technical problems encountered in the development of the radioimmunoassay, such as difficulty in preparing radioactively labeled CCK. It is expected that these problems will be resolved eventually and that reliable estimates of blood CCK levels will become available.

Secretin

In 1902 Bayliss and Starling showed that a chemical substance extractable from small-intestinal mucosa stimulated pancreatic secretion when injected into dogs. They named this substance secretin. The structure of porcine secretin was deduced in 1966 by Jorpes and Mutt (Table 8.5). It is a linear peptide of 27 amino acid residues and shows no chemical similarity to the CCK/gastrin family of peptides. The entire molecule is required for full biological activity. Secretin in the small intestine and in blood seems to exist in only one biologically active molecular form.

Secretin has multiple biological effects when administered experimentally by injection, but the number of its normal physiological actions is considered to be small. The principal action of secretin seems to be stimulation of water and bicarbonate ion secretion by the exocrine pancreas. In addition, secretin augments the secretion of pancreatic enzymes elicited by CCK stimulation. It will be remembered that CCK similarly enhances the secretion of bicarbonate ions in response to secretin. This interaction (synergism) is thought to be significant, because the secretion of small amounts of both hormones in response to eating a meal produces pancreatic responses greater than could have been achieved by either hormone alone.

The stimulus for the release of secretin is the presence of acid in the lumen of the upper small intestine. The physiological significance of the diffuse distribution of gastrointestinal endocrine cells is clearly evident in the quantitative aspect of acid-stimulated release of secretin. For example, the amount of bicarbonate secreted by the pancreas in response to intestinal acidification in the dog depends on the quantity rather than the concentration of acid in the intestinal lumen. That is, the amount of secretin released is determined by the mass of acid delivered to the intestine and the total length of intestine that is acidified. Of course, the pancreatic bicarbonate ions entering the small intestine in response to secretin stimulation help neutralize the acid chyme delivered from the stomach, and thus help to provide a luminal pH environment suitable for the catalytic action of the pancreatic digestive enzymes.

Measurement of circulating levels of secretin by radioimmunoassay has been reported, but there are wide discrepancies among the values obtained by different workers. It does seem clear, however, that circulating secretin concentrations under normal conditions are lower than the concentrations of most other gastrointestinal hormones.

Other Active Peptides of the Gut

In addition to gastrin, cholecystokinin, and secretin, a number of other peptides with potent biological activities have been identified in mammalian gut extracts. The amino acid sequences and potential physiological significance of most of these substances are unknown. Because many of the actions

TABLE 8.5. Amino acid sequences of porcine GIP, glucagon, secretin, and VIP and of chicken VIP

	GIP	Glucagon	Secretin	VIP	Chicken VIP
1.	Tyr	His	—[a]	—	—
2.	Ala	Ser	—	—	—
3.	Glu	Gln	Asp	—	—
4.	Gly	—	—	Ala	—
5.	Thr	—	—	Val	—
6.	Phe	—	—	—	—
7.	Ile	Thr	—	—	—
8.	Ser	—	—	Asp	—
9.	Asp	—	Glu	Asn	—
10.	Tyr	—	Leu	Tyr	—
11.	Ser	—	—	Thr	Ser
12.	Ile	Lys	Arg	—	—
13.	Ala	Tyr	Leu	—	—
14.	Met	Leu	Arg	—	—
15.	Asp	—	—	Lys	—
16.	Lys	Ser	—	Gln	Glu
17.	Ile	Arg	Ala	Met	—
18.	Arg	—	—	Ala	—
19.	Gln	Ala	Leu	Val	—
20.	Gln	—	—	Lys	—
21.	Asp	—	Arg	Lys	—
22.	Phe	—	Leu	Tyr	—
23.	Val	—	Leu	—	—
24.	Asn	Gln	—	Asn	—
25.	Trp	—	Gly	Ser	—
26.	Leu	—	—	Ile	Val
27.	Leu	Met	Val-NH$_2$	Leu	—
28.	Ala	Asp		Asn-NH$_2$	Thr-NH$_2$
29.	Gln	Thr			
30.	Gln				
31.	Lys				
32.	Gly				
33.	Lys				
34.	Lys				
35.	Ser				
36.	Asp				
37.	Trp				
38.	Lys				
39.	His				
40.	Asn				
41.	Ile				
42.	Thr				
43.	Gln				

[a] —, indicates amino acid residue identical to the amino acid in the preceding column.

attributed to some of these "candidate" gastrointestinal hormones overlap with other, better studied gastrointestinal hormones, it seems likely that some of them will eventually be found to be identical with previously identified substances. We have already seen an example of this in the case of cholecystokinin and pancreozymin. It seems just as probable, however, that gut tissue contains many as yet undiscovered hormones. It has been estimated that the digestive tract has the largest mass of endocrine cells and the greatest diversity of hormones of any organ in the body. This section will describe briefly the candidate hormones of the gut. It seems likely that some of them will soon be accorded true hormonal status.

Two further members of the secretin/glucagon family of hormones have been characterized structurally. The amino acid sequences of porcine gastric inhibitory peptide (GIP) and vasoactive intestinal peptide (VIP) are shown in Table 8.5. The original action ascribed to GIP was inhibition of gastric acid secretion. So far, it has not been possible to demonstrate that this is a physiologically important action of the peptide. More recently, however, the ability of GIP to enhance glucose-stimulated insulin release from the

TABLE 8.6. Amino acid sequences of some candidate gastrointestinal hormones

	Motilin	Bombesin	Substance P	Neurotensin
1.	Phe	Glp[a]	Arg	Glp[a]
2.	Val	Gln	Pro	Leu
3.	Pro	Arg	Lys	Tyr
4.	Ile	Leu	Pro	Glu
5.	Phe	Gly	Gln	Asn
6.	Thr	Asn	Gln	Lys
7.	Tyr	Gln	Phe	Pro
8.	Gly	Trp	Phe	Arg
9.	Glu	Ala	Gly	Arg
10.	Leu	Val	Leu	Pro
11.	Gln	Gly	Met-NH_2	Tyr
12.	Arg	His		Ile
13.	Met	Leu		Leu
14.	Gln	Met-NH_2		
15.	Glu			
16.	Lys			
17.	Glu			
18.	Arg			
19.	Asn			
20.	Lys			
21.	Gly			
22.	Gln			

[a] Glp = pyroglutamyl.

pancreatic islets has been discovered. A major physiological role for GIP as the agent that causes increased insulin release in response to oral compared to intravenous glucose administration is now appreciated. Accordingly, it has been suggested that the acronym *GIP* might be applied more appropriately to *Glucose-dependent Insulinotropic Peptide*. The insulinotropic effect of GIP has been demonstrated *in vitro* using isolated rat pancreatic islets, suggesting that GIP acts directly on the insulin-secreting B cell.

Vasoactive intestinal peptide was originally identified by virtue of its ability to cause vasodilation, probably a pharmacologic action. Subsequently, VIP was shown to have diverse actions in mammals when tested by injection or infusion. Attempts to measure increases in circulating immunoreactive VIP levels after food ingestion have been unsuccessful; so the potential role of VIP as a gastrointestinal hormone is doubtful. However, because VIP is found in nerves as well as in endocrine cells in the gut, it is possible that its secretion is stimulated by nervous activity, that it acts locally, and thus it does not appear in the blood stream in appreciable amounts. Some demonstrable actions in response to VIP injections in mammals include inhibition of gastric acid secretion, stimulation of pancreatic bicarbonate ion secretion, stimulation of bile flow, stimulation of small-intestinal water and electrolyte secretion, decreased systemic blood pressure, relaxation of gut smooth muscle, release of insulin and glucagon, stimulation of lipolysis in fat cells, and stimulation of glycogenolysis in the liver. It is not surprising, in view of the structural similarities among members of this peptide hormone family, that some of the biological effects of VIP overlap with the physiological actions of other hormones of this family.

Motilin has been characterized chemically (Table 8.6) and shown capable of increasing gastric motility and initiating periodic interdigestive waves of small intestinal smooth muscle contractions in dogs. Whether endogenous motilin regulates these processes is unknown.

Intestinal peptides that exhibit immunological cross-reactivity with some pancreatic glucagon antisera have been known to exist for some time. The amino acid sequences of these "enteroglucagons" (gut glucagons, or glucagon-like immunoreactants) have not been established, but recent evidence indicates that they contain pancreatic glucagon as a fragment of their full structure. As might be expected, enteroglucagon can mimic the action of pancreatic glucagon as a stimulant of glycogenolysis in the liver. However, the potency of enteroglucagon is extremely weak compared with pancreatic glucagon, and its physiological role, if any, is uncertain.

Extracts of gastric and intestinal tissues contain substances that react with antisera to somatostatin, TRH, LHRH, bombesin, substance P, enkephalin, and neurotensin. The chemical natures of the immunoreactive substances have not been determined, except for substance P and neurotensin. All of these peptides have demonstrable actions on the gut and its

TABLE 8.7. Active factors extractable from the gastrointestinal tract

Factor	Tissue of Origin	Action
Bulbogastrone	Anterior (bulbar) small intestine	Inhibition of gastric acid secretion
Chymodenin	Small intestine	Stimulation of pancreatic chymotrypsinogen secretion
Duocrinin	Small intestine	Stimulation of Brunner's gland secretion
Enterocrinin	Small intestine	Stimulation of intestinal secretion
Enterogastrone	Small intestine	Inhibition of gastric acid secretion
Entero-oxyntin	Small intestine	Stimulation of gastric acid secretion
Gastrone	Gastric juice	Inhibition of gastric acid secretion
Gastrozymin	Small intestine	Stimulation of pepsin secretion
Incretin	Small intestine	Stimulation of insulin secretion
Pancreotone	Small and large intestines	Inhibition of exocrine pancreatic secretion
Villikinin	Small intestine	Stimulation of motility of villi

associated organs, but whether they are of any physiological significance is unknown.

Crude extracts of the gut with diverse actions on gastrointestinal functions have been described (Table 8.7). It is obvious that some of the actions attributed to these extractable factors overlap with actions of more fully characterized peptides. For example, the listed actions of enterogastrone and incretin can be duplicated by GIP. Whether the active substance in enterogastrone and incretin extracts is GIP awaits clarification.

BRAIN/GUT/SKIN DISTRIBUTION OF PEPTIDES

In 1931 von Euler and Gaddum discovered substance P in extracts of both intestine and brain. Since then, and with increasing occurrence in recent years, many other peptides have been found in both brain and gut. In addition, many peptides of the brain and gut have also been found in extracts of amphibian skin. This diverse tissue distribution of peptides may be reflected in the cellular distribution of active peptides in the mammalian gastrointestinal tract. In the gut, peptides are not limited only to true endocrine cells. Some gastrointestinal peptides are in nerve cells and some are in endocrine-like cells that do not seem to secrete their products into the blood. These "paracrine" cells are presumed to secrete their peptides into the surrounding intercellular spaces to influence target cells within the range of diffusional distribution (see Fig. 8.2).

Only substance P and neurotensin have been shown to be chemically identical in the brain and gut. Thyrotropin-releasing hormones from mammalian brain and amphibian skin have been shown to have the same amino acid sequences. Most other peptides of the so-called brain/gut/skin triangle have been characterized chemically from only one of these sites and then shown by immunological techniques to have cross-reacting counterparts in the other sites.

Peptides first isolated from the gut and subsequently shown to have counterparts in the brain include CCK, VIP, gastrin, and motilin. Of these, factors resembling the first two have been identified also in frog skin. Caerulein, the CCK-like peptide in the skin of certain frogs (see Table 8.4), has been localized in the dermal glands of the skin, which discharge their contents to the environment under adrenergic stimulation. Bombesin, a peptide first isolated from frog skin (for structure, see Table 8.6), has been found in the brain and gut as well. Peptides first isolated from the brain and later shown to have immunological counterparts in the gut include somatostatin, enkephalin, TRH, and neurotensin. Each peptide has a specific pattern of distribution at each of the sites at which it is found. Not every peptide found in the brain, gut, or skin is present also at the other sites.

The finding that the same peptide may be present in neurons of the brain and gut, in gut endocrine cells, and in skin exocrine cells, suggests that the same peptide may serve as a neurotransmitter, hormone, and paracrine agent. The functions of these peptides in the skin and the brain are not understood. It is clear that the gastrointestinal hormones are a subset of a large group of peptides produced by diverse tissues with no obvious phylogenetic, embryological, or functional relationships. Dockray has suggested that these molecules evolved early in phylogeny and have been conserved in widely different groups. He further speculates that once an organism has developed the capacity to produce a particular peptide, this capacity can be drawn on independently by different cell types by changes in the pattern of gene expression. This implies that an organism can use the same chemical to mediate different functions by segregating the chemical mediator by using neurocrine, endocrine, or paracrine routes of delivery to target cells.

MECHANISMS OF ACTION OF GASTROINTESTINAL HORMONES

Saturable and specific binding of radioactively labeled VIP to isolated preparations of liver, fat, intestinal epithelial, and pancreatic acinar cells has been demonstrated. Plasma membranes from liver and fat cells appear to possess a single class of receptors that have a high affinity for VIP and a low affinity for secretin and do not interact appreciably with glucagon. Furthermore, these receptors probably are physiologically meaningful because there was a good correlation between the abilities of VIP and secretin to inhibit the binding of radioactively labeled VIP and their abilities to activate the second messenger system (adenylate cyclase).

Pancreatic acinar cell preparations have proven to be useful for studying the properties of the receptors for the CCK and secretin families of hormones because hormone binding, second-messenger changes, and biological responses can all be measured using identical incubation conditions. Pancreatic acinar cells seem to possess two classes of binding sites for the secretin family of peptides, in contrast to the single class of binding sites found on liver and fat cells. Each class of receptor interacts with VIP and secretin, but not with glucagon. One class of binding sites has a high affinity for VIP and a low affinity for secretin; the other has a high affinity for secretin and a low affinity for VIP. It has been pointed out that changes in either the number or the specificity of different receptor populations on pancreatic acinar cells could explain the differences in responses of the avian and mammalian pancreas to secretin and VIP (see below). This is an example of the importance of studying changes in receptor properties as well as changes in hormone properties in comparative endocrinology. As yet, there are no data available on the properties of the avian pancreatic acinar cell VIP/secretin receptors.

Studies of binding of secretin to target cell preparations are few in number, mainly because of difficult technical problems encountered in preparing radioactively labeled secretin of high specific activity.

Pancreatic acinar preparations also have proven to be excellent systems in which to examine the properties of CCK receptors. The binding of radioactively labeled CCK in such preparations has been shown to be reversible, temperature dependent, saturable, specific, and localized in the plasma membrane. There is a close correlation between the relative potencies with which several different CCK-related peptides inhibit the binding of labeled CCK and the relative potencies with which these same peptides increase amylase secretion. This is an important finding, since it indicates that the sites on pancreatic acini that bind labeled CCK are the receptors with which CCK interacts to produce changes in acinar cell function.

Rat gastric mucosal membrane preparations have been shown to bind radioactively labeled gastrin specifically and saturably. This preparation seems to contain a single class of binding sites whose binding capacity is related to the feeding history of the animal. Fasting decreases the number of gastrin receptors, and either refeeding or treatment with gastrin brings the receptor concentrations back to the control levels. This suggests that gastrin stimulates the production of its own receptor and that this "up regulation" may be involved in the normal biological response to gastrin. These gastrin receptor studies must be interpreted with caution, however, because of the lack of demonstration of a relationship between receptor binding properties and biological responses. This is due to the cellular heterogeneity of gastric mucosal preparations, the inability to study acid secretion *in vitro*, and ignorance of the second messenger for gastrin in acid-secreting cells.

The second messengers used by the various gastrointestinal hormones provide some interesting comparisons. For example, in the rat and the guinea pig, secretin, VIP, bombesin, and acetylcholine, in addition to CCK, are capable of stimulating digestive enzyme release from pancreatic acinar cells *in vitro*. Secretin and VIP seem to interact with the same receptor site, but the other stimulants each appear to have a specific receptor. However, CCK, bombesin, and acetylcholine, on the one hand, and secretin and VIP, on the other, stimulate different maximal rates of enzyme secretion. Moreover, within each group of stimulants (we may call them the CCK and secretin groups for convenience), no additive effects are observed when two factors are tested in combination at maximal concentrations, suggesting that they stimulate the same intracellular mechanism. When two stimulants of opposite groups, such as CCK and secretin, are tested together, the secretory response is greater than the additive effects of either agent alone (synergism), which suggests that they stimulate different intracellular mechanisms.

The intracellular events mediating these interesting interactions have been worked out. Cholecystokinin, bombesin, and acetylcholine release calcium intracellularly in acinar cells, and this is followed by a prompt increase in cyclic GMP (cGMP) levels. This transient rise in cGMP allows a prolonged enzyme secretory response via the activation of a cGMP-dependent protein kinase and a sustained phosphorylation of proteins directly involved in exocytosis.

In contrast, binding of secretin and VIP leads to prolonged elevation of intracellular cAMP and the activation of cAMP-dependent kinases. Calcium and cGMP do not seem to be involved.

The pancreatic acinar cell is thus an interesting example of a hormonal target in which distinct second-messenger systems, stimulated by different first messengers (the hormones and acetylcholine), can mediate the same final cellular response. These relationships are summarized in Fig. 8.3.

Another area of interest is the mechanism of the regulation of gastric acid secretion. Hydrochloric acid is secreted by the parietal cells of the mammalian stomach. Agents that can stimulate the parietal cell to secrete acid *in vivo* include gastrin, acetylcholine, histamine, and amino acids. Thus, there are neurocrine (acetylcholine), endocrine (gastrin), paracrine (histamine), and direct secretagogue (amino acids in the gastric lumen) pathways for stimulation of parietal cells. Not surprisingly, the overall regulation of gastric acid secretion is complex.

It has long been known that the stimuli for gastric acid secretion interact when tested *in vivo*. For example, certain antihistaminic drugs, such as cimetidine, inhibit the response to acetylcholine and gastrin as well as histamine. This observation and others led to the proposal that histamine is the final common mediator for all stimulants of the parietal cell. According to this theory, gastrin and acetylcholine release histamine in the vicinity of parietal cells (presumably from paracrine histaminocytes, although these cells have not yet been identified with certainty), and parietal cells have

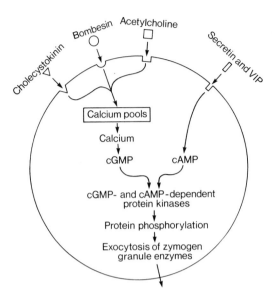

FIGURE 8.3. A summary of the actions of several secretagogues on the pancreatic acinar cell. See text for details.

receptors only for histamine. The interactions of gastric secretagogues are of clinical as well as academic interest, because peptic ulcer disease is effectively treated by reducing gastric acid output.

Experimental tests *in vivo* of the final common mediator hypothesis have yielded conflicting results. For example, it has been possible to demonstrate an effect of gastrin on histamine metabolism only in the rat stomach. However, the recent development of *in vitro* preparations of viable parietal cells, isolated from the other cell types of the gastric mucosa, has allowed more definitive assessment of the hypothesis.

In studies of canine parietal cells *in vitro*, Soll has shown that gastrin, acetylcholine, and histamine each have specific receptors on this cell type. This contradicts the final common mediator hypothesis. The main findings leading to this conclusion can be summarized as follows:

1. Gastrin, histamine, and acetylcholine each stimulated the isolated parietal cells when tested alone *in vitro*.
2. The histamine response under such test conditions was blocked by cimetidine, the acetylcholine response was blocked by atropine, but the gastrin response was not blocked by either inhibitor.
3. The response to a combination of histamine and gastrin far exceeds the sum of the responses to the single agents.
4. Cimetidine markedly inhibits this histamine–gastrin interaction, leaving a residual response equivalent to that produced by gastrin alone.

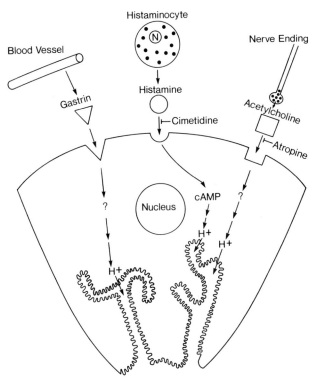

FIGURE 8.4. A summary of the actions of several secretagogues on the gastric parietal cell. See text for details.

5. A similar pattern of interaction and independence of action is found between histamine and acetylcholine.

Such data indicate that the apparent lack of specificity of the inhibitors atropine and cimetidine observed *in vivo* may be explained by effects of these drugs on secretagogue interactions at the level of the parietal cell. In the intact gastric mucosa, the parietal cell may be exposed to the constant tonic influence of histamine and acetylcholine, so that when gastrin interacts with the parietal cell, the acid secretory response represents the result of the interaction of all three substances and therefore can be inhibited by both antagonistic drugs. These interactions are illustrated in Fig. 8.4. It is interesting to note that these recent findings, while not compatible with the final common mediator hypothesis, nevertheless implicate histamine and acetylcholine as important substances in the control of gastric acid secretion.

The second messenger for the action of histamine on the parietal cell seems to be cAMP. The second messengers for the actions of gastrin and acetylcholine on the parietal cell are unknown, but probably are not cAMP.

COMPARATIVE ASPECTS OF GASTROINTESTINAL HORMONES

The existence of families of interrelated gastrointestinal peptide hormones is good reason to expect that the chemical and biological similarities of the peptides reflect common evolutionary histories. Until recently, however, comparative studies of the gut hormones were few in number.

We may consider the two main families of gastrointestinal peptide hormones to be the CCK and secretin families. The CCK family includes the various molecular forms of CCK and gastrin as well as the amphibian skin peptide caerulein (see Tables 8.3 and 8.4). The secretin family includes secretin, VIP, GIP, and glucagon (see Table 8.5). With few exceptions, the amino acid sequences of only the mammalian peptides of these families are known. Therefore, it is not possible yet to construct a meaningful outline of the molecular evolution of the structure of these hormones.

More complete comparative information exists at the level of studies of the presence of active factors, resembling the mammalian peptides in their biological and immunological properties, extractable from various tissues of lower vertebrates and invertebrates. These studies, coupled with much new information gained from immunostaining of gut endocrine cells, allow a preliminary assessment of the distribution of some members of the CCK and secretin peptide families in nonmammalian species.

Secretinlike biological activity has been identified in crude extracts of intestines from representative species of every vertebrate class, and even from an invertebrate species, the octopus. VIP-like activity has been described in extracts of shark, teleost, and avian tissues. The species distribution of GIP has not been studied in depth. Glucagonlike factors have been found in tissue extracts of all vertebrate groups, a protochordate, and several invertebrate species. For none of these peptides has the study of species distribution been performed in a systematic way. Hence, it is impossible to discern yet the pattern of evolution of the individual peptides. From the information above, we might speculate that secretin and glucagon may have evolutionary precedence, and thus closely resemble the hypothetical peptide of ancestral origin in this family.

It will be remembered that VIP is capable of stimulating secretion of water and electrolytes from the mammalian small intestine. The rectal gland in sharks is an outgrowth of the hindgut and thus may be considered to be functionally analagous, and perhaps homologous, to the mammalian intestine. Recently, it has been shown that porcine VIP stimulates the dogfish shark rectal gland to secrete a fluid rich in sodium chloride. Furthermore, it was found that plasma VIP levels in the dogfish were elevated by an increase in intraluminal gastrointestinal osmolality, leading to the speculation that VIP may be used in this species as an osmoregulatory hormone. Before the discovery of the effect of VIP on the dogfish rectal gland, Dockray had speculated that, in view of the likelihood that primitive vertebrates did not possess a discrete exocrine pancreas (see Chapter 9), the action of peptides of the secretin family on water and electrolyte secretion by the intestine could have foreshadowed their actions on pancreatic water and electrolyte secretion. The recent dogfish shark findings certainly support this concept. Whether VIP affects the dogfish pancreas as well is unknown.

The relationships between secretin and VIP as stimulants of pancreatic secretion in various species has been examined by Dockray (Table 8.8). He finds that avian and mammalian VIPs are more potent stimulants of the avian pancreas than are either avian or mammalian secretins, in contrast to the situation in mammals. Furthermore, extracts of teleost intestines more closely resemble VIP than secretin in their patterns of biological activity. Dockray theorizes that a peptide chemically resembling VIP more closely than secretin may be the physiologically important regulator of pancreatic juice secretion in lower vertebrates.

CCK-like peptides have been detected in intestinal extracts prepared from species representing all of the vertebrate classes as well as several invertebrate species. In view of the fact that the intestine is more ancient than the stomach in vertebrate phylogeny, we might predict that CCK is a more primitive peptide than gastrin in animals. In vertebrates this seems to be the case. It is not yet clear whether the active material in invertebrates is more like CCK or gastrin.

It would appear that gastrin first arose at the time of the divergence of reptiles and amphibia in vertebrate evolution. Larsson and Rehfeld found only CCK-like peptides in the stomachs of teleosts and amphibians, whereas reptile, bird, and mammalian stomachs seemed to contain gastrinlike peptides. How fishes and amphibians may differentially regulate gastric versus

TABLE 8.8 Relative potencies of some vertebrate gastrointestinal peptides in stimulating the flow rate of pancreatic juice in rat and turkey[a]

Stimulant	Pancreatic Juice Flow	
	Rat	Turkey
Porcine secretin	+ + +	+
Chicken secretin	+ +	+
Porcine VIP	+	+ +
Chicken VIP	+	+ + +
Cod intestinal extract	+	+ + +

[a] After G. J. Dockray, *Gen. Comp. Endocrinol.*, **25**:203 (1975).

intestinal digestive processes without separate gastrin- and CCK-like hormones is unknown.

Clearly, these families of hormones arose early in animal evolution. They must play important roles in physiology to have persisted so long and in such diverse animal species. The antiquity of the gastrointestinal hormones and the diversity of adaptations of the feeding and digestive processes evident in vertebrates and invertebrates suggest that detailed studies of the comparative endocrinology of the peptides of the gut will yield rich insights into understanding the evolution of regulatory mechanisms in general.

ADDITIONAL READING

1. Bloom, S. R., ed. (1978). *Gut Hormones*. Churchill Livingstone, Edinburgh.

2. Dockray, G. J. (1975). Comparative studies on secretin. *Gen. Comp. Endocrinol.* **25**:203–210.

3. Dockray, G. J. (1977). Molecular evolution of gut hormones: application of comparative studies on the regulation of digestion. *Gastroenterology* **72**:344–358.

4. Dockray, G. J. (1979*a*). Comparative biochemistry and physiology of gut hormones. *Ann. Rev. Physiol.* **41**:83–95.

5. Dockray, G. J. (1979*b*). Evolutionary relationships of the gut hormones. *Fed. Proc.* **38**:2295–2301.

6. Fujita, T., and S. Kobayashi (1977). Structure and function of gut endocrine cells. *Int. Rev. Cytol.* Suppl. 6:187–233.

7. Glass, G. B. J., ed. (1980). *Gastrointestinal Hormones*. Raven, New York.

8. Grossman, M. I. (1977). Physiological effects of gastrointestinal hormones. *Fed. Proc.* **36**:1930–1932.

9. Grossman, M. I. (1979). Neural and hormonal regulation of gastrointestinal function: an overview. *Ann. Rev. Physiol.* **41**:27–33.

10. Makhlouf, G. M. (1974). The neuroendocrine design of the gut. The play of chemicals in a chemical playground. *Gastroenterology* **67**:159–184.

11. Soll, A. H., and J. H. Walsh (1979). Regulation of gastric acid secretion. *Ann. Rev. Physiol.* **41**:35–53.

12. Stoff, J. S., R. Rosa, R. Hallac, P. Silva, and F. H. Epstein (1979). Hormonal regulation of active chloride transport in the dogfish rectal gland. *Am. J. Physiol.* **237**:F138–F144.

9

The Endocrine Pancreas

We have seen in the preceding chapter how gastrointestinal peptides control the flow of ingested food down the digestive tube and the assimilation of nutrients into the body from the intestinal lumen. The efficient distribution of these absorbed ''fuels'' to body tissues is of critical importance to the economy of the organism. After all, life depends on keeping the metabolic fires burning. In this chapter we will consider some of the endocrine substances that regulate the distribution of absorbed nutrients within the body.

The pancreas develops as a glandular outpocketing of the intestine. Embryologically, then, the hormone-secreting cells of the gut and pancreas arise from different parts of the same continuous epithelium. Furthermore, several hormones and active peptides are found in both the gut and pancreas of adult vertebrates (see Table 8.1). If we consider that the endocrine gut regulates the entry of metabolic fuels into the organism and that the endocrine pancreas regulates the disposal of these fuels within the organism, we may perhaps appreciate that the similarities in origin between the two endocrine systems can reflect their functional interrelationships.

ANATOMY AND CYTOLOGY OF THE ENDOCRINE PANCREAS

In most vertebrates the endocrine pancreas consists of individual islets of hormone-secreting cells encapsulated by connective tissue and embedded in the acinar exocrine tissue of the pancreas. These structures are called *islets of Langerhans* in honor of the 19th century scientist who first described them. Islets of Langerhans are ductless, have a rich blood supply, and are innervated in many species.

Classically, islet endocrine cells were at first distinguished morphologi-

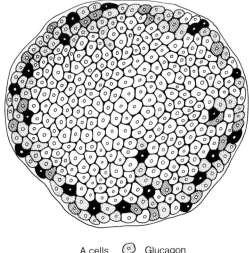

A cells	⊙	Glucagon
B cells	⊙	Insulin
D cells	●	Somatostatin
PP cells	⊘	Pancreatic polypeptide

FIGURE 9.1. Diagrammatic representation of the endocrine cell distribution in a typical mammalian islet of Langerhans. PP cells are found in exocrine pancreatic acini as well. A cells and PP cells are distributed also in the gut epithelium.

cally by their affinities for certain histochemical dyes. Because tinctorial staining properties of islet cells do not necessarily reflect any specific property of the hormones they contain, these histochemical criteria for identifying islet endocrine cells have proven inadequate, and their application has resulted in much confusion over the years. Modern immunocytochemical techniques have allowed less equivocal identification of the islet endocrine cells and have provided the basis for their rational classification.

There are four well-characterized islet endocrine cell types in mammals: A cells (glucagon), B cells (insulin), D cells (somatostatin), and PP cells (pancreatic polypeptide). In mammalian islets of Langerhans, B cells often are located centrally, surrounded by a mantle of A, D, and PP cells (Fig. 9.1). In addition, PP cells are scattered individually among acinar cells in the exocrine pancreas. A cells secreting pancreatic-type glucagon (distinct from enteroglucagon), D cells, and PP cells are also found in the gastrointestinal tract proper in many species.

Certain gastrointestinal hormones (gastrin, CCK, VIP, GIP, and others) have been identified in the pancreas of some species and in some pancreatic tumors. Some of these peptides (for example, CCK and VIP) may be acting as neurotransmitters, since they are found in axonal terminals, and are not pancreatic hormones at all. Others seem to be contained in true endocrine cells but are found only in some species (for example, endocrine gastrin-containing cells are found in cat but not hog pancreases). In view of the close ontogenetic, phylogenetic, and functional relationship of the gut and the pancreas, it may well be that all gut hormones in some species and during some periods of development are also present in the pancreas and, conversely, that all pancreatic hormones can be found in gut endocrine cells. However, because the physiological status of these minor components of the endocrine pancreas requires further study, their possible functions will not be considered here.

Not all vertebrates conform to the mammalian pattern of pancreatic anatomy and cytology. In the cyclostomes (Agnatha), the exocrine pancreas does not exist as an anatomically discrete gland, but instead is represented by individual "acinar" cells diffusely distributed in the intestinal epithelium. In the agnathan hagfishes, the endocrine pancreas (the islet organ) is located in the submucosa of the intestine and is visible externally as a whitish bulge surrounding the intestinal entry of the bile duct. In the lampreys, islet tissues (the follicles of Langerhans) are more widely distributed as small clumps of cells that may be found within the intestinal mucosa. The two largest clumps of endocrine pancreatic tissue are found, according to Hardisty, at the junction of the esophagus and the intestine and at the level where the intestine passes and is in contact with the liver.

There are differences in islet organ cytology between hagfishes and lampreys. In both groups, insulin-containing B cells and somatostatin-containing D cells are found. While this is apparently the full complement of hagfish pancreatic hormones, two other cell types appear in the lamprey endocrine pancreas during the anadromous (upstream) final migration of some species. The nature and function of the presumed hormones of these latter two cell types have not been established. However, they do not seem to contain either glucagon or PP. Therefore, the agnathan endocrine pancreas differs from that of the gnathostomes in the absence of typical A and PP cells. In addition, the agnathan endocrine pancreas does not seem to be innervated and is relatively poorly vascularized.

The pancreases of the gnathostomes are similar in anatomy and cytology, with a small number of striking variations. The similarities include the invariable association of the endocrine with exocrine tissue and the presence of A, B, D, and PP cells. Furthermore, it appears that all gnathostome pancreases may contain a distinct fifth type of granular islet cell of unknown content and function.

Instead of existing as a discrete glandular organ, the teleost endocrine pancreas in many species is disseminated in the abdominal cavity along with small clumps of exocrine pancreatic tissue. In some teleosts much of the endocrine tissue is gathered together into so-called Brockmann bodies or principal islets (Fig. 9.2), which are still associated with some exocrine pancreatic tissue. The lungfish pancreas exhibits yet another anatomic arrangement: the endocrine (islets) and exocrine tissues are located within the wall of the intestine. In certain tetrapod species, the tendency of islets to aggregate into a particular area or lobe of the pancreas is evident. This tendency is especially notable in certain reptiles and birds, in which many islets are gathered in the "splenic lobe" of the pancreas. Furthermore, in

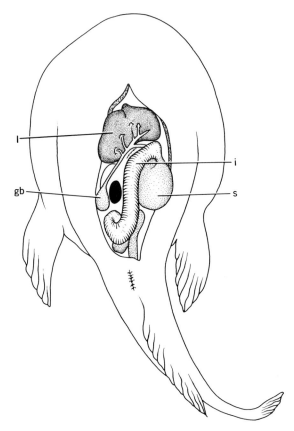

FIGURE 9.2.   Ventral view of a partially dissected angler fish (*Lophius piscatorius*). The liver (*l*) has been displaced forward, revealing the gallbladder (*gb*), intestine (*i*), and lower end of the stomach (*s*). Running obliquely anterior from the gallbladder is the long cystic duct. The Brockmann body, or principal islet of endocrine pancreatic tissue, is shown as solid black just median to the gallbladder. [After W. Bargmann, *Handbuch mikr. Anat. Menschen,* **6:**2, 1939.]

birds there seem to exist separate A and B islets—large A-cell and smaller B-cell islets; both types contain D and PP cells.

The innervation of endocrine pancreatic tissue among the vertebrates is variable. The agnathan endocrine pancreas is not innervated. As a group, the gnathostomes in general possess innervated islets. The exceptions include most birds, a few reptiles, and possibly the Holocephali (Chondrichthyes). The degree of islet innervation is especially great among the teleosts, providing a striking parallel with the degree of innervation of the teleost pars distalis (see Chapter 2). Aminergic, cholinergic, and peptidergic nerve terminals have been reported in islets of Langerhans. The identities of the possible peptide neurotransmitters in the endocrine pancreas have not been established with certainty, and there may be species differences.

Nevertheless, VIP and CCK have been detected in islet nerves of some mammals by immunocytochemical techniques.

Finally, we may ask when the hormones of the typical vertebrate endocrine pancreas first arose in the evolution of animals. Substances having the immunological and, in some instances, the physiological properties of insulin- and glucagonlike factors have been identified in the intestines of invertebrate species, and they probably first arose in the common ancestors of both protostomes and deuterostomes. No organs resembling the pancreas or islets of Langerhans have been found in invertebrates, but mammalian insulin has been shown capable of affecting glucose metabolism in several invertebrate species (e.g., molluscs). These observations, together with the fact that glucagon is present in the agnathan gut but not in the pancreas, suggest that the vertebrate pancreatic hormones are of ancient heritage and arose first as gastrointestinal hormones. Their subsequent evolutionary migration from the intestinal epithelium to an extramural gland allowed an

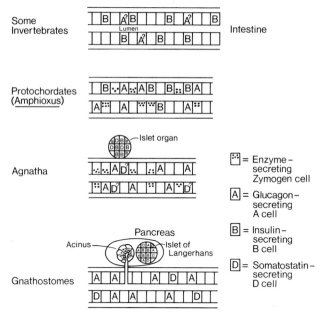

FIGURE 9.3. Hypothetical scenario of the evolution of the endocrine and exocrine pancreas. Glucagon-secreting A cells and insulin-secreting B cells have been identified in the intestinal epithelium of some invertebrate species. In *Amphioxus* the endocrine cells are intermingled with enzyme-secreting zymogen cells in the intestinal epithelium. In the agnathan hagfishes, B cells and somatostatin-secreting D cells are removed from the intestinal epithelium, whereas A cells, possibly some D cells, and zymogen cells remain in the intestine. In gnathostomes, zymogen cells and A cells are found in the remote pancreas. Note that some A cells and D cells remain in the intestinal epithelium. It is not known whether D cells are present also in invertebrate and protochordate intestinal epithelia. PP cells are omitted from this scenario because there is not enough information available about their species distribution.

enormous increase in the mass of endocrine tissue while simultaneously generating an increase in the absorptive surface area of the intestine. Whether the close association between pancreatic endocrine and exocrine tissue (which was retained in the move from the gut to the pancreas) reflects a functional interaction or just a common embryological origin remains a controversial question. Figure 9.3 summarizes this hypothetical evolutionary sequence.

INSULIN

Structure and Biosynthesis

Insulin is a polypeptide hormone consisting of two disulfide-linked peptide chains (Fig. 9.4). After insulin is secreted into the circulation by the B cells of the endocrine pancreas, it plays a major role in the regulation of carbohydrate, amino acid, and fat metabolism in mammals. Insulin is the only hypoglycemic hormone; it is also an anabolic hormone in the sense that it promotes the synthesis and storage of glycogen, proteins, and lipids and inhibits the degradation (catabolism) of these substances. The key target tissues of insulin are muscle, fat, and liver. Insulin has also been found to be essential for the growth of many other tissues.

The two chains of the insulin molecule are not synthesized separately and later combined. Instead, a single proinsulin peptide, containing the A and B chains as well as an intervening C peptide, is the biosynthetic precursor of insulin (Fig. 9.5). During the intracellular transport of proinsulin from its site of biosynthesis in the rough endoplasmic reticulum of the B cell, it is slowly cleaved by specific enzymes, yielding insulin and C peptide. Recently, studies utilizing messenger RNA coding for rat proinsulin have revealed that the biosynthesis of insulin involves a precursor even larger than proinsulin. This *preproinsulin*, as it has been termed, consists of proinsulin plus a 23–amino acid extension on the N-terminal end of the B chain. Apparently, this peptide extension is removed very rapidly during biosynthesis, probably before the full proinsulin chain is completely synthesized. The biosynthesis of insulin is summarized in Fig. 9.6.

Mammalian proinsulins vary in length; these variations occur only in the C-peptide portions that link the A and B chains. Furthermore, analysis of the amino acid sequences of the mammalian C peptides indicates that these peptides exhibit a much higher rate of mutation acceptance than do the corresponding insulins. This finding is consistent with the possibility that the C peptide in the proinsulin molecule does not have any specific hormonal function.

The primary structures of insulins from more than 25 species of vertebrates have been determined. The variability of primary structures among species is depicted in Table 9.1. It appears that amino acid substitutions can

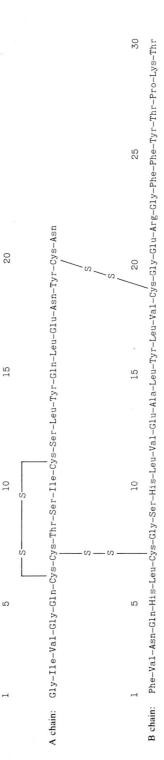

FIGURE 9.4 Primary structure of human insulin.

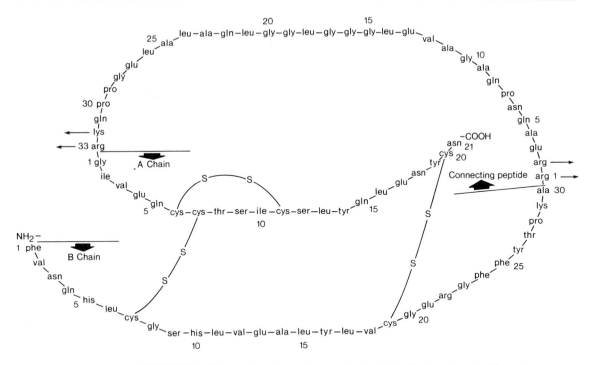

FIGURE 9.5. Primary structure of hog proinsulin. Note that hog insulin differs from human insulin (Fig. 9.4) only in the substitution of alanine for threonine at position B-30. Before secretion of insulin, the lysine and the three arginine residues at the two ends of the C peptide are removed enzymatically, resulting in the secretion of a 29-residue C-peptide fragment.

occur at many positions in either the A or B chain without destroying biological activity in a particular species. On the other hand, certain structural features are conserved throughout vertebrate evolution. In particular, the positions of the three disulfide bonds, the N- and C-terminal regions of the A chain, and the hydrophobic residues in the C-terminal region of the B chain seem to be highly conserved. This is not surprising, since chemical modifications in any of these regions tend to reduce or abolish biological activity.

Purified insulin molecules tend to aggregate spontaneously into pairs (dimers). Certain invariant residues in the A and B chains seem to be involved in maintaining the secondary and tertiary structural features that are important in the formation of these dimers. In the presence of Zn^{2+} in the gnathostome B-cell secretory granule, three insulin dimers will associate with each other to form a hexameric unit, which apparently is the storage form of the hormone in the granule. The hagfish insulin dimer seems to be incapable of forming hexamers.

The striking conservatism seen in the primary structures of vertebrate insulins is reflected also in their biosyntheses. It has been shown that translation of teleost islet messenger RNA *in vitro* in the presence of mammalian microsomal membranes led to the correct cleavage of the fish preproinsulin, resulting in the synthesis of authentic fish proinsulin. These data suggest that the mechanisms and information required for at least part of the insulin biosynthetic pathway are also highly conserved during evolution.

Regulation of Insulin Secretion

Considering the importance of islet hormones in the regulation of carbohydrate, protein, and lipid metabolism, it is not surprising that these met-

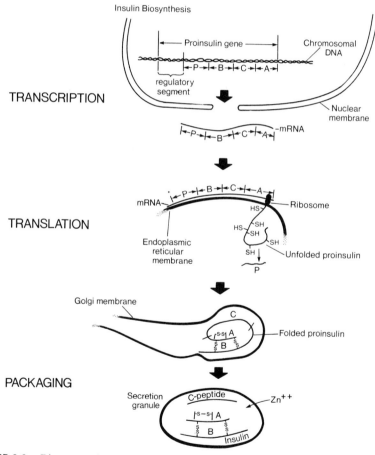

FIGURE 9.6. Diagrammatic representation of the biosynthesis of mammalian insulin. Messenger RNA (mRNA), which is produced by transcription of the proinsulin gene, consists of the "pre" segment (P), segments encoding the A and B chains, and the segment for the connecting peptide (C). The "pre" peptide of preproinsulin is cleaved even before translation is completed at the ribosome. The final cleavage of proinsulin to yield insulin occurs in Golgi vesicles. Insulin molecules spontaneously form pairs (dimers) which, in the presence of zinc ions (Zn^{2+}), form aggregates of six insulin molecules, or hexameric units.

TABLE 9.1. Amino acid sequences of insulins

	A Chain			B Chain		
	Human	Hagfish	Other Species[a]	Human	Hagfish	Other Species[a]
0.						Val, Met
1.	Gly	—[b]	—	Phe	Arg	Ala
2.	Ile	—	—	Val	Thr	Ala, Pro, Tyr
3.	Val	—	His	Asn	Thr	Ala, Lys, Pro, Ser
4.	Glu	—	Asp	Gln	Gly	Arg
5.	Gln	—	—	His	—	Arg
6.	Cys	—	—	Leu	—	—
7.	Cys	His		Cys	—	—
8.	Thr	His	Ala, Glu	Gly	—	Glu
9.	Ser	Lys	Gly, Arg, Asn	Ser	Lys	Pro
10.	Ile	Arg	Pro, Val, Thr	His	Asp	Asn, Gln
11.	Cys	—	—	Leu	—	—
12.	Ser	—	Asn, Asp, Thr	Val	—	—
13.	Leu	Ile	Arg, Lys	Glu	Asn	Asp
14.	Tyr	—	Phe, His, Asn	Ala	—	Thr
15.	Gln	Asn	Asp	Leu	—	—
16.	Leu	—	—	Tyr	—	—
17.	Glu	Gln	Met	Leu	Ile	Ser
18.	Asn	—	Ser	Val	Ala	—
19.	Tyr	—	—	Cys	—	—
20.	Cys	—	—	Gly	—	Gln, Arg
21.	Asn	—	—	Glu	Val	Asp, His
22.			Asp	Arg	—	Asp
23.				Gly	—	—
24.				Phe	—	—
25.				Phe	—	—
26.				Tyr	—	—
27.				Thr	Asp	Arg, Gln, Ile, Ser
28.				Pro	—	Ser
29.				Lys	Thr	Asn, Met
30.				Thr	Lys	Ala, Asp, Ser
31.					Met	

[a] Amino acid substitutions found in the insulins of many species of birds, mammals, and fishes.
[b] —, indicates amino acid residue identical to preceding column.

abolic fuels are important determinants of islet hormone secretion. Hyperglycemia can stimulate insulin release by directly stimulating B cells. Whether this is an effect of a membrane-bound glucose receptor or the result of intracellular glucose metabolism is unresolved. In any case, glucose seems to stimulate cAMP and Ca^{2+} accumulation, and these substances therefore are prime candidates for intracellular roles in the secretion of insulin. The threshold for glucose-stimulated insulin secretion is high enough to suggest that glucose alone does not regulate circulating insulin levels. An important function of nonstimulatory levels of blood glucose may be to modify insulin secretion in response to other stimuli (see below).

Circulating amino acids also stimulate insulin release. Individual amino acids differ in their ability to affect insulin secretion. Some amino acids are inactive, and there are species differences among mammals. In people arginine, followed by lysine and leucine, are the most potent insulin releasers.

The effects of the products of lipid metabolism on insulin secretion are confusing. There are marked species differences among mammals. Even studies in a single species comparing *in vivo* and *in vitro* responses often yield conflicting results. In general, it seems that short- and long-chain fatty acids and ketone bodies stimulate insulin secretion.

It has been observed that greater insulin secretion occurs in response to glucose or amino acids when given orally than when given intravenously. This observation has led to the proposal that one or more gastrointestinal hormones may be involved in the physiological regulation of insulin secretion. The gastrointestinal hormone GIP (see Chapter 8) seems to be the best available candidate for this action. CCK, gastrin, and VIP also have been shown capable of stimulating insulin release when given by injection. However, as we have seen, these substances are also found in pancreatic nerve terminals, and they may be acting as neurotransmitters instead of as gastrointestinal hormones. Glucagon also stimulates insulin release.

Islets of Langerhans have a rich sympathetic and parasympathetic innervation. Circulating epinephrine and the sympathetic neurotransmitter norepinephrine inhibit insulin secretion by interacting with B-cell alpha-adrenergic receptors. This is apparently part of the mechanism for the inhibition of insulin secretion during exercise. Interestingly, B cells also have a small population of beta-adrenergic receptors which, when activated by epinephrine, stimulate insulin secretion. However, this response can be demonstrated only in pharmacologic experiments and seems to be of no physiological significance. Pituitary growth hormone stimulates insulin release. This can be interpreted as a "recruitment" of the anabolic influence of insulin by growth hormone in order to promote growth.

Acetylcholine, a parasympathetic neurotransmitter, stimulates insulin release. This effect can be blocked by atropine, a muscarinic cholinergic receptor antagonist. Classical conditioning can lead to the ability to voluntarily release insulin, and this response can be blocked by atropine or vagotomy (cutting the parasympathetic vagus nerve). With so many factors—both endocrine and nervous—affecting insulin secretion, it is difficult to determine their respective roles in insulin release. At present the best interpretation is that plasma glucose and amino acid concentrations have a primary influence on insulin release. The nervous and endocrine influences appear to be modulators that apply to special physiological situations (exercise, emergency exertion, "anticipating" the intestinal absorption of carbohydrate after a meal, etc.).

Actions of Insulin

Insulin is the only hormone that lowers blood glucose concentrations, thus providing protection against the deleterious consequences of hyperglycemia and glycosuria. Insulin is an anabolic hormone because it promotes the rapid transfer of glucose from blood to tissues, activates glucose-utilizing mechanisms, and inhibits the actions of other hormones that promote gluconeogenesis.

Skeletal muscle is an important insulin target tissue. Elevated blood insulin concentrations, such as occur after eating a meal, stimulate the entry of glucose into skeletal muscle cells. Also, the synthesis of the important glucose-phosphorylating enzyme hexokinase in skeletal muscle is stimulated by insulin. Muscle cells store glucose as glycogen when circulating glucose and insulin are abundant. Insulin enhances the activities of glycogen-synthesizing enzymes and inhibits the activities of enzymes that catalyze glycogen breakdown. Insulin stimulates glycolysis in skeletal muscle by promoting synthesis of several glycolytic enzymes (in addition to hexokinase). All metabolic pathways for the utilization of glucose in skeletal muscle are enhanced in the presence of insulin.

Insulin has no direct influence on glucose uptake by the mammalian liver (in contrast to this action in muscle). However, it affects intracellular hepatic sugar metabolism in much the same way that it affects skeletal muscle cells. All the actions of insulin on both target tissues tend to reduce blood glucose concentrations and enhance macromolecule synthesis.

Skeletal muscle and the liver in mammals can store only limited quantities of glycogen between meals. Adipose tissue provides a third storage site for metabolic fuels that are regulated, in part, by insulin. When blood glucose and insulin levels rise after a meal, glucose can enter adipose cells and be utilized in the synthesis of lipid. In addition to promoting lipid synthesis, insulin opposes lipid degradation by inhibition of the enzyme lipase.

Insulin directly enhances the uptake (transport) of certain amino acids into skeletal muscle and liver cells and promotes protein synthesis. Synergism between insulin and the (protein) anabolic effects of growth hormone and androgens is probably important in the normal growth of most body tissues.

Mechanisms of Insulin Action

Many of the actions of insulin can be accounted for by an interaction of the hormone with specific cell membrane protein receptors. The properties of the hormone–receptor interaction have been studied extensively in several cell types, but have not as yet led to an understanding of the mechanism of insulin action. In the last few years, insulin binding to receptors associated with various intracellular organelles, such as Golgi vesicles and rough endoplasmic reticulum, has been described. Whether insulin has an intracellular site of action or is merely degraded inside the cells is unclear.

The search for a single intracellular second messenger for insulin has been long and controversial. Most workers now agree that cAMP or cGMP are not involved. It seems that cellular Ca^{2+} is a possible mediator of insulin action in at least some systems. Perhaps insulin utilizes several second messengers or different ones in different target tissues. Such a finding should not be surprising in view of the diverse actions of insulin on a variety of target tissues. For the moment, the molecular basis of insulin action remains unknown.

GLUCAGON

Structure and Biosynthesis

Glucagon is a straight-chain polypeptide 29 amino acid residues in length. The primary structures of all mammalian glucagons determined so far are identical, unlike the situation for insulin. Avian glucagons differ only minimally from the mammalian hormones. These relationships are depicted in Table 9.2. The isolation of anglerfish glucagon has been reported. Although its full amino acid sequence is not yet known, it appears to be about the same size as mammalian and avian glucagons, differing in primary structure at several sites.

Some evidence has been obtained that glucagon is synthesized as a larger molecule than the secreted form of the hormone and that this biosynthetic precursor is subjected to post-translational processing by limited proteolysis. Such substances have been detected in the islet tissues of mammals, birds, and fishes. Interestingly, porcine/bovine and anglerfish proglucagons seem to contain glucagon in their N-terminal segments, as opposed to the situation in many other prohormones (parathyroid hormone, cholecystokinin, gastrin, and others), in which the secreted form of the hormone is liberated from the C-terminal part of the prohormone.

Regulation of Glucagon Secretion

Falling blood glucose concentrations stimulate the islet A cell to secrete glucagon. Amino acids stimulate the release of glucagon as well as of insulin. Elevated blood free fatty acid concentrations inhibit glucagon secretion in some carnivorous mammals.

Both glucagon and insulin release are augmented by beta- and inhibited by alpha-adrenergic receptor stimulation. However, unlike the situation for insulin secretion, epinephrine and norepinephrine normally stimulate glucagon secretion. Thus it seems likely that the insulin-secreting B cells may

TABLE 9.2. Amino acid sequences of pancreatic glucagons

	Cow, Human, Camel, Hog, Rat, Rabbit	Chicken, Turkey	Duck
1.	His	—[a]	—
2.	Ser	—	—
3.	Gln	—	—
4.	Gly	—	—
5.	Thr	—	—
6.	Phe	—	—
7.	Thr	—	—
8.	Ser	—	—
9.	Asp	—	—
10.	Tyr	—	—
11.	Ser	—	—
12.	Lys	—	—
13.	Tyr	—	—
14.	Leu	—	—
15.	Asp	—	—
16.	Ser	—	Thr
17.	Arg	—	—
18.	Arg	—	—
19.	Ala	—	—
20.	Gln	—	—
21.	Asp	—	—
22.	Phe	—	—
23.	Val	—	—
24.	Gln	—	—
25.	Trp	—	—
26.	Leu	—	—
27.	Met	—	—
28.	Asn	Ser	—
29.	Thr	—	—

[a] —, indicates amino acid residue identical to preceding column.

have predominantly alpha-adrenergic receptors, whereas the A cells seem to have a higher beta-adrenergic receptor population. Acetylcholine augments glucagon as well as insulin secretion.

Actions of Glucagon

Glucagon is only one of several hormones (including catecholamines, cortisol, growth hormone, and others) that cause an elevation of blood glucose concentrations. About one-half of the glucagon that reaches the liver from the pancreas via the hepatic portal vein is degraded there. Thus it is not surprising to find that most of the actions of glucagon are limited to the liver. The hormone is most important during intervals when liver glycogen reserves have been built up from the previous meal and digestion is completed, resulting in a shift from rising to falling blood glucose concentrations. Also, because both insulin and glucagon secretion is stimulated by amino acids, glucagon prevents the hypoglycemia that would otherwise accompany increased insulin secretion after a protein meal.

Glucagon stimulates glycogenolysis in the liver via activation of the phosphorylase enzyme system. Glucagon does not regulate skeletal muscle phosphorylase. Mammalian skeletal muscle cells do not have physiologically important glucagon receptors, and circulating glucagon levels in blood after passing through the liver are very low. Regulation of skeletal muscle glycogen reserves is exerted primarily by circulating epinephrine.

Pharmacologic doses of glucagon affect many tissues. Very high glucagon

TABLE 9.3. Amino acid sequences of some vertebrate somatostatins

	Hog and Pigeon[a]		Catfish[b]	
1.			Asp	
2.			Asn	
3.			Thr	
4.			Val	
5.			Arg	
6.			Ser	
7.			Lys	
8.			Pro	
9.	Ala		Leu	
10.	Gly		Asn	
11.	Cys		—[c]	
12.	Lys		Met	
13.	Asn	S	—	S
14.	Phe		Tyr	
15.	Phe		—	
16.	Trp		—	
17.	Lys		—	
18.	Thr		Ser	
19.	Phe	S	Ser	
20.	Thr		—	S
21.	Ser		Ala	
22.	Cys		—	

[a] Hog hypothalamic somatostatin; pig pancreatic somatostatin.
[b] Catfish (*Ictalurus punctata*) pancreatic somatostatin.
[c] —, indicates amino acid residue identical to preceding column.

concentrations stimulate the heart and stimulate lipolysis. This lipolytic activity may have a physiological significance in birds.

Glucagon interacts with a high-affinity, low-capacity receptor on liver cell plasma membranes. This interaction results in the elevation of cytoplasmic cAMP, which acts as the second messenger for the first messenger, glucagon.

SOMATOSTATIN

The majority of mammalian islet D-cell somatostatin seems to be identical, or nearly so, to hypothalamic somatostatin. Catfish pancreatic somatostatin is larger and exhibits several amino acid substitutions (Table 9.3). However, while these differences in primary structure between mammalian and fish somatostatin reduce the immunoreactivity of the fish peptide as measured with antisera to mammalian somatostatin, the catfish pancreatic somatostatin has full biological activity in reducing growth hormone secretion from rat pituitaries.

Whether the secreted somatostatin acts as a blood-borne hormone or only locally (by diffusion within the islet) is unresolved. Somatostatin inhibits the secretion of both insulin and glucagon in response to all studied stimuli for their release. Under certain conditions, somatostatin is a more effective inhibitor of glucagon than of insulin secretion. Somatostatin may also inhibit PP secretion. At this time, somatostatin is mainly of research interest as a tool for manipulating circulating levels and concentration ratios of insulin and glucagon. For example, a researcher can evaluate the effects of insulin or glucagon alone in an experimental animal by infusing somatostatin to suppress endogenous islet hormone secretion and by infusing insulin or glucagon to evaluate their independent metabolic roles.

PANCREATIC POLYPEPTIDE

The primary structures of the known vertebrate pancreatic polypeptides (PPs) are depicted in Table 9.4. Pancreatic polypeptide was first identified as a contaminant in extracted insulin preparations. It does not seem to have a physiologically important role in controlling blood glucose concentrations. PP has a variety of actions on gastrointestinal functions, including stimulation of basal gastric secretion, inhibition of gastrin-stimulated gastric secretion, relaxation of the gallbladder, and inhibition of exocrine pancreatic secretion of bicarbonate and digestive enzymes. Of these various actions of PP, inhibition of pancreatic secretion has the lowest dose requirement and therefore is the best candidate for a physiological role of PP.

Pancreatic polypeptide is released into the blood after eating a meal. Protein-rich meals are most effective, and their ability to release PP depends

TABLE 9.4. Amino acid sequences of pancreatic polypeptides

	Cow (bPP)	Sheep (oPP)	Hog (pPP)	Human (hPP)	Chicken (aPP)
1.	Ala	—	—	—	Gly
2.	Pro	Ser	Pro	Pro	—
3.	Leu	—	—	—	Ser
4.	Glu	—	—	—	Gln
5.	Pro	—	—	—	—
6.	Gln	—	Val	—	Thr
7.	Tyr	—	—	—	—
8.	Pro	—	—	—	—
9.	Gly	—	—	—	—
10.	Asp	—	—	Asx[b]	Asp
11.	Asp	—	—	Asx	Asp
12.	Ala	—	—	—	—
13.	Thr	—	—	—	Pro
14.	Pro	—	—	—	Val
15.	Glu	—	—	—	—
16.	Gln	—	—	—	Asp
17.	Met	—	—	—	Leu
18.	Ala	—	—	—	Ile
19.	Gln	—	—	—	Arg
20.	Tyr	—	—	—	Phe
21.	Ala	—	—	—	Tyr
22.	Ala	—	—	—	Asp
23.	Glu	—	—	Asp	Asn
24.	Leu	—	—	—	—
25.	Arg	—	—	—	Gln
26.	Arg	—	—	—	Gln
27.	Tyr	—	—	—	—
28.	Ile	—	—	—	Leu
29.	Asn	—	—	—	Asn
30.	Met	—	—	—	Val
31.	Leu	—	—	—	Val
32.	Thr	—	—	—	—
33.	Arg	—	—	—	—
34.	Pro	—	—	—	His
35.	Arg	—	—	—	—
36.	Tyr-NH$_2$	—	—	—	—

[a] —, indicates amino acid residue identical to preceding column.
[b] It is uncertain whether this residue is Asp or Asn.

on a vagal cholinergic reflex. Bombesin also can elicit PP release via a vagal cholinergic reflex. Somatostatin can inhibit PP release.

DIABETES MELLITUS

The most common endocrine disorder in people is diabetes mellitus (sugar diabetes). This disease is characterized by an abnormally high glucose concentration in the blood. The complications of diabetes include heart disease, blindness, cataracts, blood vessel damage, nervous disorders, and kidney damage.

Insufficient secretion of insulin by the pancreatic B cell characterizes the so-called juvenile-onset (insulin-dependent) form of diabetes mellitus. This hypoinsulinemia seems to be associated with hyperglucagonemia. It is easy to understand how this bihormonal or "double-trouble" hypothesis could explain the cause of juvenile-onset diabetes. About 10% of American diabetics suffer from this severe form of the disease. Juvenile-onset diabetics must be treated with exogenous insulin to control their symptoms.

More than 90% of American diabetics suffer from maturity-onset (insulin-resistant) diabetes mellitus. It most often occurs in people who are over 40 years old and overweight. The clinical manifestations of maturity-onset diabetes are often mild, and the high blood glucose concentration can sometimes be controlled by dietary restrictions alone. Interestingly, maturity-onset diabetes is characterized by normal or even excessive blood insulin concentrations. The problem, instead, seems to be a reduced sensitivity of fat and muscle cells to the effects of insulin (insulin resistance).

Recently, intriguing hypotheses have been proposed to explain the insulin-resistant, maturity-onset form of diabetes mellitus. Several groups of researchers have shown that there are reduced numbers of insulin receptors in insulin-resistant tissues. This reduction in the number of insulin receptors, in fact, seems to be caused by abnormally high blood insulin concentrations. The observation that dieting can control maturity-onset diabetes in obese patients seems to be explained by the fact that weight loss decreases blood insulin concentrations, and this in turn causes body tissues to bind increased amounts of insulin. Whether the relationship between blood insulin concentrations and the number of insulin receptors on target cells is the final explanation of maturity-onset diabetes mellitus is not clear yet.

COMPARATIVE STUDIES OF THE ENDOCRINE PANCREAS

There are conspicuous differences among the insulin responses to specific stimuli in mammalian species that produce different end products of digestion. For their supply of carbohydrates, for example, ruminants seem to rely on gluconeogenesis instead of absorbing sugars as such from the gut, as the monogastric species do. Interestingly, propionate, a fatty acid (an important gluconeogenic substrate in ruminants, produced in their gut by microorganisms), is a more potent stimulus for insulin secretion than is glucose in sheep. Propionate does not release insulin in nonruminant mammalian species. Thus, while insulin is an important anabolic hormone in all mammals, the secretory response of the B cell can be adapted to the individual feeding and digestive physiologies of specialized groups, such as ruminants.

Some very interesting results have been obtained recently in comparative studies of the insulin receptor. Insulins from a wide variety of vertebrate species, when tested in mammals, differ in biological potency by as much as 50- to 100-fold. For example, guinea pig insulin is only a few percent as active as hog insulin, whereas chicken and turkey insulins are two to three times more potent than hog insulin when tested in certain mammalian bioassays. Because the intrinsic activities (efficacies) of all insulins, with the possible exception of hagfish insulin, appear to be identical, differences in the potencies of insulins of different species can be attributed entirely to differences in the binding affinity of the insulins for the insulin receptor.

A study of the properties of insulin receptors from several mammals, two birds, an amphibian, and an osteichthyean reveals remarkable similarities among the receptors with respect to pH and temperature optima, negative cooperativity, immunological reactivity, and specificity of hormonal binding. The similarities in specificity of binding of various insulins by the different species was most striking. It was found that the insulin receptors of all species studied had similar absolute affinities as well as the same relative affinity for insulins of different species. In contrast, the insulins of the various species had widely different affinities for the insulin receptor. In other words, the homologous insulin in a given species often bound less well to its own receptor than did insulins of other species. Because the affinity of the insulin receptor is more or less fixed in a given species, animals with insulins of low affinity (and therefore low biological potency), such as the guinea pig, appear to compensate by increasing the concentrations of receptors and circulating insulin, whereas animals with more ''potent'' insulins, such as chickens and turkeys, have relatively lower concentrations of receptors and circulating insulin.

These findings suggest that the insulin receptor is functionally highly conserved, more highly conserved, in fact, than insulin itself. They also strongly suggest that the receptor is a more ancient molecule than the hormone. Perhaps this may help explain the finding that responses to insulin have been observed in invertebrates, protozoa, and even plants!

Hagfish insulin and insulin receptors deserve special mention for several reasons: (1) the hagfish islet organ is the most primitive ''endocrine pancreas'' extant; (2) hagfish insulin exhibits the greatest divergence in amino acid sequence from mammalian insulins; (3) the hagfish insulin receptor is unique in that it does not seem to have the same affinity for homologous insulin as it does for insulins of heterologous species.

In bioassays using mammalian tissues, hagfish insulin has a potency of 5 to 10% of that of porcine insulin, but it can stimulate the same maximal responses at high doses. In some experiments hagfish insulin is also 5 to 10% as potent as porcine insulin in binding to insulin receptors on mammalian cells. However, in other experiments hagfish insulin exhibits about 25% binding potency relative to porcine insulin. If substantiated, this would be the first known discrepancy between insulin receptor binding and biological activity. The possible explanations for the dissociation of these two cellular events in target cell response is unknown, but surely will prove interesting.

The hagfish insulin receptor exhibits the same absolute affinity and rank order of preference for insulins of other species as found in receptors of more advanced vertebrates, thus supporting the conclusion that the insulin receptor is functionally better conserved than the hormone during evolution. However, it is interesting that hagfish insulin bound better to the homologous hagfish insulin receptor (25% as potent as porcine insulin) than it did to mammalian receptors (5 to 10% as potent as porcine insulin).

In separate studies it has been found that blood insulin concentrations in hagfishes are low compared to other fishes and mammals. The hagfishes, then, may represent an exception to the rule that a species with an insulin of low potency when tested in mammals will compensate by having increased circulating insulin concentrations. It seems that hagfishes have compensated for having low blood insulin concentrations by somehow increasing the affinity of their own receptors for insulin, whereas all other vertebrates with relatively low blood insulin concentrations appear to compensate by increasing the number or concentration of insulin receptors on their cells. Detailed comparative studies of the structure and properties of the hagfish insulin receptor versus the insulin receptors of other vertebrate species may reveal the basis for these apparently different adaptive solutions to a common endocrinological problem.

The vigorous defense of blood glucose levels by insulin and glucagon seen in mammals is not observed in many lower vertebrates. In mammals the brain relies on a supply of glucose from the blood as the principal source of metabolic energy. Interruption of this supply even for minutes leads to irreparable damage of central nervous tissue. Many fishes and some amphibians, on the other hand, are able to withstand prolonged intervals when their blood glucose concentrations are zero without deleterious consequences. Furthermore, in many of these species pancreatectomy does not lead to significant derangement of glycemia. Nor does glucose seem to be an important regulator of insulin and glucagon secretion in many of these animals. How can we account for these observations?

In hagfishes, lampreys, and osteichthyeans, the regulation of amino acid metabolism may be the primary functional role of insulin. In these animals insulin shows a profound effect on the level of circulating amino acids, and their B cells show a secretory response to increased levels of amino acids. Furthermore, insulin stimulates the active uptake of amino acids into muscle and their incorporation into proteins.

Chondrichthyeans have received scant attention, but regulation of lipid metabolism is a strong candidate for a physiological function of pancreatic hormones in these fishes. The absence of adipose tissue raises a problem that must be solved in studies of the potential role of the endocrine pancreas in lipid metabolism in chondrichthyeans. It may very well be that these hormones influenced lipid metabolism in the liver or some other site long before they took on the adipocyte as a target cell type.

It has often been stated that pancreatectomy in birds leads to hypoglycemia, as opposed to the hyperglycemia (diabetes mellitus) seen with the same operation in mammals. However, it is extremely difficult to prove that surgical pancreatectomy is complete, especially in birds. Even microscopic remnants of pancreatic tissue can influence the glycemia observed after such intervention. This is a difficult problem in birds, which as a group are characterized by regional differences in islet hormone content within the pancreas. Nevertheless, the pancreatic endocrinology of birds does show several striking features. Avian blood glucose levels depend much more on glucagon than on insulin, in contrast to mammals, and this is reflected also in the ratio of circulating glucagon and insulin. Birds have been found to be relatively insensitive to insulin, tolerating doses many times higher than would be needed in a large mammal to provoke fatal hypoglycemia. Glucagon is a potent lipolytic hormone in birds, and this action appears to be unopposed by insulin, suggesting that the regulation of lipid metabolism may be the most important function of avian glucagon.

Epple has argued that careful interpretation of comparative studies indicates that among the gnathostomes the importance of both insulin and glucagon is greatest in the tetrapods and that the control of blood amino acid levels is an ancient function of insulin, whereas its role in maintaining a constant blood glucose concentration is more recently evolved and best developed in mammals. In lower vertebrates insulin seems to be a more important regulator of intracellular glycogen formation, and its effects on blood glucose originally may have been only a secondary role. The extreme sensitivities of mammalian fat cells to insulin and of avian fat cells to glucagon are specializations that developed rather late in vertebrate evolution. Finally, the role of glucagon in cold-blooded (heterothermic) vertebrates is poorly understood.

There have been very few comparative studies of the functions of pancreatic somatostatin and PP. Mammalian somatostatin has been shown capable of inhibiting insulin release from the hagfish islet organ. Furthermore, extracts of hagfish islet organs contain somatostatinlike substances that cross-react with antisera against mammalian somatostatin. Whether the endogenous hagfish somatostatin has a physiological role in the control of insulin release is unknown. However, the lack of specificity between mammalian and hagfish somatostatins as revealed by these studies suggests that the structure and function of pancreatic somatostatins among vertebrates has been strongly conserved.

Studies of PP in birds reveal some differences in action when compared to mammals. In chickens, avian pancreatic polypeptide (aPP) stimulates gastric juice secretion, including pepsinogen and HCl, as well as total volume. At much higher doses, aPP causes liver glycogen depletion, increased blood uric acid levels, and decreased blood glycerol and free fatty acid levels. Interestingly, aPP does not seem to influence exocrine pancreatic secretion in chickens, in contrast to the findings in mammals. Whether aPP stimulates gastric acid secretion in chickens indirectly, via release of antral gastrin from the gut, remains to be investigated. Ingested protein and secreted acid in the gut seem to stimulate the release of aPP in chickens. Studies of the effects of PPs in other lower-vertebrate species will be of interest in light of these apparently divergent roles of the hormone in birds and mammals.

ADDITIONAL READING

1. Emdin, S. O., S. Gammeltoft, and J. Gliemann (1977). Degradation, receptor binding affinity, and potency of insulin from the Atlantic hagfish (*Myxine glutinosa*) determined in isolated rat fat cells. *J. Biol. Chem.* **252**:602–608.

2. Epple, A., J. E. Brinn, and J. B. Young (1980). Evolution of pancreatic islet functions. In *Evolution of Vertebrate Endocrine Systems* (P. K. T. Pang and A. Epple, eds.), Texas Tech Press, Lubbock, pp. 269–321.

3. Falkmer, S., and S. O. Emdin (1981). Insulin evolution. In *Structural Studies on Molecules of Biological Interest* (G. Dodson, J. P. Glusker, and D. Sayre, eds.). Oxford University Press, London, pp. 420–440.

4. Falkmer, S., J. F. Cutfield, S. M. Cutfield, G. G. Dodson, J. Gliemann, S. Gammeltoft, M. Marques, J. D. Peterson, D. F. Steiner, F. Sundby, S. O. Emdin, N. Havu, Y. Östberg, and L. Winbladh (1975). Comparative endocrinology of insulin and glucagon production. *Am. Zool.* **15**(Suppl. 1):255–270.

5. Grillo, T. A. I., L. Leibson, and A. Epple, eds. (1976). *The Evolution of Pancreatic Islets.* Pergamon, Oxford.

6. Hardisty, M. W. (1979). *Biology of Cyclostomes.* Chapman & Hall, London.

7. Muggeo, M., B. H. Ginsberg, J. Roth, D. M. Neville, P. De Meyts, and C. R. Kahn (1979*a*). The insulin receptor in vertebrates is functionally more conserved during evolution than insulin itself. *Endocrinology* **104**:1393–1402.

8. Muggeo, M., E. Van Obberghen, C. R. Kahn, J. Roth, B. H. Ginsberg, P. De Meyts, S. O. Emdin, and S. Falkmer (1979*b*). The insulin receptor and insulin of the Atlantic hagfish. Extraordinary conservation of binding specificity and negative cooperativity in the most primitive vertebrate. *Diabetes* **28**:175–181.

9. Oyama, H., R. A. Bradshaw, O. J. Bates, and A. Permutt (1980). Amino acid sequence of catfish pancreatic somatostatin. *J. Biol. Chem.* **255**:2251–2254.

10. Shields, D., and G. Blobel (1977). Cell-free synthesis of fish preproinsulin, and processing by heterologous mammalian microsomal membranes. *Proc. Natl. Acad. Sci. USA* **74**:2059–2063.

11. Spiess, J., J. E. Rivier, J. A. Rodkey, C. D. Bennett, and W. Vale (1979). Isolation and characterization of somatostatin from pigeon pancreas. *Proc. Natl. Acad. Sci. USA* **76**:2974–2978.

12. Steiner, D. F., and N. Freinkel, eds. (1972). The Endocrine Pancreas. In *Handbook of*

Physiology, Sect. 7 (R. O. Greep and E. B. Astwood, section eds.). American Physiological Society, Washington, D. C.

13. Steiner, D. F., and H. S. Tager (1979). Biosynthesis of insulin and glucagon. In *Endocrinology* (L. J. DeGroot, G. F. Cahill, Jr., W. D. Odell, L. Martini, J. T. Potts, Jr., D. H. Nelson, E. Steinberger, and A. I. Winegrad, eds.). Grune & Stratton, New York.

14. Stewart, J. K., C. J. Goodner, D. J. Koerker, A. Gorbman, J. Ensinck, and M. Kaufman (1978). Evidence for a biological role of somatostatin in the Pacific hagfish, *Eptatretus stouti. Gen. Comp. Endocrinol.* **36**:408–414.

15. Unger, R. H., and L. Orci (1976). Physiology and pathophysiology of glucagon. *Physiol. Rev.* **56**:778–826.

10

The Adrenal Medulla

The adrenal glands in mammals are compound endocrine glands consisting of an inner medulla and an outer cortex. The adrenal medulla secretes catecholamine hormones, whereas the adrenal cortex secretes steroid hormones (see Chapter 12). The medullary portion differentiates in the embryo from neural crest cells and represents a modified ganglion of the sympathetic division of the autonomic nervous system. The cortical component arises from the lateral mesoderm near the developing gonadal primordia. The adrenal medulla retains an extensive innervation throughout life, whereas the adrenal cortex is poorly innervated, if at all.

The neural crest–derived cells, which comprise the bulk of the adrenal medulla, are homologous not only as to origin, but also in their biochemical properties, to the postganglionic sympathetic nerves that extend to many organs in the body. These endocrine cells, as well as the postganglionic sympathetic nerve cells, are directly innervated by preganglionic sympathetic nerves that utilize acetylcholine as their neurotransmitter. The adrenal medullary cells, under this neural cholinergic regulation, secrete either epinephrine (adrenaline) or norepinephrine (noradrenaline) directly into the blood.

In mammals the adrenal medulla consists of cords and clumps of endocrine cells interspersed with a rich sinusoidal blood supply. Certain chromate compounds stain medullary cells yellow-brown. Thus these cells are often termed *chromaffin cells*. Some cells outside of the adrenals also stain with chromates, including the so-called enterochromaffin cells of the gut epithelium. These enterochromaffin cells contain serotonin (5-hydroxytryptamine)—an indole amine, not a catecholamine. This illustrates the nonspecificity of staining of the chromaffin reaction Nevertheless, "chromaffin tissue" has been used as a synonym for the adrenal medulla by many authors.

The mammalian adrenal medulla is involved in the regulation of carbohydrate metabolism and it serves as a functional adjunct to the sympathetic division of the autonomic nervous system. It is not necessary for life. The mammalian adrenal cortex, on the other hand, is essential for life, mainly because its secretions are involved in the regulation of salt and water metabolism. The functions of the adrenal cortex are detailed in Chapter 12. Both the adrenal medulla and the cortex are important in the physiological adaptation of the organism to certain demands of the environment and to stress.

GROSS COMPARATIVE ANATOMY

The name adrenal implies a close anatomical and embryological relationship with the kidneys (Fig. 10.1). In birds and mammals the adrenals are located

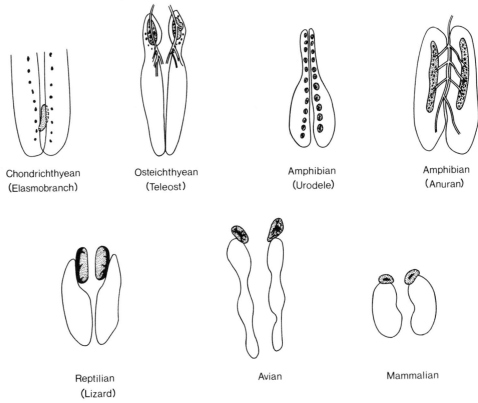

Chondrichthyean
(Elasmobranch)

Osteichthyean
(Teleost)

Amphibian
(Urodele)

Amphibian
(Anuran)

Reptilian
(Lizard)

Avian

Mammalian

FIGURE 10.1. Types of vertebrate adrenals and their association with the kidneys, in ventral view. Solid black indicates catecholaminergic tissue, and stippling indicates corticosteroidogenic tissue. Teleost kidneys show postcardinal venous drainage; anuran kidneys show postcaval venous drainage. Teleost catecholaminergic and corticosteroidogenic tissues are embedded in "head" kidneys. Adrenals are shown as if in section.

bilaterally at the anterior poles of the metanephric kidneys. In osteichthyean fishes the anatomical association is more intimate, and the adrenal tissues are embedded in renal structures. In the chondrichthyeans and some amphibians the adrenal tissues are often found outside the elongated kidney masses and themselves may be elongate structures on the surfaces of the adult (mesonephric) kidneys. In reptiles the adrenals are located anterior to the kidneys, often at some little distance from the adult (metanephric) kidney. The adrenal–renal relationship is not only of morphological significance, but, as will appear later, it is also of physiological significance.

In the typical mammal, as we have seen, the two quite distinct endocrine components are organized into the surrounding external cortex and the internal medulla. Not only in mammals, but in vertebrates generally, many authors refer to "cortical" and "medullary" tissues, even though the cortex–medulla relationship does not exist in nonmammalian forms. As a result, use of the terms *adrenocortical* or *interrenal* for the cortical homologues and of *adrenomedullary* or *chromaffin* for the medullary homologues in lower vertebrates is popular. All of these terms are objectionable for one reason or another; so perhaps it is simplest to use the terms *corticosteroidogenic tissue* and *catecholaminergic tissue* to refer to the homologues of the mammalian adrenal glands in other vertebrates.

In agnathans catecholaminergic cells are associated with the large veins in the peritoneal cavity and are also found in the wall of the heart. Interestingly, these cardiac catecholaminergic cells in lampreys and hagfishes seem to lack innervation. Their control and physiological significance is not known.

In chondrichthyeans clusters of catecholaminergic cells are arranged segmentally along the medial borders of the kidney (Fig. 10.1). This is the only vertebrate group in which the glands are truly "interrenal." In osteichthyeans there are many group and species differences, but, in general, the catecholaminergic cells are associated with the corticosteroidogenic tissue near the kidney veins (Fig. 10.1). In teleosts the corticosteroidogenic and catecholaminergic tissues often are embedded in the anterior poles of the kidneys, the so-called head kidneys. The head kidney, where it exists, is sometimes literally in the head, with strands of tissue projecting even into the foramina of the skull. In many species this structure is not actually a kidney, representing instead a pronephros transformed into a lymphoid organ in the adult.

In amphibians catecholaminergic cells are associated with the mesonephric kidneys. The salamander adrenal tissue generally appears as irregular accumulations on the ventral surfaces of the kidneys, between the kidneys, or embedded in the kidneys (Fig. 10.1). In frogs and toads they form a pair of elongate bodies on or partly surrounded by the ventral surface of the kidneys (Fig. 10.1).

The adrenals in reptiles consist of intermingled corticosteroidogenic and catecholaminergic tissue. In many lizards the bulk of the catecholaminergic

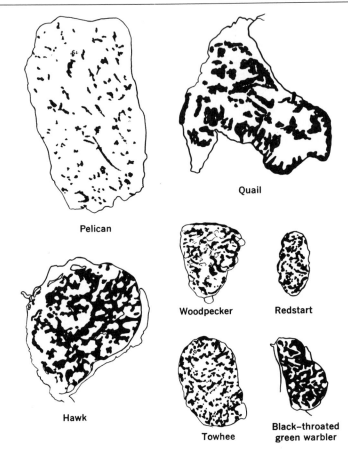

FIGURE 10.2. Drawings of sections through the adrenal glands of seven bird species to show relative amounts of catecholaminergic tissue (black) and corticosteroidogenic tissue (white). In the case of the black-throated green warbler, the corticosteroidogenic tissue appears to be distributed within the catecholaminergic tissue. [From F. A. Hartman and K. A. Brownell, *The Adrenal Gland*, Lea & Febiger, Philadelphia, 1949.]

tissue tends to form a kind of dorsal capsule on the corticosteroidogenic tissue without much interpenetration (Fig. 10.1). Here, any tendency toward a cortex—medulla relation is exactly the opposite from that typically seen in mammals. In crocodilian reptiles catecholaminergic islands are scattered throughout the corticosteroidogenic tissue, much as in birds, suggestive of the relationship between these two groups surviving from the archosaur line.

In birds the adrenals have a location similar to that in mammals—at the anterior poles of the kidneys (Fig. 10.1). The catecholaminergic tissue is completely dispersed in the corticosteroidogenic tissue, although where there is a high ratio of catecholaminergic to corticosteroidogenic tissue (e.g., the green warbler *Dendroica virens*), the converse statement would appear to be more accurate (Fig. 10.2). At any rate, no cortex—medulla type of arrangement is obvious among the birds.

There is, thus, abundant evidence in the lower vertebrates for the interspersion of catecholaminergic and corticosteroidogenic tissues. In most fishes the two tissues remain separate. Many teleosts, however, show complete intermingling. The interspersion of the two components is considerable in most amphibians and reptiles, except for lizards, which have a peripheral concentration of catecholaminergic tissue. In birds interspersion is also the rule. In most mammals the cortex–medulla relationship again represents a division into two separate though contiguous components. However, even in mammals a vascular connection between the corticosteroidogenic and catecholaminergic tissue is retained, which may be of some physiological significance, as we shall see later.

CATECHOLAMINES

Catecholamines are derivatives of catechol (Fig. 10.3), which, in turn, is a derivative of the amino acids phenylalanine and tyrosine. The biosynthetic pathway of the catecholamines is outlined in Fig. 10.4. Adrenal medullary cells differ from central and sympathetic adrenergic nerves in that some medullary cells possess the enzyme phenylethanolamine-N-methyltransferase (PNMT) and can thus synthesize epinephrine. The rate-limiting step in catecholamine biosynthesis is the conversion of tyrosine to dopa (dihydroxyphenylalanine), catalyzed by the enzyme tyrosine hydroxylase. Endproduct feedback inhibition of this enzyme by dopamine and norepinephrine serves as a control mechanism of the synthetic process.

Catecholamines are stored in membrane-bound granules in adrenal medullary cells. The granules contain catecholamines, lipids, ATP, Ca^{2+}, Mg^{2+}, and proteins called chromogranins. The inner surface of the granular membrane also contains dopamine-β-hydroxylase and ATPase. The ATPase is involved in the transport of catecholamines from the cytoplasm into the granule. In fact, the retention of catecholamines inside the granule depends on the continuous activity of this ATPase in the presence of ATP and Mg^{2+}. The drug reserpine inhibits this system and results in catecholamine depletion. In the biosynthesis of epinephrine, norepinephrine leaves the granules, is converted to epinephrine in the cytoplasm by PNMT, and then enters a

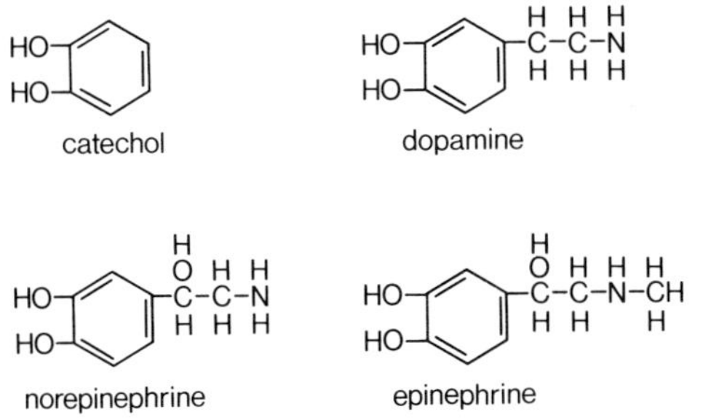

FIGURE 10.3. Structures of catechol and three catecholamines.

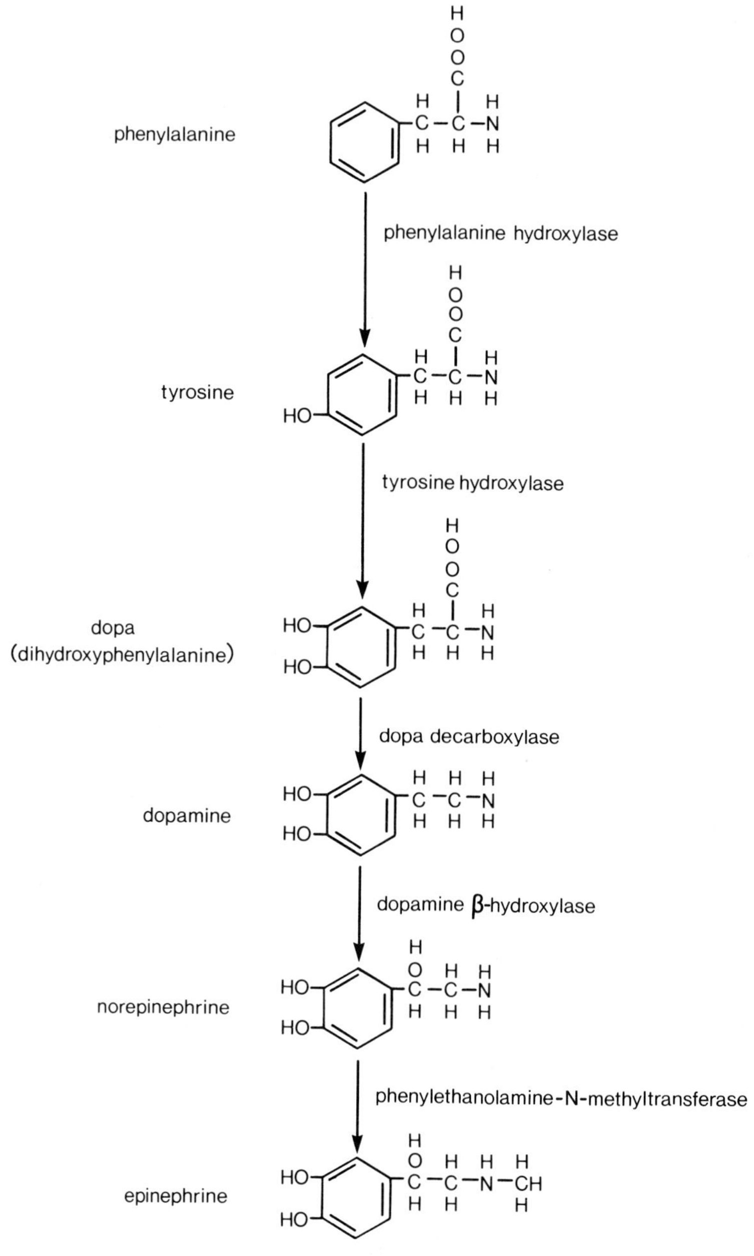

FIGURE 10.4. Biosynthesis of catecholamines. Phenylalanine hydroxylase is found mainly in the liver, and so catecholamine biosynthesis normally begins with tyrosine as the substrate. L-isomers are normally involved, and therefore L-epinephrine and L-norepinephrine are produced. Each of the enzymatic steps requires particular cofactors, which are not shown.

different set of granules where it is stored. Neural stimulation of the adrenal medulla results in catecholamine release by exocytosis.

It has been shown that epinephrine and norepinephrine are stored in two separate adrenal medullary cell types (Fig. 10.5), even though norepinephrine is a biosynthetic precursor of epinephrine. Furthermore, selective release of the two hormones occurs, and the selectivity is related to the nature of the stimulus. However, it is thought that norepinephrine released at postganglionic sympathetic nerve endings is quantitatively much more important than that secreted into the blood by the adrenal medulla in mammals.

Catecholamines are metabolized to physiologically inactive molecules by oxidative deamination and methylation. Of these, methylation is the fate of most of the circulating catecholamines in people. Catechol-O-methyltransferase (COMT), found mostly in the liver and kidneys, catalyzes the methylation of epinephrine and norepinephrine to the inactive metabolites metanephrine and normetanephrine, respectively (Fig. 10.6). COMT is not found in adrenergic nerve endings. Instead, the enzyme monoamine oxidase (MAO) is present in mitochondria in sympathetic nerves. Monoamine oxidase oxidatively deaminates epinephrine and norepinephrine to the inactive metabolite 3,4-dihydroxymandelic acid (VMA; Fig. 10.6). It has been estimated that about 25% of the circulating catecholamines in people are oxidatively deaminated before being methylated and excreted in the urine.

Reliable determinations of the circulating levels of catecholamines have been difficult to achieve both for technical reasons and because the very act of drawing a blood sample can elevate blood catecholamine concentrations above basal. Nevertheless, there is evidence to suggest that the basal

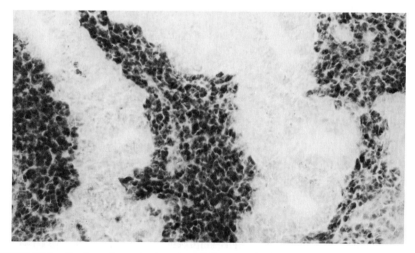

FIGURE 10.5. Region of a cat adrenal medulla treated with postassium iodate. Medullary tissue is homogeneous in appearance by ordinary histological methods; however, iodate stains norepinephrine-containing cells, thus distinguishing them from the nonstaining, epinephrine-containing cells. [From N.-Å. Hillarp, University of Lund.]

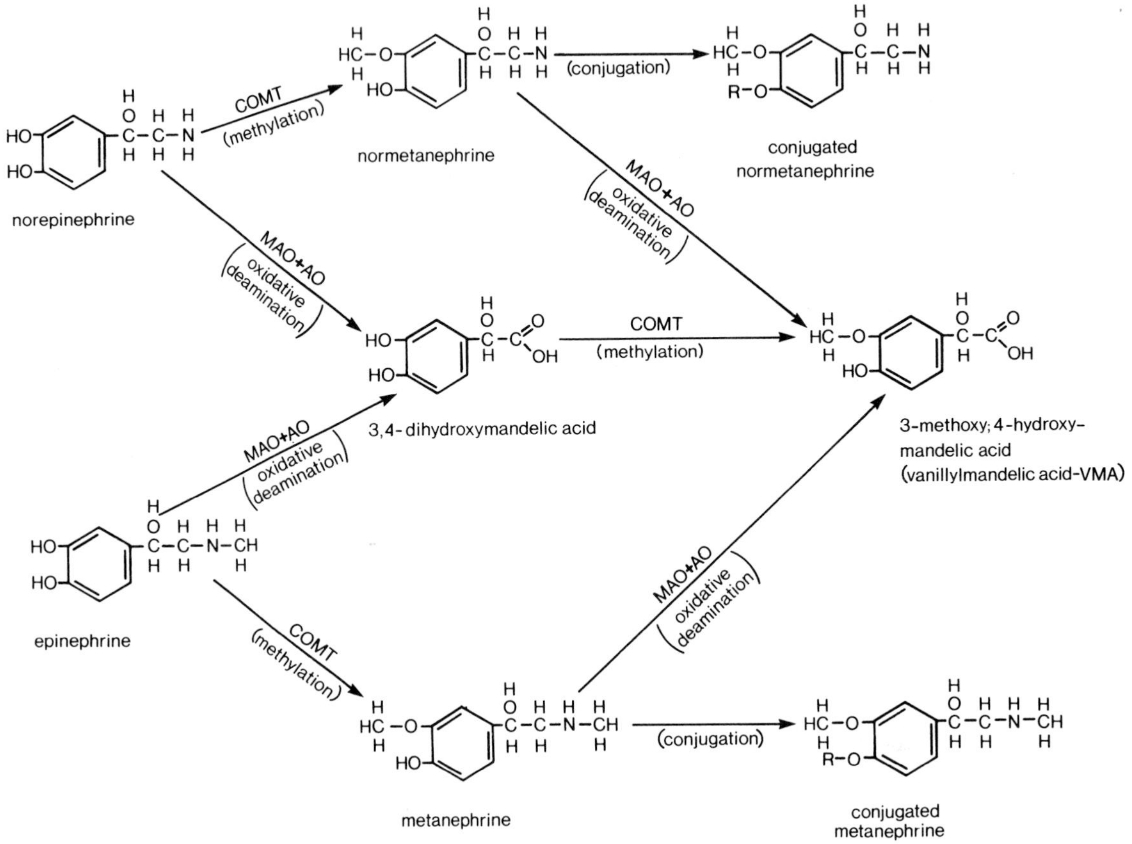

FIGURE 10.6. The major metabolic pathways for epinephrine and norepinephrine. COMT is catechol-*O*-methyltransferase; MAO + AO is monoamine oxidase and aldehyde oxidase. Because metanephrine and normetanephrine have higher affinities for MAO than do epinephrine and norepinephrine, respectively, methylation more efficiently precedes oxidative deamination.

levels of epinephrine and norepinephrine in normal people are about 50 pg (1 pg = 10^{-12}g) and 300 pg per ml of blood plasma, respectively. Circulating catecholamines are removed from the blood very rapidly compared to most other hormones, the half-lives of epinephrine and norepinephrine amounting to only a few minutes in mammals. These short half-lives are functions of the enzymatic conversion of the catecholamines to inactive metabolites and of the uptake and recycling of secreted catecholamines by sympathetic adrenergic nerve endings.

Nearly all of the epinephrine in blood disappears after adrenalectomy in mammals, but the norepinephrine remains about the same. The plasma norepinephrine originates mostly in sympathetic adrenergic nerve endings in almost all parts of the body. Apparently, some norepinephrine of neural origin escapes degradation by COMT and MAO, escapes reuptake by adrenergic nerve terminals, and "overflows" into the systemic circulation.

The adrenal medulla also contributes to circulating norepinephrine, but to a variable degree, depending on a variety of factors. First, there are species differences in the ratio of secreted epinephrine to norepinephrine, even among species in a single vertebrate class (Table 10.1). Second, there are intraspecies differences related to age, sex, and physiological condition. In particular, developmental studies have indicated that during fetal life the catecholamine content of the adrenal glands of people, cattle, rabbits, rats, and guinea pigs consists exclusively of norepinephrine. Epinephrine first appears postnatally and is correlated with increasing adrenal PNMT content and adrenal cortex development. The sympathetic nervous system is not well developed at birth in most mammals. It has therefore been suggested that vascular tone in the fetus and neonate may be under the endocrine control of norepinephrine from the adrenal medulla and that later in life, as epinephrine becomes the predominant adrenal hormone, this function is taken over by the sympathetic nervous system. It has been shown that ACTH and glucocorticoids can enhance PNMT activity in the mammalian adrenal medulla. In a real sense, then, the adrenal medulla may be considered as a target organ for adrenal cortex mediated stress responses.

These considerations suggest that the increasing tendency for the association of corticosteroidogenic and catecholaminergic tissues in vertebrate phylogeny (Fig. 10.1) may be related to a correspondent increasing tendency to secrete epinephrine rather than norepinephrine (Table 10.1). The mammalian adrenal gland, when viewed from this perspective, represents the highest degree of association between the two endocrine tissues in that the blood supply of the adrenal medulla comes directly from the cortex; thus

TABLE 10.1. Percentage of norepinephrine in the adrenal glands of various vertebrates

Group	Norepinephrine (%)
Chondrichthyeans	66–100
Amphibians	40–60
Reptiles	60
Birds	0–80
Mammals	
Whale	83
Ungulates	15–50
Carnivores	27–60
Rodents	2–50
Lagomorphs	0–12
Primates	0–20

the catecholaminergic cells are exposed to the highest concentrations of glucocorticoids of any cells in the body. Whether the involvement of epinephrine in mammals in "fight-or-flight" responses to certain environmental conditions has contributed to the current success enjoyed by this group of animals is certainly worth consideration. This is an attractive hypothesis, but it should not be considered as fully established. The influences of ACTH and glucocorticoids on PNMT activity in lower vertebrates have not been studied extensively.

Adrenergic Receptors

The concept of adrenergic receptors was introduced by Ahlquist in 1948 after an examination of the structure–activity relationships among several sympathomimetic drugs (substances that can mimic the effects of sympathetic nerve stimulation). He classified these receptor sites as either alpha or beta. His basic observations were that all adrenergic receptors were sensitive to epinephrine, norepinephrine, and related chemicals, but that there were quantitative differences in the order of potencies of these substances in their actions on different receptors. Furthermore, certain competitive antagonistic drugs were capable of blocking the actions of catecholamines on alpha receptors or beta receptors, but not on both.

Table 10.2 summarizes some of the properties of alpha, beta, and dopamine receptors. Note that isoproterenol in particular has been useful in experimentally distinguishing adrenergic receptors because, unlike the naturally occurring catecholamines, it is a much more potent beta-adrenergic agonist than it is an alpha-adrenergic agonist. Isoproterenol is not known to be a naturally occurring catecholamine, but it has proven to be very valuable as a pharmacologic tool for understanding adrenergic receptors. Note also that it has recently been possible to differentiate beta receptors into $beta_1$ and $beta_2$ categories, each subtype subject to competitive antagonism by different drugs. Finally, dopamine receptors have been identified in the central nervous system and in the blood vessels of the kidneys; in the latter site they cause vasodilatation when activated.

Physiologically epinephrine can stimulate both $beta_1$ and $beta_2$ receptors; in most cases it is a relatively weak alpha-receptor stimulator compared to norepinephrine. Norepinephrine, on the other hand, is quite potent at both $beta_1$- and alpha-receptor sites; it is much less effective at $beta_2$-adrenergic receptors.

In our discussion of adrenergic receptors, we must clearly recognize the difference between agonists and antagonists. Agonists include the naturally occurring catecholamines epinephrine, norepinephrine, and dopamine, as well as certain synthetic analogues such as isoproterenol. These substances are agonists because, when they interact with adrenergic receptors, they cause a response. That is, adrenergic agonists can elicit a target cell response when acting alone, and this response may be excitatory or inhibitory. Ad-

TABLE 10.2. Classification of adrenergic receptors[a]

Basis of Classification	Receptor Types			
	Alpha	Beta$_1$	Beta$_2$	Dopamine
Potency of agonists	NE $\geq$ E $>$ D $>$ I[b]	I $>$ E $\geq$ NE $>$ D	I $>$ E $\geq$ NE $>$ D	D $\gg$ EN
Selective blockade				
Alpha antagonists (phentolamine, phenoxybenzamine, ergot alkaloids, and others)	Block	No block	No block	No block
Beta antagonists				
General (propranolol, dichloroisoproterenol, and others)	No block	Block	Block	No block
Beta$_1$ type (practolol and others)	No block	Block	Weak block	No block
Beta$_2$ type (butoxamine and others)	No block	Weak block	Block	No block
Dopamine antagonists (haloperidol and others)	No block	No block	No block	Weak block

[a] Adapted from Moran, *Handbook of Physiology*, Vol. 6, Sect. 7 (H. Blaschko, G. Sayers, and A. D. Smith, eds.), American Physiological Society, Washington, D.C., p. 447 (1975).

[b] NE, norepinephrine; E, epinephrine; D, dopamine; EN, epinine; I, isoproterenol.

renergic antagonists, on the other hand, do not occur naturally; they are simply pharmacologic tools. Furthermore, they do not themselves alter target cell responses but only inhibit responses that would occur in the presence of an appropriate agonist. Thus the effects of adrenergic antagonists may also be either stimulatory or inhibitory, depending on the normal response of the adrenergic target cell to an agonist. These concepts are useful in the interpretation of the responses of adrenergic target cells that contain more than one type of adrenergic receptor.

Insulin-secreting B cells in the mammalian endocrine pancreas have both alpha- and beta-adrenergic receptors. Normally, alpha receptors predominate, and the overall physiological response observed after catecholamine stimulation is an inhibition of insulin release. However, if alpha receptors are experimentally blocked by administration of an alpha-adrenergic antagonist such as phentolamine, catecholamine stimulation leads to enhanced insulin release because of activation of the minor population of beta-adrenergic receptors, which are "unmasked" by the pharmacologic manipulation. By contrast, glucagon-secreting A cells of the mammalian endocrine pancreas have an excess of beta- over alpha-adrenergic receptors, and the normal response to catecholamines is stimulation of glucagon release. Another example of opposite responses mediated by alpha- and beta-adrenergic receptors on single cells is the skin melanophore response in some amphibians and reptiles. These examples and other responses known to be mediated by adrenergic receptors are listed in Table 10.3.

Adrenergic receptors are located in the cell membranes of target cells. The activation of both types of beta-adrenergic receptors is associated with increased intracellular production of cAMP via increased adenylate cyclase activity. Not all beta responses have been studied yet, so that it is premature to conclude that all beta-adrenergic responses are mediated by cAMP as the second messenger. Of course, glucagon acts on liver cells to increase their content of cAMP and produces metabolic effects similar to those of catecholamines. Glucagon also activates adenylate cyclase, but not via beta-adrenergic receptors.

Alpha-adrenergic receptors are not associated with the activation of adenylate cyclase. In fact, a large body of experimental evidence suggests that alpha-receptor activation is associated with decreased production of cAMP.

As with the beta-adrenergic receptors, dopamine receptors in the brain appear to be coupled to adenylate cyclase. Dopaminergic agonists promote the accumulation of cAMP in membrane preparations derived from dopamine-sensitive brain regions.

When catecholamine-sensitive target cells containing beta-adrenergic receptors are exposed to beta agonists for several hours either *in vivo* or *in vitro*, there is a selective desensitization, or "down regulation," of the membrane-bound adenylate cyclase to the stimulatory effects of catecholamines. It appears that catecholamines can regulate their own receptors in much the same manner as has been observed for other hormone–receptor interactions,

TABLE 10.3. Classification of adrenergic receptor-mediated responses[a]

Tissue and Action[b]	Receptor Type
Heart	
Increased contractility	$Beta_1$
Increased pacemaker frequency	$Beta_1$
Increased conduction velocity	Beta[c]
Blood vessels	
Arteriolar constriction	Alpha
Arteriolar dilatation	$Beta_2$ in skeletal muscle and perhaps in heart; dopamine in kidney
Venoconstriction	Alpha
Bronchioles	
Dilatation	$Beta_2$
Gastrointestinal tract	
Decreased motility	Alpha at intramural ganglia; $beta_1$ in smooth muscle
Contraction (sphincters)	Alpha and beta[c]
Uterus	
Relaxation	$Beta_2$, influenced by estrous state and pregnancy
Contraction	Alpha
Spleen	
Contraction	Alpha
Relaxation	Beta[c]
Nictitating membrane	
Contraction	Alpha
Relaxation	Beta[c]
Iris	
Radial muscle contraction	Alpha
Skin	
Erector piliae contraction	Alpha
Melanosome dispersion (darkening), amphibians and reptiles	Beta[c]
Melanosome aggregation (lightening), amphibians and reptiles	Alpha
Secretion of skin glands, amphibians	Alpha
Exocrine glands	
Salivary amylase secretion	Beta[c]
Sweat	Alpha
Inhibition of milk ejection	Beta (?)
Skeletal muscle	
Fast muscle, augmented contraction	Beta[c]
Slow muscle, decreased contraction	Beta[c]
Extraocular, induced contraction	Alpha
Neuromuscular transmission, enhanced	Alpha

TABLE 10.3. *(Continued)*

Tissue and Action[b]	Receptor Type
Central nervous system	
Consummatory behavior	
Thirst	Beta[c]
Water satiety	Alpha
Hunger	Alpha
Satiety	Beta[c]
Metabolism	
Hepatic glycogenolysis	$Beta_2$
Lipolysis	$Beta_1$, plus alpha in some species
Calorigenesis	Beta[c]
Endocrine pancreas	
Insulin secretion inhibition (predominates)	Alpha
Insulin secretion stimulation	Beta[c]
Glucagon secretion inhibition	Alpha
Glucagon secretion stimulation (predominates)	Beta[c]

[a] Adapted from Moran, *Handbook of Physiology*, Vol. 6, Sect. 7 (H. Blaschko, G. Sayers, and A. D. Smith, eds.). American Physiological Society, Washington, D.C., p. 447 (1975).
[b] Actions are in mammals unless noted otherwise.
[c] Differentiation into $beta_1$ or $beta_2$ has not yet been accomplished.

such as for insulin (see Chapter 9) and endogenous opiates. It may be that such desensitization represents a mechanism to protect sensitive target tissues from chronically elevated levels of hormones. These responses may be of clinical significance as well, because down regulation may limit the therapeutic effectiveness of administered drugs and hormones.

Down regulation of beta-adrenergic receptors has been shown to be accompanied by a decrease in the number of beta-type binding sites per cell without a change in the binding properties of individual binding sites. Interestingly, beta-adrenergic antagonists, such as propranolol, do not induce down-regulation. However, they block the ability of agonists to do so. These observations suggest that chronic beta-receptor occupancy by agonists leads to changes (conformational or other) in the beta-adrenergic receptors that in some way inactivate a portion of the receptor population. Whether these receptors are lost from the cell membrane or in some way inactivated *in situ* is not known. However, it is thought that chronic receptor occupancy by an agonist, rather than an active process of receptor loss, is responsible for the decreased receptor number. Down regulation of catecholamine receptors is reversible, though the mechanism by which this happens is unknown.

The results of some studies suggest that alpha- and beta-adrenergic receptors are interconvertible and may represent allosteric conformations of the same structure. Changing the temperature of frog hearts changes the properties of adrenergic receptors mediating inotropic (strength of contraction) responses to catecholamines. The characteristics of these receptors change from beta to alpha when the temperature of the isolated hearts is reduced. Simple temperature-dependent ''unmasking'' of separate alpha- and beta-receptor pools was ruled out in these studies. As another example, hypothyroidism can induce in frog hearts the appearance of alpha-adrenergic receptors, which are absent or unreactive in euthyroid animals. Finally, it has been shown that stimulation of alpha receptors in rat kidney membranes causes a specific decrease in the affinity of beta receptors for agonists. Clearly, more research is needed to sort out the relationships and interactions among the various kinds of receptors for catecholamines.

Catecholamine Actions

Table 10.3 lists some of the actions of catecholamines and the specific adrenergic receptors mediating these actions. The so-called sympathoadrenal system is both a nervous system, releasing norepinephrine as a neurotransmitter in mammals, and an endocrine system, releasing epinephrine and norepinephrine as hormones. Therefore, one must consider the effects of neurotransmitters as well as blood-borne mediators in assessing the adrenergic responses of an organism to such perturbations of homeostasis as exercise, anxiety, fear, anger, and other forms of stress.

Epinephrine is a potent activator of $beta_1$ and $beta_2$ receptors, and a moderate activator of alpha receptors. In contrast, norepinephrine is a more selective activator of alpha and $beta_1$ receptors than of $beta_2$ receptors. These observations provide clues to the relative importance of hormonal versus neural control of the adrenergic responses listed in Table 10.3. In most mammals epinephrine is the primary adrenal medullary hormone and is more able to elicit a generalized response than is norepinephrine; that is, epinephrine is capable of activating all adrenergic receptors that are accessible from the bloodstream. Norepinephrine, on the other hand, is mainly a neurotransmitter whose influence is restricted to alpha and $beta_1$ receptors.

An increase in blood epinephrine concentration sets in motion a large number of physiological mechanisms required to sustain vigorous physical activity. Epinephrine causes hyperglycemia by several mechanisms, including stimulation of hepatic glycogenolysis, stimulation of hepatic gluconeogenesis from lactate produced in skeletal muscle, inhibition of insulin release, stimulation of glucagon release, and stimulation of ACTH release (and, consequently, of glucocorticoids by the adrenal cortex). Glucocorticoids further accelerate hepatic gluconeogenesis. The effects of epinephrine-stimulate glucocorticoids are not as rapid as the other hyperglycemic actions of epinephrine.

Epinephrine increases cardiac output and elicits a redistribution of the blood supply. Blood vessels in parts of the body not involved in muscular activity, such as in the skin and gut, are constricted, thus decreasing blood flow to these areas. Blood vessels in skeletal muscles are dilated (probably indirectly, by stimulatory action on the skeletal muscles themselves, resulting in a local hyperemic reflex). Direct actions of epinephrine on skeletal muscle include facilitation of neuromuscular transmission and augmentation of contractile processes in white (fast) muscle fibers.

Epinephrine also stimulates pulmonary ventilation, mainly by dilatation of bronchioles. In addition to diverting blood away from the gut, epinephrine directly inhibits gut motility. Physiological levels of epinephrine also mediate many other adjustments made in preparation for physical activity, including reduction of urine formation, accelerated blood coagulation, spleen contraction, increased sweating, and piloerection.

It was first pointed out many years ago by Cannon that adrenal medullary secretions can be considered as hormones leading to fight-or-flight emergency responses. These responses to short-term stress are distinguishable from the response to chronic stress associated with glucocorticoids and the general adaptation syndrome described by Selye (see Chapter 12). However, the emergency reaction of Cannon can be considered as being closely related to the alarm reaction of the Selye hypothesis, and we have seen how epinephrine can directly affect ACTH secretion.

The usefulness of epinephrine in preparing mammals for physical responses to emergency situations is undeniable, but the hormone is important in responses to other forms of stress as well. In addition to fear, emotional stress, such as anxiety and apprehension, and physical stresses threatening homeostasis, such as hypoxia, hypotension, hypoglycemia, and cold, also are effective activators of adrenal medullary hormone secretion in mammals.

Exercise can be thought of as a form of physiological stress, and so it is not surprising that physical activity itself leads to adrenal medullary hormone secretion. All of the adjustments brought about by epinephrine in emergency situations also occur in response to exercise and have been shown to be mediated by catecholamines.

Comparative Studies of Catecholamines

The comparative anatomy and the relative amounts of catecholamines in vertebrate catecholaminergic tissue were discussed earlier in this chapter. Burnstock has pointed out that circulating catecholamines, released from diffusely distributed catecholaminergic cells, appear to play a much more significant role in lower than in higher vertebrates, in which direct nervous control has been developed to a more extensive degree. This concept has been supported by the demonstration that the total concentration of catecholamines in the plasma of a chondrichthyean, the dogfish shark (a species that lacks direct sympathetic innervation of catecholamine target tissues), is 40 to 50 times greater than in the plasma of people.

There is only fragmentary information available regarding the physiological actions of catecholamines in lower vertebrates. However, it seems clear that the cardiac-stimulating and hyperglycemic actions of catecholamines are almost universally distributed in vertebrates.

There are intriguing differences in the responses to administered epinephrine versus norepinephrine in particular species. For example, when injected in dogfish sharks, epinephrine and norepinephrine have opposite effects on cardiac stroke volume; the former causes an increase, whereas the latter causes a reduction. It is not clear whether these are direct effects of the catecholamines or whether one or both responses are results of reflex adjustments in peripheral vasomotor tone.

Catecholamines elicit hyperglycemia in representatives of all vertebrate groups. Here again, however, interesting departures from the typical mammalian situation are evident. Epinephrine produces hyperglycemia in two chondrichthyeans, the dogfish shark and the ratfish. Norepinephrine has no effect on blood glucose in dogfish sharks but is hypoglycemic in ratfishes. To further complicate the picture, norepinephrine has been shown to be a potent hyperglycemic agent in skates—about twice as potent as epinephrine. It would seem that the interpretation of these perplexing species differences among the chondrichthyeans might be facilitated by investigations of the types of adrenergic receptors mediating these responses.

In osteichthyeans generally, epinephrine seems to be a more potent hyperglycemic and glycogenolytic agent than norepinephrine. Also, epinephrine has been clearly demonstrated to stimulate gluconeogenesis in carp.

The general patterns of action of the catecholamines in the tetrapods (amphibia, reptiles, birds, and mammals) seem to be similar. In the cold-blooded vertebrates, however, it may be that catecholamines rather than glucocorticoids are the primary regulators of hepatic gluconeogenesis.

Some comparative information is beginning to appear regarding the properties of adrenergic receptors in vertebrates. The order of potencies of agonists, the susceptibility to antagonists, and the stereospecificity of the beta-adrenergic receptors in frog and turkey erythrocytes and in human lymphocytes appear to be very similar. It may be that adrenergic receptors, like the catecholamines themselves, appeared early in vertebrate evolution and have not changed much since that time.

Exercise and stress have been shown to be effective in causing an increase in circulating catecholamines in rainbow trout and dogfish sharks. Taken together, it appears that catecholamines, adrenergic receptors, and the physiological responses of catecholamine target tissues evolved early and have persisted relatively unchanged throughout vertebrate phylogeny. Perhaps this endocrine system was first concerned with tonic influences on cardiovascular and metabolic systems under resting conditions as well as with acute responses to stressful conditions. Later in vertebrate evolution, sympathetic nerves took over most of the tonic control of these systems, freeing the adrenal medulla to become more specialized in its involvement in responses to acute stressful situations in higher vertebrates. Much more comparative research must be accomplished before these ideas can be considered as anything more than pure speculation.

ADDITIONAL READING

1. Ahlquist, R. P. (1948). A study of the adrenotropic receptors. *Am. J. Physiol.* **153**:586–600.

2. Burnstock, G. (1969). Evolution of the autonomic innervation of visceral and cardiovascular systems in vertebrates. *Pharmacol. Rev.* **21**:247–324.

3. Butler, P. J., E. W. Taylor, M. F. Capra, and W. Davison (1978). The effect of hypoxia on the levels of circulating catecholamines in the dogfish *Scyliorhinus canicula. J. Comp. Physiol.* **127**:325–330.

4. Kunos, G., M. S. Yong, and M. Nickerson (1973). Transformation of adrenergic receptors in the myocardium. *Nature New Biol.* **241**:119–120.

5. Lefkowitz, R. J. (1976). β-Adrenergic receptors: recognition and regulation. *New Engl. J. Med.* **295**:323–328.

6. Moran, N. C. (1975). Adrenergic receptors. In *Handbook of Physiology*, Vol. 6, Sect. 7, (H. Blaschko, G. Sayers, and A. D. Smith, eds.), American Physiological Society, Washington, D. C., pp. 447–472.

7. Patent, G. J. (1970). Comparison of some hormonal effects on carbohydrate metabolism in an elasmobranch (*Squalus acanthias*) and a holocephalan (*Hydrolagus colliei*). *Gen. Comp. Endocrinol.* **14**:215–242.

11

Steroid Hormones
and Steroidogenesis

Steroid hormones are members of a group of closely related lipid compounds that are secreted by several endocrine organs. The major steroidogenic endocrine glands of vertebrates are the interrenal glands (adrenal cortex of mammals), the gonads (testis in the male and ovary in the female), and the placenta of mammals. The steroid hormones of these glands are essential for the continued existence of the individual (adrenocortical steroids) and of the species (gonadal steroids). Steroids have a wide variety of effects on the organism, including morphogenic, metabolic, and behavioral effects.

Since the functions of various steroids overlap, depending on their structural relatedness, and since so many different naturally occurring steroids have been identified, this chapter is devoted to some of their general chemical and biological features. Adrenocorticosteroids are dealt with in Chapter 12; gonadal steroids are covered in Chapter 13.

OCCURRENCE OF STEROIDS

Steroids consist of a tetracyclic nucleus (Fig. 11.1), which is named cyclopentanoperhydrophenanthrene. The rings are labelled A, B, C, and D, as shown in Figure 11.1b. The phenanthrene portion of the nucleus is comprised of rings A, B, and C, while ring D is the cyclopentane portion. *Perhydro* refers to the fact that this hypothetical parent molecule (gonane or sterane) is not an aromatic compound, but is completely saturated. All the individual carbon and hydrogen atoms usually are not shown in the symbolic representation of steroid compounds (Fig. 11.1b).

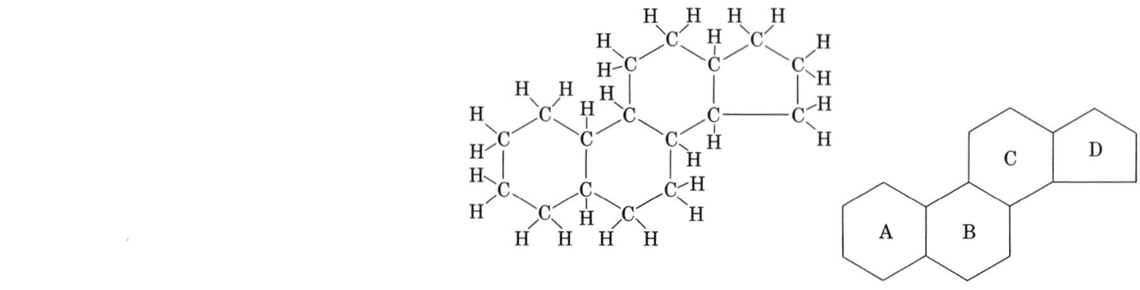

FIGURE 11.1. Complete structural formula (*a*) and symbol (*b*) of the steroid nucleus. The rings of the steroid nucleus are referred to individually by the letters indicated in *b*.

Steroid compounds with this nucleus are ubiquitous in living organisms. In addition to vertebrate and invertebrate animals, steroids have been identified in bacteria, blue-green algae, fungi, molds, and higher plants. Not only is it remarkable that mammalian-type adrenocortical and gonadal steroids can be found in these other organisms, but the steroid biosynthetic mechanisms are similar throughout the biosphere. Sandor and colleagues have proposed that both the types of steroids produced and their synthetic pathways have changed little during the evolution of life. They further hypothesize that the first cyclopentanoperhydrophenanthrene nucleus was synthesized abiotically and that the steroids were later adapted as bioregulators. Regardless of the exact mechanism of evolution, the presence of mammalian-type steroids in diverse organisms suggests that it was not so much the hormones themselves that evolved, but rather the steroid hormone receptors developed adaptively in vertebrate target tissues.

Hundreds of naturally occurring steroids have been identified in extracts of living matter, although many of these compounds are metabolites with little or no biological activity. We can add to this list hundreds of steroid compounds synthesized in the organic chemical laboratory and not identified in nature. Some synthetic steroids exhibit profound biological or pharmacologic activity and are useful in the treatment of disease or in the control of physiological processes (e.g., birth control pills). A complete survey of all the steroids and their synthetic pathways is beyond the scope of this chapter.

Steroid hormones are responsible for a multitude of important effects in vertebrates. The variety of these effects defies simple schemes for their classification. However, a general classification of the physiological and pharmacologic activities of steroids in humans and other mammals has emerged. The two major groups, adrenocortical and gonadal steroids, are so named because of their principal organ source. Adrenocorticoids are further grouped into glucocorticoids and mineralocorticoids; gonadal steroids consist of androgens, estrogens, and progestogens. Glucocorticoid activity is the ability to facilitate the formation of carbohydrates from noncarbohydrate sources (gluconeogenesis from protein and fat). Typical glucocorticoids are cortisol, corticosterone, and cortisone. Mineralocorticoids are defined by their ability to affect water and electrolyte metabolism (favoring retention of Na^+ and excretion of K^+). Androgens are steroids with the ability (typified by the male hormone from the testis) to stimulate male characteristics and maintain male sex accessory glands and ducts. Examples of androgens are testosterone, 5α-dihydrotestosterone, and androstenedione. Estrogens have the ability (typified by the primary female steroids secreted by the ovarian follicle) to stimulate female secondary sex characteristics and to help maintain the female reproductive tract. Estrone, estradiol, and estriol are among the estrogens. Progestogens have the ability (typified by hormones of the corpus luteum of the ovary) to stimulate the uterus and maintain uterine development during pregnancy. These steroids include progesterone and 17α-hydroxyprogesterone.

By no means should it be understood that these are the only actions of steroids in vertebrates. This classification has remained in general usage because of its convenience rather than its precision. It is convenient to be able to designate a class of steroids as having a principal activity without referring to the names of specific compounds. For example, one might make the statement that "glucocorticoids are immunosuppressants." This would be understood to mean that cortisol, corticosterone, cortisone, and some other compounds suppress the immune system.

A number of examples could be listed to point out the limits of this classification scheme. Many steroids have no significant biological activity; they may be present as intermediate structures or steroid hormone metabolites. The scheme does not consider relative biological potencies of the different steroids within a group. Furthermore, there may be significant overlap of function. For example, aldosterone is usually classified as a mineralocorticoid, but it is a potent glucocorticoid in some animals. The functional overlap of these steroid groups is particularly apparent in nonmammalian vertebrates. Glucocorticoids stimulate aspects of female reproduction in bony fishes. Clearly the usefulness of this classification scheme is limited to some mammalian species. Thus this scheme may be appropriate only for mammalian and clinical endocrinology.

STRUCTURE AND NOMENCLATURE OF STEROIDS

The basic nucleus of steroids has seventeen carbon atoms numbered as indicated in Fig. 11.2a. This nucleus has six asymmetric carbon atoms located where the rings are joined: carbon atoms 5 and 10 link rings A and B, carbon atoms 8 and 9 link rings B and C, and carbon atoms 13 and 14 link rings C and D. Each asymmetric carbon atom has one hydrogen atom that can be attached in one of two possible positions relative to the rest of the molecule. The nucleus can be visualized as a relatively flat structure lying in the plane of the page; a hydrogen atom attached to an asymmetric carbon can project out of the plane either toward or away from the observer. If the hydrogen projects toward the observer, it is said to be in the cis or β position. A hydrogen that projects away from the observer is in the trans or α position. The positions of the hydrogens on asymmetric carbons of naturally occurring steroids are shown in Fig. 11.2b, where a solid line indicates the β position and a broken line the α position. In this example, attachment of the hydrogen to carbon 5 by a wavy line indicates that it may be in either the α or β position in different series of steroids (stereoisomers). The position of the hydrogen on carbon 5 has a profound effect on the shape of the molecule; the nucleus is flatter when this hydrogen is in the α position (Fig. 11.3). This may have significant consequences for its interaction with carrier proteins and receptors.

Additional carbons can be attached to the 17-carbon (or C_{17}) nucleus to form other classes of steroid compounds (Fig. 11.4). When a methyl group is attached to carbon 13 (in the β position), a new, C_{18} compound, known as *estrane*, is formed. If a second methyl group is added to carbon 10, again in the β position, a C_{19} compound with the parent name *androstane* is formed. The methyl groups on carbons 10 and 13 are usually depicted as straight lines (Fig. 11.2c). The final parent compound we will consider—*pregnane*—is formed by the addition of an ethyl group (in the β position) to carbon 17. In this series of C_{21} compounds, the carbon nearest the D ring is carbon 20, while the further carbon is carbon 21 (Fig. 11.2c). Note that this addition of an ethyl group makes carbon 17 asymmetric.

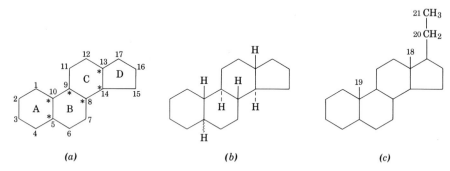

(a)   (b)   (c)

FIGURE 11.2. Numbering system and position of hydrogen atoms on asymmetric carbons in steroid compounds. (*a*) Numbering of carbon atoms in the steroid nucleus and hypothetical steroid parent compound (gonane or sterane), a 17-carbon cyclic hydrocarbon. Asterisks indicate the six asymmetric carbon atoms. (*b*) Position of hydrogen atoms on the asymmetric carbon atoms. The hydrogens on carbons 8, 10, and 13 are in the cis or β position (placed on the side of the molecule nearer the observer), and the hydrogens on carbons 9 and 14 are in the trans or α position (placed on the side of the molecule away from the observer). The hydrogen on carbon 5 may be either α or β, depending upon the steroid (see Fig. 11.3). (*c*) The numbers given the carbon atoms of the methyl groups attached to carbons 10 and 13 and of the ethyl group attached to carbon 17.

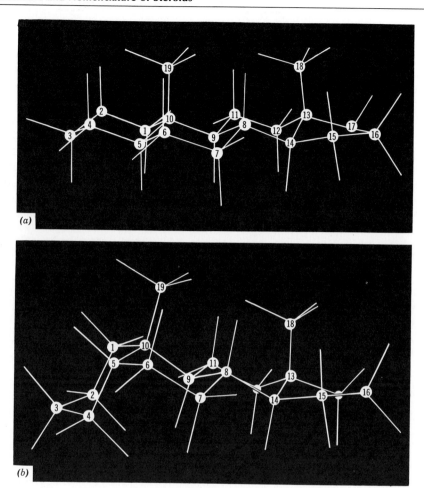

FIGURE 11.3. Models of two stereoisomers of the androstane molecule. The numbered spheres represent the carbon atoms; note the two methyl groups attached to carbons 10 and 13. Change of the position of the H atom attached to carbon 5 from the side opposite the 10-methyl (*a*) to the same side (*b*) changes the shape of most of the molecule. In the upper compound, 5α-androstane, the H on carbon 5 is in the trans position; in the lower compound, 5β-androstane, it is in the cis position. [From L. F. Fieser and M. Fieser, *Steroids*, Reinhold, New York, 1959.]

Additional modification of the C_{18}, C_{19}, and C_{21} compounds is achieved through the attachment of functional groups (hydroxyl, carbonyl, etc.) to various carbon atoms. As in the case of the hydrogen on carbon 5, functional groups may be in the α or β position to form stereoisomers. Considering all the possible attachments of functional groups and stereoisomers, millions of different steroid compounds of the three classes are possible. However, only a small fraction of the theoretically possible steroids occur in vertebrates. In general, naturally occurring vertebrate steroid hormones may

sterane (gonane) 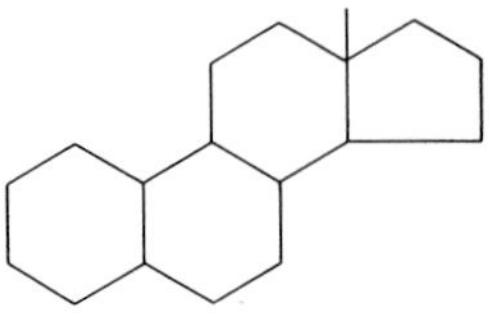   estrane

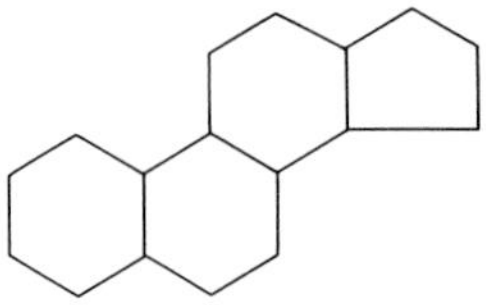

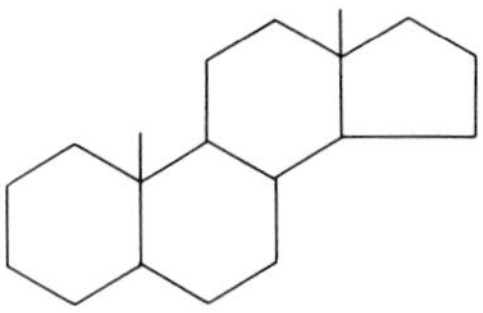

androstane 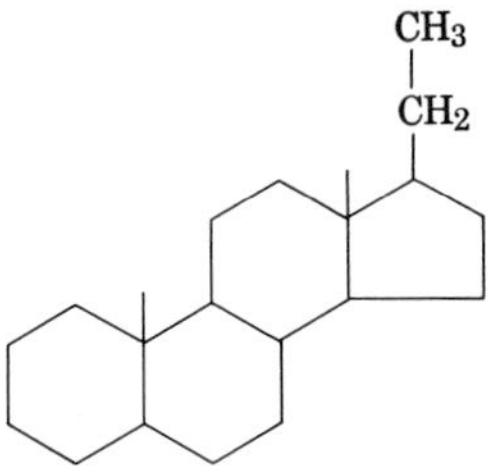   pregnane

FIGURE 11.4. Structures of the hypothetical steroid hydrocarbons upon which the nomenclature is based. Gonane is the steroid nucleus. Estrane has a methyl group on carbon 13 and is a C_{18} steroid; androstane has an additional methyl group on carbon 10 and is a C_{19} steroid.

have functional groups attached to carbon 18 of the methyl group; carbons 20 and 21 of the ethyl group; and carbons 1, 3, 11, 16, and 17 of the nucleus.

Another means of modifying steroids is by removal of hydrogen atoms to form double bonds between carbon atoms. Although a large number of theoretical compounds can be created in this manner, unsaturation of vertebrate steroids occurs primarily only in rings A and B. Frequently, vertebrate steroids have a double bond between carbons 4 and 5 or carbons 5 and 6. Most naturally occurring C_{18} compounds have three double bonds (complete unsaturation) in the A ring.

It is not entirely clear why the identified vertebrate steroid hormones usually have functional groups attached only to certain carbon atoms and often have double bonds in only the A and B rings. There must be some selective pressure against forming or retaining other possible steroid compounds. On the other hand, structures of steroids are known only for a very small fraction of the extant vertebrate species. Certainly, investigation of additional species will reveal novel steroid structures. Understanding the evolution of steroid compounds is difficult, since single-point mutations in the genetic code are not necessarily translated into different forms of steroid hormones, as is the case for peptide hormones. Mutations may modify the structure of the enzymes involved in steroid synthesis without seriously affecting enzyme function. Presumably, many mutations must occur to modify an enzyme so that it will produce a new steroid. One may speculate further that the particular requirements of steroid hormone receptors have restricted the types of steroid compounds that are functional hormones. Only the useful steroids are retained. Whatever the reason for these trends in the location of functional groups and unsaturation, the structural trends of naturally occurring vertebrate steroids are helpful organizing principles for the student to keep in mind.

Rules of Steroid Nomenclature

Modern steroid nomenclature has strict rules to which workers in the field try to adhere, with varying success. Biologists should understand these rules and be able to visualize the structure of a steroid from its accurate scientific name. Fortunately, since the systematic names are usually long, certain trivial names for commonly occurring steroid hormones, such as estrone, testosterone, cortisone, and progesterone, are accepted in the literature and denote only one compound. The rules referred to in this chapter are based on the recommendations of the International Union of Pure and Applied Chemistry and the International Union of Biochemistry. Some confusion exists, especially in the older literature, since other schemes of nomenclature have been used in the past.

The hypothetical parent compounds upon which steroid nomenclature is based are given in Fig. 11.4. Removal of hydrogens to form double bonds (unsaturation) is indicated by changing the ending of the parent compound name. Replacement of hydrogens with other groups is indicated by suffixes and prefixes. The number of the carbon that was modified and the position (α or β) of the modification, if applicable, is also indicated. The commonly used groups with their prefixes, suffixes, and order of suffix preference are indicated in Table 11.1.

If the compound has no double bonds (completely saturated), the parent compound name ends with *-an(e)*. Removal of a hydrogen to form a double bond is indicated by changing the ending of the parent name to *-en(e)*. Two double bonds change the ending to *-dien(e)*, and three make it *-trien(e)*. The location of the double bond is indicated by giving the number where the bond starts before the name of the parent compound. Thus a double bond between carbons 4 and 5 of the parent compound pregnane would be identified as *4-pregnene*. If the double bond is between nonconsecutively numbered carbons, the second carbon is indicated in parentheses after the first— e.g., *5(10)-pregnene* for a double bond between carbons 5 and 10. When multiple double bonds occur, their locations are indicated starting with the lowest number. Thus double bonds between carbons 1 and 2, 3 and 4, and

TABLE 11.1. Some symbols used in indicating modifications of parent steroids

Group	Prefix	Suffix	Suffix Preference
Double bond (C=C)		-en (e)	
Carboxylic acid (COOH)	Carboxy-	-oic acid	1
Ester (OCOR)	Acetoxy-	-yl acetate	2
Aldehyde (CHO)		-al	3
Carbonyl (C=O)	Oxo-	-one	4
Hydroxyl (OH)	Hydroxy-	-ol	5
Chloro (or other halogen)	Chloro- (etc.)		

5 and 10 (complete unsaturation of the A ring) of estrane would be identified as *1,3,5(10)-estratriene* (Fig. 11.5*b*).

The stereochemistry of the asymmetric carbon 5 is indicated after the carbon number and before the family name; *5α-androstane* indicates that the hydrogen on carbon 5 is in the α position. When both double bonds and stereochemistry must be identified, the ending of the parent name becomes a suffix showing the location of unsaturation. Thus androstane with the hydrogen on carbon 5 in the β position and a double bond between carbons 16 and 17 would be named *5β-androst-16-ene*. Many of the natural steroids have a double bond between carbons 4 and 5, or 5 and 6, or 5 and 10. This eliminates the hydrogen on carbon 5, so the steric difference between 5α and 5β need not be considered.

A single-group attachment is indicated as a suffix (except for halogen compounds). When several different groups are attached, only one group is a suffix while the others become prefixes. The group that should be the suffix is determined by this decreasing order of preference: acid, ester, aldehyde, ketone, alcohol. This preference is shown in Table 11.1. Accordingly, the addition of a hydroxyl on carbon 11 (β position) and an oxygen on carbon 20 of pregnane would be indicated as *11β-hydroxypregnan-20-one*. The addition of the hydroxyl only would give us *pregnan-11β-ol*. Note

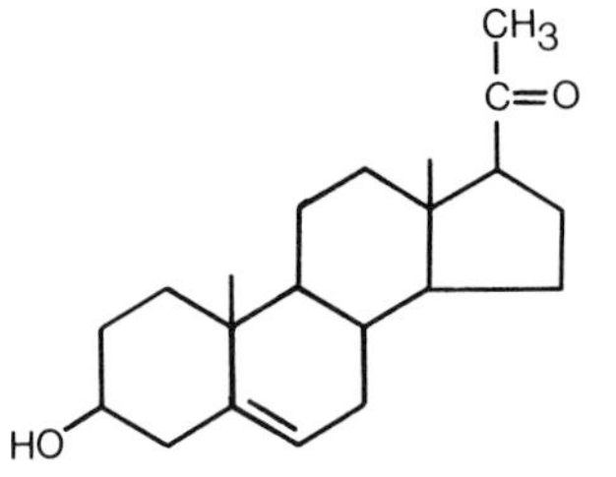

(a) Pregnenolone
(3β-hydroxy-5-pregnen-20-one)

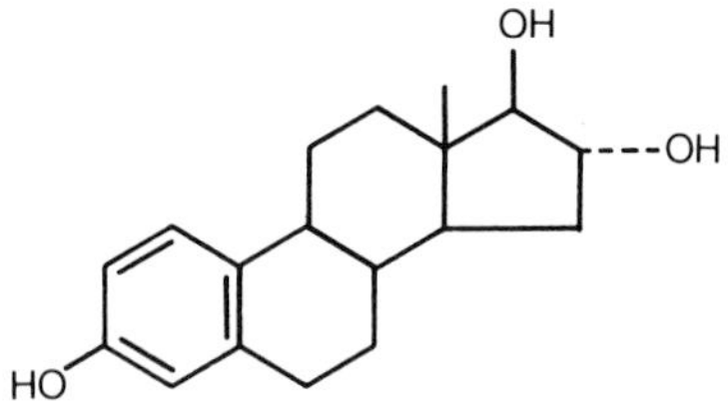

(b) Estriol
(1,3,5(10)-estrotriene-3β,16α,17β-triol)

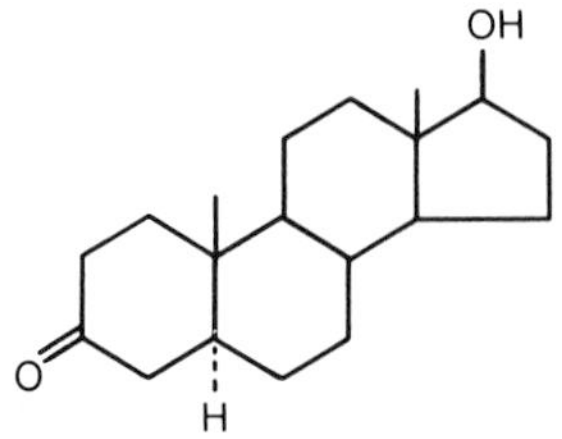

(c) 5α-Dihydrotestosterone
(17β-hydroxy-5α-androstan-3-one)

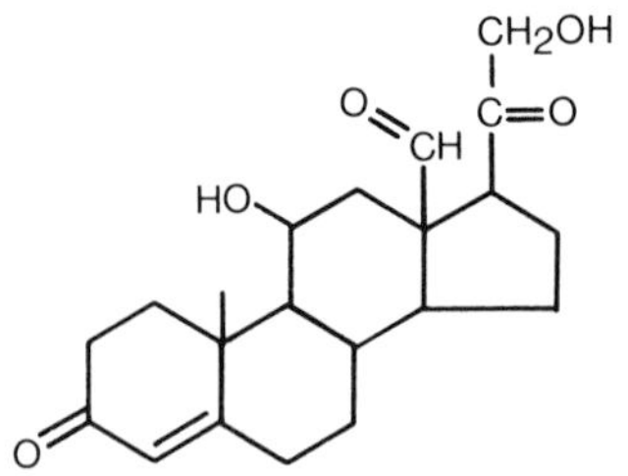

(d) Aldosterone
(11β, 21-dihydroxy-3, 20-dioxo-4-pregnen-18-al)

FIGURE 11.5. The chemical structures of four naturally occurring steroids. Both trivial and systematic names are shown.

that in these examples the terminal *e* has been dropped from the parent name. This is according to the rule that the *e* should be dropped when the suffix begins with a vowel. Thus pregnane with oxygens on both carbons 11 and 20 would be *pregnane-11,20-dione*. The introduction of the oxygen on carbons 11 and 20 does not introduce asymmetry. When there is more than one prefix, they should be put in alphabetical order (e.g., *3β-acetoxy-16α-hydroxy-11-oxopregnan-18-al*).

Both the systemic and trivial names for four naturally occurring steroids are shown in Fig. 11.5. Obviously, the trivial names are easier to say and remember. Sometimes trivial names are modified by prefixes indicating substituents on other steroids (e.g., *1α-hydroxycorticosterone* for 11β,21-dihydroxypregnane-3,20-dione). Many of the synthetic steroids also have trivial names (e.g., dexamethasone, prednisolone).

The following sequence should be followed to facilitate the systematic identification of a steroid:

1. Is it a C_{18}, C_{19}, or C_{21} compound? Choose family name.
2. Are α or β hydrogens indicated? Identify location and position.
3. Are there any double bonds? Choose the ending of the family name and indicate location of bond(s).
4. Are there any groups attached? Decide on suffix according to types of groups. Decide on prefix(es).
5. Indicate all locations and positions, where applicable. Put prefixes in alphabetical order. Decide on terminal *e* of family name.

These rules for steroid nomenclature are becoming more widely accepted. However, disagreement can be found in steroid names in the literature. Some British publications have retained the system in which double bonds are always indicated before the ending of the family name of the steroid. An older system used a △ symbol as a prefix to identify double bonds.

METABOLISM OF STEROIDS

In considering the formation of steroids in the organism, it must be kept in mind that the several steroidogenic tissues (ovary, testis, adrenal, placenta) have the ability to produce small amounts of related steroids. Common metabolic pathways are present to some extent in all of these organs. Apparently, a particular synthetic pathway is favored by the trophic hormone (ACTH, LH, FSH, PRL) and its receptor in the target tissue. Similarly, the steroids themselves may act on enzyme-mediated steps in a pathway, either to stimulate or inhibit them. Thus the types of steroids produced by a tissue will depend on both the types and activities of enzymes present in the tissue. Furthermore, it is probable that one steroid-secreting organ can modify a steroid originally secreted by another organ, thus changing its physiological activity. For example, the mammalian adrenal cortex may take up and modify chemically the progesterone secreted by the ovary, in order to make corticoids. This is not surprising, since these tissues normally take up some cholesterol (a nonhormonal precursor steroid) from the blood. Uptake and modification of steroids also occurs in tissues that are not normally considered steroidogenic. For example, the prostate gland of some mammals can convert circulating testosterone to dihydrotestosterone. Chemical modification of plasma steroids also occurs in the brain, skin, salivary glands, and other tissues.

In order to allow an overall picture to emerge, we will present in a single scheme (Fig. 11.6) the steps in biosynthesis of hormonally active steroids that may be present in adrenocortical or gonadal tissues. The actual pattern or pathway will vary in different organs, in different species, and at different stages of development so that only one or a few of the related steroids are produced. In one tissue at any given time alternative pathways may be available but are considered minor routes of steroid biosynthesis. A comprehensive coverage of the comparative aspects of steroidogenesis in non-mammalian vertebrates is beyond the scope of this chapter. Therefore, the picture presented here is applicable primarily to laboratory and domestic animals.

Cholesterol Biosynthesis and Distribution

Steroid hormones are synthesized from a C_{27} precursor steroid, cholesterol. About half of the cholesterol in the human body comes from the diet, while the rest is synthesized from acetate, which is essentially a two-carbon fragment. Virtually all tissues have some capacity for cholesterol synthesis, although most of the circulating cholesterol that is synthesized is made in the liver. Adrenocortical and gonadal tissues can synthesize cholesterol, and they can take it up from the blood when circulating levels are sufficiently high. Thus there are multiple sources of this steroid hormone precursor: *de novo* synthesis within the endocrine organ, and uptake from the circulating pool that is maintained by the liver or supplied in the diet.

Bloch, Dauben, and others have demonstrated the biochemical pathway of cholesterol synthesis. Cholesterol is made from 18 molecules of acetate in about 30 enzymatic steps occurring in the cellular cytoplasm. Some of these steps are illustrated in Fig. 11.7. These steps may be categorized into four processes. First, three acetyl units are converted into a six-carbon intermediate, mevalonic acid. A part of this conversion involves the reduction of 3-hydroxy-3-methylglutaryl-CoA (HMG-CoA) by the enzyme HMG-CoA reductase, which is the rate-limiting step in cholesterol biosynthesis. In the next process, six mevalonic acid molecules are each phosphorylated and decarboxylated, and then polymerized to form the linear C_{30} compound, squalene. Cyclization of squalene forms lanosterol, which undergoes de-methylation and reduction to yield cholesterol.

In most steroidogenic tissues cholesterol that is not directly needed for hormone production is stored within the cell in the form of cholesteryl esters. Electron microscopy of steroidogenic cells reveals lipid droplets that contain fatty acid esters of cholesterol, principally cholesteryl oleate in some mammals (Fig. 11.8). At times of high demand for steroid hormonogenesis, cholesteryl esters are cleaved to yield free cholesterol (Fig. 11.9).

In many situations, particularly after prolonged stimulation of steroidogenesis, a significant amount of cholesterol may be taken up from the blood. Cholesterol circulates in the form of cholesteryl esters bound to low- and high-density lipoproteins (LDL and HDL). In most mammalian adrenal cells that have been studied, LDL or HDL particles containing cholesteryl esters are bound to membrane receptors and taken up into the cells to contribute to the intracellular pool of cholesterol (Fig. 11.9). In some cases of sustained high rates of steroidogenesis, cellular uptake of these cholesterol-containing lipoprotein particles is necessary for maximal steroid hormone synthesis.

Biogenesis of Steroid Hormones

The initial step in converting cholesterol to a steroid hormone is the breaking off of the six-carbon side chain attached to carbon 20. This step occurs in the mitochondria and therefore requires transport of free cholesterol into mitochondria. The inner membrane of mitochondrial cristae contains an enzyme system belonging to the family of mixed-function oxygenases known as the cytochrome P450s. Side-chain cleavage (scc) of cholesterol by $P450_{scc}$ requires a reducing cofactor (NADPH) and results in the formation of the C_{21} compound pregnenolone. Pregnenolone is then transported out of the mitochondria to the endoplasmic reticulum, where it is either oxidized to form progesterone or hydroxylated to form 17-hydroxypregnenolone. Progesterone is an important steroid hormone in itself and is secreted in large amounts by the corpus luteum of the ovary (Chapter 13). Depending on the animal species and tissue, progesterone or 17-hydroxypregnenolone are converted to the androgens, estrogens, and corticoids by alternative biochemical pathways. In the adrenal tissue of some mammals and birds, the 17-hydroxylation pathway is not a major route of biosynthesis, since corticosterone is the major product in these species. However, in the human adrenal an active 17-hydroxylating pathway results in the synthesis of cortisol as the major glucocorticoid. Similar species differences in major and minor pathways occur in other tissues; for example, the rat testis produces primarily androstenedione, while the human testis produces testosterone. These differences are undoubtedly due to genetic regulation of the types of steroid-converting enzymes synthesized in steroidogenic tissues.

The C_{19} steroid hormones (androgens) are usually produced from C_{21}

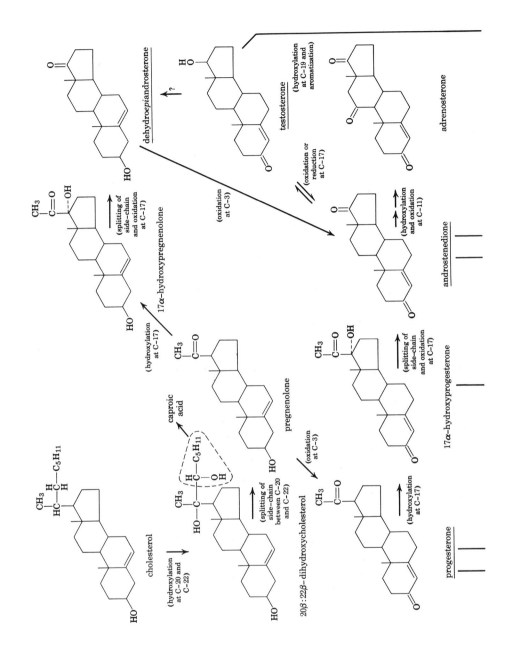

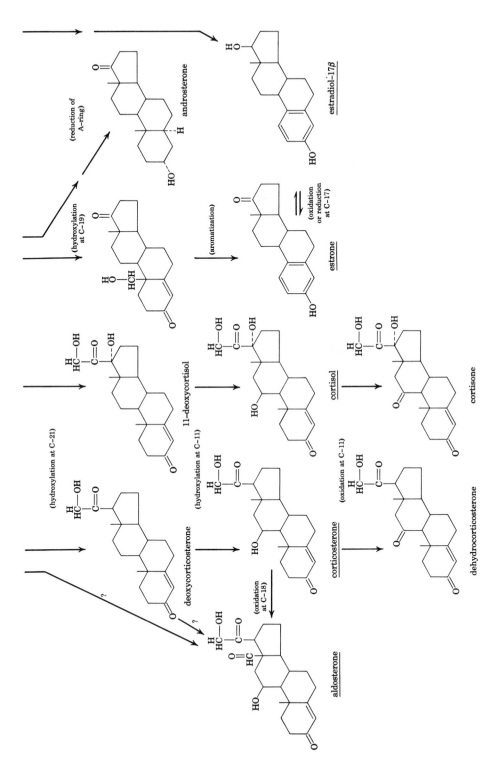

FIGURE 11.6. Major metabolic pathways involved in the biogenesis of steroid hormones. The principal secretory products of the steroidogenic organs are underlined. Specific enzymes have been characterized, and mitochondrial or microsomal participation has been determined for many of the steps shown. The 17- and 21-hydroxylations appear to require mitochondria; the 11-hydroxylation, microsomes. Also, various cofactors have been specified for many of the steps. For example, reduced triphosphopyridine nucleotide (TPNH) and molecular O_2 are required for the various hydroxylations and for the side-chain splitting (desmolase enzyme activity). In addition, certain ions are known to be required for the conversion of corticosterone to aldosterone by the zona glomerulosa cells of the adrenal cortex.

403

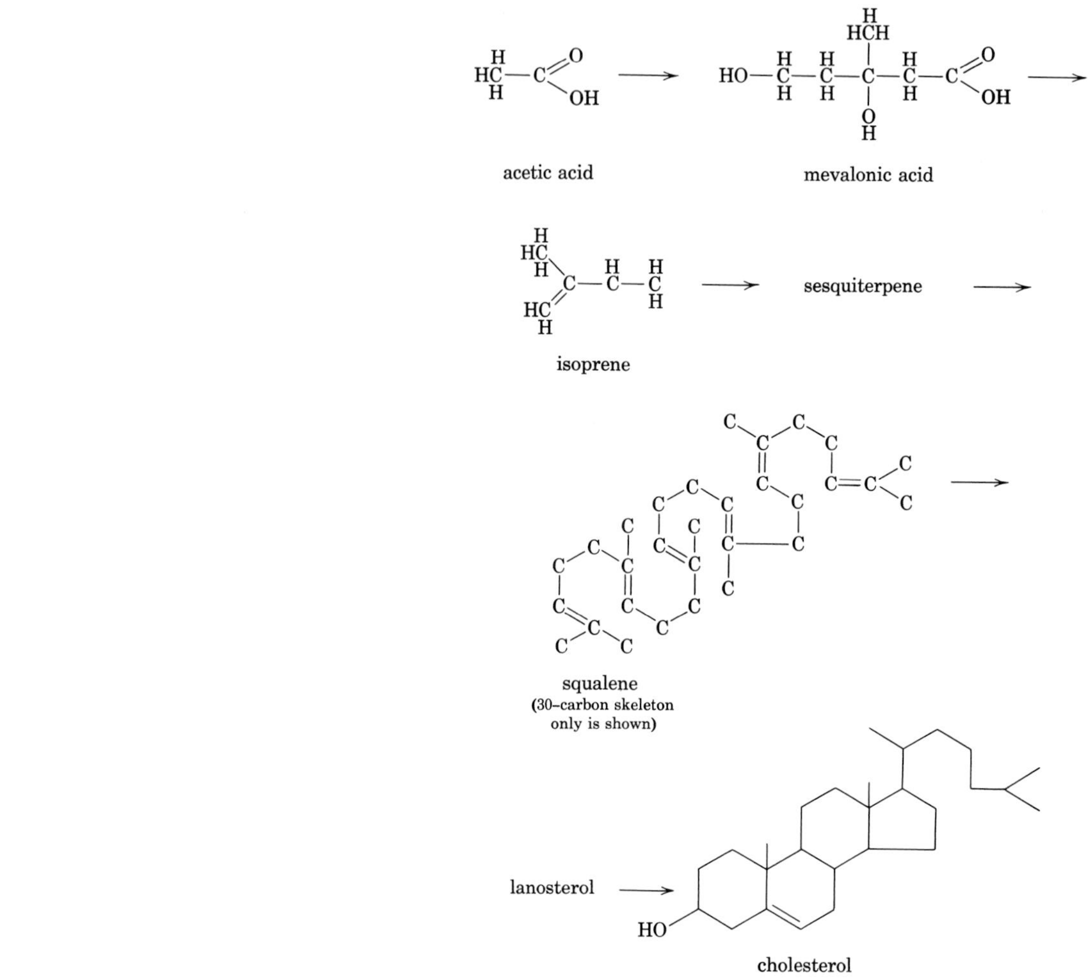

FIGURE 11.7. Steps in the synthesis of cholesterol from acetate via the linking of small units to form the unsaturated aliphatic hydrocarbon squalene and the closure of rings to form the cyclic sterols.

compounds that have a hydroxyl on carbon 17 and no functional group on carbon 21. Thus 17α-hydroxypregnenolone and 17α-hydroxyprogesterone are precursors of androgens, while corticosteroids are not generally converted to androgenic hormones. Side-chain cleavage of corticosteroids to form C_{19} compounds in mammals occurs mainly in the testis and adrenal cortex and to a limited extent in the ovary and placenta.

The C_{18} steroid hormones (estrogens) are most often produced from androgens through several enzymatic steps. Initially, a hydroxyl group is attached to carbon 19. Subsequently, carbon 19 is removed and double bonds are introduced into ring A, which thereby becomes aromatized. The adrenal cortex produces only small amounts of estrone, while the testis may secrete as much as 30% of the total estrogen formed in males.

There is considerable information available concerning the properties and subcellular localization of enzymes involved in steroidogenesis. Some of the enzymes, as mentioned earlier, appear to be members of the cytochrome P450 class and require NADPH and molecular O_2 for full activity. Enzyme systems responsible for the formation of progestins, androgens, and estrogens are localized in the cell cytoplasm, associated with the microsomal fraction. Part of the corticosteroidogenic pathway is located in the mitochondrion. The compartmentalization of cholesterol and steroid hormone utilization and synthesis in a human adrenal cortical cell is shown in the scheme in Fig. 11.9. The complexity of the pathways leading to the formation of free cholesterol and steroid hormones and the number of organelles involved provide many possible points for the control of steroidogenesis. Stimulation of the adrenal cortex by ACTH affects many of these processes either directly or indirectly. A clearly recognized primary effect of ACTH is stimulation of the side-chain cleavage system that converts cholesterol to pregnenolone. The mechanism of ACTH action in this system appears to involve the elevation of intracellular cyclic AMP and the phosphorylation–dephosphorylation cycle of a regulatory protein (see Fig. 1.14). Some

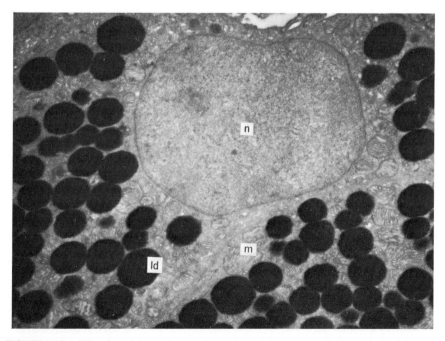

FIGURE 11.8. Electron micrograph of an outer zona fasciculata cell of an adult male mouse ($\times$ 12,000). Note intensely osmophilic lipid droplets (*ld*), mitochondria (*m*), and nucleus (*n*). [From T. Zelander, *J. Ultrastr. Res.*, Suppl. 2, 1959.]

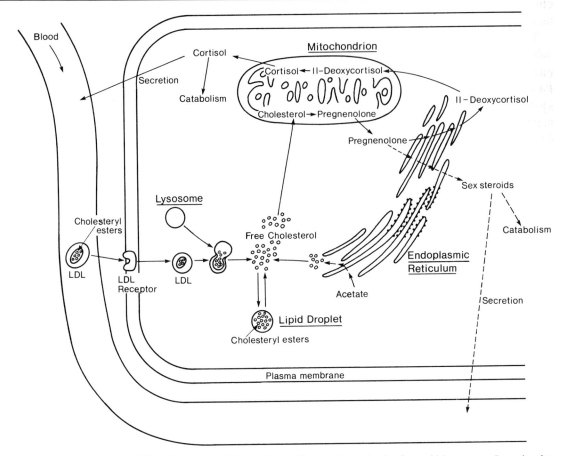

FIGURE 11.9. Intracellular pathways for the biosynthesis of steroid hormones. Low-density lipoprotein (LDL) particles containing cholesteryl esters in the blood combine with a LDL receptor on the plasma membrane and are taken up by the cell. LDL particles within the cell interact with lysosomes, which liberate the cholesteryl esters. Cholesteryl esters from LDL particles or from lipid droplets may be de-esterified to yield free cholesterol. Steroidogenic cells may synthesize cholesterol from acetate. Cholesterol molecules are taken up by the mitochondria and converted to pregnenolone. Pregnenolone enters the cell cytoplasm and is acted upon by steroidogenic enzymes located on or near the endoplasmic reticulum. In the adrenal cell, the enzyme that converts 11-deoxycortisol to cortisol is located within the mitochondrion. Steroids produced within the cell may be either secreted into the blood or catabolized within the cell.

ACTH effects may be blocked by treating adrenal cells with inhibitors of protein and mRNA synthesis, although the precise involvement of transcription and translation in ACTH action is not known. One might presume that part of the response to ACTH may involve synthesis of enzymes in the corticosteroidogenic pathway. Additional primary effects of ACTH seem to be species related. For example, ACTH promotes conversion of corticosterone to aldosterone in the rat adrenal cortex. In the dog, however, this conversion seems to be independent of ACTH stimulation. Presumably, control of steroidogenesis is adapted to the requirements of the particular species. Furthermore, the ACTH effects on the adrenal cortex may be dependent on the functional state of the gland. During the initial phase of ACTH stimulation, the conversion of cholesteryl esters to free cholesterol from lipid droplet stores is accelerated. After prolonged stimulation and concomitant depletion of stored cholesterol, the synthesis of cholesterol from acetate and uptake of cholesterol-containing lipoprotein particles are accelerated. Other hormones may modify ACTH action indirectly. In the rat adrenal, PRL inhibits 5α-reductase and 20α-hydroxysteroid dehydrogenase, enzymes that degrade corticosterone and progesterone, respectively. Thus PRL, given together with ACTH, does not affect total steroid production but increases the relative amounts of corticosterone and progesterone secreted by blocking their catabolism. The mechanisms of gonadotropin (LH and FSH) stimulation of steroidogenesis by the ovary and testis are similar to those of ACTH action on the adrenal, although the secreted steroids are, of course, different. The gonadotropins elevate intracellular cyclic AMP and also influence mRNA and protein synthesis. The conversion of cholesterol to pregnenolone is stimulated markedly. The supply of free cholesterol is increased by synthesis from acetate, hydrolysis of cholesteryl esters from lipid storage droplets, and uptake of lipoprotein particles. Furthermore, the gonadotropins may enhance the activity of particular progestins. Although the mechanisms of ACTH, LH, and FSH stimulation of steroidogenesis are similar in their respective target organs, the specificity of the steroidogenic response is imposed by the hormone receptor. Thus ACTH has no effect on steroidogenesis in gonads, and gonadotropins are ineffective for direct stimulation of the adrenal cortex.

STRUCTURE–FUNCTION RELATIONSHIP OF STEROIDS

Analysis of the structures of steroids and their physiological activity has revealed certain structural requirements for particular functions. These studies have aided the development of synthetic steroids that are more potent than the naturally occurring hormones. For example, the addition of a methyl group to carbon 2 and a fluoro group to carbon 9 of cortisol results in a compound with 40 times the glucocorticoid activity of cortisol.

For a pregnane compound to have progestogen activity it must have a 4-en-3-one configuration in the A ring, an oxygen on carbon 20, and the terminal carbon (carbon 21) must be a methyl group. The requirements for glucocorticoid activity of the pregnane nucleus include oxygens on carbons 17 and 11. Mineralocorticoid activity is determined by an oxygen on carbon 21 but no oxygen on carbon 17 of the pregnane nucleus. Seemingly minor modifications of a steroid may have profound effects on biological activity.

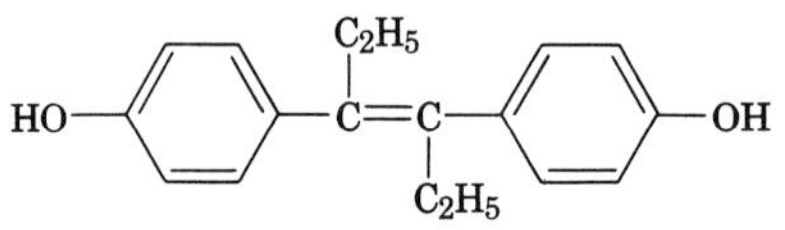

C_2H_5

HO—⬡—C=C—⬡—OH

C_2H_5

(a)

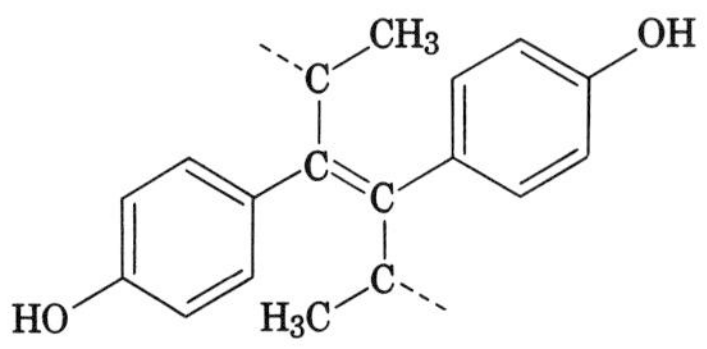

CH_3 OH

C

C=C

HO—⬡ H_3C—C

(b)

FIGURE 11.10. Diethylstilbestrol, a nonsteroid synthetic estrogen. (a) Conventional representation of the structural formula; (b) steroidlike representation of the structural formula. Note the resemblance to naturally occurring estrogenic steroids (Fig. 11.6). The broken lines in b represent the actual position of the methyl groups, rather than the hypothetical positions that give the molecule a semblance of B and C rings.

For example, the only structural difference between the strong progestogen progesterone and the strong mineralocorticoid deoxycorticosterone (DOC) is the presence of a hydroxyl group on carbon 21 of DOC.

Androgens, in addition to being C_{19} steroids (androstane), have oxygens on carbons 3 and 17. Estrogens also have oxygens on carbons 3 and 17, but are C_{18} steroids, and usually have a phenolic A ring (aromatic ring with a hydroxyl group on carbon 3). It is interesting that many synthetic estrogenic compounds do not have a steroid nucleus. For example, diethylstilbestrol (DES) is a synthetic compound with estrogenic activity, but it does not resemble a steroid in its usual representation. Except for the methyl groups, which actually point away from the rest of the molecule, DES may be drawn in a conformation that is reminiscent of naturally occurring steroids (Fig. 11.10).

STEROID CATABOLISM AND EXCRETION

Metabolism of hormonal steroids to physiologically less active or inactive compounds occurs both in steroidogenic and peripheral tissues. The major peripheral site of catabolism is the liver; the kidney and other tissues may catabolize circulating steroids to some extent. The major catabolic enzymes are involved in reductive reactions, particularly in the A ring and at carbons 3 and 20. The reduced steroids are usually conjugated to form steroid sulfates and glucuronides, which, in addition to being biologically inactive, are more water soluble and easily excreted in aqueous fluids. The principal routes of elimination are through the urine or through bile fluid, with ultimate excretion in the feces. There are many catabolic pathways for the various steroids, and numerous metabolites have been identified. Often, alternative pathways of catabolism are active simultaneously, so that a range of metabolic products are formed. Here we will consider only a few representative examples of steroid hormone catabolism.

A major route of catabolism of corticoids in humans is reduction of the double bond in the A ring and the keto group on carbon 3 to form tetrahydrocortisol and tetrahydroaldosterone (Fig. 11.11). Alternatively, about 10% of the corticoids are inactivated by removal of the ethyl side chain to form a C_{19} compound. A less significant pathway is hydroxylation of carbon 6 to form 6β-hydroxycortisol, which is such a polar (water soluble) compound that it can be excreted in the urine without conjugation. Progestogens and androgens are inactivated by reductions in the A ring and at carbon 3 (and carbon 20 of progestogens), similar to the inactivation of corticoids. In humans pregnanediol is a principle metabolite of progesterone.

In contrast to the other steroids, estrogens are not catabolized by reduction in the A ring. Instead, hydroxylation or ketone formation may occur at several positions, including carbons 2, 6, 7, 14, 15, 16, 17, and 18. Most of these hydroxylations increase the water solubility of the estrogens. Estradiol-17β is converted to estrone, which is then metabolized to estriol (Fig. 11.11). These metabolites of estradiol have some biological activity, since they can stimulate uterine growth. Estrogens that have been hydroxylated at carbon 2 may be further modified by methylation of the hydroxyl group to form a catechol estrogen (Fig. 11.11). It is not clear whether catechol estrogens perform a physiological function.

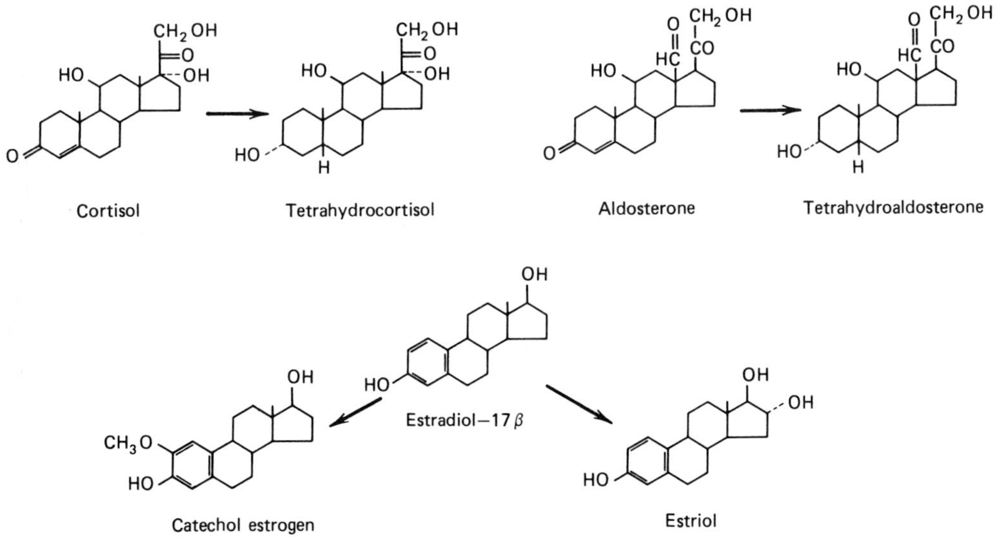

| Cortisol | Tetrahydrocortisol | Aldosterone | Tetrahydroaldosterone |

Catechol estrogen   Estradiol—17β   Estriol

FIGURE 11.11. Examples of catabolic pathways for some steroids. Reduction of the A ring is a common pathway for the inactivation of C_{21} and C_{19} steroid hormones. Estrogens may be modified by hydroxylation and methylation.

STEROID BINDING IN THE BLOOD

Steroids may be bound in a reversible, noncovalent fashion to several constituents in blood plasma; usually, these are albumin or globulin proteins. This binding to plasma proteins is a consequence of the low water solubility of steroid hormones and is important physiologically in several ways. Plasma protein–binding of newly secreted steroids helps carry the steroids away from the steroidogenic organ and facilitates transport of the steroids throughout the body. Another consequence of protein binding is the maintenance of a large pool or reservoir of steroids in the blood. Steroid molecules bound to blood proteins are not free to be diluted in the extravascular body fluids and are not available for degradation and clearance in the liver or kidneys. The plasma proteins favor the accumulation of steroids in the blood. The protein-bound reservoir of steroid hormones in the blood minimizes wide oscillations in the blood concentration of the steroid.

Steroid binding to albumins is relatively nonspecific and of low affinity. All steroid hormones bind weakly to albumin. Steroid-binding globulins, on the other hand, have relatively high affinities for specific steroid hormones. Steroid-binding globulins have been classified into two categories: corticosteroid-binding globulin (CBG, also referred to as *transcortin*) and sex hormone-binding globulin (SHBG). The specificity of these binding globulins in terms of which steroids will be bound varies from species to species. The steroid-binding specificities of human CBG and SHBG are shown in Table 11.2. Human SHBG has a high binding affinity for estradiol, testosterone, and dihydrotestosterone but does not bind estrone, progesterone, or cortisol. Human CBG has a high binding affinity for cortisol, but does not bind aldosterone. Plasma concentrations of cortisol in humans are about 1000

TABLE 11.2. Approximate affinities of steroids for serum proteins and tissue receptors in humans[a]

	Dissociation Constant, K_D ($M \times 10^9$)		
	Serum Binder		Target Tissue Receptor[b]
Steroid	SHBG	CBG	
Estradiol	5	>10	0.1 (E)
Estrone	>10	>100	0.3 (E)
Testosterone	2	>100	1 (A)
Dihydrotestosterone	1	>100	1 (A)
Progesterone	>100	2	1 (P)
Cortisol	>100	3	3 (G)

[a] From P. K. Siiteri and F. Febres, *Endocrinology*, Vol. 3 (DeGroot et al., eds.), Grune & Stratton, New York, pp. 1401–1417 (1979). (by permission).
[b] E, estrogen receptor; A, androgen receptor; P, progesterone receptor; G, glucocorticoid receptor.

times the plasma concentration of aldosterone. Part of this difference in circulating corticosteroids is due to the binding of cortisol to CBG. Aldosterone is not bound to CBG and, as a result, is removed from the circulation very quickly by the liver. Human CBG also has a high binding affinity for progesterone and may function as a blood carrier of this hormone. CBGs of other mammalian species do not have a high affinity for progesterone.

Although steroids have a high affinity for steroid-binding globulins, it is important that the affinity of the steroid for the hormonal receptor in the target tissue be at least equal to or greater in magnitude (Table 11.2). In other words, the attraction of the steroid to the steroid receptor in responsive cells should be great enough to overcome the binding of the steroid to the globulins in the blood.

The fact that a certain portion of the steroids in the blood are bound to plasma components is important to keep in mind. Only free steroids are available for binding by the hormonal receptor. The amount of bound and free steroid hormones in the blood can vary depending on the levels of plasma-binding proteins. Women have about twice the concentration of SHBG in their blood as do men. Since testosterone is bound very strongly to SHBG, a greater proportion of the total testosterone in the circulation will be bound in women than in men. Conversely, men have a greater proportion of free testosterone in their blood.

Plasma steroid-binding glycoproteins are widely distributed among vertebrates, although high-affinity binding proteins are found less frequently in fishes. Wingfield (1980) has reviewed the phylogenetic distribution of CBG and SHBG and has suggested a scheme for the evolution of these proteins. Elasmobranchs and perhaps some cyclostomes may represent the primitive condition where there is a single protein-binding system that is not highly specific. Bony fishes usually have a binding system specific for C_{18} and C_{19} steroids (SHBG), although some species have a CBG-like protein. Amphibians, reptiles, and most mammals have both SHBG and CBG, while birds appear to have lost the SHBG protein during their evolution.

APPENDIX

The following trivial names for steroids have been approved for use in journal publications by The Endocrine Society (*Endocrinology* **106**:13A, 1980):

Aldosterone	(11β,21-Dihydroxy-3,20-dioxo-4-pregnen-18-al
Androstenedione	4-Androstene-3,17-dione
Androsterone	3α-Hydroxy-5α-androstan-17-one
Cholesterol	5-Cholesten-3β-ol
Cortisol	11β,17α,21-Trihydroxy-4-pregnene-3,20-dione

Cortisone	$17\alpha,21$-Dihydroxy-4-pregnene-3,11,20-trione
Corticosterone	$11\beta,21$-Dihydroxy-4-pregnene-3,20-dione
Dehydroepiandrosterone	3β-Hydroxy-5-androsten-17-one
Deoxycorticosterone	21-Hydroxy-4-pregnene-3,20-dione
5α-Dihydrotestosterone	17β-Hydroxy-5α-androstan-3-one
17β-Estradiol	1,3,5(10)-Estratriene-3,17β-diol
Estriol	1,3,5(10)-Estratriene-3,16α,17β-triol
Estrone	3-Hydroxy-1,3,5(10)-estratrien-17-one
Etiocholanolone	3α-Hydroxy-5βandrostan-17-one
Pregnenolone	3β-Hydroxy-5-pregnen-20-one
Progesterone	4-Pregnene-3,20-dione
Testosterone	17β-Hydroxy-4-androsten-3-one).

Other trivial names of steroids may be used provided they are defined systematically.

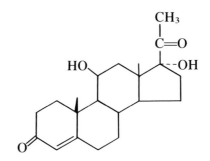

What is the systematic name of this steroid?

1. C_{18}, C_{19}, or C_{21} compound?	Decide on family name	Pregnane
2. α or β hydrogens indicated?	Identify location and position	None indicated
3. Double bonds?*	Choose the ending of the family name and indicate locations of bonds	4-Pregnene

* If both stereochemistry of hydrogen and unsaturation are indicated, location and position of hydrogen come before family name, and unsaturation is identified before family name ending; e.g., 5α-pregn-1-ene.

4. Other groups attached to carbons?	Decide on suffix according to types of groups (Table 11.1)	4-Pregnene-3,20-dione
	Decide on prefixes and put in alphabetical order	11β, 17α-Dihydroxy-4-pregnene-3,20-dione
5. Does the suffix begin with a vowel?	Decide on terminal *e* of famile name	*e* remains

1β-Chloro-16α,17β-dihydroxy-3-oxo-5β-androst-6-ene-18-al
What does this steroid look like?

(1)

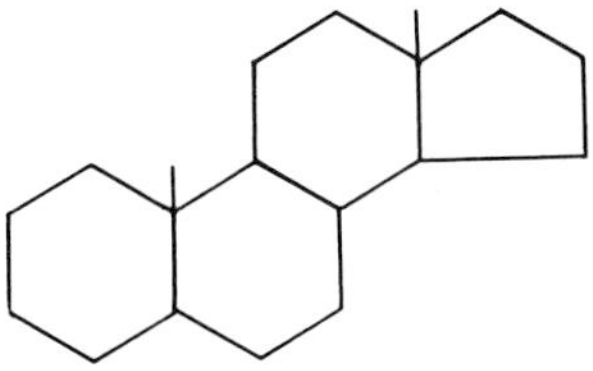

(2)

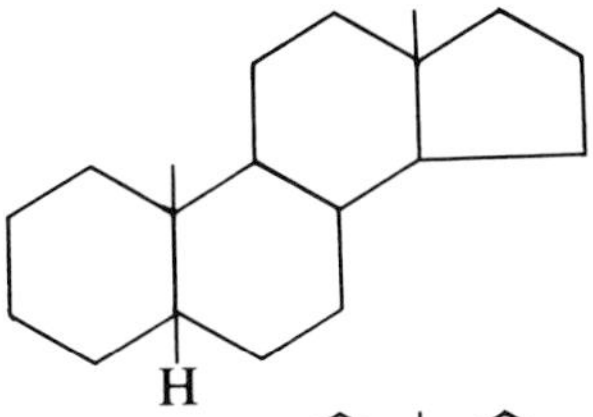

(3)

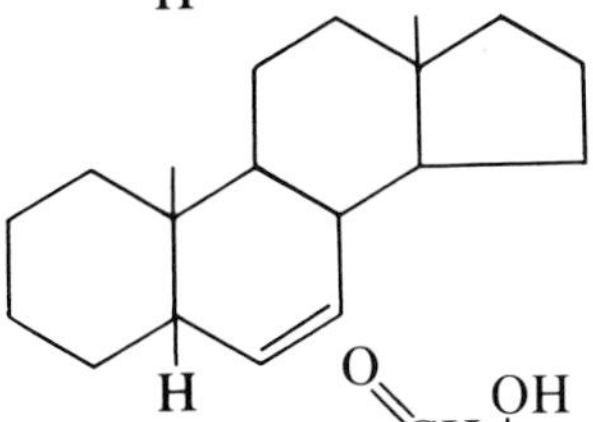

(4)

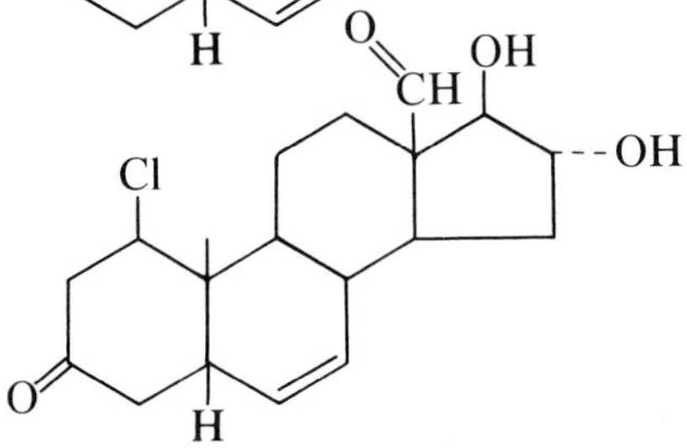

1.	What is the family name?	Androstane
2.	α or β hydrogens?	5β-
3.	Double bonds?	6-ene
4.	Other groups attached?	1β-Chloro, 16α,17β-dihydroxy, 3-oxo, 18-al

ADDITIONAL READING

1. Brown, M. S., P. T. Kovanen, and J. L. Goldstein (1979). Receptor-mediated uptake of lipoprotein-cholesterol and its utilization for steroid synthesis in the adrenal cortex. *Recent Progr. Horm. Res.* **35**:215–257.

2. Delrio, G., and J. Brachet, eds. (1980). *Steroids and Their Mechanism of Action in Non-mammalian Vertebrates*. Raven, New York.

3. Freedman, M. A., and S. N. Freedman (1970). *Introduction to Steroid Biochemistry and its Clinical Application*. Harper & Row, New York.

4. Makin, H. L. J., ed. (1975). *Biochemistry of Steroid Hormones*. Blackwell, Oxford/Lippincott, Philadelphia.

5. Sandor, T., S. Sonea, and A. Z. Mehdi (1975). The possible role of steroids in evolution. *Am. Zool.* **15** (Suppl. 1):227–253.

6. Wingfield, J. C. (1980). Sex steroid-binding proteins in vertebrate blood. In *Hormones, Adaptation and Evolution* (S. Ishii, T. Hirano, and M. Wada, eds.) Springer-Verlag, Berlin, pp. 135–144.

12

The Adrenal Cortex and Interrenal Gland

The adrenal gland is a compound structure with diverse functions. As we have seen in Chapter 10, one portion of the gland, the adrenal medulla or chromaffin tissue, is responsible for the systemic release of catecholamines. In this chapter we will consider the functions of the steroidogenic part of the gland: the adrenal cortex of mammals and the interrenal tissue of non-mammalian vertebrates. The major functions of adrenal steroids can be categorized as either metabolic (glucocorticoid), or regulating salt balance (mineralocorticoid). The adrenal glands are essential for life. Removal of the adrenals results in the inability of the kidneys to retain sodium. This loss of sodium causes dehydration and a collapse of the peripheral circulation, so that not enough oxygen is supplied to the tissues and death ensues. The glucocorticoid activities of adrenal steroids are not as essential for life as are the mineralocorticoids. The adrenal cortex is important also in various phases of the life cycles of animals. The adrenal of the mammalian fetus is quite active in producing steroids which are converted to estrogens by the placenta. Adrenal secretion of steroid precursors of androgens in the female is important in reproduction. Adrenal steroids appear to play a role in the migration of animals. In addition to such specific functions of the adrenal cortical tissue, there are important interactions of cortical and adrenal medullary tissues. Both the cortical and medullary portions of the adrenal gland function in the physiological adaptation of the organism to certain demands of the environment. The adrenal gland as a whole is important in helping the animal deal with stressful situations. In 1855 Addison described the fairly uncommon clinical disorder of adrenal insufficiency, a disease that now bears his name. The low levels of blood glucocorticoids in humans with Addison's disease are associated with symptoms of weakness, fatigue, weight loss, nausea, vomiting, and low blood pressure because of the loss of sodium and water. Addison associated these symptoms with lesions of the adrenal glands. In 1856 Brown-Séquard investigated the functions of the adrenals by performing an adrenalectomy in dogs. He concluded (correctly) from these experiments that the adrenals were essential for life, although some have suggested that the dogs in his experiments may have died from surgical trauma rather than from adrenal insufficiency. The involvement of the adrenals in carbohydrate metabolism was first indicated in 1910 when it was discovered that patients with Addison's disease had low blood sugar. During the late 1920s and early 1930s, the importance of the adrenals in salt balance was recognized by the observation that the life of adrenalectomized dogs or patients with Addison's disease could be prolonged by supplying NaCl. The 1930s through the 1950s was a period in which the steroid hormones of the adrenals were isolated, identified, and synthesized. In more recent times the identification of the diverse functions of adrenal steroids has continued. Much research has focused on the mechanisms of action of adrenal steroids and of the endocrine systems that control adrenocortical function.

Adrenocortical function in the tetrapod vertebrates is controlled predominantly by two systems. The synthesis and secretion of the glucocorticoids are controlled by the pituitary peptide adrenocorticotropin (ACTH), which is controlled in turn by the hypothalamus. The mineralocorticoids may be controlled directly by blood K^+ levels and also by a "diffuse" hormonal system, the renin–angiotensin system (RAS). The RAS is considered a diffuse system because the peptides and enzymes in the system are located in the blood and in such tissues as kidney and lung. However, as we shall see, pituitary ACTH is not without effect on mineralocorticoid synthesis. It should be kept in mind that the control of salt and water balance is also influenced by the neurohypophysis (Chapter 3). The adrenal and neurohypophyseal functions appear to be integrated in some interesting ways.

Although a large amount of information has accumulated from studies of the comparative endocrinology of adrenocortical function, these studies are not as advanced as those of mammals. On the other hand, comparative studies have demonstrated the adaptiveness of corticosteroid function, as evidenced by the fact that in nonmammalian vertebrates the steroids control the functions of such diverse structures as the nasal or orbital salt glands of birds and reptiles, the urinary bladder of amphibians, and the gills of fishes. In view of the range of functions of corticosteroids in mammals, the comparative endocrinology of these hormones is—and will continue to be—a particularly challenging area of research.

COMPARATIVE ANATOMY AND HISTOLOGY

The gross and comparative anatomy of the adrenal gland has been discussed in detail in Chapter 10 (see Fig. 10.1). In general, adrenocortical tissue is found associated with the kidneys. In fishes and amphibians the adrenals are associated with the mesonephric kidney, while in reptiles, birds, and mammals they are associated with the metanephric kidney. Both types of kidneys are the functional kidneys in the respective adult species in which they are found. The metanephric kidney is a more recently evolved structure that is present in higher vertebrates. The mesonephric kidney of higher vertebrates is functional only early in development. In lower vertebrates interrenal tissue is usually comprised of cells that are dispersed in kidney tissue. In birds, reptiles, and mammals the adrenals are compact structures located anterior to the kidney. The significance of the association of the adrenals with the kidneys is apparent in view of the regulatory actions that these organs have on each other.

The vascularization of the adrenal gland provides some basis for the close association of cortical and medullary tissues, at least in mammals. The blood supply may come from many major arteries; in the rabbit and some other mammals, including humans, the adrenal arteries branch off from the renal artery (Fig. 12.1). Once inside the adrenals, there are three possible routes for arterial blood. The vascular pathway may be either confined to the capsule or confined to the cortex. Alternatively, blood may flow within the cortex from the periphery toward the inner layers of the cortex, and then continue from the cortical sinusoids into the large blood sinusoids of the medulla. This particular route of blood flow from the cortex to the medulla may be of functional significance for two reasons. It has been observed that epinephrine secretion causes a constriction of the medullary arteries and a diversion of blood into the cortical sinusoids. This increased cortical blood results in increased output of corticoid hormones. Blood flow in the cortico-medullary direction may influence catecholamine production, since gluco-corticoids stimulate the methylation of norepinephrine to produce epine-phrine.

The interrenal cells of nonmammalian vertebrates are arranged in cords that can form interlacing networks, coils or loops. Generally, the cords of cells are not well organized into obvious patterns. In birds and some reptiles, however, the cords of cells form loops at the periphery of the gland directly below the well-formed capsule. These cords extend toward the interior of the gland in a parallel fashion. Although this pattern of cell organization in the bird or reptile adrenal is suggestive of zonation, functional zonation of the adrenal has not been observed in nonmammalian vertebrates.

The adrenal cortex of eutherian (placental) and metatherian (marsupial) mammals shows a well-organized pattern of cells. The cords of adreno-cortical tissue extend outward from the outer border of the adrenal medulla to the capsule, where they form loops of cells. In 1866 Arnold showed that the cortex consists mainly of three zones (Fig. 12.2): (1) an outer *zona glomerulosa* where the cells are arranged in whorls and often have an acinar appearance in sections, (2) a *zona fasciculata* where the cells are arranged rather strictly in columns, and (3) an innermost *zona reticularis* where the cells are arranged in network fashion. Other zones, such as the X zone of

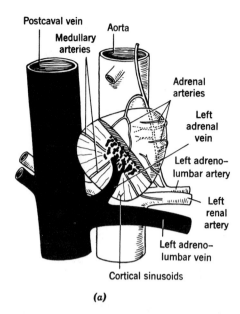

Postcaval vein

Aorta

Medullary arteries

Adrenal arteries

Left adrenal vein

Left adreno-lumbar artery

Left renal artery

Left adreno-lumbar vein

Cortical sinusoids

(a)

FIGURE 12.1. Circulation of the mammalian adrenal gland. (*a*) Diagram of the left adrenal of a normal rabbit with the lower half removed. Note direct blood supply to the medulla via the medullary arteries. Adrenaline administration causes constriction of these arteries, along with the rest of the blood vessels shown, resulting in a filling of the cortical sinusoids. Harrison suggests that these vascular changes account for the increased corticoid output seen after activation of the adrenal medulla. [Modified from R. G. Harrison, *J. Endocrinol.*, **15**:64, 1957.] (*b*) Cross section of an injection-corrosion preparation of the adrenal gland of the rhesus monkey. The fresh gland was perfused with a plastic compound, and the tissue was then dissolved away, leaving a complete replica of the vascular bed. Note the rich supply of cortical sinusoids emptying into the large medullary sinuses; two medullary arteries, which carry blood directly to the medulla from the adrenal arteries (not shown) have been exposed by removal of parts of the cortical vascular bed (*upper middle* and *upper right*). The blood vessels of the adrenal capsule are not shown. [From T. W. Williams and C. C. Boyer, *Stereo-Atlas of Microanatomy.*]

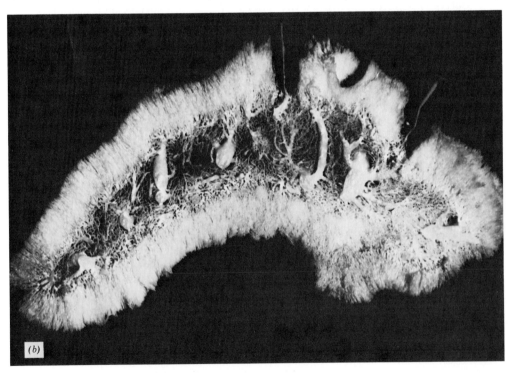

(b)

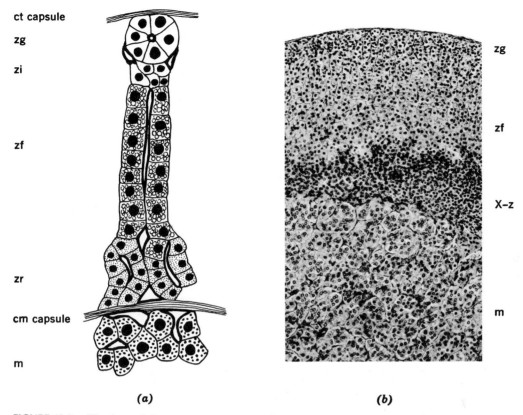

ct capsule	zg
zg	
zi	zf
zf	
	X–z
zr	
cm capsule	m
m	

(a)   **(b)**

FIGURE 12.2. Histology of the mammalian adrenal gland. (*a*) Diagram to show zonation of the adrenal cortex. Sinusoids are outlined by heavy black lines. (*b*) Section through the adrenal cortex of a male mouse (BALB/c strain), 1 month after castration at 3 months of age (× 120). X-zone of densely staining small cells has reappeared between the zona fasciculata and the medulla, in the region of the zona reticularis. *ct Capsule,* connective tissue capsule of adrenal gland; *cm capsule,* circummedullary connective tissue capsule separating the cortex from the medulla, penetrated by cortical sinusoids which drain into medullary venous sinuses; *m,* medulla of chromaffin cells arranged in lobules; *X-z,* X zone characteristic of mouse adrenal cortex in absence of androgen; *zf,* zona fasciculata, consisting of more or less vacuolated cells ("spongiocytes"); *zg,* zona glomerulosa, poorly defined in the mouse; *zi,* zona intermedia, prominent in the rat and other mammals, but not in the normal mouse; *zr,* zona reticularis (replaced by X zone in the castrated mouse).

the mouse, or the fetal zone, can be observed in the cortex of mammals before puberty or early in development. The *zona intermedia* is a variable feature that is located between the glomerulosa and fasciculata zones. The histological picture of the zonation of the cortex is due to differences in the staining properties of the steroidogenic cells in the respective zones. The glomerulosa cells are smaller and contain less lipid than the fasciculata cells. The reticularis cells are relatively small and have a densely staining cytoplasm.

The zones of the mammalian adrenal cortex can be further distinguished on the basis of functional criteria. The zona glomerulosa cells secrete aldosterone, the major mineralocorticoid hormone. Glucocorticoids are secreted by cells located in the fasciculata and reticularis zones. Apparently, the fasciculata and reticularis cells lack the enzyme responsible for the oxidation of steroids at carbon 18 (see Fig. 11.6) and therefore do not convert precursor steroids into aldosterone. The question of the origin of the different zones of the mammalian adrenal cortex is not entirely settled, although two theories have been proposed. In 1883 Gottschau suggested the escalator or "cell migration theory" in which zona glomerulosa cells divide and then migrate centrally toward the fasiculata and reticularis zones, where these cells assume the production of glucocorticoids. Alternatively, the "zonal theory," proposed by Swann, Sarason, Dean, and Greep in the 1940s, holds that cells in each zone can divide and develop steroid-synthesizing abilities that are characteristic of their zone of origin. It should be pointed out that these theories are not mutually exclusive, and there is evidence to support both. Cells that lie near the border of the glomerulosa and fasciculata zones show a high mitotic rate. Cells originating in this border area may migrate outward, to become mineralocorticoid-producing cells, or they may migrate inward to the fasciculata and reticularis zones. On the other hand, mitosis of cells has been observed in the zona reticularis. Interesting observations from *in vitro* studies of adrenocortical cells provide evidence regarding the maintenance of the steroid-synthesizing characteristics of the respective zones. Cultured zona glomerulosa cells quickly lose the capacity to secrete aldosterone and become like fasciculata and reticularis cells, which secrete glucocorticoids. This may be due to contamination of the cultured glomerulosa cells with fasciculata cells, since glucocorticoids from fasciculata cells may inhibit aldosterone production. Furthermore, treatment of the cultures with ACTH accelerates the conversion of mineralocorticoid-producing to glucocorticoid-producing cells. This observation is interesting in view of the direction of blood flow in the cortex from the glomerulosa to the inner zones. Thus the glomerulosa cells *in situ* are not exposed to high blood concentrations of glucocorticoids. Also, any cells that may migrate from the glomerulosa zone would quickly become converted to glucocorticoid producers.

In addition to the three cortical zones discussed above, other zones have been described in certain mammalian species. In the young laboratory mouse (1 or 2 weeks of age), there is a zone of small, densely staining cells in the area where the zona reticularis should be. This zone, which has a low lipid content, has been called the X zone (Fig. 12.2). The X zone disappears during the first pregnancy in female mice and on the attainment of sexual maturity in males. It has been suggested that the X zone may be the source of adrenal androgens in young mice. The disappearance of this zone can be slowed by castration and accelerated by injection of androgens in some species of mice. This evidence supports the idea that the X zone is maintained by a gonadotropic hormone, probably luteinizing hormone (LH), rather than ACTH. In several mammalian species, including humans, there is an extensive inner cortical layer that occupies the bulk of the gland in the fetus and neonate. This large inner zone, the *fetal zone*, is surrounded by a thin zone of cells, referred to as the *definitive zone*, which constitutes only about 20% of the volume of the adrenal cortex of the full-term fetus. The human fetal zone grows rapidly during the second and third trimester of pregnancy, so that at birth the adrenal gland is about the size of that of an 18-year-old. Most remarkably, the fetal adrenal gland may produce about four to five times the amount of steroid produced by an adult adrenal gland under unstressed conditions. The major steroids produced by the fetal zone are dehydroepiandrosterone (DHA) and dehydroepiandrosterone sulfate (DHAS; see Fig. 11.6). The production of these steroids may be dependent upon both ACTH from the fetal pituitary and human chorionic gonadotropin from the placenta. DHA and DHAS are secreted by the fetal zone into the fetal circulation, carried to the placenta, and converted to estrogens by steroid-metabolizing trophoblast cells in the placenta. The placenta is capable of removing the sulfate group from DHAS to form DHA, which is then converted to estriol, an important steroid for the maintenance of pregnancy. This system illustrates one interesting aspect of the function of the fetoplacental unit. The fetus supplies a significant amount of steroid precursors (DHA, DHAS), which are converted to estriol to maintain pregnancy. The fact that much of this steroid precursor is conjugated as a sulfate is important, since the unconjugated steroid could easily be converted to an androgenic steroid, which could have harmful consequences on the sexual differentiation of the fetus. Thus the fetus is protected from high androgen levels by metabolism of the steroid in the placenta, outside of the fetus.

Shortly after birth the fetal zone involutes, so that the adrenal size diminishes by about 50%. The fetal zone completely disappears within the first year or two after birth. The peripheral definitive zone of the cortex increases in size during the first few months after birth and continues to grow and differentiates into the three zones characteristic of the adult cortex.

In addition to helping maintain pregnancy by the secretion of precursor steroids for estriol synthesis, the fetal adrenal gland may provide a signal for the termination of pregnancy through secretion of glucocorticoids. In studies of sheep it has been shown that the fetal adrenal gland produces a rise of cortisol in the fetal circulation shortly before parturition. Infusions of cortisol or ACTH into the fetus can cause premature parturition. Whether

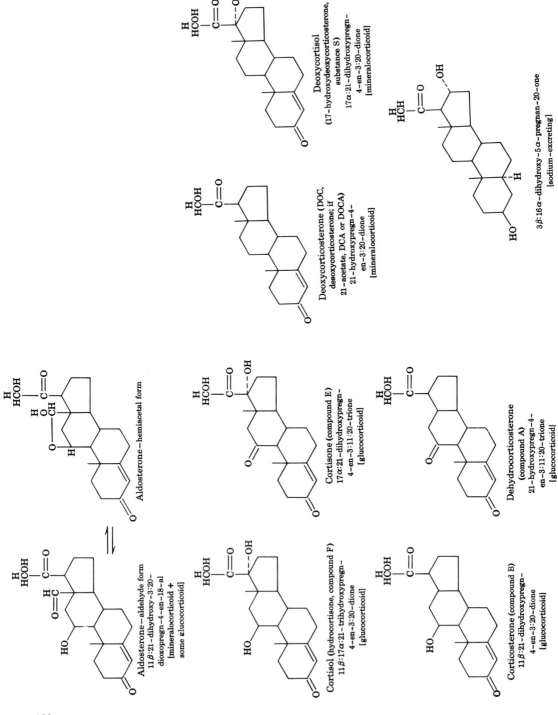

FIGURE 12.3. Structural formulae of some important corticosteroids. Common ("trivial") names, synonyms, and correct scientific names are given.

ACTH and cortisol are important for parturition in humans is not yet settled, although it has been observed that pregnancy is prolonged in women with anencephalic fetuses, which have a reduced capacity for pituitary ACTH release.

CORTICOSTEROID HORMONES

Glucocorticoids and Mineralocorticoids

The hormones from the adrenal cortex were classified by Selye as either glucocorticoids, regulating carbohydrate metabolism, or mineralocorticoids, regulating sodium metabolism. Glucocorticoids are characterized by having an oxygen ($=O$ or $-OH$ group) on carbon 11. Mineralocorticoids are 11-deoxy compounds (no oxygen on carbon 11). The best known glucocorticoids are cortisol, cortisone, and corticosterone (Fig. 12.3). Aldosterone and 11-deoxycorticosterone are the principal mineralocorticoids. However, there is some overlap in the activities of almost all of the naturally occurring corticosteroids. The adrenal cortex also secretes androgens, estrogens, and progestogens in some species, and these steroids may have important physiological functions. The differentiation between gluco- and mineralocorticoids is less meaningful to the comparative endocrinologist because this classification is based on steroid activities in mammals. In bony fishes, for example, cortisol appears quite active as a regulator of sodium ion exchange across the gill and could be considered as a mineralocorticoid.

Distribution of Corticosteroids

The study of the distribution of corticosteroids in vertebrates has been carried out in a relatively few representative species in each class. Still, enough species have been examined to allow some generalization. The definitive identification of steroids in animal blood is not a simple task. The most reliable data are obtained from studies in which extracts of plasma are subjected to a series of physicochemical tests, such as steroid crystallization, chromatography, and double-isotope derivative assay. Radioimmunoassay or simple chemical tests can often give incorrect results. Radioimmunoassay is a dependable method if it is coupled with some physical means (e.g., chromatography) of isolating the steroid of interest. One reason for the difficulty in identifying a steroid hormone in the blood is that blood may contain several steroids in a range of concentrations at the same time. This situation is further complicated by the fact that stressing an animal during blood sampling may change the relative amounts of the different circulating steroids. Despite these problems, the types of circulating corticosteroids in representative species of different vertebrate classes can be summarized (Table 12.1). The steroids included in Table 12.1 have been reliably identified

TABLE 12.1.   Major corticosteroids of vertebrates

Class	Corticosteroid in Blood
Agnatha (hagfish and lamprey)	Cortisol, 11-deoxycortisol, cortisone, corticosterone, 11-dehydrocorticosterone
Chondrichthyes	
Elasmobranchii (sharks and rays)	1α-Hydroxycorticosterone,[a] corticosterone, 11-deoxycorticosterone, 11-deoxycortisol
Holocephali (ratfish)	Cortisol
Osteichthyes (bony fishes)	Cortisol, cortisone, 11-deoxycortisol, corticosterone
Sarcopterygii	
Dipnoi (lungfish)	Cortisol, aldosterone, 11-deoxycortisol, corticosterone, 11-deoxycorticosterone
Amphibia	Corticosterone, 18-hydroxycorticosterone, aldosterone, 11-deoxycorticosterone, cortisol
Reptilia	Corticosterone, 18-hydroxycorticosterone, aldosterone
Aves	Corticosterone, aldosterone, 11-deoxycorticosterone
Mammalia	
Prototheria	Cortisol, corticosterone, aldosterone
Metatheria	Cortisol, 11-deoxycortisol, corticosterone, aldosterone
Eutheria	
Most orders	Cortisol, cortisone, corticosterone, 18-hydroxycorticosterone, aldosterone
Rodentia, Lagomorpha (some species)	Corticosterone, 18-hydroxycorticosterone, 11-deoxycorticosterone, 18-hydroxy-11-deoxycorticosterone, aldosterone

[a] Underlined steroids are the major corticosteroids secreted in that group. In the Agnatha, Holocephali, Dipnoi, and Prototheria not enough information is available for generalization.

in most species that have been examined in each class. Other steroids may be present in minor amounts in some species within a class. It has been suggested that if one looks hard enough and uses sensitive methods, one could probably find all of the natural steroids in species of all vertebrate classes. The remainder of this discussion will concentrate on the distribution of the steroids that appear to be of major significance within each vetebrate grouping.

Cortisol is the major corticoid of the fishes in general. In the jawless fishes (Agnatha) corticosteroid levels in the blood are relatively low. Furthermore, there is almost no information on the physiological actions of corticosteroids in hagfishes and lampreys. Therefore, it is difficult to determine which steroid is most important. An unusual feature of the elasmobranchs is the presence of high blood levels of 1α-hydroxycorticosterone. This steroid is not produced by adrenal tissue of other vertebrate classes, since they appear to lack the enzyme 1α-hydroxylase in their adrenal tissue. The 1α-hydroxylase enzyme is usually found in the kidney of other vertebrates, where it functions in the metabolism of vitamin D (see Chapter 7). 1α-Hydroxycorticosterone could not be found in the ratfish, which belongs to the other major subclass of the chondrichthyean fishes. The major mineralocorticoid of higher vertebrates, aldosterone, is typically absent or present in very low concentrations in the fishes. Interestingly, however, aldosterone has been shown to be present in significant quantities in the blood of at least one species of lungfishes, which are most closely related to the tetrapod vertebrates. Amphibians, reptiles, and birds are similar in that they have corticosterone as the major corticoid; aldosterone is also present in these groups, but its levels are usually low, except in amphibians. The adrenals of mammals secrete primarily cortisol, except for some species of rodents and rabbits, which secrete corticosterone.

Steroid Production

The most detailed information on the types of steroids secreted by the adrenals are available for mammals. The rates of production and plasma concentrations of steroids from the adult human adrenal glands are shown in Table 12.2. As in the fetus the major steroid secreted by the adult adrenal glands is DHAS. DHAS and DHA can be converted to more active androgens, and these, along with androstenedione and testosterone, form the

TABLE 12.2. Typical production rates and plasma levels of some adrenal steroids in a normal human adult

Steroid	Adrenal Production Rate (mg/day)	Plasma Concentration (ng/ml)
Cortisol	20	100
Cortisone	—	25
Corticosterone	2	5
11-Deoxycortisol	0.5	1
11-Deoxycorticosterone (DOC)	0.2	0.1
18-Hydroxycorticosterone	0.3	—
18-Hydroxy-11-deoxycorticosterone	0.1	—
Aldosterone	0.1	0.1
Dehydroepiandrosterone (DHA)	1.3	6
Dehydroepiandrosterone sulfate (DHAS)	20	1000
Androstenedione	0.5	1
Testosterone	0.01	0.5 (female)

majority of the circulating androgens in females. Most circulating androgens in males originate from the testes. In women adrenal androgens increase during puberty; they facilitate the growth of pubic hair and play a role in libidinal behavior (sex drive). After menopause, adrenal androgens are the main source of circulating estrogens. Adrenal androgens are of importance in several human pathologies. Adrenal tumors may produce high levels of androgens and cause hirsutism in women. Congenital adrenal hyperplasia is often due to enzymatic defects that cause excessive secretion of androgens in the fetus. These androgens may adversely affect sex differentiation and cause pseudohermaphroditism and ambiguous external genitalia.

The major glucocorticoid secreted by the human adrenal glands is cortisol. Minor amounts of corticosterone and 11-deoxycortisol are also released. Significant amounts of cortisone are found in the circulation. Cortisone has about 70% of the glucocorticoid activity of cortisol. It is unclear how much cortisone is produced by the adrenal cortex, but it is likely that most circulating cortisone arises from the peripheral metabolism of cortisol.

The major mineralocorticoids—found in about equal amounts in the human circulation—are deoxycorticosterone (DOC) and aldosterone. DOC is a potent mineralocorticoid and has about one-thirtieth the activity of aldosterone. However, much of the circulating DOC is bound to corticosteroid-binding globulin (CBG), while most of the aldosterone is free. Therefore, aldosterone is the most important mineralocorticoid in mammals physiologically.

The rates of production of steroids by the human adrenal are not exactly proportional to the concentrations in the blood. This is due to different rates of clearance of steroids from the plasma. Cortisol which has a high affinity for CBG is cleared from the plasma slowly (half life of 90 minutes) while aldosterone is removed rapidly from the blood (half life of 8 minutes).

PHYSIOLOGICAL EFFECTS OF CORTICOSTEROIDS IN MAMMALS

The actions of glucocorticoids in mammals may be categorized as metabolic or developmental. Some of the metabolic activities include gluconeogenesis, lipolysis, and protein breakdown. Among the developmental effects are differentiation of the neural retina and mammary gland and induction of surfactants in the fetal lung. In many of these glucocorticoid actions other hormones are the principal actors against the background of basal levels of glucocorticoids. Thus glucocorticoids are often thought of as having a "permissive" role in actions of other hormones.

Metabolism

One of the consequences of adrenalectomy in mammals is the inability to maintain blood glucose and tissue glycogen levels during such a stress as fasting. This is due to the lack of glucocorticoids, which promote the breakdown of proteins and fats, which, in turn, are converted into carbohydrates (gluconeogenesis). In the liver cortisol stimulates enzymes involved in the conversion of glucose and precursors of glucose to glycogen (see Chapter 15); at the same time, it inhibits the activities of enzymes involved in the breakdown of glucose. Cortisol also induces the breakdown of proteins in the liver, skeletal muscle, and lymphoid tissue. The resulting amino acids can be converted to pyruvate or oxaloacetate, which are substrates for the synthesis of glucose and the subsequent formation of glycogen. This catabolic effect of glucocorticoids on proteins results in an increase in urinary nitrogen excretion. Additional substrates for glucose synthesis are provided by cortisol's lipolytic action. Cortisol mobilizes fatty acids and inhibits the uptake of glucose by adipose tissue. Glucocorticoids also inhibit glucose, amino acid, and nucleotide uptake in fibroblasts, leukocytes, skin, and bone. In general, the metabolic activity of glucocorticoids results in provision of energy in the form of a readily usable carbohydrate (glycogen) at the expense of anabolic activities of various peripheral tissues.

Any consideration of hormonal control of intermediary metabolism must include the synergistic and permissive actions of hormone combinations. Lipolysis and fatty acid mobilization in adipose tissue stimulated by growth hormone and catecholamines are dependent on the presence of low levels of glucocorticoids. The calorigenic effects of catecholamines and glucagon also require glucocorticoids. The multihormonal control of intermediary metabolism is considered in detail in Chapter 15.

The mechanism of glucocorticoid action appears to be typical of steroid hormones. The corticoid binds to a cytoplasmic receptor that is translocated to the nucleus, where gene transcription takes place to provide RNA for protein synthesis. Most of the glucocorticoid effects can be blocked by the use of protein synthesis inhibitors such as actinomycin D. Interestingly, this mechanism is involved even in those tissues where glucocorticoids have what could be considered inhibitory effects. The glucocorticoid-evoked inhibition of glucose and amino acid uptake by lymphoid tissue and skin is associated with inhibition of RNA synthesis. This inhibition occurs only after stimulation of RNA and protein synthesis directed by corticoids.

Development

Corticosteroid effects on development have received increasing attention in recent years. Glucocorticoids have been shown to induce the expression of the enzyme glutamine synthetase in the neural retina of the chick. This is of interest because it is an example of genetic derepression by glucocorticoids allowing for the synthesis of a new product rather than an increase in the rate of expression of a gene product in an already differentiated cell. A similar differentiative effect of glucocorticoids is apparent in the mammary gland. The growth and differentiation of the mammary gland is a multihormonal phenomenon involving insulin and prolactin as well as glucocorticoids. Insulin promotes mammary epithelial cell proliferation, while prolactin and cortisol are responsible for gene expression allowing the synthesis of milk. Cortisol is important for the differentiation of mammary epithelial cells. Glucocorticoids stimulate the synthesis of both DNA and RNA in the mammary gland.

The developmental effects of corticosteroids on the fetal lung involve differentiation of pulmonary epithelial cells and the synthesis and secretion of surfactant by these cells. The surfactant reduces the surface tension in pulmonary alveoli so that individual alveolar sacs will retain their expanded state when the lungs are inflated. The deposition of surfactant in the lining of the lung occurs during the last trimester of pregnancy, a period when the circulating levels of corticosteroids in the fetus are increasing. This is an interesting example of economy in the endocrine system—the use of increasing corticosteroid levels for the final differentiation of the lung and the termination of pregnancy (see above). Unfortunately, in premature delivery the surfactant levels in the lungs often are not sufficient, and a condition known as *respiratory distress syndrome* may occur. In mothers for whom premature delivery is anticipated, glucocorticoid treatment reduces the incidence of respiratory distress syndrome in the newborn if treatment is given at least one day before delivery. Glucocorticoid administration to the newborn is not effective.

Salt Metabolism

The principal mineralocorticoid of mammals is aldosterone, which favors the retention of sodium ions and the excretion of potassium and hydrogen ions. Aldosterone accomplishes the regulation of ion balance by acting variously on the kidneys, intestine, sweat glands, and salivary glands. Aldosterone's primary site of action in the kidney appears to be on the distal convoluted tubule of the nephron, although there are reports that the proximal convoluted tubule may be sensitive to aldosterone also (Fig. 12.4). Aldosterone increases the active transport of sodium from the urine in the tubular lumen across the tubular epithelial cells to the blood plasma. The amount of sodium that may be reabsorbed by the distal tubule in response to aldosterone may represent only about 20% of the total amount of sodium taken up by the nephron from the filtrate produced by the glomerulus. Thus the action of aldosterone on sodium reabsorption can be considered as a "fine-tuning" mechanism for the precise regulation of blood sodium. This is not to say that aldosterone is not important. Hypoaldosteronism is associated with symptoms of hyponatremia and hyperkalemia such as abnormal cardiac rhythms, muscular weakness, paralysis, and hypotension. The ultimate consequence of excessive sodium loss is complete circulatory collapse. Excessive aldosterone levels in the blood (aldosteronism) cause loss of potassium, excessive retention of sodium, increased blood volume, increased extracellular volume, high peripheral vascular resistance, and hypertension. Aldosterone excess causes a high blood pH (alkalosis), while aldosterone deficiency produces acidosis. These actions may be due to the steroid effect

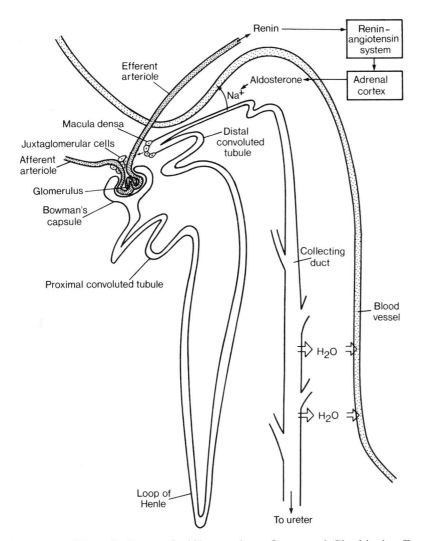

FIGURE 12.4. Schematic diagram of a kidney nephron of a mammal. Blood in the afferent arteriole enters the glomerulus of Bowman's capsule, where an ultrafiltrate of the blood plasma is formed. The ultrafiltrate passes through the proximal convoluted tubule, loop of Henle, and distal convoluted tubule. Some substances (including ions) in the ultrafiltrate are transported out of the tubule in these segments, while other substances (e.g., H^+, K^+) may be excreted into the ultrafiltrate by tubular epithelial cells. The ultrafiltrate (now called urine) is passed into the collecting duct where it is combined with urine from other nephrons to be passed to the bladder by way of the ureter. The juxtaglomerular (JG) cells are situated around the afferent arteriole. The macula densa consists of specialized cells surrounding a small portion of the distal tubule. (The macula densa is closer to the JG cells than is indicated in the figure). Low levels of sodium in the fluid in the distal tubule signal the macula densa to stimulate the release of renin by the JG cells. Renin acts on angiotensinogen in the blood to generate angiotensin, which stimulates aldosterone secretion. Aldosterone promotes sodium uptake by the distal tubule. Sodium reenters the blood through diffusional processes. Water may be transported from the urine to the blood by the action of arginine vasopressin on the collecting duct (see Chapter 3).

on acid secretion by the kidney tubule. Since aldosterone has a very minor role in the physiological regulation of acid–base balance, the hormone's influence on hydrogen ion secretion will not be considered in detail.

Regarding sodium transport, the mechanism of action of aldosterone on the epithelial cells of the distal tubule of the nephron is typical of a steroid; a cytoplasmic receptor is bound by the hormone and translocated to the nucleus for DNA transcription and synthesis of RNA and proteins. The synthesized proteins may be involved in regulating the sodium pump activity in the cell membrane, causing an increase in sodium permeability or providing additional energy (ATP) to run the sodium pump. As might be expected from this model, inhibitors of RNA or protein synthesis block the action of aldosterone on sodium uptake. In contrast, aldosterone stimulation of potassium or hydrogen ion secretion is not blocked by inhibitors of RNA or protein synthesis. Apparently, the mechanism for the excretion of these ions is unlike that for sodium reabsorption.

In addition to promoting sodium retention by the kidney, aldosterone stimulates sodium uptake from the feces along the large intestine and decreases the amount of sodium in the secretions of sweat glands and salivary glands. Clearly, aldosterone has a widespread sodium-conserving action in the body.

In evaluating the role of mineralocorticoids in the control of salt metabolism and the associated movement of water, one should be aware of other factors that influence ion movements and cell permeability. Principal among these is the neurohypophyseal factor vasopressin, or ADH (Chapter 3), and mineralocorticoid function must be considered in relationship to ADH function. ADH increases water permeability in the epithelial cells of the collecting ducts of the kidney nephron (Fig. 12.4). This allows water to be drawn out of the urine in the ductal lumen into the high-sodium environment of the renal extracellular space. Aldosterone regulation of sodium levels in the body affects ADH-mediated water reabsorption by the collecting ducts.

Other Effects of Corticosteroids

Glucocorticoids affect calcium metabolism through actions on the intestine and the skeletal system. Cortisol inhibits calcium uptake in the proximal region of the small intestine. This may be accomplished through the antagonism of vitamin D action on the gut (Chapter 7). Cortisol also induces osteoporosis or calcium resorption from bones. Patients suffering from Cushing's syndrome (high blood cortisol) for long periods of time often lose height as a result of osteoporotic collapse of the vertebral column. Bone fracture may be very common in Cushing's syndrome patients. Calcium loss into the urine may also be facilitated by cortisol.

A consequence of the catabolic action of glucocorticoids on proteins is atrophy of the skin in Cushing's syndrome. Cortisol favors the breakdown of collagen and the mucoprotein matrix of connective tissue. The skin is thin and may be marked by purple striae as a result of excess cortisol.

One of the most important pharmacologic uses of glucocorticoids is in the reduction of inflammation. Cortisol or synthetic glucocorticoids inhibit swelling by reducing histamine release and the vascular transudation of fluid. Corticosteroids reduce the movement of leukocytes into the area of the wound and block phagocytic activity. Glucocorticoids inhibit the production of kinins and prostaglandins, which are local chemical mediators of early events in swelling, pain, and leukocyte infiltration during inflammation. Subsequent events involve the release by lysosomes of proteolytic enzymes that digest dead or dying cells in the wound. Cortisol stabilizes lysosomal membranes and prevents liberation of their enzymes. Finally, glucocorticoids inhibit fibroblast growth and proliferation and the deposition of collagen during repair of the wound. Because of their potent anti-inflammatory actions, corticosteroids have been used extensively in medicine to treat a wide variety of problems. However, the use of exogenous corticosteroids can be dangerous. The prevention of inflammation counteracts the normal biological response of isolation and destruction of material (bacteria) in a wound, followed by repair. In other words, the pharmacologic use of corticosteroids ameliorates symptoms but does not correct the cause of inflammation. Thus infections may be allowed to spread without the usual indications of their spreading.

Inadvertantly promoting the spread of infection by the clinical use of corticosteroids is an example of iatrogenic or physician-induced disease. Long-term (months or years) treatment with corticosteroids can increase susceptibility to disease by suppressing the immune system. The exogenously administered glucocorticoid may suppress the secretion of ACTH and cause adrenal atrophy, so that glucocorticoid secretion is insufficient when the steroid treatment is discontinued. Corticosteroid treatment may disturb intermediary metabolism. Long-term treatment may cause muscular weakness as a result of protein catabolism. Corticosteroids elevate blood glucose levels by their actions on carbohydrate metabolism. High blood glucose stimulates insulin release. Over long periods of time, diabetes mellitus can be induced because of the inability of pancreatic β cells to maintain high rates of insulin production or because of decreased sensitivity of peripheral tissues to insulin action. Bone disorders may also develop during long-term glucocorticoid therapy. Clearly, patients receiving glucocorticoids for extended periods should be monitored carefully.

EFFECTS OF CORTICOSTEROIDS IN NONMAMMALIAN VERTEBRATES

Fishes

In vertebrates corticosteroids exert a wide range of physiological actions—from osmo- or ionoregulation to migratory behavior. Many of the steroid actions are accomplished through permissive or synergistic relations with other hormones, particularly ADH and prolactin.

Little is known about the function of corticosteroids in cyclostomes. Low and variable levels of corticosteroids are present in the blood of both hagfishes and lampreys, and these animals respond to ACTH by elevating their circulating levels of corticoids. Hagfishes maintained in 60% seawater show shifts in the body distribution of sodium in response to deoxycorticosterone or aldosterone. The significance of this observed reduction in tissue sodium is difficult to evaluate, since hagfishes normally live in 100% seawater and do not regulate blood sodium or potassium.

Lampreys either live in fresh water or migrate between fresh water and the sea. Treatment of lampreys in fresh water with aldosterone, but not with cortisol, reduces their sodium loss. This suggests a sodium-conserving role for corticosteroids, although aldosterone has not been identified in lampreys and there is no information on circulating levels of corticosteroids in lampreys in fresh water versus seawater.

Elasmobranchs are predominantly seawater residents that maintain high blood osmolarity by the production of urea and trimethylamine oxide. Therefore, blood ions are regulated against an environmental concentration gradient but not an osmotic gradient. Blood sodium and water concentration are controlled by the actions of the gills, kidney, and a salt-excreting rectal gland. The major corticosteroid 1α-hydroxycorticosterone, stimulates fluid and sodium excretion by the rectal gland. Little is known about corticosteroid actions on the kidney or gill, although gill cells appear to have a cytosolic protein that binds 1α-hydroxycorticosterone. It is interesting that in fishes and, as we shall see, in some other vertebrates, corticosteroids have a salt excreting-action rather than a salt-conserving action, as they do in mammals. The evidence for corticosteroid action on carbohydrate metabolism is contradictory. It has been suggested that corticosteroids may be important in regulating lipid metabolism in elasmobranchs.

Much interest has been focused on the function of corticosteroids in teleosts. However, it is difficult to generalize for this group, since the effects of corticosteroids seem to vary in different species. The goldfish (*Carassius auratus*) and the anadromous eel (*Anguilla sp.*) have received the most attention. Osmoregulation and ionoregulation in teleosts is accomplished by the activities of the gill, gut, kidney, and urinary bladder. All of these structures appear to be influenced by cortisol.

Freshwater teleosts tend to lose ions and gain water through the gills and skin. These challenges to salt and water balance are counteracted by the intake of salt across the gut, gills, and urinary bladder. Cortisol stimulates sodium uptake in these tissues in fish in fresh water. The pituitary hormone prolactin facilitates adaptation to fresh water by decreasing the water permeability of the skin, gills, gut, and urinary bladder. The prolactin effect on some of these tissues appears to be dependent on the simultaneous presence of cortisol. The coordinated actions of prolactin and cortisol allow the uptake of sodium without the diluting effects of water, which might follow the sodium ions across the membranes of the transporting tissues.

Marine teleosts are in an environment in which they tend to lose water, since seawater is hyperosmotic in relation to their body fluids. Seawater-adapted fishes must maintain body water by removing the salts from ingested seawater. To accomplish this, sodium is taken up across the gut, and water follows passively. Since fishes in seawater have low levels of prolactin, the gut is permeable to water. The sodium that is taken up across the gut is pumped out through the gill. Cortisol stimulates sodium transport inward across the gut (as it does in freshwater-adapted fishes) and also outward across the gill. It is interesting that cortisol stimulates sodium uptake by the gills of fishes in fresh water, while it stimulates sodium excretion by the gills of fishes in seawater. The mechanism of this reversal in the direction of sodium transport by the gill is poorly understood.

This description of corticosteroid control of osmoregulation is based primarily on studies of three species of *Anguilla*. Other teleosts certainly have different endocrine control mechanisms for osmoregulation, although the information is not as complete as for anguillids.

Studies of fishes adapted to either fresh water or seawater for long periods have shown little difference in the circulating cortisol levels. However, in fishes in seawater both the production rate and the plasma clearance rate of cortisol are elevated. When eels are transferred from fresh water to seawater, there is an elevation of plasma cortisol for several days. Transfer of eels from seawater to fresh water has no affect on plasma cortisol levels. The situation, apparently, is different for another euryhaline teleost, *Sarotherodon mossambicus*. Transfer of this fish from seawater to fresh water or vice versa causes a transient rise in blood cortisol. Presumably, the sensitivity and responses of the various cortisol target organs change in fishes under conditions of different environmental salinity. These aspects of corticosteroid function in teleosts are largely unexplored.

The metabolic effects of cortisol in teleosts appear to be similar to those in mammals. Cortisol produces hyperglycemia and maintains liver glycogen levels in bony fishes. It also has a catabolic effect on proteins. Perhaps the most striking example of the metabolic actions of cortisol in fishes is that of the Pacific salmon in its spawning migration. Pacific salmon stop eating long before they arrive at the spawning grounds. The interrenal gland is activated, and plasma cortisol levels increase sixfold. Cortisol promotes the breakdown of body proteins (skeletal muscle), thus providing enough substrate for gluconeogenesis so that the liver glycogen content may double. This glucocorticoid-directed alteration in protein and carbohydrate metabolism provides ample energy for reproduction, which is the final effort in the life of the Pacific salmon.

Amphibians

Mineralocorticoids promote sodium transport primarily in the amphibian skin and urinary bladder. Amphibians take up water from their environment across the skin. This inward transport of water depends on the transepithelial osmotic gradient. Active uptake of sodium across the skin increases this gradient and increases water flow into the animal. As we have seen in Chapter 3, the water permeability of frog skin depends on the presence of arginine vasotocin (AVT). Therefore, maximal transport of water across the skin occurs in the presence of both mineralocorticoids and AVT.

The amphibian urinary bladder serves as a water reservoir to be used when the animal is in a desiccating environment. Again, as we have discussed in Chapter 3, water in the urinary bladder is made available for regulation of blood and extracellular volume by the action of AVT. The urinary bladder may be called upon to replenish blood sodium levels as well. Mineralocorticoids stimulate the transport of sodium out of the urinary bladder and thereby reduce urinary sodium levels. Furthermore, mineralocorticoids can acidify the urine by promoting hydrogen ion secretion by the urinary bladder. The mechanisms of mineralocorticoid action on sodium uptake and hydrogen ion secretion appear similar to those in the distal tubule of the mammalian kidney. Aldosterone-mediated sodium uptake requires the synthesis of RNA and proteins, while hydrogen ion secretion seems to be independent of these events. This similarity between the mammalian distal tubule and the amphibian urinary bladder, together with the relative ease of experimenting with the urinary bladder, has made the urinary bladder a popular model for studying mineralocorticoid effects on ion transport. The urinary bladder is of interest in a phylogenetic sense because it is the first tissue to show a differentiation between the mineralocorticoid and glucocorticoid activities of steroids. Aldosterone is more potent than corticosterone or cortisol in inducing sodium transport in frogs.

Some studies of frog tadpoles have shown that aldosterone is not active in promoting sodium or water retention, while cortisol and corticosterone are effective. Other studies have shown that aldosterone levels in the blood of bullfrog tadpoles are low or nondetectable but that both cortisol and corticosterone are present in approximately equal concentrations. These observations have led to the suggestion that there may be shifts in the types of corticosteroids produced and in the effects of mineralocorticoids during amphibian metamorphosis.

The metabolic activities of corticosteroids in frogs appear to be similar to those in mammals. Glucocorticoids elevate blood sugar levels and tend to increase liver and muscle glycogen levels. Presumably, these responses to glucocorticoids have some relationship to protein anabolism and lipolysis in amphibians. Not a great deal is known about the metabolic effects of steroids working in association with other metabolic hormones in amphibians. Changes in corticosteroid activities during different seasons and during metamorphosis require further study.

Reptiles

Of all the major classes of gnathostome vertebrates in which corticosteroid function has been studied, reptiles have received the least attention. Despite this fact, reptiles are an important group in the overview of the evolution of mineralocorticoid function. The reptiles were the first completely terrestrial vertebrates, and they are the first to have a metanephric kidney. Thus they face a great need for salt and water regulation, and, compared to amphibians, the reptilian kidney may take on a more important role in osmoregulation. On the other hand, such extrarenal sites of electrolyte excretion as nasal or orbital salt glands evolved with the reptiles.

The activity of the reptilian adrenal glands may vary with the season and may be associated with changes in temperature, hibernation, and reproductive state. Reptiles have exploited such a wide variety of habitats that corticosteroid actions which may be important to a desert lizard may not be physiologically significant to a freshwater turtle. These considerations, and the fact that relatively few reptilian species have been studied, make it difficult to generalize about corticosteroid function in reptiles.

Salt and water balance in reptilian species may be regulated by the kidney, urinary bladder, cloaca, and nasal salt glands. In responsive species corticosteroids favor the retention of salt and water by the kidney. In the terrestrial tortoise *Testudo*, plasma levels of aldosterone decrease after loading the animal with salt and increase after administration of a diuretic. This suggests that circulating aldosterone is physiologically significant in the control of salt and water balance. Interestingly, in the snake *Natrix* aldosterone stimulates sodium uptake by the proximal tubule of the kidney nephron. It has been suggested that the proximal tubule may be the primitive site of steroid action on the kidney. Perhaps during the evolution of the mammalian kidney, with its long loop of Henle and important distal convoluted tubule, the major site of corticosteroid action switched from the proximal to the distal segment.

Little evidence is available on corticosteroid control of the cloaca. It appears that aldosterone stimulates sodium transport out of the bladder and into the blood at least in the turtle. In marine or desert reptiles the nasal gland may be responsible for most of the salt excretion by the animal. In the nasal gland it appears that both acetylcholine and corticosteroids work together to promote the excretion of fluid containing sodium and chloride.

The role of corticosteroids in controlling the intermediary metabolism of reptiles has received little attention. However, there is evidence that steroid action is similar to that of other vertebrates. Corticosteroids cause hyperglycemia, increase liver glycogen, and may have a catabolic effect on proteins.

Birds

As in other vertebrates, corticosteroids in birds function to control salt balance and some metabolic activities. The importance of corticosteroids in the regulation of electrolytes in avian species is reflected by the fact that the adrenal gland in marine birds is larger than in birds living in terrestrial or freshwater habitats. The adrenals have been implicated in the reproduction and migration of birds, since the size of the gland may vary seasonally in accordance with these activities. Additionally, corticosteroids may have immunosuppressive activities in birds, since they cause involution of the bursa of Fabricius, which is one of the avian lymphoid organs.

Although few studies of the effects of corticosteroids on the bird kidney have been made, it is clear that in the duck cortisol decreases sodium excretion and increases potassium excretion by the kidney. As in reptiles, the nasal gland in marine birds in particular is an important site of salt excretion. Nasal gland function in birds is regulated by parasympathetic innervation (acetylcholine) and by corticosteroids. Cortisol and corticosterone are potent stimulators of salt excretion by the nasal gland of the duck; aldosterone appears less effective in this regard.

Administration of corticosteroids causes hyperglycemia and fat deposition in birds. The effect on fat deposition is important, particularly in migratory birds. The possibility that corticosteroids play a role in the migration and premigratory fattening of birds may be an example of the economical use of a hormone for several coincidental physiological processes.

CONTROL OF ADRENOCORTICAL FUNCTION

Adrenocortical function is under the control of two major systems: one system regulates the glucocorticoids, while the other controls the release of mineralocorticoid. The release of glucocorticoids by the zona fasciculata and zona reticularis is under the influence of pituitary adrenocorticotrophin (ACTH), which, in turn, is controlled by the hypothalamic factor (or factors) termed *corticotrophin-releasing factor* (CRF). The activity of the CRF–ACTH axis is regulated by a negative feedback system, so that high levels of circulating glucocorticoids, which are induced by ACTH, act on the hypothalamus and/or pituitary to inhibit the further release of ACTH. Although the production of aldosterone by the zona glomerulosa may be influenced to some degree by ACTH, the major regulators of mineralocorticoid release are the renin–angiotensin system (RAS) and plasma potassium levels. The peptide precursor of angiotensin is produced by the liver and released into the blood circulation where it is converted to angiotensin by the enzyme renin, which is produced by the kidney. Under an appropriate stimulus, such as low blood sodium, renin is released by the kidney to elevate blood levels of angiotensin, which stimulates the production of aldosterone by the zona glomerulosa.

The patterns of change in circulating levels of glucocorticoids may be divided into three categories: (1) diurnal rhythms, (2) episodic release, and (3) stress-related release. The basal levels (unstressed condition) of glucocorticoids are known to fluctuate during a 24-hour period. In humans, basal glucocorticoids in the blood are highest between 3:00 and 8:00 in the morning and lowest between 6:00 in the evening and midnight. In such nocturnal animals as the rat this diurnal rhythm is shifted so that the lowest levels of glucocorticoids occur between 8:00 in the morning and 4:00 in the afternoon. Therefore, it appears that basal glucocorticoids are highest toward the end of the sleep cycle, just before and during the time when the greatest daily activity begins. Studies of the diurnal rhythm of glucocorticoids in humans suggest that the cycle is not entrained by feeding or sleep–wakefulness cycles, and the rhythm does not appear to be affected by stress. On the other hand, studies of the first appearance of daily glucocorticoid fluctuations in young rat pups indicate that the rhythm first develops in relation to feeding cycles rather than to light–dark cycles. Regardless of the mechanism of entrainment of the cycles, it is clear that some environmental clues are important. When a person travels to a significantly different time zone, as may be encountered after an overseas flight, it takes about 5 to 10 days for the circadian corticosteroid rhythm to shift its pattern to correspond to the new time.

The endocrine mechanism responsible for the circadian rhythm in glucocorticoids includes the brain, pituitary, and adrenal glands. It is believed that the biological clock controlling the cycle lies somewhere in the central nervous system outside of the hypothalamus. The concentration of ACTH in the pituitary gland and the secretion of ACTH into the blood varies according to the cycle. Thus the elevation of blood levels of glucocorticoids is due to stimulation of the adrenal by ACTH. An additional factor contributing to the diurnal fluctuation is the adrenal gland's sensitivity to ACTH, which is greatest at the time of the highest level of circulating glucocorticoid. The heightened sensitivity of the adrenal to ACTH may be an intrinsic property of the gland, since it is not influenced by denervation of the gland or by varying the pattern of previous exposure to exogenous ACTH. Although the diurnal pattern is not influenced by elevated glucocorticoid levels resulting from stress, there is no diurnal pattern in patients with high blood glucocorticoid levels resulting from Cushing's disease. Although most of the studies of circadian rhythms of glucocorticoid release have been done in mammals, such rhythms have been observed in birds, reptiles, and fishes. This suggests that daily rhythms of interrenal activity may be a common occurrence in vertebrates.

Episodic releases of corticoids are the relatively brief fluctuations of blood levels of the steroids that can be observed in humans if blood is sampled every five minutes. The function of these small fluctuations is not known; however, they appear to be a result of minute-to-minute changes in the rate of steroid secretion by the adrenal gland. Episodic release occurs for both glucocorticoids and mineralocorticoids. Furthermore, the episodic changes of the two types of adrenal steroids are synchronized in time. Episodic release of glucocorticoids can be prevented by the administration of dexamethasone, which is a potent inhibitor of ACTH release. Episodic release of mineralocorticoids can be eliminated by denervation of the kidney, a maneuver that eliminates the stimulation of mineralocorticoid release by the renin-angiotensin system. The evidence that episodic releases of glucocorticoids and mineralocorticoids are synchronized but can be eliminated independently implies that this type of release is controlled by the central nervous system acting through the hypothalamo-hypophyseal axis for glucocorticoids, and through the renin–angiotensin system for mineralocorticoids.

The release of glucocorticoids during stress results in rather high circulating levels of glucocorticoids, which may last for several hours or longer. These large outpourings of corticosteroids may occur within minutes after an acute stress. Chronic stress may result in a sustained elevation of blood corticosteroid levels. The significance of stress-related secretion of corticosteroids will be discussed later in connection with Selye's general adaptation syndrome.

CRF–ACTH

The control of adrenal function by ACTH has received much attention. The action of ACTH may be considered either trophic or steroidogenic. The trophic action refers to the ability of ACTH to maintain the size and differentiated state of the adrenal gland. ACTH stimulates cell division and supports the synthesis of protein and nucleic acids and the multiplication of mitochondria in adrenal cells.

The steroidogenic action of ACTH involves increasing the levels of precursors for steroid synthesis and the synthesis and activation of enzymes in pathways leading to the formation of steroid hormone molecules. ACTH binds to its membrane receptor on adrenal cells and causes an elevation of intracellular cyclic AMP. Calcium ions are required for this initial action of ACTH. The availability of free cholesterol within the adrenal cell is increased by the activation of cholesterol esterase, which liberates cholesterol from its storage in liposomes. ACTH facilitates the uptake of circulating cholesterol that is bound to low-density lipoproteins (LDL) in the blood by increasing the number of LDL receptors on the adrenal cell membrane. Specific enzymes that are activated by ACTH include those for cholesterol side-chain cleavage, 3β-hydroxysteroid dehydrogenase, and 11- and 18-hydroxylases, among others. Although the understanding of the mechanisms of ACTH actions in nonmammalian vertebrates is not as detailed as for mammals, the available information suggests that similar mechanisms are present in all vertebrates—from cyclostomes through birds. An interesting aspect that deserves additional study is the possible synergistic effect of other hormones on ACTH action. Prolactin may be involved in the regulation of steroidogenesis by maintaining the levels of steroid precursors in adrenal cells. Recent evidence indicates that LPH and endorphin, which are hormones of the same molecular family as ACTH (see Fig. 4.1), may potentiate the action of ACTH.

The release of ACTH by the pituitary is controlled by hypothalamic CRF.

The identity of the physiological CRF is not entirely settled. Extracts of hypothalamic tissue contain at least three substances that elicit the release of ACTH. The smallest of these substances is arginine vasopressin, the antidiuretic hormone of the pars nervosa. Most researchers doubt the physiological significance of the ACTH-releasing activity of vasopressin. However, it may be premature to discount the significance of this activity, since vasopressin from the pars nervosa may gain access to ACTH cells in the pars distalis through retrograde blood flow from the pars nervosa to the hypothalamus and then back to the pars distalis of the pituitary. Direct release of vasopressin into hypophyseal portal blood may occur, since vasopressin has been shown to be present in the external layer of the median eminence of the hypothalamus. Furthermore, Zimmerman and colleagues (1973) have shown vasopressin to be present in the hypophyseal portal blood of a monkey at concentrations that would be sufficient to induce release of ACTH. If vasopressin by itself is not a functional CRF, it is likely that it potentiates the effect of the authentic CRF.

The other hypothalamic substances with CRF activity are larger than vasopressin. The amino acid sequence of the smaller of these substances from sheep hypothalamus has been determined by Vale and colleagues (Fig. 12.5). Interestingly, this putative CRF also releases β-endorphin from the pituitary. Further work will be necessary to confirm the physiological significance of this CRF. The CRF peptide, which Vale's group has characterized is structurally related to a 40–amino acid peptide—sauvagine—which has been isolated from frog skin, and to urotensin I, which is a peptide present in the urophysis of fishes.

The release of CRF and/or ACTH is subject to feedback inhibition by glucocorticoids. This negative feedback in some mammals has been divided into two components. One component is a fast or rate-sensitive mechanism, while the other is a slower-acting, proportional type of control. These mechanisms can be demonstrated by imposing a stress on an animal and measuring the secretory response of the adrenal in the presence or absence of high, constant levels of glucocorticoids, which may be infused into the animal's bloodstream. The untreated animal responds to stress quickly with a high elevation of blood glucocorticoids. If a large amount of cortisol is infused into an animal within 5 minutes before a stress is applied, the secretion of glucocorticoids in response to a stress can be eliminated almost entirely. However, if the same amount of cortisol is infused over a period of 5 to 20 minutes, there is no inhibition of glucocorticoid release in response to stress. This demonstrates the rate-sensitive feedback mechanism that monitors rapid increases in blood glucocorticoids to inhibit ACTH release in response to stress. The proportional feedback mechanism can be shown by another experiment. Cortisol is infused into the blood of an animal at a slowly increasing rate, so that an elevated circulating level is attained after 20 minutes. This high blood level of cortisol is then maintained constantly for 20 minutes to several hours. During this period the animal is stressed, and

Ser-Gln-Glu-Pro-Pro-Ile-Ser-Leu-Asp-Leu-Thr-Phe-His-Leu-Leu-Arg-Glu-Val-Leu-Glu-Met-Thr-Lys-Ala-Asp-Gln–

10 20

Leu-Ala-Gln-Gln-Ala-His-Ser-Asn-Arg-Lys-Leu-Leu-Asp-Ile-Ala

30 40

FIGURE 12.5. The amino acid sequence of a corticotropin-releasing factor isolated from sheep hypothalamic tissue. [From Vale et al. *Science* **213**:1374, 1981.]

the response of the adrenal is measured. The results show that there is no inhibition of the stress response in the presence of high circulating cortisol until 2 hours after the infusion was begun. Thus the feedback inhibition of the stress response by high, constant levels of cortisol is delayed by about 2 hours. The details of these two types of mechanisms are poorly understood. However, it is suspected that there are separate hypothalamic sensors for circulating glucocorticoids, since corticosterone and cortisol exert both fast and delayed feedback actions, while deoxycorticosterone and 11-deoxycortisol are active in delayed feedback only. It is speculated that the fast, rate-sensitive feedback mechanism is responsible for the control of ACTH release during acute stress and that the delayed, level-sensitive feedback mechanism is important in regulating the basal activity of the pituitary–adrenal axis. Negative feedback is operative in the pituitary–adrenal axis of nonmammalian vertebrates, but whether multiple feedback mechanisms are common in vertebrates in general has not been determined.

The Renin–Angiotensin System

Release of mineralocorticoids by the zona glomerulosa is regulated by the renin–angiotensin system (RAS), by plasma potassium concentrations, and, to a lesser extent, by ACTH. The RAS has been called a *diffuse* hormonal system, since the production of the most active hormonal substance in the system, angiotensin II, occurs through the concerted action of several enzymes in a variety of tissues.

In mammals the main structural components of the RAS are the juxtaglomerular cells and the macula densa, which are located in the kidneys. Juxtaglomerular (JG) cells are situated on the afferent and, sometimes, efferent arterioles associated with the glomerulus of Bowman's capsule (Fig. 12.4). The JG cells appear to have evolved from smooth muscle or epithelial cells of the arteriole. JG cells contain the enzyme renin, which, when released into the blood, converts angiotensinogen (synthesized and secreted by the liver) into angiotensin I. The macula densa consists of specialized epithelial cells of the distal convoluted tubule of the kidney nephron (Fig. 12.4). Macula densa cells monitor the sodium content of the distal tubule fluid and may regulate the release of renin by the JG cells. The distal tubule of the mammalian nephron winds back toward the glomerulus to encounter the glomerular arterioles. The JG cells and macula densa are closely apposed at this junction.

Angiotensinogen is a high–molecular weight (50,000 to 100,000) glycoprotein that is synthesized in the liver and released into the blood circulation. Mammalian angiotensinogen is similar to serum albumin or to the α_1- or α_2-globulins, depending on the animal species. When angiotensinogen in the blood is subjected to the action of renin released by the JG cells, the decapeptide angiotensin I is formed (Fig. 12.6). Angiotensin I may be converted into smaller peptides, which are more active biologically, by enzymes lo-

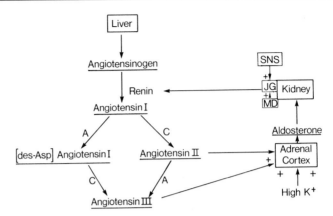

FIGURE 12.6. Diagram of components in the renin-angiotensin system. The liver secretes renin substrate (angiotensinogen) into the blood, where it is enzymatically converted to angiotensin I by renin. Angiotensin I may be converted to angiotensin II by converting enzyme (*C*) located in the lung or the blood. Alternatively, angiotensin I may be converted to [des-Asp]angiotensin I by an angiotensinase (*A*) in the blood plasma. Angiotensin II and [des-Asp] angiotensin I may be converted, respectively, to angiotensin III by angiotensinase or converting enzyme. Angiotensin II and angiotensin III stimulate secretion of aldosterone by the adrenal cortex. High blood levels of potassium ion (K^+) may stimulate direct secretion of aldosterone. Aldosterone stimulates sodium uptake in the kidney. The release of renin by the juxtaglomerular (*JG*) cells is stimulated by low blood pressure, the macula densa (*MD*), or the sympathetic nervous system (*SNS*). See Fig. 12.4 for comparison.

cated in the lung, liver, and the general vascular bed. A converting enzyme removes the two amino acids on the carboxyl terminus of angiotensin I to yield angiotensin II (Fig. 12.7). Alternatively, an angiotensinase might cleave off the amino-terminal asparagine of angiotensin I to produce [des-Asp] angiotensin I (Fig. 12.6). The combined action of both enzymes produces the heptapeptide angiotensin III. Angiotensin II is considered to be the most active of these peptides in stimulating aldosterone release, although angi-

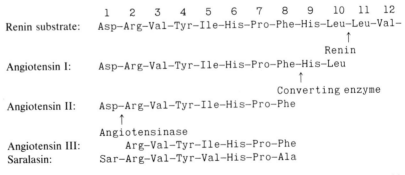

FIGURE 12.7. Structures of peptides of the renin–angiotensin system and of the peptide saralasin, which blocks angiotensin action.

otensin III also appears to be a potent secretagogue for aldosterone. Angiotensin I and [des-Asp] angiotensin I have slight or no action on aldosterone release.

A key point in the regulation of the RAS is the release of renin, since the renin substrate (angiotensinogen) and various other enzymes for the generation of angiotensins are usually present. Renin release by the JG cells is controlled by blood pressure in the renal arterioles, sodium level in the distal tubule fluid, the sympathetic branch of the autonomic nervous system, and such blood humoral factors as epinephrine, arginine vasopressin, potassium, and some steroids. Changes in arteriolar blood pressure appear to be sensed directly by JG cells, so that a decrease in pressure causes release of renin and subsequent generation of angiotensins. Since angiotensin II is a potent pressor substance, its presence in the circulation will contribute to the elevation of blood pressure. The macula densa monitors the concentration or load of sodium in the distal tubular lumen and brings about renin release by JG cells. Lowered tubular sodium is a stimulus for renin release, which ultimately causes an elevation in aldosterone, which, in turn, stimulates transport of sodium from the distal tubule lumen to the blood. Low levels of sodium in the nephron tubules are usually indicative of low blood sodium. The macula densa, operating through the RAS and the adrenals, corrects the sodium imbalance by favoring sodium retention. Participation of the sympathetic system in the control of renin release may be in response to low blood pressure. The sympathetic system is active in alarm situations; it regulates blood flow by shunting blood away from such tissues as the stomach and intestines and toward skeletal muscle and the brain. Increased sympathetic activity stimulates renin release by JG cells through a beta-adrenergic mechanism.

The width of the zona glomerulosa and the blood levels of potassium are often significantly correlated. Furthermore, it has been shown *in vitro* that potassium ions in the extracellular spaces of the adrenals have a direct effect on aldosterone release. High levels of potassium favor the secretion of aldosterone, which acts on the distal tubule of the kidney nephron to increase potassium secretion. Low levels of sodium may also stimulate aldosterone secretion; however, the low sodium levels required for this effect seem to be lower than physiological. Therefore, the importance of the low sodium effect has been questioned. It has been suggested that adrenal glomerulosa cells may monitor the ratio of potassium to sodium and respond accordingly.

All of the various secretagogues for aldosterone release appear to be working through some common mechanisms within the adrenal cell. Angiotensin II, potassium ions, and ACTH—all contribute to elevated levels of cyclic AMP and increased activity of the cholesterol side-chain cleavage enzyme in zona glomerulosa cells. Potassium and angiotensin II appear to activate the 18-hydroxylase that is responsible for the conversion of corticosterone to aldosterone. The specific action of angiotensin II can be inhibited by the octapeptide analogue saralasin (Fig. 12.7). Presumably, this peptide occupies the angiotensin II receptor on the glomerulosa cell membrane, thereby blocking occupancy by angiotensin II, but does not induce the change in the receptor molecule necessary for a biological response.

In addition to the stimulation of aldosterone release and the elevation of blood pressure, angiotensin II has other effects which will be mentioned here briefly. For example, angiotensin II may have a direct effect on the uptake of sodium across the proximal portion of the kidney nephron. Angiotensinogen can be acted upon by enzymes located within the kidney, and local effects of angiotensins can be realized. Angiotensin II may act on the preoptic area of the brain to induce drinking behavior. It is not clear whether this dipsogenic action on the brain is due to angiotensin that may have entered the brain from peripheral blood through circumventricular organs or whether the effect is due to angiotensins produced locally within the brain. Certain areas within the brain produce an enzyme (isorenin) that is similar to kidney renin. Other tissues containing isorenins include the placenta and uterus. Some evidence suggests that angiotensin produced in the uterus may be involved in stimulation of contraction of the uterine musculature. A provocative observation is that angiotensin II stimulates the release of arginine vasopressin by the pars nervosa. This is an interesting example of the coupling of salt and water balance. Angiotensin stimulates sodium uptake either through aldosterone or by itself and also facilitates water retention through vasopressin action. The physiological significance of many of the observed actions of angiotensins still needs confirmation. Most of the varied actions of the RAS seem to be concerned with salt and water balance and with regulation of blood pressure, two interdependent physiological phenomena. The level of such regulation by the RAS ranges from promoting drinking behavior to control of mineralocorticoid release.

Comparative Aspects of the RAS.   The RAS appears to be present in all classes of jawed vertebrates but is absent in cyclostomes and elasmobranchs. The lack of a RAS in the elasmobranchs is curious, since the system seems to be present in the other major group of chondrichthyeans, the holocephalans. The JG cells may have evolved early, since they are present in the kidneys of teleosts. However, the macula densa is absent in fishes and most amphibians, and probably evolved later relative to the evolution of the JG cells.

The structures of angiotensin I from representatives of several vertebrate classes have been determined (Table 12.3). Angiotensin I is quite similar in structure in all the vertebrates. Variation in amino acid sequence is present at amino acid positions 1, 5, and 9. The substitutions of asparagine for aspartic acid and of valine for isoleucine at positions 1 and 5, respectively, would produce relatively minor changes in the structural conformation of the peptide. On the other hand, amino acid substitutions at position 9 are most common and extreme. However, changes at position 9 might have

TABLE 12.3. Amino acid sequences of Angiotensin I from various vertebrate species[a,b]

Species	Amino Acid Sequence									
	1	2	3	4	5	6	7	8	9	10
Human, pig, horse, dog, rat	Asp	Arg	Val	Tyr	Ile	His	Pro	Phe	His	Leu
Ox, sheep	Asp	Arg	Val	Tyr	Val	His	Pro	Phe	His	Leu
Fowl (*Gallus domesticus*)	Asp	Arg	Val	Tyr	Val	His	Pro	Phe	Ser	Leu
Snake (*Elaphe climocophora*)	Asx[c]	Arg	Val	Tyr	Val	His	Pro	Phe	Tyr	Leu
Bullfrog (*Rana catesbeiana*)	Asp	Arg	Val	Tyr	Val	His	Pro	Phe	Asn	Leu
Japanese goosefish (*Lophius litulon*)	Asn	Arg	Val	Tyr	Val	His	Pro	Phe	His	Leu
Chum salmon (*Oncorhynchus keta*)	Asn	Arg	Val	Tyr	Val	His	Pro	Phe	Asn	Leu

[a] From Nakajima, T., M. C. Khosla, and S. Sakakibara, Comparative biochemistry of renins and angiotensins in the vertebrates. *Jpn. Heart J.* **19**:799–808 (1978).
[b] Rectangles enclose the unvarying portions of the decapeptide.
[c] It is uncertain whether this residue is Asp or Asn.

little effect on the physiology of the RAS, since this residue is removed during the generation of the most active angiotensin II octapeptide.

The steroidogenic action of angiotensin II has been seen in teleosts, amphibians, reptiles, and mammals, but not in birds. Studies of the RAS in teleosts during adaptation to seawater or fresh water have shown transient or sustained increases or decreases in RAS activity, depending on the species. Most investigators have interpreted these changes as evidence for control of cortisol secretion by angiotensin. However, since angiotensins elevate blood pressure in fishes, the observed increases in blood cortisol levels may be due to increased perfusion of the interrenal gland rather than to a specific increase in the synthesis of cortisol. In teleosts plasma renin activity either decreases or does not change in response to sodium depletion. In contrast, renin activity increases after sodium depletion in mammals. This discrepancy cannot be resolved without additional studies. The lack of effect of angiotensin on corticosteroidogenesis in birds may not be indicative for this group as a whole, since only a few species have been studied.

Although additional studies of the RAS in nonmammalian vertebrates is needed, Nishimura (1980) has summarized the functions of the RAS in various classes of vertebrates based on the available data. Increase in blood pressure in response to angiotensin seems to be a universal response in jawed vertebrates, elasmobranchs included. Stimulation of drinking behavior and direct effects on the kidney have been observed in teleost fishes, birds, mammals, and some reptiles. Nishimura has speculated that the RAS evolved primarily as a blood pressure-regulating mechanism and that other functions, such as steroidogenesis and sodium regulation, may be features that were acquired secondarily. This hypothesis is attractive when one considers that the macula densa is absent from the kidneys of lower vertebrates. It has been speculated that the blood pressure effects of angiotensins in mammals may be a relic of the primitive function of the RAS, since these effects are unimportant relative to other blood pressure-regulating mechanisms in mammals.

SELYE'S CONCEPT OF STRESS AND THE GENERAL ADAPTATION SYNDROME

Adrenal secretion of glucocorticoids is activated by a variety of stimuli, including hemorrhage, infectious diseases, burns, exposure to cold or heat, exercise, lack of oxygen, and severe or mild emotional involvements. Selye was the first to recognize the fact that all of these stimuli—so different qualitatively and quantitatively—elicited a similar response in the animal subject. He defined *stress* as "the nonspecific response of the body to any demand made upon it." All of the various stimuli that cause the stress response are termed *stressors*. Selye's concept of stress has been popular, since it organizes a group of seemingly unrelated environmental stimuli into one category. However, the stress concept frequently has led to much confusion, most often because the particular stressor being considered has not been clearly defined. For example, stressors have been mistakenly defined as any stimuli that activate the pituitary–adrenal system. Furthermore, stress agents have often been considered to have a negative connotation only. In fact, such an emotional state as extreme joy can be just as "stressful" as extreme sorrow. In spite of these problems, the stress concept has been useful in provoking a great deal of thought and research.

In the late 1930s, Selye began a series of experiments that led to the hypothesis that the pituitary–adrenal system plays a central role in homeostasis. While searching for a new ovarian hormone, Selye injected rats with crude extracts of cattle ovaries and observed adrenal enlargement, atrophy of the thymus and lymph nodes, and gastric ulcers. In subsequent experiments the same responses were noted after the injection of extracts from other organs or after injection of toxic drugs. Although Selye did not find a new ovarian hormone, his observation that a characteristic set of symptoms developed in response to any toxic substance formed the basis for the idea of the general adaptation syndrome (GAS).

The concept of the general adaptation syndrome is a unifying theory that attempts to explain how an organism tries to adapt to stress through activation of the pituitary–adrenal system and how the benefit of any acquired adaptation may be lost under conditions of prolonged stress. The syndrome consists of three stages: (1) the alarm reaction, (2) resistance, and (3) exhaustion. The alarm reaction is the immediate response after exposure to a stressor. During the alarm, large amounts of corticosteroids are released to protect the organism from possible damage. Blood levels of glucose are maintained at the expense of body protein. Inflammatory reactions are suppressed to guard against excessive responses to tissue wounding or infection. If the organism continues to be exposed to the stressor, the resistance stage is entered. Resistance to the stressor is the successful adaptation of the organism. Many of the metabolic and other changes that occurred during the alarm reaction return to the normal, prestress condition. After prolonged exposure to the stressor, the adaptation that had occurred is lost. This is the exhaustion stage. Extreme exhaustion leads to the death of the organism. In Selye's original concept the adrenals were believed to be active throughout the alarm reaction and resistance stage; their activity decreased during exhaustion as resistance to the stressor was lost.

This concept has been modified in more recent times to include the participation of the autonomic nervous system in the alarm reaction and probably during other stages. Measurements of circulating levels of corticosteroids during chronic stress of animals have shown that there is an initial increase in corticosteroid levels, followed by a decrease and then a prolonged elevation. Selye and colleagues have also shown that many diseases that develop as a result of chronic stress may be induced by treating animals with glucocorticoids in combination with sodium salts, lipids, and other agents. In spite of such evidence, the general adaptation syndrome concept has received considerable criticism. The question has been raised whether the stage of resistance is a period of adaptation or is in fact a time of maladaptation of the organism. Furthermore, it has been found that even minor disturbances may elicit an adrenal response that is characteristic of the alarm reaction. This has necessitated the reevaluation of criteria for the definition of a stressor. Others have argued that inducing a disease by treating animals with corticosteroids and other substances does not constitute a demonstration of a causal relationship between corticosteroids and disease during stress.

Regardless of such controversy, the general adaptation syndrome and the stress concepts have been useful for several groups of researchers. The relationship between stress and population dynamics is an interesting example. As populations of animals increase in size, and especially in density, there is increased interaction and competition for living space, resources, and mating privileges. There are a variety of mechanisms, both behavioral and physiological, that come into play in conditions of crowding. In some species territorial behavior gives way to the establishment of social hierarchies when the available living space becomes limited. Disease, starvation, and failure to achieve reproductive maturity are factors that act to limit the number of individuals in a population. The pioneering work of J. J. Christian implicated the adrenal gland in the adaptation of animals to high population densities. Subsequent work has confirmed the importance of the pituitary–adrenal system in both behavioral and physiological control over the size of animal populations, and this field of study continues to be an interesting and challenging area of research.

Christian's initial observation that the size of the adrenal glands of laboratory mice increased with the population density has been extended to include populations of monkeys, wild rats, deer, and rabbits. High blood levels of corticosteroids may either induce or be a consequence of behaviors that are present in animals at high population densities. The size and secretory rate of the adrenal glands are increased greatly in lemmings during times of peak population density, when the lemmings embark upon their mass migrations. In animals that form dominance hierarchies, the size of the adrenal gland is negatively correlated with social rank, so that the adrenals of subordinate individuals are larger than those of the dominant animals.

Several physiological mechanisms, probably mediated by corticosteroids, may operate to limit population size. Immunosuppressive and anti-inflammatory actions of corticosteroids may increase the susceptibility of individuals to disease. Mortality due to disease may be a major determinant in controlling the size of some animal populations. High blood levels of corticosteroids inhibit the release of gonadotropins by the pituitary and prevent normal reproduction. Thus the pituitary–adrenal system acts as a natural birth control mechanism in some animal populations at high density.

Most studies of adrenal involvement in population dynamics have concentrated on mammals. Application of the stress concept to population regulation of nonmammalian species is an attractive area for further research. Interrenal activity during the life cycle of the Pacific salmon is an interesting example for comparison. During the spawning migration of the salmon, the interrenal gland produces large amounts of corticosteroids. In contrast to some mammals, the hyperadrenocorticalism of salmon does not seem to interfere with reproduction. The limited data available suggest that the high levels of corticosteroids cause the death of Pacific salmon shortly after spawning. Corticosteroids may limit the population of Pacific salmon by removing the adults from the population after they have spawned.

ADDITIONAL READING

1. Chester Jones, I., and I. W. Henderson (1976, 1978, 1980). *General, Comparative and Clinical Endocrinology of the Adrenal Cortex*, Vols. 1–3.

2. Christian, J. J. (1975). Hormonal control of population growth. In *Hormonal Correlates of Behavior*. Vol. 1 (B. E. Eleftheriou and R. L. Sprott, eds.). Plenum, New York, pp. 205–274.

3. Holt, W. F., and D. R. Idler (1975). Influence of the interrenal gland on the rectal gland of a skate. *Comp. Biochem. Physiol.* **50C:**111–119.

4. Idler, D. R., and B. Truscott (1980). Phylogeny of vertebrate adrenal corticosteroids. In *Evolution of Vertebrate Endocrine Systems* (P. K. T. Pang and A. Epple, eds.). Texas Tech Press, Lubbock, pp. 357–372.

5. James, V. H. T., ed. (1979). *The Adrenal Gland.* Raven, New York.

6. Laragh, J. H., and J. E. Sealey (1973). The renin-angiotensin-aldosterone hormonal system and regulation of sodium, potassium and blood pressure homeostasis. In *Handbook of Physiology: Renal Physiology* (J. Orloff and R. W. Berliner, eds.). American Physiological Society, Washington, D. C., pp. 831–908.

7. Lichardus, B., R. W. Schrier, and J. Ponec, eds. (1980). Hormonal regulation of sodium excretion. In *Developments in Endocrinology,* Vol. 10. Elsevier/North-Holland, Amsterdam.

8. Liggins, G. C. (1976). Adrenocortical-linked maturational events in the fetus. *Am. J. Obstet. Gynecol.* **126:**931–941.

9. Nishimura, H. (1980). Evolution of the renin-angiotensin system. In *Evolution of Vertebrate Endocrine Systems* (P. K. T. Pang and A. Epple, eds.). Texas Tech Press, Lubbock, pp. 373–404.

10. Thomas, D. H. (1980). Aldosterone effects of electrolyte transport of the lower intestine (coprodeum and colon) of the fowl (*Gallus domesticus*) *in vitro. Gen. Comp. Endocrinol.* **40:**44–51.

11. Truscott, B. (1980). Corticosteroids of the Coelacanth *Latimeria chalumnae* Smith: A provisional study on their identity. *Gen. Comp. Endocrinol.* **41:**287–295.

12. Uva, B., M. Vallarino, A. Mandich, and G. Isola (1982). Plasma aldosterone levels in the female tortoise *Testudo hermanni* Gmelin in different experimental conditions. *Gen. Comp. Endocrinol.* **46:**116–123.

13. Vale, W., J. Spiess, C. Rivier, and J. Rivier (1981). Characterization of a 41-residue ovine hypothalamic peptide that stimulates secretion of corticotropin and β-endorphin. *Science* **213:**1394–1397.

14. Zimmerman, E. A., P. W. Carmel, H. K. Husain, M. Ferin, M. Tannenbaum, A. G. Frantz, and A. G. Robinson (1973). Vasopressin and neurophysin: high concentrations in monkey hypophyseal portal blood. *Science* **182:**925–927.

13

Endocrine Control of
Sexual Reproduction

The management of the process of sexual reproduction in higher vertebrates is undoubtedly the most complicated phenomenon in integrative physiology. Not only are the roles of each of the hormones involved in this integration themselves complex, but there also are systems for coordinating or gearing the actions of the separate hormones with each other as well as with environmental cues. Moreover, the mechanisms in the two sexes are different.

The strategies, timing, and patterns of the reproductive process in the evolution of vertebrates have been highly adaptive in order to make possible maximum reproductive success in a variety of habitats and specialized life cycles. Even between closely related species there are differences in reproductive mechanisms that may be obvious or subtle to the human observer. In fact, it is quite usual for small differences in reproductive patterns to create the kind of reproductive isolation that makes possible the evolution of separate species within a sympatric population.

Although the orientation of this textbook is along comparative lines, it is clearly impossible to remain faithful to this orientation in treating the endless variety of patterns of comparative reproductive endocrinology. Accordingly, while retaining the comparative approach, we will concentrate on the reproduction of mammals, particularly that of rats and humans.

First, the general features of sexual reproduction will be described. The major part of this chapter will be devoted to the endocrine regulation of reproduction in the rat and human being, with occasional mention of appropriate and pertinent phenomena in other species.

GENERAL FEATURES OF SEXUAL REPRODUCTION

The Biological Value of Sexual Reproduction and Sexual Adaptation

Male and female organisms and sexual reproduction in animals and plants are so universally familiar that it often comes as a surprise when the biologist asks why reproduction needs to be sexual. There are numerous patterns of vegetative, nonsexual reproduction; yet, most asexually reproducing organisms also have a sexual phase of reproduction. The persistence and success of a biological mechanism such as sexual reproduction, in keeping with evolutionary doctrine, implies that it endows the *species* that possesses it with some kind of advantage for long-term survival.

The special advantage conferred by sexual reproduction is that at every mating of two individuals a series of new combinations of genetic factors is formed in the offspring. This, as Charles Darwin recognized, produces a population of organisms with an infinite variety of properties and combinations of properties (temperature tolerance, size, metabolic characteristics, resistance to disease organisms, pigmentation, details of neuromuscular function, etc.). In a given environment the genes that yield properties that are most appropriate to that environment will produce organisms that are most likely to reproduce themselves. Hence the incidence of "favorable" genes will increase, and the incidence of "unfavorable" or inappropriate genes will decrease. As a species gradually "adapts" to a changing environment, or to a new environment, sexual reproduction allows the environment during each generation to gradually "select" the most favorable average genetic constitutions for the species. On the other hand, in a species that reproduces exclusively by asexual mechanisms, there is only a single parent organism that merely reduplicates a given set of genetic factors. An asexual species obviously cannot adapt its genetically controlled features to a cataclysmic or continuous environmental change, nor could a species with a fixed set of genetic determinants "invade" a novel environment.

Accordingly, the basis for the success of sexually reproducing species is the maintenance of a degree of variability among individuals that comprise a population and a continuous recombination of the groups of genetic determinants that cause this variability. If the recombination of genetic factors (breeding) did not occur *often enough* to assure a variety of recombined gene groups, this also (almost like asexual reproduction) would impair the genetic plasticity or adaptability of a species. This would occur, for example, if the same individuals reproduced forever. For this reason, there is adaptive advantage to the species in limiting the reproductive life of an individual organism. Thus we can understand the biological function of senescence and of the limitation of reproductive potency to a phase in the life cycle of a species. Indeed, in this context one can understand the biological function of death of individuals in the postreproductive phase of the life cycle: such individuals contribute nothing further to the genetic features of a species, and they may only compete with the reproductive members for the limited resources of the environment.

Patterns of Sexual Reproduction

As was stated above, some of the most highly adapted and ingenious biological mechanisms that have been evolved are those that are directly concerned with the assurance of success in reproduction. Indeed, what we see today are those mechanisms that have maintained the species that evolved them. The less successful species, obviously, were eliminated.

Number of Offspring. Perhaps the simplest and most obvious of mechanisms is the production of vast numbers of offspring per parental pair. For example, the American eel (*Anguilla rostrata*) produces 5 to 20 million young per spawning. The eggs are fertilized externally in seawater. There is no parental care of the young, and continuance of the species depends solely upon the statistical chances of survival of sufficient young (concealment and escape from predators). Other species of teleost fishes have evolved mechanisms of various degrees of complexity—perhaps at greater cost of energy to the parent—that permit the formation of fewer eggs but guarantee a greater survival rate of offspring. For example, fishes such as the bluegill (*Lepomis*) and the salmon (*Salmo salar* or species of *Oncorhynchus*) are behaviorally adapted to lay their eggs in simple nests in which they are more or less covered by sand or gravel. In *Lepomis*, the male guards the eggs and newly hatched young against predators. In such species the numbers of eggs per breeding pair is only a few thousand. In still other species (as in the stickleback *Gasterosteus aculeatus*), more elaborate, enclosed nests and guarding behavior reduce the number of spawn to a few hundred. In some cichlids (e.g., *Tilapia*), the eggs are generally fewer than 100 and are incubated and irrigated in the mouth of the male until well past hatching; the parent during this time is behaviorally adapted not to feed. In the sea horse (*Hippocampus*) there is a special pocketlike structure, the marsupium of the male, in which the young—generally about 100—can safely develop to a relatively mature stage.

Reproductive Patterns that Require Structural Adaptations. A common adaptive feature among the lower vertebrates is the inclusion of a relatively large amount of nutritive yolk in a relatively small number of eggs. Often this is combined with a deposition around the egg of protective coatings of jelly or harder materials. These two features—in oviparous (egg-laying) vertebrates like the hagfishes, some elasmobranchs (sharks, rays, skates), and most reptiles and birds—permit the embryo to develop to a relatively large size before hatching, at which time it becomes independent relatively quickly. The formation of large amounts of yolk is a metabolic adaptation

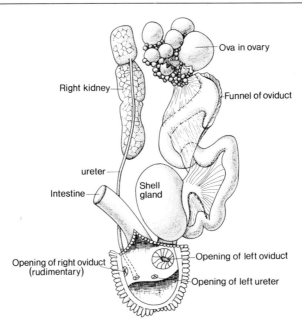

Right kidney

ureter

Intestine

Shell gland

Opening of right oviduct (rudimentary)

Ova in ovary

Funnel of oviduct

Opening of left oviduct

Opening of left ureter

FIGURE 13.1. Female urogenital system of the chicken. There is only one ovary and one functional oviduct on the left. The left kidney is not shown. Eggs in their follicles in all stages are shown. See also Fig. 13.10. [Adapted from L. A. Adams and S. Eddy, *An Introduction to the Vertebrates,* Wiley, New York, 1951.]

in which the liver is the synthetic organ, and the yolk lipids and proteins are transferred to the developing eggs via the blood.

The formation of protective or nourishing deposits around the eggs requires structural modifications of the oviduct and/or uterus of the mother. In the walls of these organs, glands secrete the extraoval layers around the eggs as they pass toward the cloaca (Fig. 13.1). In the domestic hen, for example, as many as five membranes or layers surround the fully formed egg (Fig. 13.2). These are successively added as coatings by different glandular areas as the egg moves down the oviduct during a period of about 24 hours after ovulation. The innermost layer is the vitelline membrane, which is actually produced in the ovary. This is followed by two layers of albumen of different densities. Next are two tough, keratinous shell membranes, and finally, the shell itself, which consists largely of $CaCO_3$ (about 5 gm). The yolk and the albumen are the primary substrates for nutrition and development during the three weeks of incubation. The shell membrane and shell are not only protective, but are so constructed (by inclusion of pores) as to allow for the respiratory needs of the embryo. When the complex avian egg (or any other large, protected, yolky egg), together with the anatomical, endocrine, and metabolic features that fabricate it, is considered from a mechanistic perspective, it must arouse the full admiration of a systems engineer.

Internal fertilization is a common adaptation in vertebrates that greatly increases the chances for contact between eggs and spermatozoa. While internal fertilization is a special development in some aquatic vertebrates, it is obligatory in vertebrates that live on land. It is probably one of the major reproductive adaptations that permitted the vertebrates to emerge from the aquatic to the terrestrial environment. Generally, internal fertilization requires the development in the male of a special intromittent organ or organs in order to introduce the spermatozoa into the female. Such male organs are known in all vertebrate groups except the cyclostomes and Amphibia. In some urodele amphibians internal fertilization is accomplished without an intromittent device. Here, in the course of a mating behavior ritual, the male deposits a packet of spermatozoa called a spermatophore. The female follows the male and, using the lips of the cloaca by an imperfectly understood means, ''picks up'' the spermatophore. Many female vertebrates have developed specialized areas in the lower female tract where the sperm may be stored, sometimes for periods longer than a year (fishes, amphibians, reptiles), to be used eventually for fertilization of eggs at appropriate times.

Ovoviviparity and *viviparity* are systems of greater and greater adaptive complexity that permit the developing young to remain within the maternal parent to complete a part of their development in this protected environment. Ovoviviparous animals retain the developing eggs and embryos in the ovary (teleost fishes) or in the oviduct or uterus of the mother until the yolk is partly or almost completely used up. Ovoviviparity requires relatively little anatomic adaptation on the part of the mother, although there are some structural accommodations in the ovary, oviduct, or uterus to facilitate re-

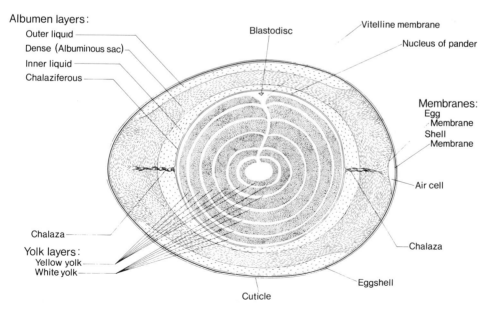

FIGURE 13.2. Structure of a hen egg as though cut through the long axis. [From A. L. Romanoff and A. J. Romanoff, *The Avian Egg,* Wiley, New York, 1949.]

tention of the young. The degree to which there is maternal nutritional or metabolic support of developing ovoviviparous young is still not well understood. However, there clearly is an exchange of respiratory gases, excretory products, and some important ions between embryo and mother in this condition.

In some ovoviviparous teleosts, such as the rockfish *Sebastes*, there is very little apparent structural specialization on the part of either the mother or the embryo to make possible internal development. In other teleost species, such as the family Goodeidae, there are elaborate prolongations and modifications of tissue (gills, cloaca, pericardium, etc.) that extend away from the embryo and have the obvious temporary purpose of facilitating metabolic exchange between mother and embryo. The shells of the large eggs of ovoviviparous elasmobranch fishes are still laid down, but in a very thin membranous form that provides a minimal barrier to respiratory gas exchange.

Viviparity is a condition in which the young are retained in the maternal reproductive tract until a relatively advanced state of development, depending almost entirely during this time on a specialized, highly vascular organ (the placenta) for nutrition. In analyzing the relationship between the embryo and the mother, it often is very difficult to decide whether the condition that exists should be called ovoviviparity or viviparity. The distinction is often made on the basis of the derivation of "nourishment" from the mother, particularly when the egg has little or no yolk supply to depend upon.

Some teleostean yolky embryos, supported by complex vascularized tissue extensions (as mentioned above) from the gut, the gills, the cloaca, or the pericardium, clearly absorb more than respiratory gas and perhaps supplement their yolk supply from maternal blood. These are generally defined as ovoviviparous. But, in fact, do they differ from those species in which the vascular embryonic yolk itself is in intimate contact with maternal uterine tissue, as in some elasmobranchs? The same intimate relationship may exist between the teleostean yolk sac and the ovarian follicle wall. There is not enough information available about what is exchanged between the mother and the embryo in ovoviviparous and "viviparous" species of fishes.

In some teleost species (*Anableps*) and in certain "viviparous" salamanders (*Salamandra atra*), only one or a small number of an originally larger number of embryos survive in the maternal reproductive tract. The survivors feed on their brothers and sisters. In such cases of sibling cannibalism it is fruitless to be concerned with whether this best fits the definitions of ovoviviparity or viviparity.

However difficult it may be to decide whether a given adaptive reproductive mechanism in a lower vertebrate is or is not viviparous, there is no question that the original intention of the term was to specify the system in mammals. Here a definitive but temporary organ, the placenta, is formed by vascularized extraembryonic tissues of the embryo and vascular tissues

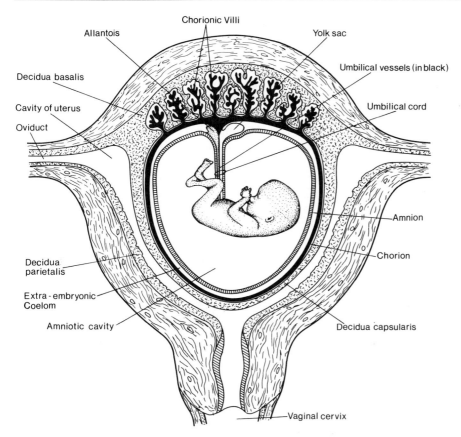

FIGURE 13.3. The human fetus surrounded by its fetal membranes within the uterus. The membranes and layers have been simplified and emphasized for easier understanding of their relationships. There is an actual space (the extraembryonic coelom) between the amnion and chorion. However, there is no actual space between the chorion (an embryonic layer) and the surrounding maternal decidua basalis and capsularis (though one is shown). [Adapted from A. F. Huettner, *Comparative Embryology of the Vertebrates*, Macmillan, New York, 1949.]

of the maternal uterus. The interdigitation of these tissues is quite intimate, and there are various degrees of destruction of maternal tissue by the embryonic component to increase this intimacy.

In placentas such as the pig's there is minimal destruction of maternal tissue. In the human placenta (Fig. 13.3) there is maximal destruction of maternal tissue, so that maternal blood bathes the outermost embryonic placental layers. These examples represent degrees of adaptation to enable more efficient metabolic exchange between maternal and fetal blood in the placenta. The placenta has other functions of an endocrine nature that will be described later in this chapter; these, too, are facilitated by the unrestricted access to the maternal blood.

Behavioral and Nervous Management of Organisms for Efficient Reproduction

Sexual reproduction has created a number of difficult biological problems whose solution has required some remarkable and admirably precise mechanisms, particularly among such large animals as the vertebrates. The major problem is that the two kinds of sex cells are housed in separate animals. This calls for one animal to signal to the other (1) its presence and location, and (2) its readiness for mating. What follows is a machinelike series of responses that bring the two individuals together and dispose them with respect to each other so that sexual coupling can take place, enabling the gametes to mix and fertilization to occur. G. W. Corner (1963) has expressed this beautifully:

> This is the sexual urge, the totality of impulses that serve to bring the sexes together for mating. It is the most important coordination of all, for without the union of the sexes all the other intricate processes are useless. It, too, is partly regulated by the hormones, but we know too little about this as yet to discuss it profitably here. The way of an eagle in the air, the way of a man with a maid . . . are still in part beyond the reach of science. In view of the fact that we are still ignorant of the means by which the simplest one-celled animal is impelled to conjugate with another of its kind, we can only wonder at the complexity of sex psychology in the higher animals, and at all the lures that nature has provided to insure the union of the sexes. What marvels of color and fragrance, bird song and firefly radiance, have been lavished to this end! And for mankind what emotions are bound up with it, of young romance and mature devotion, hope and fear, selfishness, slyness and cruelty. To the fanatic, sex is a snare of the devil, to a Casanova a heartless game; to Stephen Dedalus as a young man it was torment; to some happier lad, it is a rosy dream. All these have much to gain by seeing it also, with the biologist, as part of the inevitable process of animal life. To understand is not to demean ourselves, nor to rob the human heart of virtue and the love of beauty.

The signals used to trigger reproductive behavior are numerous and utilize almost all of the senses—visual, olfactory, auditory, and tactile. When the signal is a chemical one, usually detected as an odor, it is called a sex pheromone. Auditory clues include bird calls. The commonest and easiest sex signals for the human observer to appreciate are the visual ones. The visual signal may be ritual or reflex movements (courtship) by one or the other sex, or it may make use of a structural device. Structures used in this way include skin pigments that appear at mating time, excrescences on the head (pearl organs of fishes, comb of the rooster) or other body parts, tall fins on the tails of certain salamanders, and others.

Mating behavior of many species, including humans, has been a frequent subject for study, and there are many fascinating descriptions of the specific form it takes for a given species. Here it is important to observe that each species has evolved its own behavioral pattern, which is adapted to its own ecological situation and guarantees the continuity of the genetic line. The timing of mating behavior in vertebrates is regulated by the brain. The brain center that governs mating behavior is sensitive to sex hormone titers. When a gonad becomes active (at the appropriate time of the year, or of the reproductive cycle) and contains ripe gametes, it secretes sex hormones which act upon the nervous system to arouse the appropriate mating behavior. There are, of course, exceptions to this generalization. Human reproductive activity is relatively—but not completely—independent of sex hormone levels in the blood.

The brain center for mating behavior is localized to a large extent in the hypothalamus and there are, apparently, anatomic relations between it and the ''reward'' or ''pleasure'' center, as well as the center for aggressive behavior. It can be selectively stimulated electrically or by implanting small amounts of male or female sex hormones near it, evoking the typical mating activity.

THE GONADS AND REPRODUCTIVE STRUCTURES

The gonads in vertebrate embryos are mesodermal structures that differentiate from sexually indifferent rudiments. Eventually, the genetic sex of the embryo manifests itself, and the initially bipotential gonad normally develops in the male or in the female direction. Adult gonads of both sexes play a double role: (1) they are the centers for the production of germ cells, the testis producing spermatozoa and the ovary producing ova; and (2) they are the primary sources of the sex steroid hormones that regulate the postnatal development of the reproductive ducts and glands as well as the secondary sex characteristics. Thus the gonads not only produce the sex cells (holocrine secretions), but also, through their endocrine secretions, ensure the fulfillment of the reproductive potencies of the sex cells. The gonadal hormones do this by conditioning all of the ducts through which the sex cells must pass and by contributing to the arousal of behavioral responses in male and female organisms that will bring them together at the precise time when the sex cells have matured; thus these hormones make successful fertilization possible.

Endocrine Factors Regulating Reproductive Cycles

The principal steroidal products of the testis are *androgens* (testoids), so called because they stimulate the development of structures associated with ''maleness.'' The principal ovarian hormones fall into two groups: *estrogens* (folliculoids), which are capable of stimulating female reproductive activity and ''femaleness'' generally, and *progestogens* (luteoids), which play a secondary role in modifying the female reproductive tract, particularly for its functions in pregnancy. The gonads and their steroidal secretions are not essential for the continued existence of the individual organism, and in some species there is little obvious external change if they are removed. However, the need for normally functioning gonads for the continued existence of the species is apparent. Gonadal function is almost exclusively under the control of the pars distalis of the pituitary. The periodic interactions of the several gonadotropins from the pituitary with the functioning gonad provide the complex control mechanism that allows the establishment of reproductive cycles and of extended periods for care of the young.

One expression of the cyclic nature of female reproductive activity in vertebrates is in periodically recurring mating behavioral patterns. The female is relatively receptive of the male only at certain times. In mammals the time of maximum receptivity is known as *estrus* (rut, heat), and the female reproductive cycle is referred to as the *estrous cycle*. These behavioral changes are paralleled by changes in the structure and function of the genital tract; the changes in the mammalian vagina and uterus in particular have been studied thoroughly.

The genital changes are dependent on cyclic changes in the ovary and on the pattern of hormone production. Unlike the male gonad, which presents a relatively consistent histological picture during activity, the female gonad has "several faces," depending upon the degree of maturation of the ova. The ovary is a complex of endocrine and gametogenic structures that are not all present or functional at the same time.

The ovarian cycle depends upon the cyclic production of several adenohypophyseal factors (gonadotropins) that determine the composition of the ovary over time and the functioning of its several parts. It is the brain itself (especially the hypothalamus) that controls the length of the phases of cyclic pituitary function. Furthermore, the difference between male and female gonadal cyclic activity is in the hypothalamus. If the hypophysis of a noncyclic male mammal (e.g., the laboratory rat) is transplanted into the sella turcica of a female, it will function as if it were a cyclic female hypophysis, and vice versa.

The hypothalamus, in turn, is responsive to controlling influences originating from various other areas of the central nervous system. The environment—especially variations in light, temperature, rainfall, and diet—exerts its influences on reproductive activity through higher nervous centers which eventually communicate with the hypothalamus. Impinging upon the hypothalamus are fiber tracts from all over the brain and spinal cord, and many of these pathways ultimately regulate the activity of the hypophysiotropic neurosecretory neurons that can release LHRH at the median eminence. In mammals the limbic system, including the amygdala and the hippocampus, is concerned with both the physiological and psychological aspects of sexual function. The hypothalamic center regulating mating behavior is in the preoptic nucleus. Presumably it is a target of sex hormone action.

Typical Structure of the Mammalian Ovary

The mature mammalian ovary (Fig. 13.4) consists of five principal histological components: (1) a *germinal epithelium*, covering most of the surface of the ovary; (2) hollow, spherical *follicles*, which arise initially from the germinal epithelium; (3) solid, spherical *corpora lutea* (singular, *corpus luteum*), into which ripe follicles generally transform, usually after discharge of the contained ovum; (4) *interstitial tissue*, homologous to that of the testis in the male, very prominent in some species; and (5) *ovarian stroma*, connective tissue in which the epithelioid structures mentioned above are embedded and which gives rise to the tunics (thecae) of the follicles and to the fibrous connective tissue that eventually replaces the corpora lutea. A dense layer of connective tissue, the tunica albuginea, underlies the germinal epithelium.

The germinal epithelium gives rise to small nests of cells, one of which enlarges and becomes located centrally. A primordial follicle (Figs. 13.4 and

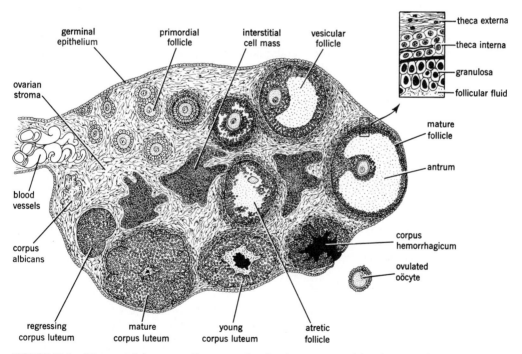

FIGURE 13.4. Diagram of the mammalian ovary showing the sequence of development of the primordial follicle into a mature follicle, as well as the formation of the corpus luteum and its regression to leave a corpus albicans. A follicle undergoing atresia is also indicated. A section of the wall of a vesicular follicle is shown under higher magnification at the upper right. It should be understood that for purposes of illustration all phases of follicular and luteal development are shown as though they occurred at the same time. However, in the normal ovary these phases are consecutive, not contemporary with each other. [Based in part on B. Patten and on R. M. Eakin, in Gorbman and Bern, 1962.]

13.5) is thus formed, consisting of an oogonium surrounded by a layer of *granulosa cells*. Nuclear meiotic changes convert the oogonium to a primary oocyte. The follicle grows largely as a result of granulosa cell proliferation, and the oocyte increases in size as yolk is accumulated. The cellular sheath that surrounds the early follicle becomes differentiated into two layers: (1) an internal epithelioid layer, highly vascular, called the *theca interna*; and (2) an external, more fibrous layer, called the *theca externa*. A fluid-filled cavity—the *antrum*—begins to form in the mass of granulosa cells, and the follicle is now referred to as a *vesicular follicle* (Fig. 13.6). The usually vesicular follicle enlarges as fluid accumulates and as the granulosa cells continue to proliferate. Eventually, at the proper phase of the ovarian cycle, sufficient pressure is exerted at the surface of the ovary to cause local ischemia (deficiency in circulation) and necrosis of a part of the follicular wall. As a result, the follicle ruptures, and the secondary oocyte is released, surrounded by a layer of granulosa cells. This is the process of *ovulation*.

The ruptured follicle often becomes filled with blood, to form the *corpus hemorrhagicum* or *Blutpunkt* (the early pregnancy tests depend upon finding recently ovulated follicles in the ovary of a rat, evidenced as bloody spots or *Blutpunkte*). The granulosa cells begin to accumulate a yellow pigment and transform into *lutein* cells; some theca interna cells also become pigmented and, as *paralutein* cells, contribute to the histogenesis of a new organ—the yellow body, or *corpus luteum*. This structure grows and is maintained for a period whose length depends on the species and its phys-

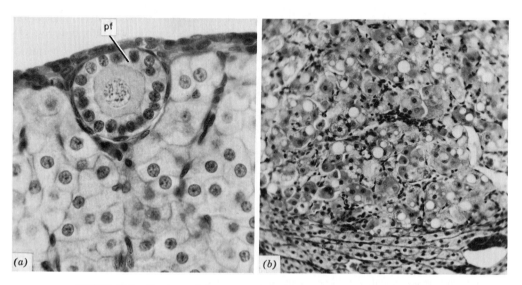

FIGURE 13.5. Portions of the ovary of the lump-nosed bat. (*a*) Primordial follicle (*pf*) surrounded by maximally developed interstitial tissue, from a lactating female; (*b*) portion of a maximally developed corpus luteum from a pregnant female. [From O. P. Pearson, M. R. Koford, and A. K. Pearson, *J. Mamm.*, **33**:273, 1952.]

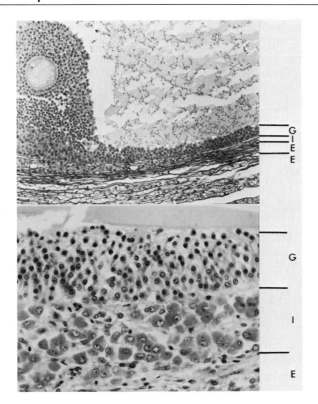

FIGURE 13.6. Follicular walls in ovaries of two mammals. *Above*: the scaly anteater or pangolin (*Manis sp.*). The ripe follicle has a large antrum and the oocyte is located in a hillock of granulosa cells (*G*). The granulosa cells nearer the edge of the follicle appear differentiated from those in the hillock (the cumulus oophorus). The theca is divided into two zones: the more cellular theca interna (*I*) and the more fibrous theca externa (*E*). The theca externa is separable into a denser and looser layer. The theca interna is better developed in the neighborhood of the cumulus oophorus. *Below*: a more highly magnified view of the fully developed ovarian follicular wall of the mare. Labels for the three layers are the same as above. [Photographs provided by Professor H. W. Mossman from his collection.]

iological state. If fertilization occurs, the corpus may last for part or all of the duration of pregnancy, again varying with the species. Whether associated with pregnancy or not, it eventually degenerates and is invaded by connective tissue. A small connective tissue scar—the *corpus albicans*—often marks the site of a degenerated corpus luteum.

The ovarian cycle can be divided into a follicular phase, marked by large vesicular follicles, and a luteal phase, characterized by large, healthy-appearing corpora lutea. The follicles are considered to be the primary source of estrogen, and the corpora lutea of progestogen. Most follicles undergo degeneration before ovulation; this process is known as *atresia*. Atretic follicles have no gametogenic significance, but may add to estrogenic and other hormone levels to an important degree. In the human female such atretic follicles often have unusually well-developed thecae internae. The relation of the cells of this theca to ovarian interstitial cells, as well as their steroidogenic potencies, are as yet imperfectly understood.

Analytic studies on the rat have shown that combinations of either theca interna cells or interstitial cells with either mature granulosa cells or corpus luteum cells will produce estrogen, but the pure cell types will not do so separately. This observation allows one to account for estrogen production by preovulatory and atretic follicles and also by the corpus luteum. After ovulation in some forms, small follicles begin to develop, but most become atretic. However, they contribute to estrogen production in the luteal phase.

Complete ovarian cycles, including the transformation of follicles into corpora lutea, can occur without ovulation. Such anovulatory cycles can be produced experimentally by destruction of the developing ova by X-irradiation.

In addition to the production of estrogen by the follicle and the production of both estrogen and progestogen by the rat corpus luteum, the ovary also may secrete androgen. In some forms this is a notable phenomenon. In female moles (insectivores) there is a persistent medullary gland (derived from the male component of the embryonic gonad; see below) in the ovary, which normally and constantly secretes androgen without appreciably impairing fertility. Witschi believed that the interstitial tissue of both ovary and testis produces androgens; in the human ovary a special group of hilar epithelioid cells has been assumed to be the major source of ovarian androgen. The synergistic role of this steroid in the normal female mammal in such events as uterine growth or mammary development has never been defined. Nor has its possible effect on pituitary regulation of ovarian function been determined.

Other Mammalian Ovaries

Most textbook descriptions of *the* mammalian ovary, including the foregoing one, are based largely on the rat and the human, because they are studied the most. However, generalizations based on these two species, while convenient, are not really justifiable. For example, we must include among mammalian ovaries those of the oviparous monotremes, in which the yolky egg fills the entire follicle, and the granulosa is a uniform perioval layer. In some mammals (the mole *Condylura*) the antrum is greatly reduced (Fig. 13.7b). There are some mammals (the Malagasy hedgehog *Setifer*) (Fig. 13.7c) in which there is no antrum in the follicle, the entire follicle being filled with granulosa cells. In this animal, furthermore, it is remarkable that fertilization occurs while the egg is buried in the cell-filled follicle, and ovulation occurs after fertilization. How do the spermatozoa "find" the egg in this insectivore? How can ovulation occur with the burden of granulosa cells blocking it?

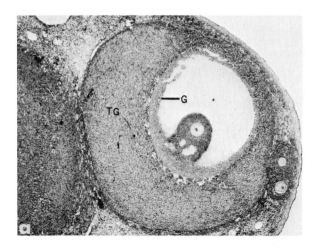

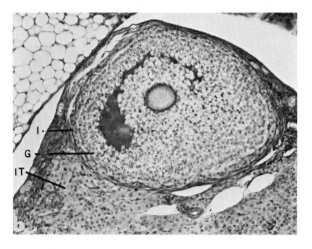

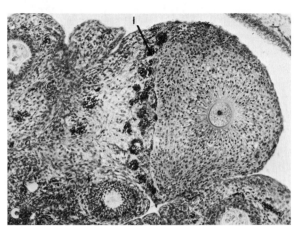

FIGURE 13.7. Ripe follicles with specialized features in three mammals. (*a*) The pocket gopher (*Geomys*). The theca interna (*I*) becomes greatly hypertrophied and, even before ovulation, forms a mass called a *thecal gland* (*TG*). *G* is the granulosa layer. The oocyte is borne upon a hillock of granulosa cells, the cumulus oophorus, which in this follicle is beginning to dissociate itself from the follicular wall prior to ovulation. (*b*) The star-nosed mole (*Condylura*). The ripe follicle has only a small antrum and a clear but modest theca interna (*I*) and theca externa (not labeled, but just outside of the theca interna). There is a well-developed mass of interstitial tissue (*IT*) of the adrenocortical type. Compare this with other ovarian photographs. The granulosa layer (*G*) has a "secretory" appearance. (*c*) The Madagascar hedgehog (*Setifer setosus*). The ripe follicle has no antrum. Fertilization in this species is intrafollicular (the state shown here); thus spermatozoa must penetrate the solid granulosa mass around the ovum, and ovulation must occur under the burden of overlying granulosa. Note that there is no connective tissue layer (tunica albuginea) over the outer side of the follicle as in other mammals (above). The follicle projects outward from the ovary, so that there is a theca only on the basal (attached) side of the follicle. Here the theca interna (*I*) can be distinguished by the numerous blood vessels containing groups of darkstaining red blood cells. [Photographs provided by Professor H. W. Mossman from his collection.]

Another remarkable mammalian ovary—in light of what we know from the rat and human—is that of the South American vizcacha, a form that produces a very large number of small follicles with antra. At each cycle 300 to 700 eggs are ovulated, but of these only two can successfully complete the term of pregnancy, if fertilized! Still another unusual ovarian phenomenon is the occurrence of polyovular follicles, as in the striped skunk. Here, apparently by division of the oogonium-oocyte *after* follicle formation, as many as 20 oocytes may occur within one follicle (Fig. 13.9c). The utility of this mechanism can be questioned, like that in the vizcacha.

H. W. Mossman has pointed out that it is wrong to think of "interstitial

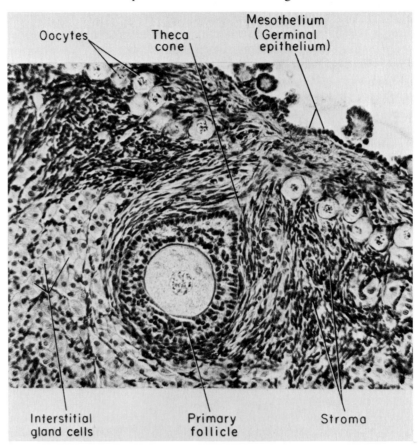

FIGURE 13.8. High magnification of a rabbit ovary. Primordial follicles containing small oocytes are in a zone near the surface of the ovary separated from the germinal epithelium by a fibrous layer. A single small follicle (primary follicle), with about three layers of granulosa cells, contains a larger oocyte. Around the small follicle is a layer of theca cells, which initially form a cone toward the edge of the ovary. The interstitial cells resemble the corpus luteum cells seen in Fig. 13.5b. [Photograph provided by Dr. R. J. Blandau, University of Washington.]

tissue'' of all mammalian ovaries as being equivalent, and he classifies at least seven types. In all cases interstitial cells are those found between follicles and functional corpora lutea. The most common type is derived from the *theca interna* of atretic follicles. The abundance of such generally rounded masses of apparently hormone-secreting tissue is correlated with cycles of follicular formation and atresia (Fig. 13.7a). Stromal-type interstitial tissue often is seen as regular cords of cells that seem to take origin from the ovarian cortex and extend inward. This type is most abundant in rabbits (Fig. 13.8) and hyraxes (Fig. 13.9). Cytologically, Mossman considers stromal interstitial tissue similar to thecal cells. A third type of ovarian interstitial tissue is the medullary cord-type seen typically in the mink and shrew (Fig. 13.9a). This type forms rows or groups of cells that seem to arise from the inner (medullary) part of the ovary, which is characteristically concerned with testicular structures. However, there is no evidence that ovarian medullary cords secrete anything but estrogenic or possibly progestational steroids. A fourth type of interstitial cell is the corticoadrenal cell type found commonly in the ovaries and nearby structures of the equine mammals, the armadillo, and ground squirrel. Definitive proof that these structures secrete corticosteroids is not yet at hand, but corticosteroids are known to be important in reproductive phenomena of some female mammals (e.g., monkey). Other types of interstitial tissue found in the fetal ovary only, and those derived from rete tubules (male structures near the attachment of the mesovarium; Fig. 13.9a) or from nervous tissue can be mentioned.

At any rate, the diversity of types of ovarian interstitial hormone-secreting cells is indicative of the range of pliability and modification of the endocrine functions of the mammalian ovary in evolutionary adaptation of reproductive mechanisms. Since little is yet known of the cyclicity, amounts, and exact nature of the ovarian hormones, or their precise tissues of origin, we can do little more than speculate in the following pages about endocrine mechanisms in female mammals other than the human and rat.

An example of this rather academic speculation concerns the need for an antrum in the follicle. One interpretation is that as the ovum has shrunk in most placental mammals because unneeded yolk is no longer deposited in it, the follicular wall could not shrink, because this would lessen its endocrine secretory capacity. In the South American vizcacha, for example, in which ovarian follicles remain only a little larger than the ovum itself, hundreds of follicles are formed, probably because their periodic hormonal production is needed. In the human ovary, which normally matures only one follicle and one ovum per cycle, there are many atretic follicles produced during the same cycle. These cannot ovulate, but their theca internas proliferate to form numerous cyclic ''thecal glands'' (see Fig. 13.7a, which illustrates an eccentrically proliferated thecal gland) whose steroid secretion is essential in precipitating ovulation (to be explained later) and in regulating the sex accessory structures to a state appropriate to receive the ovulated egg.

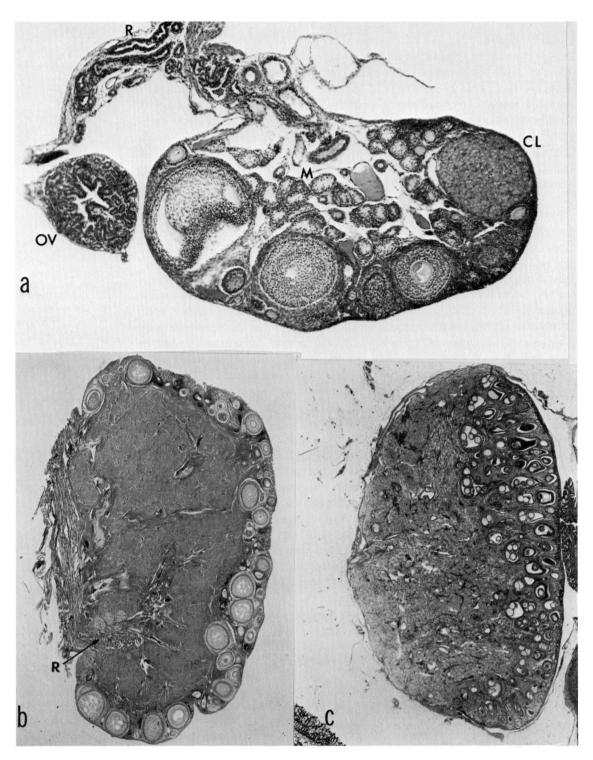

Nonmammalian Vertebrate Ovaries

Just as there is no one mammalian ovarian type, it is not really possible to typify the ovarian structures of other vertebrate groups. However, a few generalizations can be made.

In birds, generally there is only one (left) ovary (Fig. 13.1), but there are a few species (hawks, ring doves) that are bilateral. After ovariectomy, the rudimentary ambisexual right ovary, under proper experimental conditions, can be made to differentiate as a testis or as an ovary with the appropriate female or male endocrine properties. The follicle is completely filled by the avian oocyte, which develops to huge proportions by accumulation of yolk (Fig. 13.10); most of the yolk is synthesized in the liver, not by the egg or follicle itself. The avian follicle is lined by a thin granulosa and two thecal layers. Commonly the avian egg follicle grows so large that the ovary cannot accomodate it. As it matures and grows, it is suspended from the ovary by a stalk that contains the vascular supply. In several species the ovarian theca secretes estradiol and testosterone. Progesterone may be secreted by the postovulatory follicle, but no corpus luteum is formed. These hormones play particular—and usually successive—roles in the avian female reproductive process. Some follicular atresia occurs in avian ovaries. However, the endocrine status of atretic follicles in birds is unsettled.

The usual caveat must be made at this point that what is known about the endocrine properties of the parts of the bird's ovary is based on research with only a few common species, most often the chicken. Justification for making firm generalizations is lacking.

The reptilian ovary is hollow, and as eggs mature and grow, they project into the central lumen. Only suggestions of such a space can be seen in the avian ovary or that of monotreme mammals, the structure of the reptilian follicle resembles that of birds in most respects, but there is more variability in the sizes of the ova and the amounts of yolk deposited. True corpora lutea that secrete progesterone are formed in some reptilian species, particularly

FIGURE 13.9. Ovaries of three mammals showing special features. (a) Pregnant Shrew (*Sorex vagrans*). Note the corpus luteum (*CL*). The oviduct (*OV*) appears on the left. Above the oviduct is the mesentery, or mesovarium. The mesovarium contains rudiments (*R*) of the mesonephric tubules. In the male they would form the epididymis. Such embryonic remainders in the female are called epoophoron. The ovary contains three large follicles. In the medullary (inner) part of the ovary are a number of medullary cords (*M*), also probably originating from male rudiments. (b) Hyrax (*Procavia sp*). Note the great development of interstitial tissue of the adrenal type, occupying most of the gonad except for the follicles at the right margin. There is an extensive remnant of mesonephric (male) rete tubules (*R*). (× 11.5) (c) Juvenile striped skunk (*Mephitis*). Interstitial tissue, probably of medullary origin, is as well developed as in the hyrax. There are numerous oocytes in the antrums of individual follicles (a peculiarity that is difficult to account for). This is more common in young females and in the deeper (medullary) follicles. Up to five oocytes appear in the sectional plane of one follicle. The ovary is embedded in fat, except for the surface at the right where the oviduct is visible. (× 27) [Photographs provided by Professor H. W. Mossman from his collection.]

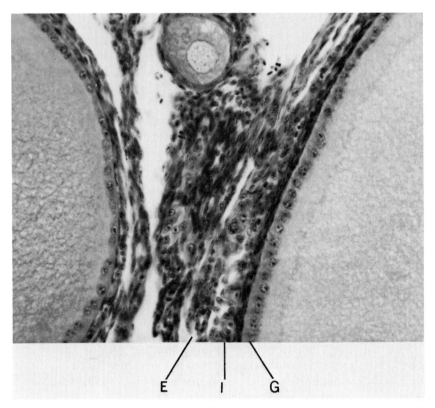

E   I   G

FIGURE 13.10. Section of a small portion of the ovary of the white-crowned sparrow (*Zonotrichia leucophrys*). The edges of two developing eggs and their follicles are shown. For the follicle on the right, the granulosa layer (*G*), theca interna (*I*) and theca externa (*E*) are labeled. A small (primordial) follicle appears between the two larger ones. In the loose connective tissue below the small follicle some interstitial cells can be seen (not labeled). [Photograph provided by Professor M. D. Kern, College of Wooster.]

the viviparous and ovoviviparous species. These latter are species in which eggs are retained in the oviduct or uterus and develop placentalike organs of metabolic exchange between embryo and mother. Thus in reptiles there is a much broader range of modes of reproduction than in birds—from purely oviparous (e.g., alligators) to viviparous (e.g., rattlesnake).

The amphibian ovary also is paired and hollow (Fig. 13.11), like that of reptiles. Ovulation of matured eggs is into the general coelomic cavity. The yolky oocyte fills the entire follicle, and the stretched, thin granulosal and thecal layers are reduced to a minimum, but are steroidogenic. Possibly steroidogenic interstitial tissue, as well, occurs in the amphibian ovary, and in some species postovulatory follicles have a "glandular" histological structure. Most amphibians are oviparous; but, as mentioned earlier in this chapter, types of viviparity may be found in some species. Corpus luteum–like structures have been described in the ovaries of viviparous salamanders (e.g., *Salamandra atra*) as well as in viviparous toads (e.g., *Nectophrynoides*). The corpora lutea of *Nectophrynoides* are active (in histochemical tests) in steroid hormone production, and there is some evidence that the steroid is progesterone. Corpus luteum-like structures are lacking in ovaries of oviparous amphibians.

An odd adaptation for care of developing eggs is found in some anuran oviparous amphibians, in which the eggs are carried on the back of the female (e.g., *Pipa pipa*). The eggs at first adhere by virtue of the sticky character of the external jelly coat. Then they gradually sink into individual integumentary pits that form around them. This tendency is carried to a further extreme in tree frogs of the genus *Gastrotheca*, in which the eggs are placed within marsupiumlike folds of skin on the back of the female for development. The involvement of hormones in these phenomena is unknown. It should be obvious that aside from the anatomic adaptations, this reproductive pattern requires that there must be complex behavioral adaptations as well.

The ovary of teleostean fishes is paired, as a rule (but not always), and hollow, but otherwise it is variable enough to resist generalizations about it. Commonly, the oviducts are attached to the ovary in such a way that the ovarian lumen is continuous with that of the oviduct. Ovulation in such species must be inward, into the ovarian lumen. In the salmonids, on the other hand, there is no oviduct. Here eggs are shed outward, into the coelomic cavity. A duct that is open from the posterior, narrowed end of the abdominal cavity to the urogenital papilla leads the eggs to the exterior. Most of the species of bony fishes are oviparous. However, viviparity is reasonably common. In most viviparous teleosts, embryos develop in the oviducts. However, in other groups fertilization and development occur in the ovarian lumen (Fig. 13.12). In Poeciliids fertilization and most of the

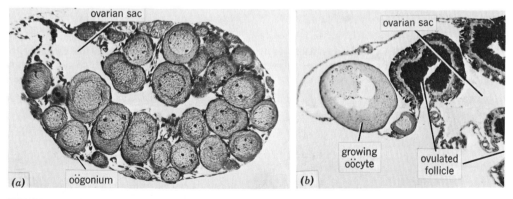

FIGURE 13.11. Ovaries of the wood frog: (*a*) at the metamorphosis stage; (*b*) in the adult after ovulation. (Adult ovary is at half the magnification of the younger ovary.) [From E. Witschi, *Development of the Vertebrates*, Saunders, Philadelphia, 1956.]

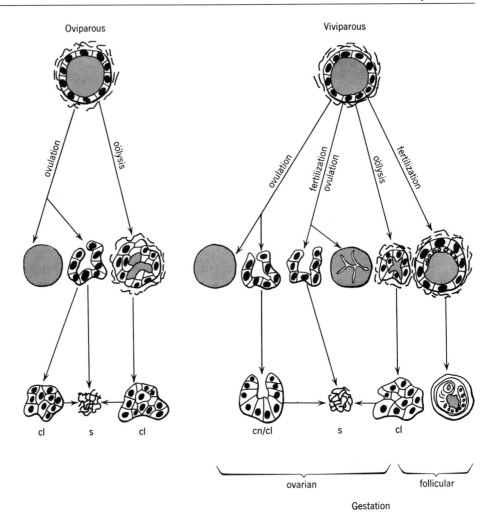

FIGURE 13.12. Possible fates of the ovarian follicle in different teleost species. Ova (yolk masses) are shown in gray. Embryos develop in the ovaries of some species (for example, sea perches); here the ovarian epithelium (and, occasionally, the postovulatory follicle) may form a partially luteinized nutritive structure: the calyx nutricius (*cn/cl*). *cl*, Corpus luteum; *s*, scar. [Redrawn from W. Hoar, *Memoir of the Society for Endocrinology*, No. 4, Cambridge University Press, London, 1955.]

development of the embryo occur in the ovarian follicle itself. Some of the additional adaptations required for viviparity in teleosts were described earlier in this chapter.

The ovarian follicle of teleosts is relatively simple. Most often there is a thin granulosa layer that surrounds the yolky egg cell. The theca does not usually contain obvious secretory cells but is thin and fibrous. After ovulation the granulosa layer of oviparous species may either degenerate or

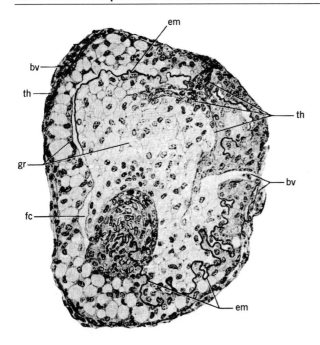

FIGURE 13.13. Preovulatory corpus luteum (formed from an unovulated atretic follicle) of a bony fish (the bitterling). The only recognizable remainder of the degenerated oocyte is the fragmented vitelline membrane (*em*). Both granulosa (*gr*) and theca cells (*th*) grow into the area formerly occupied by the oocyte. Experimental evidence indicates that the corpus luteum of the bitterling secretes a progesteronelike hormone. *bv*, Blood vessel; *fc*, follicular cavity. [From J. H. Bretschneider and J. J. Duyvené de Wit, *Sexual Endocrinology of Non-mammalian Vertebrates*, Elsevier, New York, 1947.]

undergo hypertrophy and hyperplasia to form a corpus luteum–like structure (Fig. 13.12). In some species corpus luteum–like structures may form from atretic follicles. In viviparous teleosts the same kinds of alternatives are found. That is, the granulosa of the ovulated follicle may degenerate or form a presumably secretory corpus luteum. Corpora lutea may also form from atretic follicles (Fig. 13.13). In some viviparous species the follicle may develop structures into which extensions of embryonic tissue grow. The function of such follicular derivatives is nutritive and satisfies other vital needs (respiration, excretion) of the retained embryos.

Among the elasmobranch species (sharks, skates, and rays), some have one ovary, and some two ovaries. All have two oviducts into which there is a common opening (ostium) at the anterior extremity of the body cavity. The oviducts each enlarge posteriorly to become uteri, which open into the cloaca. Characteristically, the elasmobranchs produce extremely large yolky eggs in their ovaries. The follicles investing these eggs consist of granulosa and thecal layers (Fig. 13.14). The ovulated follicles characteristically transform into corpora lutea (*Scyliorhinus*, the dogfish shark), for which there is good evidence of progesterone formation. Corpora lutea also may form from atretic follicles. In fact, in some species (*Torpedo*) all corpora derive from atretic follicles, and apparently none from ovulated follicles. Generally, between the oviduct and uterus there is a shell gland. In oviparous elasmobranch species the shell gland, oviduct, and uterus secrete layers of nutritive materials and a leathery shell around the yolky egg. The shells often have fantastic shapes and long tendrils that entwine and attach the

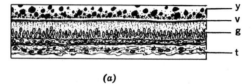

(a)

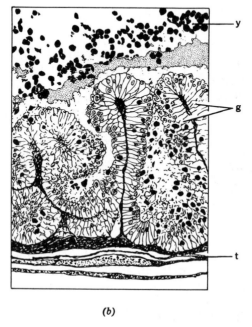

(b)

FIGURE 13.14. Sections through the walls of ovarian follicles from the spiny dogfish ($\times$ 68). (a) From a large follicle, showing active secretion of yolk by normal granulosa cells; (b) from a large atretic follicle, showing phagocytic granulosa cells ingesting yolk; this structure represents the beginning of corpus luteum formation and illustrates the primitive phagocytic function of the corpus luteum. g, Granulosa; t, theca; v, vitelline membrane; y, yolk granules. [After F. L. Hisaw, Jr. and F. L. Hisaw, *Anat. Rec.*, **135**:296, 1959.]

eggs to underwater plants. In viviparous species, which retain the fertilized egg in the uterus, there is either no shell or one that is so thin as to appear like a transparent film.

There is special interest in the gonads of cyclostomes (lampreys and hagfishes), since they are modern representatives of the most primitive vertebrates. However, aside from the fact that both have only a single ovary and no sex ducts, there is little similarity between the ovaries of the two cyclostome groups. Both are oviparous, but the lamprey lays large numbers of small eggs in the gravel of running streams, while the hagfish forms only about 20 to 30 large, oval, yolky eggs at one time (Fig. 13.15). Hagfish eggs have a leathery shell with a tuft of hooks at each end. The function of these hooks seems to be to attach eggs to each other or to objects near where they are deposited. In both types of cyclostomes the ovarian follicle consists of a granulosa and theca layer that surround the egg. The unusual feature of the hagfish egg follicle is that it secretes the eggshell. This means that the ovarian granulosa itself at the narrow ends of the eggs must be folded into highly complex patterns to secrete the numerous hooks. No other vertebrate

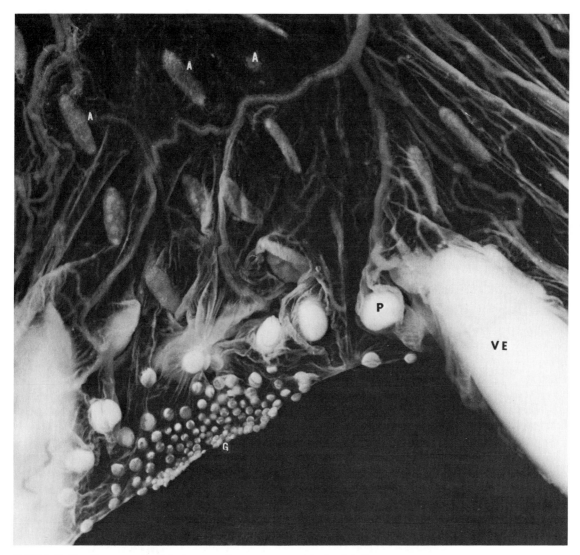

FIGURE 13.15. One segment of the long membranous ovary of the hagfish (*Eptatretus stouti*). The germinal epithelium is restricted to the free ventral edge (*G*) of the ovary. Oocytes multiply in this region and grow as they move dorsally (upward). The largest previtellogenic oocyte in its follicle is labeled *P*. Vitellogenesis begins as the follicles and their eggs elongate. However, only 20 to 30 eggs continue vitellogenesis (*VE*) to maturity; all the others undergo atresia (*A*). Because the process of folliculogenesis is continuous, the number of atretic follicles increases as normal eggs continue vitellogenesis. The rather uniform atretic follicles are 4 to 5 mm long and can be used to gauge the sizes of other structures in this photograph.

ovarian follicle has such a function or intricate form. The endocrine properties of the cyclostome ovary are virtually unknown.

Structure of the Male Reproductive System

The large number of alternatives in female reproductive patterns (yolky versus nonyolky eggs, oviparity versus viviparity, extraoval nutritive layers, production of a second type of steroid hormone, etc.) has resulted in a wide spectrum of structures of female systems, not only in the vertebrates at large, but even within the mammalian group. The tasks of the male system are certainly more uniform: the production of spermatozoa and their delivery through ducts at the proper time. As a consequence, male reproductive systems are much more comparable among mammals, and even among males of the entire vertebrate group.

Compare, for example, the male reproductive system of the rat (Fig. 13.16) with that of a bird or salamander (Figs. 13.17 and 13.18). In all cases there are two testes. Spermatozoa, the testicular *external "secretion,"* pass into a usually complexly folded tube—the epididymis—and from there into

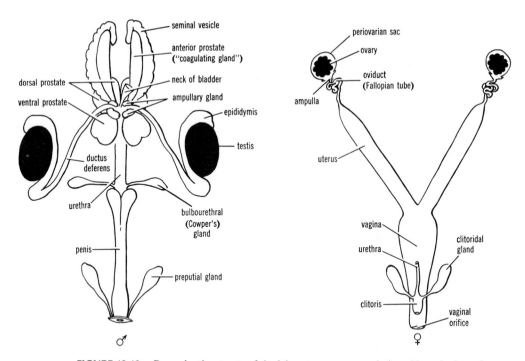

FIGURE 13.16. Reproductive tracts of the laboratory rat, ventral view. Note the homologous ambisexual preputial and clitoridal glands. In the female rat, each uterus (right and left) projects into the upper vagina via a separate cervix. The male sex accessory glands show considerable variation among different mammalian species. [Based on C. D. Turner, *General Endocrinology*, Saunders, Philadelphia, 1960.]

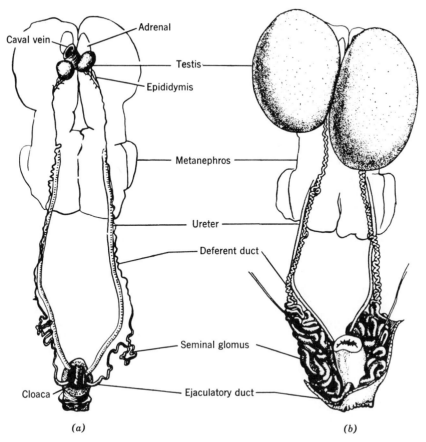

Caval vein
Adrenal
Testis
Epididymis
Metanephros
Ureter
Deferent duct
Seminal glomus
Cloaca
Ejaculatory duct

(a)   (b)

FIGURE 13.17. Male reproductive tract of orange weaver finch (*Euplectes franciscanus*) (*a*) in March (sexually inactive) and (*b*) in September (sexually active). [From E. Witschi, *Comparative Endocrinology* (A. Gorbman, ed.), Wiley, New York, 1959.]

a straighter tube—the vas deferens (or deferent duct). This duct is generally joined by the ureter from the same side at its lower end, and together they drain to the outside through the urethra. The principal differences in male systems mostly pertain to the amount (and region) of coiling of the vas deferens, the addition of glands at the lower end of the vas deferens, and modification of the tissues around the urethra to form an intromittent organ. The intromittent organ (penis) enables the transfer of sperm to the female for internal fertilization. In mammals in particular, a variety of glands become associated with the lower end of the vas deferens (Fig. 13.16). These secrete fluids (semen) in which the spermatozoa become suspended, and they have different functions: nutrition, control of pH, volume. Seminal volume becomes an important factor when sperm must transverse uteri of large diameter (e.g., horse, elephant) on the way to the ovum in the oviduct.

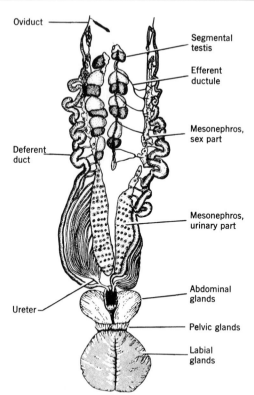

FIGURE 13.18.   Urogenital organs of an adult male salamander (*Taricha torosa*). Note segmental testis and rudimentary oviduct. Light area of each testicular lobe contains mature sperm; dark area contains immature stages. [From E. Witschi, *Development of Vertebrates*, Saunders, Philadelphia, 1956.]

As will be described below, the functions of all of these accessory structures are regulated by the testicular androgens. Thus the testis not only produces spermatozoa, but—through its hormonal endocrine secretion—it ensures the functional adequacy of the ducts through which the spermatozoa must pass, the glands in whose secretions the sperm are contained, and the behavior than ensures the delivery of the spermatozoa to the site of fertilization.

Structure of the Testis.   In mammals the testes are typically oval and are surrounded by a fibrous coat, the tunica albuginea (Fig. 13.19). The organ is filled completely by a complex of seminiferous tubules, in which the spermatozoa form by multiplication and differentiation of stem cells—the spermatogonia—which remain next to the basement membrane (Figs. 13.19, 13.20). As the spermatogonia enter the process of spermatogenesis, they grow in size, and meiotic changes can be seen in their nuclei (leptotene and pachytene stages are visible in Fig. 13.20). Such a cell is called a primary spermatocyte. After two quick divisions, during which the chromosome number is reduced to haploid, the spermatid stage is produced. Spermatids then undergo radical cytoplasmic changes (spermiogenesis) that result in the formation of mature spermatozoa. At least the latter stages of spermiogenesis are in part regulated by testosterone. The process of spermiogenic maturation continues even as the sperm move through the seminiferous tubules into the epididymis.

The tubular structure of the testis varies slightly in different mammals. In the rat at least some of the tubules end blindly distally. In humans, however, the distal ends of the seminiferous tubules anastomose, forming loops (Fig. 13.21). The attached ends of the seminiferous tubules empty into the rete, a maze of interconnected nonspermatogenic tubules, which in turn are drained by short vasa efferentia into the epididymis. When sperm first enter the epididymis, they are relatively low in fertility (i.e., the ability to successfully fertilize an egg). It has been estimated that sperm require about three weeks (both in humans and rodents) to traverse the epididymis. During this time they continue to mature, and gradually become increasingly more fertile. However, this completion of extratesticular maturation requires an appropriate concentration of male hormone in the medium suspending the spermatozoa. This concentration of androgen in the epididymal lumen is made possible by an androgen-binding protein (ABP) secreted by the Sertoli cells.

The Sertoli cells (Fig. 13.20) are another cellular constituent of the seminiferous tubule. They are anchored to the basement membrane and extend toward the lumen of the tubule. The Sertoli cell is obviously (number of

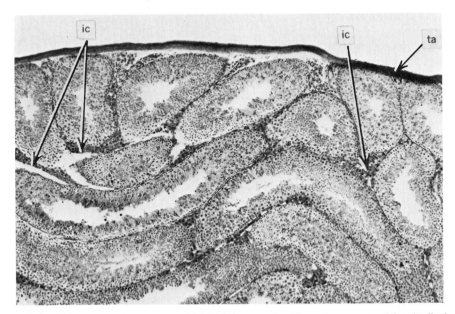

FIGURE 13.19. Testis of 9-month-old laboratory mouse. Note transverse and longitudinal sections through seminiferous tubules. Between tubules are islands and strands of dark-staining interstitial cells (*ic*). Testis is enclosed in a dense connective tissue capsule, the tunica albuginea (*ta*).

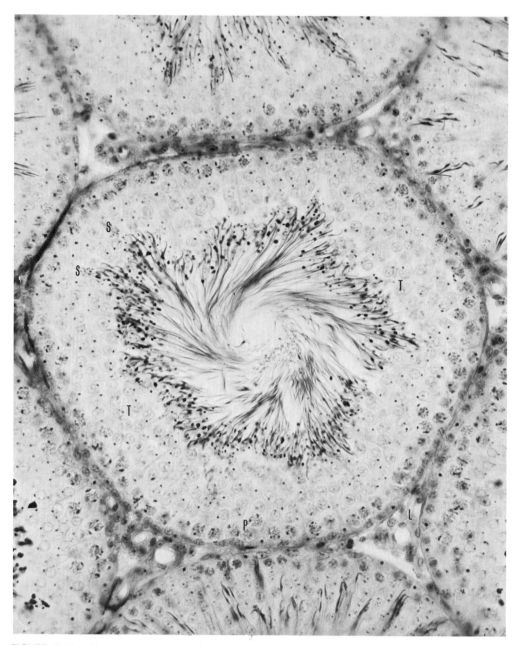

FIGURE 13.20. *Center*: cross section of a single seminiferous tubule of the rat. Maturing sperm fill most of the lumen. The heads of most of these are still buried in the Sertoli cells (*S*). Most of the cells forming a broad zone between the spermatozoa and the outer edge of the tubule are spermatids (*T*). Against the basement membrane, at the outer edge of the tubule, is a slightly darker zone of oval nuclei belonging to the spermatogonia (not labeled). Between these cells and the spermatids is a zone (1 to 2 cells broad) of large nuclei containing granular, threadlike material or dense pachytene chromosomes. These (labeled *P*) are the primary spermatocytes. The triangular areas between the tubules contain interstitial Leydig cells (*L*). These generally surround a blood capillary. [Photograph provided by Professor Edward Roosen-Runge, University of Washington.]

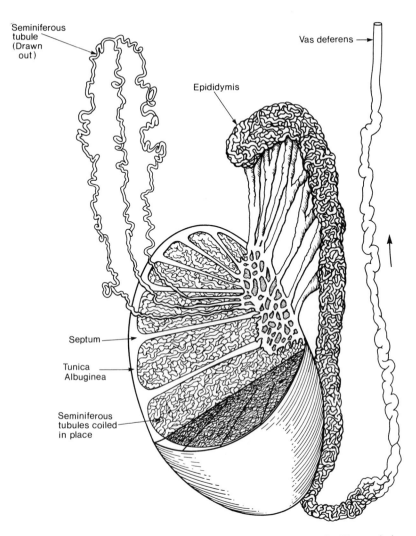

Seminiferous
tubule
(Drawn
out)

Vas deferens →

Epididymis

Septum

Tunica
Albuginea

Seminiferous
tubules coiled
in place

FIGURE 13.21. General organization of the human testis. The testis is divided into compartments by connective tissue septa extending inward from the tunica albuginea. The incomplete septa allow for continuity of the rete tubular network at one side of the human testis. The rete is drained by vasa efferentia (unlabeled) into the epididymis and thence into the vas deferens. One seminiferous tubule complex is shown as though it were drawn out to one side to illustrate the anastomosis of the distal ends of three tubules. [After G. W. Corner, *The Hormones in Human Reproduction*, Atheneum, New York, 1963.]

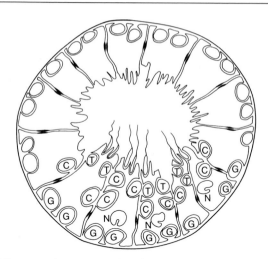

FIGURE 13.22. Diagrammatic representation of the relationships between Sertoli cells and the spermatogenic cell line in a cross section of the seminiferous tubule of the rat. The Sertoli cells form a continuous ring, with cell-to-cell contact. Tight junctions of Sertoli cells are shown as thickened black structures at the contact cell surfaces. Against the basement membrane are the spermatogonia (G). The spermatocytes (C) and spermatids (T) derived from the spermatogonia are shown closer to the lumen. Some spermatozoa, still embedded in the Sertoli cells, are shown at the luminal extremities. The relative detail of sperm line relationships is shown only at the bottom of the figure. N, nuclei of Sertoli cells.

mitochondria, development of endoplasmic reticulum, etc.) a metabolically active cell with a complex of functions. In addition to secreting ABP, it apparently synthesizes enzymes for metabolizing steroids to form testosterone or testosterone steroid derivatives. A less well-established function of Sertoli cells is the synthesis and secretion of a substance named *inhibin*. This substance, for which there appears to be a chemical counterpart in the ovary, is a nonsteroidal inhibitor of FSH release from the pars distalis. More will be said about inhibin later in this chapter.

An interesting structural feature of the Sertoli cell is illustrated diagrammatically in Fig. 13.22. A short distance inward from the basement membrane, the cell membranes of adjacent Sertoli cells appear tightly joined. Parallel and adjacent to these tight junctions are arrays of rough endoplasmic reticulum and microfibrils. In experimental tests of the movement of marker substances injected into the blood or into the space between seminiferous tubules, it has been found that these inter-Sertoli cell junctions form a block to the free movement of chemical materials from an outer or basal "compartment" into the adluminal compartment (Fig. 13.23). This has been named the *blood–testis barrier*. In effect, it ensures that the only substances that can penetrate into the lumen of the seminiferous tubule must be taken up and/or secreted by the Sertoli cell. Also, as Fig. 13.22 shows diagrammatically, the cells of the spermatogonial series are more or less deeply embedded in the Sertoli cells and partly encased in their plasma membranes. The spermatogonia and early primary spermatocytes are in the basal compartment, while the later primary spermatocytes, spermatids, and spermatozoa are within the adluminal compartment. How entire cells penetrate the blood–testis barrier, while chemical metabolites do not, is not yet clear. However, it is clear that spermatozoa complete their development in an environment whose chemical composition is selectively controlled by the Sertoli cells.

Sites of Synthesis of Androgenic Hormones.   A variety of approaches have been used to help decide where in the testis the synthesis of male hormone occurs. Cytological features generally associated with an ability to synthesize steroids (abundant smooth endoplasmic reticulum and tubular "cristae" in the mitochondria) can be sought, and such structures have been described both in the Leydig (interstitial) cells and the Sertoli cells. His-

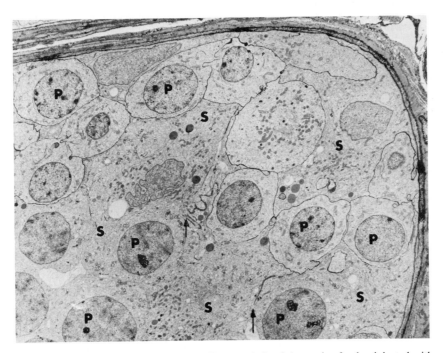

FIGURE 13.23.   Section of part of a seminiferous tubule of the testis of a dog injected with a lanthanum salt, used as a staining agent. The stain has diffused between the external tubular cells and is visible as a clear thin black line in the intercellular spaces. The fine black lines end at a particular distance from the basement membrane, adjacent to Sertoli cells (two such places are marked by arrows). These points are where the tight junctions between Sertoli cells are located. Labels: S, Sertoli cell; P, primary spermatocyte. Note that some primary spermatocytes (younger stages) are outlined by lanthanum stain and, therefore, are outside the blood–testis barrier. Other primary spermatocytes (deeper in the tubule) lack the lanthanum outline, and thus are beyond the blood–testis barrier. [Photograph was supplied by Dr. Carolyn J. Connell.]

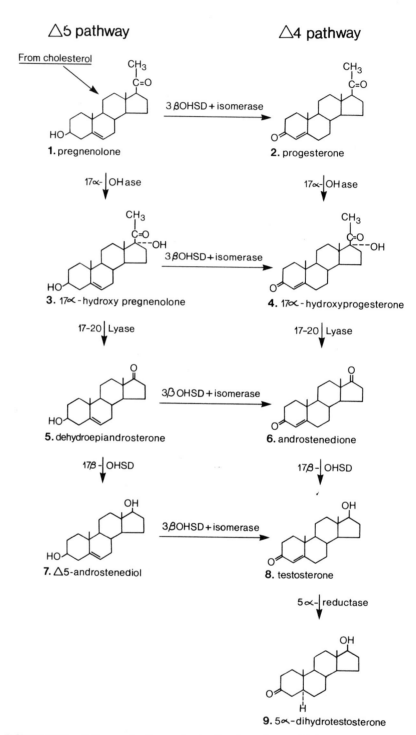

FIGURE 13.24. Pathways for the synthesis of androgenic steroids by testicular tissue.

tochemical tests for enzymes such as 3β-hydroxysteroid dehydrogenase can be done, and these enzymes can be found in both Leydig and Sertoli cells. There are some procedures for the separation of testicular cell types that will yield almost pure interstitial cells, or pure tubules, or even "enriched" Sertoli cell preparations. Such cell preparations can be incubated with isotopically labeled precursors such as cholesterol, pregnenolone, or progesterone (Fig. 13.24), and later analysis shows whether labeled testosterone has been produced. In such *in vitro* tests Leydig cells can produce testosterone from cholesterol. However—though there is disagreement on this point, particularly as regards different species—Sertoli cells appear to lack the ability to form testosterone from cholesterol, by side-chain cleavage although they can do this from labeled pregnenolone or progesterone. It must be said, however, that in the human or rat testis, in quantitative terms, the Sertoli cells contribute only a small fraction to the total testosterone and androstenedione formation.

SEX HORMONES

Testicular Hormones

Testosterone is without question the most frequently encountered male sex steroid. However, in different mammalian species the concentrations and distributions (in mitochondria and smooth endoplasmic reticulum) of the steroidogenic enzymes is such that still other androgenic hormones may be produced in considerable proportions. For example, the rat testis has been found to secrete pregnenolone and progesterone as such. The rabbit testis secretes androstenedione and androstenediol as well as dihydrotestosterone (Fig. 13.24) in addition to testosterone. The stallion testis is well known as a source of estrogens. The testes of some fishes and amphibians secrete 11-ketotestosterone.

It is of some interest that testosterone can be formed from pregnenolone by a variety of metabolic pathways. The two major pathways are called the Δ4 and Δ5 pathways, respectively, depending upon whether the intermediate compounds utilized have the unsaturated bond in the A or B ring. As Fig. 13.24 shows, part of one pathway may be used, shifting to the other if the appropriate enzymes are present. Using (for brevity) the numbers of the intermediate compounds as they appear in Fig. 13.24, we may summarize the *major* pathway to testosterone used in the rabbit as **1, 3, 5, 7, 8**—thus primarily a Δ5 pathway. In the rat the major pathway is **1, 3, 4, 6, 8**. However, such studies are generally done with the testis *in vitro*, and the pathway *in vivo* might be different. Nevertheless, this kind of study illustrates the possibility of differences in rates and patterns of gonadal steroidogenesis, depending upon the genomic control of the amounts and kinds of enzymes transcribed and translated in the hormonogenic cells.

Another variable in this picture is the fact that some cells, because of the nature of their enzyme content, can perform only later or limited steps in hormone synthesis. This is seen in the inability of Sertoli cells to synthesize testosterone from cholesterol. Sertoli cells thus are obliged to depend upon neighboring Leydig cells for pregnenolone, the earliest steroid intermediate they are able to utilize for the production of testosterone. Another interesting illustration of this is the fact that some "targets" of androgen action (brain, seminal vesicle, prostate) cannot synthesize testosterone, but, because they contain 5α-reductase, they can convert testosterone within their cytoplasms to 5α-dihydrotestosterone (DHT). Some brain cells contain the enzymatic machinery to convert testosterone to estradiol (Fig. 13.25).

Ovarian Hormones

The typical hormones produced in the ovary are estradiol-17β and progesterone. However, judging from their ultrastructure and histochemical properties, there are four kinds of steroid-secreting cells in the ovary: interstitial, thecal, granulosa, and corpus luteum cells. These tissues are developed to different degrees according to the time in the life cycle, in the seasonal cycle, and in the reproductive cycle. Since these tissues may—and probably do—have different steroidogenic and secretory properties, depending upon their enzymatic equipment, this creates an array of possibilities for the secretion of different ovarian steroids at different phases of the sex cycle.

In the preceding paragraphs some of these possibilities have already been mentioned; thus, in addition to estradiol and progesterone, variable amounts (depending on the species) of corticosteroids, androgens, and estrone may be found in the ovary and in the blood (Fig. 13.25) of female mammals. In addition to estradiol, equilin and equilenin (Fig. 13.25) are produced in lesser quantities by the horse. If such relatively different ovarian estrogens can be formed in the equine ungulates, one wonders what steroids might be found by chemical "exploration" in still other vertebrate species. The currently used methods of radioimmunoassay do not lend themselves to chemical identification of steroids, so that further progress in this area may be slow. Estriol in fairly large amounts is found in the human placenta.

Considerable attention recently has been directed to the relative steroid synthetic abilities of the ovarian theca and granulosa cells. Conclusions are based on separating the two cell types from each other and culturing them with various isotope-labeled steroid hormone precursors, sometimes in the presence of gonadotropic hormones. At the end of culture the steroid products formed from the precursors are identified. By such procedures it has been found that theca cells readily synthesize progesterone and androgens from precursors, but in several species they have insufficient aromatase enzyme to produce much, if any, estrogen from the androgens (Fig. 13.26). Granulosa cells, on the other hand appear to lack the enzymes that split off carbon 20 and carbon 21 and hydroxylate carbon 17. Thus progesterone will

Abbreviated Summary
Ovarian Steroidogenesis

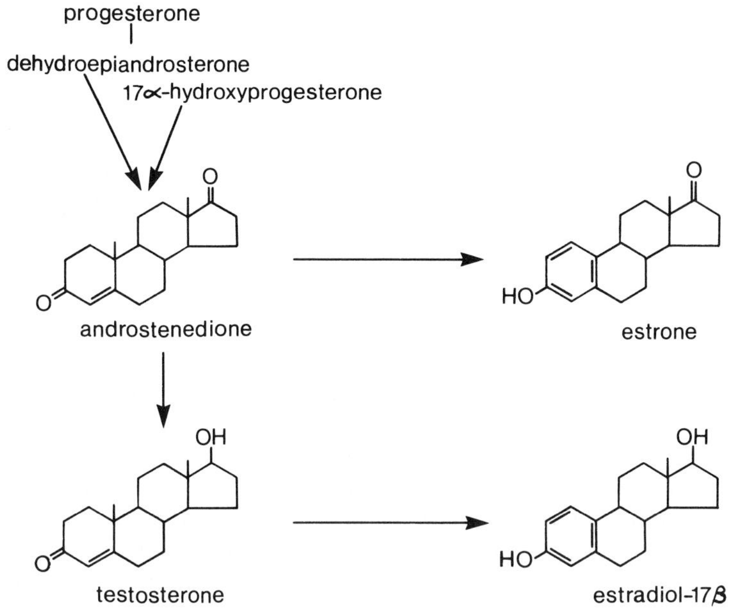

progesterone

dehydroepiandrosterone

17α-hydroxyprogesterone

androstenedione

estrone

testosterone

estradiol-17β

Other Estrogens

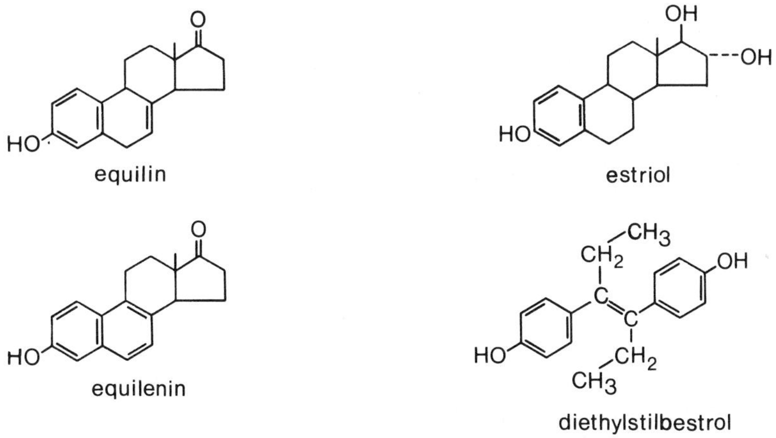

equilin

estriol

equilenin

diethylstilbestrol

FIGURE 13.25. Brief summary (leaving out intermediate steps) of the metabolism of steroids in ovarian and other tissues. The conversion of androgens to estrogens involves the removal of one methyl group (carbon 19) and unsaturation of the A ring. This process is generally referred to as aromatization, though, properly, aromatization should refer only to the ring change. Aromatization can occur in tissues outside the ovary and is considered especially significant in the brain. See text for further discussion.

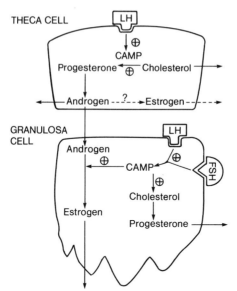

FIGURE 13.26. Scheme of steroid synthesis in cells of the wall of the mammalian ovarian follicle. [Based principally on P. C. K. Leung and D. T. Armstrong, *Ann. Rev. Physiol.*, **42**:71–82, 1980.]

form in the granulosa cells from precursor cholesterol (Fig. 13.26), but not androgen. However, the granulosa cells often contain a high concentration of aromatase and, utilizing androgen that diffuses from the nearby theca cells, convert it to estrogen. FSH has been found in the rat to augment or even to induce the formation of ovarian follicular aromatase. This pattern of collaborative distribution of synthetic follicular function is not universal. In the rhesus monkey, for example, isolated theca cells produce estradiol readily; granulosa cells appear to have the same properties as those mentioned above. Unfortunately, much of this analytic work is open to the criticism that separated ovarian follicular cell types in culture do not function in the same way as they do in the whole organ.

Ovarian Inhibin. A nonsteroid substance has been reported that is extractable from the antra of large follicles of pigs and cows. It inhibits secretion of FSH by cultures of rat pituitary cells. Chemically it appears to resemble *inhibin* from the Sertoli cell of the testis. Its function is uncertain, but it may play a role in regulating the reproductive cycle.

Relaxin. Relaxin is a water-soluble polypeptide substance only recently purified, but known as a biological entity for many years. Its source appears to be the corpus luteum of pregnant animals. Its typical action, after which it is named, is a softening of the ligament that connects the lower ends of the pelvic bones to each other. This permits enlargement of the space enclosed by the pelvic bones. Such separation of the pelvic bones facilitates the movement of large fetuses through the birth canal at the time of parturition. There is evidence that estrogens must act first ("prime") on the collagenous tissue of the pelvic ligament before relaxin is effective. Furthermore, it appears that relaxin may have some hitherto unsuspected actions upon the uterus. The amino acid sequence of relaxin contains similarities to insulin.

Steroid-Binding Proteins in the Blood and Steroid Hormone Distribution

Steroid hormones are carried in the blood in concentrations that exceed their solubility because they are bound to particular proteins and kept out of solution. Only a small fraction of free steroid hormones exists in blood plasma and this is in equilibrium with the hormones bound to the carrier proteins. These proteins were described in Chapter 11, and a few additional remarks can be made here with particular reference to the sex steroids.

Sex steroids have been found to bind to a number of different blood proteins in different mammalian species. In nonmammalian species there has been little direct study of this question. In a presumably primitive animal such as the hagfish, for example, there is no detectable protein binding of estradiol in the blood, bringing two questions into focus. Is a lack of steroid binding by proteins in the blood a primitive feature? If it is, what are the adaptive values of such binding? The same questions can be raised concerning the lack of sex steroid-binding proteins in the blood of a fairly large number of avian species. Mammals uniformly have such plasma proteins, but for two surprising exceptions: the rodents and elephants (Table 13.1).

TABLE 13.1. Steroid hormone-binding proteins in vertebrate plasma[a]

Protein	Animal Source	Hormones Bound[b]
CBG (corticosteroid-binding protein)	All mammals (except monotremes) and birds tested; some reptiles and amphibians. Not detectable as such in bony or cartilaginous fishes or in Agnatha	P, C
SBP, SHBG, SBG, TeBG (sex steroid-binding globulin)	All mammals except rodents and elephants. Undetectable in birds. Found in some reptiles; in others a separate T-binding and E-binding protein. Found in bony fishes, but in cartilaginous fishes and lampreys only low-affinity sex hormone binding is found; no binding in hagfishes	E, T
α-Fetoprotein	Rodents, just before and briefly after birth	E
PBG (progesterone-binding globulin)	Guinea pig	P

[a] From J. C. Wingfield, *Hormones, Adaptation and Evolution* (S. Ishii, T. Hirano, and M. Wada, eds.), Springer, Berlin (1979).
[b] P, progesterone; C, corticosteroids; E, estradiol; T, testosterone.

The only sex hormone-binding protein that seems to have a clearly established functional role is α-fetoprotein. Sex differentiation of both the gonad and the brain take place in the latter part of the uterine gestational period, and the brain is still sensitive to the inappropriate hormone for several days after birth. For the mammalian fetus the high concentrations of circulating female sex hormones (estradiol and progesterone) from the maternal and placental circulations at this time would seem to threaten normal male or female differentiation. The relatively high levels of α-fetoprotein would seem to protect against this by retaining estradiol in the blood.

The affinity constants of most of the blood steroid-binding proteins are approximately 10^{-8} M. The affinity constants of the tissue receptor cell proteins for the same hormones are approximately 10 times greater, or about 10^{-9} M. Thus at equilibrium the free steroid hormones will tend to diffuse from the blood into the tissues toward the responsive cells. This generalization depends on the assumption that the steroids in the tissues are being metabolized continually and that a supply of free receptors for the hormones is always available.

ACTIONS OF THE SEX STEROID HORMONES

The actions of the sex steroid hormones at the cellular level were described in Chapter 1. To recapitulate briefly, the steroid hormones diffuse into the cell, where they are fixed by specific high-affinity receptor proteins. In combination with these proteins, they move into the nucleus, where they localize at particular sites in the chromatin complex and lead to the formation of RNAs that later mediate the synthesis of particular proteins. We may infer that the particular parts of the genome whose transcriptional activities are regulated in this way by the steroid hormones are differentiated according to the target cell type. In other words, in each cell type a different spectrum of proteins will be synthesized. Among the actions stimulated by estradiol are endosteal bone formation (mice), lipovitellin synthesis in the liver (many vertebrates), exocrine secretions by a variety of glands in the oviduct and uterus, growth of ducts in the human mammary gland, pigmentary changes in the areolar skin around the human nipple, changes in behavior, changes in contractility of uterine smooth muscle, and more. It is obvious that the enzymes and structural proteins synthesized in each of these tissues in response to estrogen are different and that they are parts of the special patterns evolved in the reproduction of particular vertebrate species. Accordingly, in describing the biological actions of the different steroids, a complete list cannot be offered, but some of the chief or representative actions of the steroid hormones will be described.

It can be anticipated that the effects of the sex steroids can be grouped into particular categories: (1) actions on the gonad itself, (2) actions on the ducts through which the gametes and developing young must pass, (3) actions on accessory sex structures and metabolism, (4) feedback actions on the hypothalamo-pituitary system, and (5) other actions.

Actions of Ovarian Hormones

Actions at the Ovarian Level. Evidence that the steroid hormones produced by the gonads have actions in the gonads themselves has been accumulating, but this is still not well understood. Furthermore, in the intact test animal experiments must be conducted with care because steroids can—and do—have gonadal effects, both positive and negative, through feedback actions upon pituitary gonadotropic secretion. Therefore, some of the experiments to eliminate this possibility have been done with cultured ovarian or testicular cells, and these have other, special interpretive difficulties. However, it is now clear that there are high-affinity receptors for estrogens and progesterone as well as for corticosteroids in the ovaries of several species that have been appropriately tested.

Some ovarian follicular growth can be induced by estradiol in rats even after hypophysectomy, although under normal conditions a gonadotropic function for estradiol would not seem to be essential. A normal role for estrogen, therefore, would seem to be to potentiate the action of gonadotropin (FSH) on follicular growth. Aside from direct potentiation of follicular development, estradiol also sensitizes pituitary gonadotropic cells to LHRH so that they secrete more hormone. Thus the growing ovarian follicle, by producing estradiol, promotes its own further growth and development through several mechanisms. Progesterone has no direct action on growing ovarian follicles but, depending on the dosage in an experiment, it can stimulate ovulation or prevent it through feedback actions upon the hypothalamo–pars distalis system.

In the post ovulatory mammalian ovary that contains corpora lutea, the action of steroids seems more variable, depending on the species. Estradiol is luteotropic in rabbits, maintaining corpora lutea even after removal of the pituitary gland. Estradiol is also somewhat luteotropic in other species, such as the rat, sheep, horse, and pig, but only if the pituitary is present. In still other species estradiol is luteolytic, causing involution of the corpora lutea in cows, hamsters, and humans. The luteolytic action of estradiol in the hamster seems to require the presence of the uterus, which becomes a source of prostaglandins under estrogenic stimulation; the prostaglandins, in turn, exert the luteolytic action.

In submammalian vertebrates estrogen and progesterone, insofar as they have been studied, have actions analogous to those mentioned in the mammalian ovary; that is, estradiol can stimulate earlier phases of oogenesis. Progesterone and corticosteroids, at least in Amphibia and fishes, can stimulate final maturational changes and ovulation. To what extent these actions are independent of pituitary gonadotropins is not clear.

Actions on the Female Duct System. The first complete studies of the molecular basis of steroid hormone action were those conducted on the avian uterus in connection with the synthesis of the protein avidin. Avidin synthesis involves the successive actions of estrogen and progesterone and transcription of specific RNAs. Ultimately, avidin messenger RNA was isolated and transcribed in a cell-free (*in vitro*) system. There is considerable evidence from many species that estradiol and progesterone can influence their own and each other's cytoplasmic receptor activity in the normal target organs for sex steroids. Estradiol can "prime" (increase) the receptor activity of both hormones. Progesterone in some instances can suppress estradiol receptor activity in the female reproductive tract.

In the embryo sex steroid receptor activity is found in the Müllerian duct, the precursor of the future oviducts, uteri, and vagina. Receptor activity varies during the development of the female tract as well as during the pubertal and postpubertal periods. Furthermore, there are different concentrations of steroid hormone receptors in different regions of the tract. In mammals—at least where they have been sufficiently studied—uterine sex steroid receptors are specific for certain classes of steroids. This may not be the case in lizards, in which uterine growth and glandular secretion can be stimulated by either estradiol or testosterone. In one lizard species (*Lacerta* sp.) both of these hormones stimulate avidin synthesis. Of course, it is possible that the testosterone is being aromatized to estrogen in this reptilian uterus. This remains to be clarified.

The accessory sex organs of the female are essentially tubes through which the spermatozoa must pass toward the egg, and through which the fertilized egg and embryo must pass toward the exterior (see Figs. 13.1 and 13.16). The uppermost part of this tube is a funnel, or ostium, in which the ovary is enclosed. In the rat this funnel is completely closed over the ovary in the form of the periovarial membrane, making it impossible for eggs to escape into the abdominal cavity. In other mammals the eggs, after ovulation, are led by ciliated cells of the funnel into the oviducts, or fallopian tubes. The oviducts, uterus, and vagina all have equivalent, but somewhat different, cross-sectional, circumferentially layered structures. The innermost layer of each is epithelial. In the oviducts the epithelium is ciliated. In the mammalian uterus the epithelial layer dips downward to form frequent, simple tubular glands. In the mammalian vagina the epithelium is generally of the stratified, squamous (flakelike) cell type. Below the epithelial layer is loose connective tissue, and below this, forming the bulk of the tubular organs, is a muscularis layer composed of separate smooth muscle layers running in different directions.

The sex steroids exert a variety of regulatory influences on the tubular parts of the female system. First, there is a *trophic* influence. In an ovariectomized female the oviducts, uterus, and vagina remain undeveloped or regress to a very small size. With injections of large amounts of sex steroid, the same organs can grow to supernormal size. Other, more particular features of the female tract that are susceptible to hormonal control are the number of ciliated cells and their activity in the oviduct; the contractions of the muscularis layers of the oviducts, uterus, and vagina, and the patterns of these contractions (e.g., peristaltic, tonic, toward or away from the ovary); the degree of development and the secretions of the endometrium (glands and supporting, vascularized connective tissue of the uterus); and the multiplication of cells and their character (i.e., whether they are "cornified") in the vaginal mucosa.

Later in this chapter we will discuss the cyclic variations in sex steroid and gonadotropic hormonal concentrations that are characteristic of the reproductive careers of all female vertebrates. This ebbing and flowing of hormonal concentrations results in corresponding cyclic changes in the different regions of the tubular female reproductive tract. In the human uterine endometrium these periodic changes are particularly profound, with the highest glandular structure developed by the successive actions of follicular estrogen and of progesterone from the corpus luteum. The eventual reduction of progesterone secretion causes involutional structural changes, tissue death, and sloughing—the phenomenon of menstruation.

In general, progesterone is the hormone that provokes the kind of endometrial growth and proliferation that makes uterine pregnancy possible in mammals. In the ovariectomized rat, for example, adequate treatment with estrogen followed by progesterone sensitizes the stimulated uterus. At this point, if a surgical thread is passed through the uterus and left in place, a mass of endometrial cells forms around it by localized mitotic multiplication. This tumorlike mass of cells resembles the cells that surround an implanted embryo and form the decidual layers around it; the experimental mass is therefore called a *deciduoma*.

It is of interest that in a variety of experimental or natural situations, in which the uterus may be presumed to be adequately prepared for implantation, implantation of an embryo will not occur if estrogen is missing from the system. In such cases implantation occurs promptly after estradiol treatment. Delayed implantation of blastocyst embryos, often for months, is part of the normal breeding cycle in certain mammalian species (e.g., bears).

In the vagina the cellular actions of estradiol and other estrogens are so characteristic that for many years they were considered diagnostic of the estrous condition—the time when ovarian estrogens are secreted in significant quantities. These actions include stimulation of epithelial cell multiplication and differentiation of the more superficial cell layers. In response to estrogen these cells synthesize a fibrous protein (keratin). During the four-day estrous cycle of the rat there is a succession of changes in the cellular composition of the vaginal mucosal epithelium, reflecting the changes in ovarian hormones secreted into the blood. Before hormonal bioassay was yet possible, J. A. Long and H. M. Evans (1922) discovered that microscopic "smear" samples of the superficial cells in the rat vagina correlated well with the progression of cyclic stages in the ovary (Fig. 13.27,

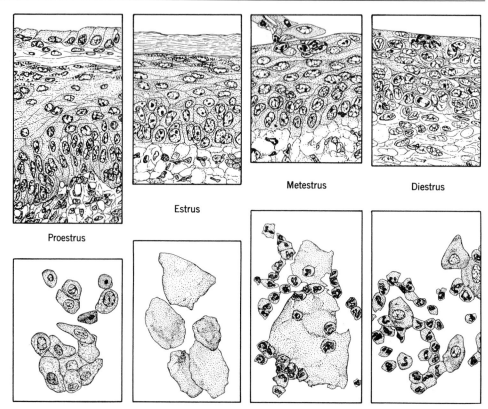

FIGURE 13.27. Vaginal cycle in the rat. *Upper row*: alteration in the lining epithelium of the vagina as visualized in histological sections. Beneath the stratified epithelium (stippled) are connective tissue and blood capillaries. *Lower row*: cells that detach from the lining when a vaginal smear is made (see Table 13.2). In proestrus the surface epithelium is underlain by the newly cornified layers; a smear shows the surface cells to be nucleated epithelium. In estrus the nucleated surface epithelium has been sloughed, and the detached cells are nonnucleated, cornified "squames" (squamous cells), as shown in the smear. In metestrus the superficial "squames" shed entirely, and the leukocytes that invade the epithelium are apparent in the smear along with the "squames". In diestrus the detached cells are nucleated, and are shed along with leukocytes in a variable amount of mucus. [Redrawn from J. A. Long and H. M. Evans, *The Oestrous Cycle in the Rat*, Memoir of the University of California, 1922.]

Table 13.2). The vaginal smear itself could then be used as the basis for the earlier bioassays of estrogens. Typically, for this purpose, unknown materials could be injected into ovariectomized mice or rats to determine the minimum amount needed to induce vaginal cornification. Another characteristic hormonal response of the rat vaginal mucosa is mucification in response to progesterone (Fig. 13.28).

Other Morphological Actions of Female Sex Steroids. Besides the tubular female sex accessory structures, which have contact with the gametes and

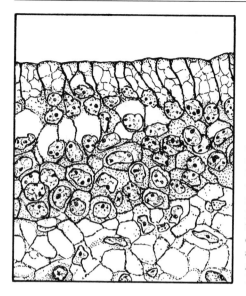

FIGURE 13.28. Section through the vagina of a rat in midpregnancy. The surface cells are columnar, and the middle cell layers are beginning to become vacuolated. The epithelium is intensely mucus-secreting. This mucification reaction is characteristic of pregnancy; it can be produced experimentally by injections of progestational or androgenic steroids. [Redrawn from J. A. Long and H. M. Evans, *The Oestrus Cycle in the Rat*, Memoir of the University of California, 1922.]

their products, there are other structures that have a role in reproduction and are regulated by the sex steroids. These can be quite varied in character, depending upon the animal species and the particular mode of reproduction. In mammals, for example, the development and growth of the mammary glands involves sex steroids. In general, estrogens stimulate duct development in these glands, and progesterone stimulates the development of the secretory alveoli, the small cellular units in which milk is synthesized and secreted. However, mammary physiology and its endocrine regulation are complex, involving corticosteroids, prolactin, growth hormone, insulin, oxytocin, and possibly other regulators. For this reason, it will be given separate consideration in a later section.

Another important and consistent target of action of estrogens is the liver. In all vertebrates that produce large, yolky eggs, most, if not all, of the yolk lipoprotein that becomes incorporated into the eggs is synthesized in the liver. In some reptiles and birds at the height of vitellogenesis as much as half of the proteins in blood are vitelloproteins being transported between the liver and ovary. This means that the transcriptive and translational processes stimulated by estrogen and the consequent lipovitelloprotein synthesis are extremely active. This response can be evoked experimentally in males (roosters), as well as in ovariectomized females, by estradiol injection. It has been assumed that in such species the ovarian follicular cells take up this material and transmit it to the ova, possibly with the permissive action of LH. In teleost fishes it has been claimed that a separate "gonadotropin" is involved in promoting the transport of vitelloprotein from the blood into the ovum, but whether there is further or obligatory endocrine intervention in this process in higher vertebrates is not clear.

TABLE 13.2. Schematic outline of changes in the reproductive organs of the rat during the estrous cycle[a]

Stage	Ovary	Living Animal	Histology of Vaginal Mucosa	Uterus
I Proestrus (12 hrs)	Follicles rapidly growing. Corpora lutea of previous cycle degenerating	Vaginal mucosa slightly dry. *Smear* of epithelial cells only. In heat toward end	Cornified layer *under* surface layer of epithelium. Epithelium thick	Uterus becomes distended with fluid increasing the diameter
II Estrus (12 hrs)	Follicles largest. Germ cells undergo maturation	Vaginal mucosa dry and lusterless. *Smear* of few cornified cells. In heat. Copulation	Cornified layer well formed and on the surface. Epithelium thick	Reaches greatest distension and thinness of epithelium
III Early metestrus (15 hrs)	Ovulation	As in stage II, but *smear* shows abundant cornified material. Animal not in heat	Cornified layer shedding and finally completely detached	Epithelium undergoing vacuolar degeneration
Late metestrus (6 hrs)	Young corpora lutea. Eggs in oviduct. Follicles smallest (next crop)	Vaginal mucosa slightly moist. *Smear* of cornified cells and many leukocytes	Cornified layer gone. Epithelium thin. Many leukocytes	Some vacuolar degeneration, but also regeneration
IV Diestrus (57 hrs)	Follicles of various sizes. Corpora lutea continue to grow	Vaginal mucosa moist, glistening. *Smear* of leukocytes and epithelial cells	Epithelium thin. No cornified layer yet. Some leukocytes	Epithelium undergoing regeneration

[a] Modified from Long and Evans, *Memoirs Univ. Calif.*, **6** (1922).

The skin is a usual but variable target of estrogenic hormones. Hair growth tends to be inhibited by estrogens and accelerated by ovariectomy. Dermal collagen is decreased by estrogen in some mammals (rat, guinea pig) and increased in primates. In certain groups of monkeys estrogens evoke a striking reddening (by pigmentary and vascular changes) in the perineal region—the "sex skin." Patterns of subdermal fat deposition that are considered characteristically "female" depend on estrogen.

Aside from their well-characterized actions on hepatic protein synthesis, the estrogens have a variety of other metabolic actions, some of them not nearly so well defined. The common denominator in many of these actions seems to be the induction of specific enzymatic changes at the cellular level, which eventually lead to the observable metabolic phenomena. One interesting class of such phenomena is the estrogen-evoked increase in plasma calcium, especially in birds, where it must support eggshell secretion. In rodents high levels of estrogen not only raise plasma calcium, but also stimulate bone structural changes. Included in these changes is the deposition of new bone on the endosteal surface, virtually eliminating the marrow cavity of long bones and producing an essentially "solid" bone.

It is of some interest also that female mammals tend to grow more slowly than males and that females grow larger after ovariectomy. Experimentally, estrogens antagonize the anabolic action of adrenal corticosteroids. At the same time, they have an anabolic action in the liver with respect to protein synthesis.

Actions at the Level of the Central Nervous System: Feedback and Reproductive Behavior.   If radioactive estradiol or progesterone are injected into a female vertebrate, they will localize in the brain in specialized functional centers that contain receptors for them. This localized binding and intracellular and intranuclear accumulation of steroid hormone can be demonstrated by the technique of autoradiography. Such information has been used to confirm the facts that estrogens exert a feedback action, either positive or negative, on pituitary gonadotropin secretion and that they can evoke the expression of female sexual behavior. Correlated with these actions is the accumulation of radioactive estrogen in the hypophysiotropic zone of the hypothalamus, especially the amygdala, and in the preoptic nucleus. The hypothalamic hypophysiotropic zone is the source of LHRH, and the preoptic area is the locus for the control of sexual behavior. Unfortunately, the distribution of radioactive estrogen and progesterone in mammalian brains is not restricted to the centers for which these functions have been indicated by physiological evidence. Another source of challenge is the difficulty of locating chemical properties in the brain with precision. High-affinity estrogen receptors can be extracted from brain tissue, but it is impossible to tell with certainty exactly from which cells they were extracted.

Progesterone receptors are even more generally distributed than estradiol receptors in terms of regions from which they are extractable. For example, progesterone receptors are found in the cerebral cortex, whereas estrogen receptors are not. However, the general level of progesterone receptors in mammalian brain is low, especially after ovariectomy. In the rat and guinea pig, estrogen injection is followed within a few hours by a prompt increase in brain progesterone receptor levels and hormone binding. This is accompanied by the appearance of accentuated female sexual behavior, which includes the assumption of a lordosis posture in the presence of a male. This posture consists of a crouch, with the back held concave and the posterior elevated, presenting the vaginal opening to the male. Progesterone treatment promptly diminishes progesterone receptor activity in the brain and causes the disappearance of lordosis behavior in the guinea pig and rat.

The hormonal regulation of female sexual behavior in other mammalian and vertebrate species varies; some species require only estrogen, while others require progesterone, with or without prior estrogen action. There is some difficulty in interpreting experiments intended to show the differences in distribution of estrogens and androgens in the brain. Generally, these distributions show much overlap, but there are ''specific'' sites in the posterior parts of the brain that accumulate more androgen than estrogen. Some of the interpretive difficulty is due to the fact that androgen-accumulating centers may contain aromatizing enzyme systems capable of converting testosterone to estradiol or other estrogens.

In most vertebrates the endocrine regulation of female reproductive behavior has been less well studied than that of males. Perhaps this is because female sexual behavior, in many instances, appears to be largely a matter of receptivity to the male. However, female sexual behavior often is a more complex manifestation, involving motor or orienting responses to odors (pheromones), vocalizations (enabling the female to seek out the male), or visual responses to courtship displays. In addition to regulating overt sexual behavioral activity in female mammals, estrogens have been shown to stimulate secretion of a vaginal pheromone in estrous animals that attracts males and evokes male sexual approach. This phenomenon is well known in, among others, pigs, sheep, dogs, and monkeys. An interesting situation arises in monkeys in which the vaginal pheromonal attractant is controlled by estrogen, while female sexual receptivity is regulated by an adrenal gland androgen. Thus, by use of surgical or chemical inhibitors, it is possible to create experimentally a female that is attractive to males but is hostile to them. The female sex pheromone of dogs has been chemically identified as a fairly simple organic substance.

More complex female behaviors, such as nest building, often are shared between the sexes, and in the female itself may have complex endocrine and neuroendocrine control. The phenomenon is found in some form in most vertebrate groups, including mammals, with the possible exception of amphibians. The sex steroids most often regulate such behaviors, although sometimes sequentially. However, prolactin also may play a role, particu-

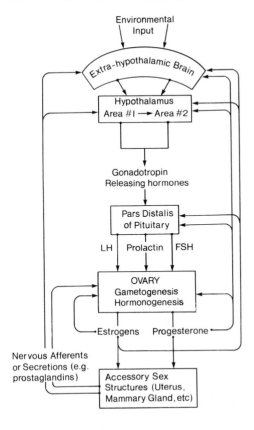

FIGURE 13.29. Diagram of the interactions of endocrine organs, hormones, and hormonal targets in the brain–pituitary–ovary system. Downward arrows indicate the normal sequence of actions of LHRH from the hypothalamus, gonadotropic hormones (FSH, LH, PRL) from the pars distalis, and sex steroids (estrogens and progesterone) from the ovary. Upward arrows indicate feedback actions of prostaglandins and nervous afferents from the vagina-uterus upon the ovary and the brain, and of estrogens and progestogens upon the ovary, pars distalis, and the brain. The various kinds of feedback actions are further discussed in the text.

larly during later phases, when egg incubation and guarding and care of the young are involved. The subject has too many adaptive complexities, especially on a comparative vertebrate basis, for adequate consideration here, and additional data are rapidly piling up.

Feedback is an interesting phenomenon in biological systems as a means of autoregulation of ongoing processes; regulation is achieved when the product of such a process influences the original reactions that generated it. Apparently simpler types of feedback are seen within the cell when a product of a metabolic process regulates the rate of the entire metabolic pathway. Endocrine feedback is considerably more complex, only superficially resembling the intracellular biochemical systems. Sex steroid hormone feedback upon gonadotropin secretion is exerted through interaction with centers in the hypothalamus that produce LHRH (Fig. 13.29). There is abundant evidence that some feedback action may be exerted directly on pituitary gonadotropic cells, at least in particular test species. The basis for steroid feedback, as mentioned earlier, is the presence in these centers of specific hormone receptors and the inducibility of the receptors by some hormones and suppression by others. It is of further interest that LHRH itself has a ''priming'' action for its own cell receptors in the pars distalis. Thus the apparent simplicity of feedback control is so riddled with modifying factors that no resemblance remains to the simple intracellular biochemical model mentioned at the start of this discussion.

An exception to the simple feedback model that challenges our understanding even more profoundly is the existence of both positive and negative feedback by the same hormone—estradiol—under slightly different circumstances. In mammals (in rats and monkeys in particular), relatively large doses of estradiol exert a negative feedback action, inhibiting the secretion of pituitary gonadotropic hormone. Relatively small levels (but not too low) have a positive feedback action, *stimulating* gonadotropic secretion by the pars distalis. In the rat, progesterone will continue the positive feedback action initiated by estradiol, but only for a limited time. An appropriate dosage pattern of estradiol, even in an ovariectomized female, will produce a peak level of LH secretion that resembles the normal preovulatory LH surge; if the ovary is present and appropriately developed, such treatment will evoke ovulatory changes in the ovarian follicles.

There is still no adequate explanation for the differences between positive and negative steroid feedback mechanisms. For that matter, there is no explanation for the general usefulness of a positive feedback mechanism that has explosive potential. In the female vertebrate organism it is fortunately self-terminating. The progesterone-secreting phase of ovarian function, which begins at ovulation, soon leads to a decrease in steroid and LHRH receptors in the brain and pituitary, ending positive feedback.

Preovulatory surges of LH or of both gonadotropins are general among mammals. Adequate studies (that is, studies based on an appropriate radioimmunoassay) to reveal this phenomenon are relatively rare in other vertebrate groups. However, in several avian species a preovulatory gonadotropic surge has been described, apparently mainly as a positive feedback response to progesterone. In the goldfish there is also a preovulatory gonadotropic surge, but in fishes generally, steroid feedback relationships around this time have not been adequately studied.

Further discussion of sex steroid hormone feedback will be included in the following sections in connection with relevant features of the female and male cycles.

The Female Reproductive Cycle and Its Regulation

The cyclicity of production of female gametes has been referred to a number of times already, and in different contexts. External evidence of the hormonal fluctuations that accompany the cycles of gametogenesis in the rat ovary are illustrated in parallel vaginal epithelial changes (Fig. 13.27). In the human vagina, although there is a characteristic complex of cellular changes in the vaginal cycle, including some cornification, these changes are not nearly as striking as those in the uterus (which during the short, four-day cycle of the rat are minimal). The human (and other primates) uterine cycle includes a relatively long period of stimulation of the endometrium by progesterone—to the point where the initially simple glands become extremely hypertrophied and complex in outline, giving the endometrium as a whole a spongy character. At the end of ovarian progesterone secretion by the corpus luteum, there is a sudden decrease in the vascular supply of this activated endometrium, leading to the death of all but the basal endometrial cells. This dead tissue, plus some blood, is shed in the process known as *menstruation*. For primates, therefore, the female cycle is known as the *menstrual cycle*.

Another accompaniment of the ovarian gametogenic cycle is hormone-dependent sexual behavior. The time of ovulation is the time of maximal ovarian follicular size and function and the beginning of corpus luteum formation. To ensure fertilization of the ovulated egg, it is highly advantageous for the female to be maximally attractive to males at this time and to be maximally receptive and responsive to sexual advances of males exhibiting mating behavior. This type of female behavior is known as estrous behavior, giving the name *estrous cycle* to the repetitive reproductive phenomena (other than pregnancy) seen in a majority of female mammals. The hormonal basis for female sexual behavior was discussed earlier.

There is considerable variety in the pattern of the various phenomena that constitute the female cycle in different mammals. In many mammalian species there is only one estrous cycle per year, generally in a clement season that is favorable for reproduction and/or for the rearing of newborn young. Such species are referred to as *monestrous*. In the dog, which is listed in Table 13.3 as monestrous, there usually are two periods of heat (estrus) each year, one in the spring and one in the autumn. However, domestication and genetic selection of breeds may disturb this pattern, yielding types of dogs with more or fewer than two cycles per year. In certain large marine mammals that live continually in the water except when they come ashore once each year for breeding, the young of the previous year's mating are born soon after the brief land phase begins. Even while the pups are being reared, mating takes place to fertilize the eggs of the single, abbreviated estrous cycle that follows.

Most of the mammals listed in Table 13.3 are indicated as polyestrous. That is, they repeat estrous cycles spontaneously until a successful fertilization results in pregnancy, interrupting the train of cycles. Some polyestrous species cycle continuously, irrespective of season. Most primates, equatorial (nonseasonal), and domesticated species are in this group. However, we may note that the galago, a primitive primate, is seasonally polyestrous, as is the sheep. The sheep, in fact, is particularly interesting because its ovarian cycles and breeding are regulated by neuroendocrine mechanisms so that they occur at times of *short* photoperiods, in the autumn and winter. This is adaptive behavior for sheep, since it ensures that lambs are born at a favorable time, in the spring or early summer.

TABLE 13.3 Estrous cycles in mammals

Species	Length of Cycle (days)	Mono- or Polyestrous	Breeding Season
Human (*Homo sapiens*)	28	P	Continuous
Gorilla (*Gorilla gorilla*)	39	P	—
Macacque (*Macaca mulatta*)	28	P	Continuous
Galago (*Galago senegalensis*)	32	P	April to October
Cow (*Bos taurus*)	14–23 (21 av.)	P	Continuous
Camel (*Camelus bactrianus*)	10–20	P	Continuous
Dog (*Canis familiaris*)	63 (av.)	M(?)	Spring to autumn (one to two heats per year)
Guinea pig (*Cavia porcellus*)	16–19	P	Continuous
Elephant (*Elephas maximus*)	21 (av.)	P	Continuous
Horse (*Equus caballus*)	19–23	P	Continuous
Platypus (*Ornithorhynchus anatinus*)	60	M	July to October
Sheep (*Ovis aries*)	14–20 (16 av.)	P	September to late winter
Rat (*Rattus norvegicus*)	4–5	P	Continuous
Pig (*Sus scrofa*)	18–24 (21 av.)	P	Continuous
Shrew (*Sorex araneus*)	13–19	P	March to September

Another pattern of female cycling is, strictly speaking, not a cycle, since at one point, just before ovulation, it becomes arrested. Such an animal will remain in estrus for a prolonged period, until mating occurs. The copulatory act itself provides the afferent nervous stimulus for a neuroendocrine response that liberates LHRH and an ovulatory level of gonadotropin from the pars distalis. This classical example of a neuroendocrine refex was first discussed in Chapter 1 as a phenomenon exhibited by the rabbit. Other species in which the female follows the same reproductive pattern are called *induced ovulators*. Known induced ovulators include members of the cat family, the ferret, and the mink. The period of estrus is not without limit, but may last from a few days to more than a month, depending upon the species. If mating has not occurred, the ripe ovarian follicles eventually become atretic without ovulation and, after a period of anestrus, another group of follicles begins development.

Induced ovulators are also subject to seasonal and photoperiodic control of gonadal development. This is true, for example, of the ferret, marten, and mink. Tropical and equatorial cats, without the climatic limitations of temperate-zone species, will reproduce at any time of the year.

The integrative agents for the various patterns of behavioral, morphological, and metabolic phenomena that, together, constitute the female reproductive cycle are the nervous and endocrine systems, often acting in coordination with certain key environmental signals. The precise patterns of hormonal secretion that evoke most of the visible features of the female cycle have been worked out relatively recently by the use of radioimmunoassys for sex steroids and gonadotropins. Some of the principal features of these hormonal patterns are illustrated in Fig. 13.30 for three polyestrous species: sheep, humans, and rats. Variation in the relative amounts of four hormones (estradiol, progesterone, FSH, LH) are shown over several cycles, as though fertilization of the ovulated eggs did not occur. The assays for human and rat FSH are better established than those for sheep. Thus FSH values are indicated in a tentative manner for sheep.

In studying Fig. 13.30, it is useful to note first the changes in plasma levels just before and just after ovulation. It is well to remember also that the cycle of rat is much shorter than that of the other two organisms. Furthermore, the approximate time of mating (that is, estrous behavior) and of ovulation in the rat are modulated by a neuroendocrine circadian rhythmic mechanism interacting with the fluctuating hormone levels, so that these events occur at certain hours (just after midnight and in the early morning hours, respectively). The one similarity in all three cycles is a peak in LH secretion—the LH surge—just before ovulation; this hormonal event is considered to be immediately responsible for the ovulatory response and luteinization of the follicle. In all three species the LH surge is preceded by a rise and peak in the level of estradiol. This, presumably, is the period of positive feedback when estradiol stimulates LH release from the pars distalis.

Progesterone concentrations during the cycle vary widely among the three species. In the human female, the progesterone concentration is relatively high after ovulation, at the time when the corpus luteum is secreting actively, supposedly to build the progestational type of uterine lining (endometrium). The sharp end of the progesterone secretory phase of the human cycle precipitates the breakdown of the endometrium and menstruation.

In the ewe, progesterone is high through most of the cycle—not only during the luteal, but also during the follicular phase. However, progesterone must decrease before estrous behavior or the LH surge can occur. In contrast, within the short female rat cycle there are two progesterone maxima—a brief preovulatory peak, believed to be secreted by the large ovarian follicles, and a lesser but more prolonged one at the time the corpora lutea are functional. In the rat, estrous behavior appears to *require* progesterone action after prior priming by estrogen. Thus, although the postovulatory ovarian sources and uterine functions of progesterone are similar in the three species, the preovulatory status of this hormone may be quite different.

The changing levels of FSH, if we consider the better-established instances of the human and the rat female cycles, are difficult to rationalize at this time, and raise several interesting problems. Teleologically, one would expect FSH levels to parallel follicular growth, since follicular stimulation

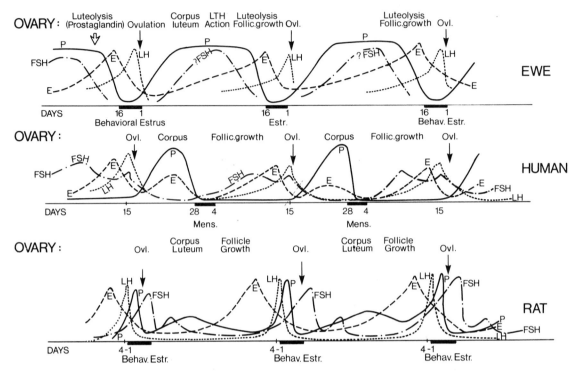

FIGURE 13.30. Variations in the relative blood levels of follicle stimulating hormone, FSH, luteinizing hormone, LH, estradiol (E) or E17β, and progesterone (P) over several successive estrous cycles in the ewe, human, and rat. It is not intended to show absolute levels of these hormones, just increases and decreases in their relative plasma concentrations. Each set of curves is over a base on which the number of days in the cycle of each species and significant external markers (estrus or menstruation) are indicated below the hormone curves. Corresponding secretory or morphological events in the pituitary and ovary are indicated above the curves. To make possible comparisons among the species, the three sets of curves have been drawn so that the times of ovulation are superimposed. That is, between ovulations the human cycle and the rat cycle are drawn to be of equal length, but one represents 28 days and the other only 4. It is important to remember this in interpreting the curves. The data on which these curves were constructed are taken from a variety of sources. For further discussion of these data, see the text.

is the demonstrable function of FSH in experiments with hypophysectomized female rats. In the human cycling female this parallelism appears to hold, and, in fact, both FSH and LH steadily increase during the postmenstrual follicular growth period. In the rat, however, there are two curious peaks of FSH, one in the immediate postovulatory period and the other during the late luteal phase. It is possible—speaking purely teleologically—that the female cycle in the rat is so short that events must be telescoped, and the earliest phases of follicular recruitment and growth must be started during the luteal phase of ovarian function. Figure 13.30 shows that during the final preovulatory period of follicular growth in the rat, FSH levels are rising again.

One of the still unsolved puzzles concerning hypothalamic control of gonadotropic secretion is that there is only one known hypophysiotropic agent, LHRH, which must regulate the release of two different gonadotropins. In the human cycle FSH and LH remain essentially parallel in their pattern of secretion, as reflected by their plasma concentrations. However, as Fig. 13.30 indicates, in the ewe and female rat FSH and LH are secreted in widely different temporal patterns. The most reasonable explanations of how one hypothalamic releasing hormone can stimulate separate secretion maxima of two different gonadotropins are based on selective negative and positive feedback, at the pars distalis level, by gonadal steroid hormones or by the inhibins that have been mentioned earlier, or by both.

Although much has been learned about the nature of the nervous and endocrine elements that interact to produce the regular cycling of the female reproductive tract, a completely satisfactory mechanistic explanation is stilll lacking. The key to the cyclicity of polyestrous species appears to reside in the brain. One hypothesis states that there are two feedback control centers in the hypothalamus, one for tonic, continuous negative feedback and the other for cyclic control of LH secretion that is subject to positive feedback (see Fig. 13.29). This implies a sexual differentiation of the hypothalamic gonadotropic feedback control centers. If a *newborn female* rat is treated with either testosterone or estradiol, it develops a normal-appearing ovary, but as an adult it remains acyclic. It may, in fact, enter a phase of continuous estrus with an extended phase of cornified vaginal epithelium. Furthermore, the animal displays various elements of male sexual behavior (Fig. 13.31). Since lack of gonadal cyclicity is characteristic of the male rat, the infantile female rat's brain is said to have been masculinized by the steroid treatment both with respect to cyclicity and behavior. Treatment at 10 days or 2 weeks of age has no permanent effect. Much of the supportive and confirmatory research that has been done with the rat and a few other mammalian species indicates that the basic pattern of sexual differentiation of the brain in the female rat, or in the male castrated in infancy, is female. Steroid treatment during the early, sensitive, or "plastic" period results in the male type of brain. There are even some subtle morphological features that accompany sexual differentiation of the brain.

Actions of the Male Hormones

Actions at the Testicular Level. Except for the Agnatha, there is clear evidence throughout the vertebrates that spermatogenesis ceases after hypophysectomy. There is also fairly well-established evidence that testosterone stimulates spermatogenesis in most vertebrates. The analysis of the relative roles of gonadotropins and androgens in regulating spermatogenesis has yielded some interesting information but is not definitively settled. The

NORMAL AND EXPERIMENTALLY ALTERED
DIFFERENTIATION OF HYPOTHALAMIC CONTROL
OF CYCLIC LH-RELEASE AND FEMALE LORDOSIS
BEHAVIOR IN THE RAT

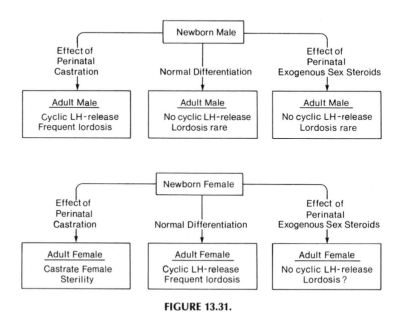

FIGURE 13.31.

analysis has been most thorough in the rat and in primates for an essentially practical reason. It has been felt that a better understanding of the hormonal regulation of male germ cell production could provide the rational procedural basis for a human fertility control program that would free the female from the full, often difficult, and possibly hazardous responsibility for contraception.

In the rat, testosterone alone, in sufficient dosage, will *maintain* active spermatogenesis even after hypophysectomy. However, if testosterone is not given to hypophysectomized rats until after spermatogenesis has halted, then even high doses are not adequate for production of fertile spermatozoa. Recent work indicates that among the "priming" actions of FSH is the sensitization of germ cells to androgens by causing them to synthesize androgen receptors. Another important action of FSH in this connection (one that testosterone also possesses in the rat, but to a lesser extent) is the stimulation of Sertoli cells to produce androgen-binding protein (ABP) and to secrete it into the lumen of the seminiferous tubules. ABP is a glycoprotein (molecular weight of about 68,000) that is similar to the androgen-binding protein in plasma (at least similar to that of rabbit plasma). Its function appears to be to aid in the transport and retention of testosterone and dihydrotestosterone in testicular tubules and in the epididymis, creating an androgen concentration in epididymal fluid that is 15-fold higher than in the blood. Without this elevated epididymal androgen level, spermatozoa are unable to complete their final development. In men with a genetic deficiency for ABP production, sterility, or at least relative infertility of the sperm, is the consequence, despite normal spermatogenesis.

Another primary function of FSH is to stimulate the synthesis of LH receptors in the Leydig cells (interstitial cells) of the testis. Androgen production by the interstitial cells is a function regulated by LH. During active spermatogenesis, androgen synthesis by the Leydig cells, in addition to the smaller amount formed by the Sertoli cells, is needed for germ cell production. Thus the role of FSH in the testis is an important one—the modulation of several different kinds of spermatogenesis-related actions.

Actions on Secondary and Accessory Male Sex Structures. The long period of time—measured in weeks—that spermatozoa spend in the upper end of the male duct system, the epididymis, should make it clear that these ducts must contribute more than a means of passage to the exterior. The cytological structure of the epithelial lining cells is that of secretory cells, and it is stimulated by testosterone and dihydrotestosterone. In castrated animals the epithelial layers of the epididymis and vas deferens (or Wolffian duct) of all vertebrates that have them undergo involution; this is promptly reversed by testosterone injection. The changes in maturing spermatozoa during their stay in the mammalian epididymis are of several kinds. There are slight but definable morphological changes. There are biochemical changes, particularly in the cellular systems having to do with energy exchange. Most important, there is a gradual increase in the viability of the spermatozoa. In this context, viability is measured by the ability of the spermatozoa to fertilize an egg if placed in the lower end of the reproductive tract of an estrous female. Spermatozoa from the upper part of the epididymis are relatively infertile; those from the lower end are relatively fertile. Among the most effective antifertility drugs in the male is α-chlorohydrin, which has an injurious effect on epididymal spermatozoa. This drug affects the epididymis itself and/or its contained sperm. The locus of action is unclear.

There is an apparent dissociation of the secretory condition of the epithelial layer of the male ducts (epididymis and vas deferens) from testicular activity in some species of mammals and reptiles. In such species, at times of seasonal atrophy of the testes or after castration, some of the male ductile structures appear actively secretory. This is true, for example, in the vole *Microtus arvalis* (Fig. 13.32). Still other male structures, such as the seminal vesicles and prostate, may undergo involution while the tubular structures remain active. In such species there is evidence that corticosteroids from the adrenal gland may be maintaining the secretory epithelia when androgen is lacking. The special adaptive value of this kind of hormonal regulation is a reproductive pattern in which spermatogenesis occurs in the autumn,

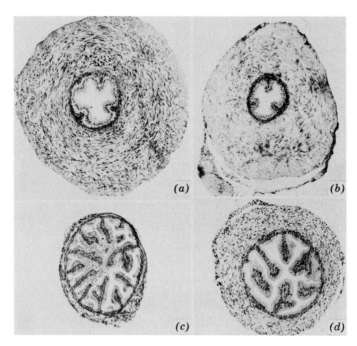

FIGURE 13.32. Sections through the ductus deferens of the male vole (*Microtus arvalis*). (*a*) From a sexually active adult; (*b*) from an adult 15 days after castration; (*c*) from a sexually inactive adult during winter; (*d*) from an adult one month after castration. Note the great epithelial hypertrophy during the period of sexual inactivity in the normal animal (*c*) and following castration (*d*). Delost suggests that the secretory state during the time of testicular inactivity is in response to adrenocorticoids. (All photomicrographs × 50.) [From P. Delost, *Ann. Sci. Nat. Zool.,* **18:**391, 1956.]

but the germ cells held in the epididymis and the ducts do not complete maturation until breeding occurs in the spring.

At the lower end of the male ductile system there generally are a number of glands that secrete fluids in which the spermatozoa are suspended at the time of or just prior to ejaculation. The best known of these are the seminal vesicles, embryonic derivatives of the Wolffian duct (vas deferens), and the prostate, an embryonic derivative of the urogenital sinus and urethra (see Fig. 13.16). In addition, there may be other glandular structures communicating with the male ducts; these include the bulbourethral, coagulating, and preputial glands, and possibly other structures. Nonmammalian vertebrates have fewer and less prominent glandular structures of this type. "Seminal vesicles" and "cloacal glands" in a number of fishes, for example, are often no more than thickened secretory sections of the lower male tract. The function of the mammalian male sex accessory glands, generally, is to secrete fluids that will maintain and protect the spermatozoa during their relatively short stay (in most species) in the lower male and female tracts.

However, the functional requirements for such glands vary considerably, depending on the reproductive mode and on the size of the animals in question. In some large mammals, it would be difficult to transport spermatozoa in a small volume of fluid to the upper end of the female tract (where fertilization takes place) without considerable loss.

The hormonal regulation of these glands, wherever studied, has been found to be by androgen. In some instances it has been shown that the glands themselves contain the enzyme (5α-reductase) needed to convert testosterone to dihydrotestosterone (DHT). In such instances we may assume that DHT is the effective androgenic regulator. In other instances both androgen and estradiol are effective. The preputial gland of the male rat has such an ambisexual hormonal response. Other male structures that appear responsive to estrogens as well as androgens include several in the rabbit (anal and inguinal glands) and the urogenital papilla of certain teleosts.

Once we enter the area of accessory male structures (those not directly connected to the male ducts), their variety is both fascinating and overwhelming. Male hormone-regulated secondary sex structures are the rule among the vertebrates, although, of course, there are exceptions. Typical of the well-studied male secondary sexual fin structures of fishes are the "sword" of the swordtail *Xiphophorus* (Fig. 13.33); the elongated spines of the dorsal fin of the filefish *Monocanthus* (Fig. 13.34); and the gonopod, the modified anal fin of the platyfish *Platypoecilus*, which is used in the act of mating. Other androgen-influenced piscine secondary sex characters are the pigmented nuptial skin coloration (*Hochzeitskleid*) of certain genera (including the stickleback *Gasterosteus*) and pearl organs on the heads of goldfishes and minnows. These structures often are important elements in the arousal of reproductive behavior of the female at the time of mating.

Among amphibians the sexually active male *Triton* salamander typically shows a dorsal crest, an enlarged tail, and a distinctive breeding pigmentary pattern. In anurans specific muscular and skeletal differences (e.g., the humerus) characterize the male (Fig. 13.35), and the enlarged thumb pad is a well-known male feature in Ranidae. In the *Rana* thumb pad, a receptor for both testosterone and DHT has been found. It is not preferential for one or the other of these androgens; it disappears by 60 days after castration and reappears—presumably synthesized anew—after DHT injection.

Among reptiles, secondary sex characters are less in evidence, although many male lizards show development of a dorsal crest, gular ("cheek") skin folds and glands, pigment changes, and, in some forms, territorial behavior. Among birds there are many characteristics controlled by androgen, such as the bill color in the English sparrow and in the black-headed gull and plumage changes in some species. The response of the comb in the chick (*Gallus domesticus*) to androgen has provided the basis for a popular biological assay for androgens. DHT receptors have been found, as one might expect for targets of androgen action, in the comb and wattles of roosters. The dependence of aggressive behavior upon androgen, including social or

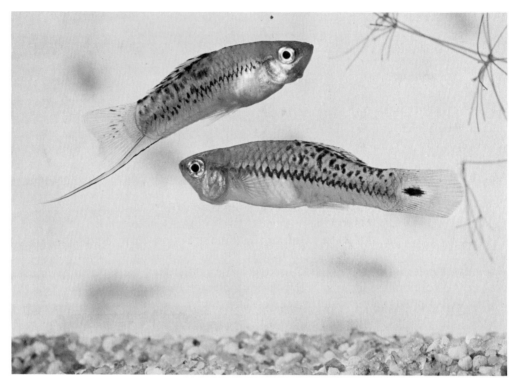

FIGURE 13.33. Sexual dimorphism in the swordtail *Xiphophorus helleri*. The "sword," evident in the male fish (*upper*), can be induced in the female fish by the administration of androgenic steroids.

"peck order" status in fowl, is well known, as is the relation of voice and song to male hormone levels in some birds.

In mammals sexually dimorphic features, including those dependent upon androgen levels, may be subtle or very striking. These can include such obvious structural features as highly developed horns or antlers, hair growth (e.g., the mane of stallions, the beard in man), and muscular and skeletal mass. In humans there are male patterns of hair distribution and androgen-dependent qualities of voice (laryngeal cartilage and vocal cord development), red blood cell concentration, size of the salivary glands, and muscular and skeletal mass. The anabolic action of androgens on human muscular development is now well known, since their use in competing athletes of both sexes has become so general, if not notorious. Testosterone and DHT receptors have been found in skeletal muscle.

Actions of Androgens on the Brain: Feedback and Reproductive Behavior. As mentioned earlier in this chapter in the discussion of the actions of estrogenic and progestational steroids on the brain, there may be considerable overlap in the distribution of nerve cells that bind estrogens and androgens. On the basis of autoradiographic technique alone, it would be difficult (though not impossible) to determine whether the same cells can bind both hormones; this then remains a possibility. However, there are some areas of the brain that bind one or the other hormone exclusively. Another confusion is introduced by the intracellular metabolism and conversion of androgens to estradiol. Aromatizing enzymes for this metabolic purpose are present in particular parts of the brain. Furthermore, certain brain responses to hormones (behavioral or functional changes) can be evoked in castrated animals by injection of *either* testosterone or estradiol. In experiments of this kind the question of whether aromatization of testosterone is *obligatory* often can be answered by injecting dihydrotestosterone, since this 5α-reduced androgen is not aromatizable.

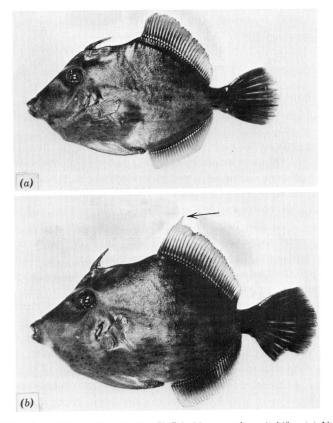

FIGURE 13.34. Sexual dimorphism in the filefish *Monacanthus cirrhifer*. (*a*) Normal adult female; (*b*) female after implantation of testosterone pellet. Note the elongation of the first spine of the dorsal fin (indicated by arrow). This example of an androgen-dependent secondary sex characteristic was selected because of the minor nature of the changes involved. Many hormone-dependent sex differences are not as dramatic as those illustrated in Figs. 13.33 and 13.35. [Photographs from S. Ishii and N. Egami.]

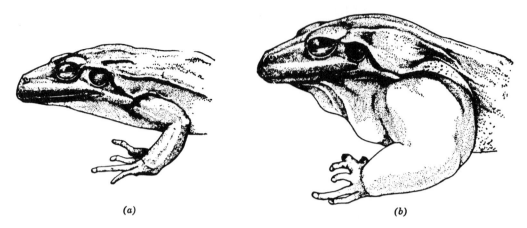

(a)   (b)

FIGURE 13.35.   Sexual dimorphism of the forelimbs of the South American frog *Leptodactylus ocellatus*. (*a*) Female; (*b*) male. The development of the muscles in the male is associated with sexual activity and results in molding of the forelimb bones to give the definitive picture seen here. [From G. Kingsley Noble, *The Biology of the Amphibia*, Dover, New York, 1931.]

With so many sites for the distribution of steroid hormone receptors in the brain, and with so much variation in the binding specificities of these receptors, we may expect that adaptation has produced numerous differences among species. To be sure, in male vertebrates there are about as many highly individualized species-specific patterns of courtship and mating as there are species. Some of these behaviors are highly complex and, to human eyes, bizarre. This being so, it is remarkable that the principal organizing locus of androgen-influenced male mating behavior in all vertebrate species that have been appropriately studied is the ventral preoptic nuclear region of the hypothalamus. There must be many differences in neuronal circuitry for the species-specific male sex behaviors, but these differences are in the sensory information used and in the motor areas that receive organizing signals from the preoptic nucleus.

Analysis of the ways in which androgenic hormones influence particular nervous elements in producing overt sexual behavior is just beginning. As yet, it is limited to the localization of sex steroid hormones in certain parts of the brain and to the localization of sexual behavior centers. The latter is accomplished by making small lesions or implanting bits of sex hormone at specific sites in the brain and noting the effects on sexual behavior. Tracing neuronal pathways to and from the sex behavior centers of the preoptic nucleus yields information that is so complex (in higher vertebrates) that it is as yet uninterpretable.

The discussion above implies that brains are sexually differentiated. This has been born out by a variety of studies. First, there are clear but subtle anatomic differences in the sizes of certain brain nuclei as well as in the numbers of dendritic spikes on neurons in certain areas. Second, there are gender differences in the type of sexual behavior generated by the action of sex steroids on the brain. Sometimes the same hormone will elicit male or female behavior characteristics in treated adults (rats). Estradiol, for example, will evoke female behavior in females (lordosis) and male behavior in males (mounting and intromission). Since we know that aromatization of testosterone to estradiol takes place in the preoptic nucleus, this is not surprising. Third, there are sex differences in feedback responses of the brain to sex steroids. Male brains respond only negatively to estradiol, whereas female brains may display positive feedback, as mentioned earlier. Estrogens are not normally secreted in significant amounts in males, except in a few species (e.g., horses). Female brains and pituitaries, in their normal relationship to the ovaries, produce a cyclic pattern of releasing hormone and gonadotropic hormone secretion, while in the male feedback yields a noncyclic, steady state of hormonal equilibrium between testicular and brain-pituitary endocrine function.

Thus it is accurate to speak of sex differentiation of the brain. In the rat permanent sex differentiation of the brain occurs just at the time of birth; so it is possible to approach this problem experimentally. Brief mention has already been made of one of the key experiments performed. Testosterone is injected into neonatal (newborn) female rats at a fairly high dose. As adults, such animals later appear normally differentiated as to gonadal sex, but they do not cycle because they do not experience an ovulatory surge of LH (see Fig. 13.31). Furthermore, their sexual behavior is shifted in the male direction. Neonatal males injected with testosterone are normal as adults. In another key experiment, the newborn rat of either sex is castrated, so that it is not exposed to gonadal sex steroids during the perinatal period. If an ovary is implanted later into *either* a male or female neonatal castrate, it cycles, and both former males and reconstituted females display lordosis behavior. If the castrations or hormone injections are done 10 days or more after birth, they have no permanent effect. Thus it is clear that the pliable period of brain differentiation ends shortly after birth. Such experiments in the rat are interpreted as follows. The infant rat of either sex is born with its brain programmed to differentiate in the female pattern (cyclic LHRH and LH secretion, lordosis, female estrous behavior). If exposed to sex steroids (either testosterone or estradiol), the brain of newborns differentiates in the male pattern (tonic or continuous LHRH and LH secretion, male mounting, and other behaviors). The steroid exposure occurs naturally from the newborn male testis, or experimentally by injection of testosterone or estradiol. Rat fetuses are protected from placental estrogens by α-feto-protein, an estrogen-specific binding protein in the blood which disappears promptly after birth. This, of course, explains why the brains of all female fetuses are not masculinized by the high levels of placental estrogens in maternal blood.

Reproductive Cycles in the Male

There is no cycle of reproductive activity in vertebrate males other than a seasonal one. There is no succession of gonadal structures in the testis as there is in the ovary, although spermatogenesis does proceed in waves along the lengths of the seminiferous tubules. At any one time, however, in almost any sexually active vertebrate male spermatogenesis is in progress and/or ripe spermatozoa are available. The endocrine control of male reproduction requires a rather steady, noncyclic secretion of gonadotropins, with a reasonably constant proportion of FSH to LH, as well as of androgen in the blood.

The reproductive strategy for most vertebrates, whether their annual reproductive periods are short, long, or continuous, is for the male to be prepared to provide fertile sperm whenever ripe eggs are available. Generally, the cooperative estrous, or mating-readiness, behavioral signals from the female will incite the male behavioral responses that ensure fertilization of the eggs.

ADDITIONAL READING

Books

1. Austin, C. R., and R. V. Short (1972–1980). *Reproduction in Mammals*, Vols. 1–8. Cambridge University Press, Cambridge.

2. Bermant, G., and J. M. Davidson (1974). *Biological Bases of Sexual Behavior*. Harper & Row, New York.

3. Bullough, W. S. (1951). *Vertebrate Sexual Cycles*. Methuen, London.

4. Burger, H., and D. De Kretser (1981). *The Testis*. Raven, New York.

5. Corner, G. W. (1963). *The Hormones in Human Reproduction*. Atheneum, New York.

6. Greep, R. O., ed. (1977). *Reproductive Physiology II*. University Park Press, Baltimore.

7. Greep, R. O., M. A. Koblinsky, and F. S. Jaffe (1976). *Reproduction and Human Welfare*. MIT Press, Cambridge.

8. Hogarth, P. J. (1978). *Biology of Reproduction*. Wiley, New York.

9. *Hormones and Reproductive Behavior, Readings from Scientific American*. Freeman, San Francisco, 1979.

10. Idler, D. R., ed. (1972). *Steroids in Nonmammalian Vertebrates*. Academic, New York.

11. James, V. H. T., M. Serio, and L. Martini, eds. (1972, 1973). *The Endocrine Function of the Human Testis*. Academic, New York.

12. Mossman, H. W., and K. L. Kuke (1973). *Comparative Morphology of the Mammalian Ovary*. University of Wisconsin Press, Madison.

13. Nalbandov, A. V. (1976). *Reproductive Physiology of Mammals and Birds*, 3rd ed. Freeman, San Francisco.

14. Parkes, A. S., ed. (1956). *Marshall's Physiology of Reproduction*, Vols. 1–3, 3rd ed. Longman's Green & Co., London.

15. Sadleir, R. M. F. S. (1973). *The Reproduction of Vertebrates*. Academic, New York.

16. Steinberger, A., and E. Steinberger (1980). *Testicular Development, Structure, and Function*. Raven, New York.

17. van Tienhoven, A. (1968). *Reproductive Physiology of Vertebrates*. Saunders, New York.

18. Zuckerman, S., and B. J. Weir (1977). *The Ovary*. Academic, New York.

Articles

1. Arrata, W. S. M., and A. Y. M. Tsai (1978). Prostaglandins in reproduction. *J. Reprod. Med.* **20:**84–89.

2. Baird, D. T., and R. J. Scaramuzzi (1976). Changes in the secretion of ovarian steroids and pituitary luteinizing hormone in the peri-ovulatory period in the ewe. *J. Endocrinol.* **70:**237–245.

3. Barraclough, C. A., P. M. Wise, J. Turgeon, D. Shander, L. Depaulo, and N. Rance (1979). Recent studies on the regulation of pituitary LH and FSH secretion. *Biol. Reprod.* **20:**86–97.

4. Brain, P. F. (1971). The physiology of population limitation in rodents—a review. *Commun. Behav. Biol.* **6:**115–123.

5. Carter, C. S., and J. M. Davis (1977). Biogenic amines, reproductive hormones and female sexual behavior: a review. *Biobehav. Rev.* **1:**213–224.

6. Catling, P. C., and R. L. Sutherland (1980). Effect of gonadectomy, season and presence of female tammar wallabies (*Macropus eugenii*) on concentrations of testosterone, luteinizing hormone and follicle-stimulating hormone in the plasma of male tammar wallabies. *J. Endocrinol.* **86:**25–33.

7. Concannon, P. W., W. Hansel, and W. J. Visek (1975). The ovarian cycle of the bitch: plasma estrogen, LH, and progesterone. *Biol. Reprod.* **13:**112–121.

8. Dorner, G. (1979). Hormones and sexual differentiation of the brain. In *Sex Hormones and Behavior*. Excerpta Medica and Elsevier/North-Holland, Amsterdam.

9. Dorrington, J. H., and D. T. Armstrong (1979). Effects of FSH on gonadal function. *Recent Progr. Horm. Res.* **35:**301–342.

10. Foster, D. L., J. A. Lemons, R. B. Jaffe, and G. D. Niswender (1975). Sequential patterns of circulating luteinizing hormone and follicle stimulating hormone in female sheep from early postnatal life through the first estrous cycles. *Endocrinology* **97:**985–994.

11. Germain, B. J., P. S. Campbell, and J. N. Anderson (1978). The role of serum estrogen-binding protein in the control of tissue estradiol levels during postnatal development of the female rat. *Endocrinology* **108:**1401–1410.

12. Greep, R. O. (1978). Reproductive endocrinology: concepts and perspectives, an overview. *Recent Progr. Horm. Res.* **34:**1–23.

13. Gustafson, A. W., and M. Shemeshi (1976). Changes in plasma testosterone levels during the annual reproductive cycle of the hibernating bat, *Myotis lucifugus lucifugus*, with a survey of plasma testosterone levels in adult male vertebrates. *Biol. Reprod.* **15:**9–24.

14. Hansel, W., P. W. Concannon, and J. H. Lukaszewska (1973). Corpora lutea of the large domestic animals. *Biol. Reprod.* **8:**222–245.

15. Horton, E. W., and N. L. Poyser (1976). Uterine luteolytic hormone: a physiologic role for prostaglandin $F_{2\alpha}$. *Physiol. Rev.* **56:**595–651.

16. Hughes, J. P., G. H. Stabenfeldt, and J. W. Evans (1975). The oestrous cycle of the mare. *J. Reprod. Fertil.* Suppl. 23:161–166.

17. Jerrett, D. P. (1979). Female reproductive patterns in nonhibernating bats. *J. Reprod. Fertil.* **56:**369–378.

18. Jöchle, W., and A. C. Anderson (1977). The estrous cycle of the dog: a review. *Theriogenology* **7:**113–140.

19. Jones, A. R., D. Stevenson, P. Hulton, and A. G. Dawson (1981). The antifertility action of α-chlorhydrin. *Experientia* **37**:340–341.

20. Karsch, F. J., and D. L. Foster (1975). Sexual differentiation of the mechanism controlling the preovulatory discharge of luteinizing hormone in sheep. *Endocrinology* **97**:373–379.

21. Karsch, F. J., S. J. Legan, K. D. Ryan, and D. L. Foster (1980). Importance of estradiol and progesterone in regulating LH secretion and estrous behavior during the sheep estrous cycle. *Biol. Reprod.* **23**:404–413.

22. Knobil, E. (1974). On the control of gonadotrophin secretion in the rhesus monkey. *Recent Progr. Horm. Res.* **30**:1–46.

23. Krutzsch, P. H. (1979). Male reproductive patterns in nonhibernating bats. *J. Reprod. Fertil.* **56**:333–344.

24. Legan, S. J., and F. J. Karsch (1979). Neuroendocrine regulation of the estrous cycle and seasonal breeding in the ewe. *Biol. Reprod.* **20**:74–85.

25. Mahesh, V. B., T. G. Molduon, J. C. Eldridge, and K. S. Korach (1975). The role of steroid hormones in the regulation of gonadotropin secretion. *J. Steroid Biochem.* **6**:1025–1036.

26. Mann, T. (1976) Relevance of physiological and biochemical research to problems of animal fertility. *Proc. R. Soc. London* **B193**:1–15.

27. O'Malley, B. W., D. R. Roop, E. C. Lai, J. L. Nordstrom, J. F. Catterall, G. E. Swaneck, D. A. Colbert, M.-J. Tsai, A. Dugaiczyk, and S. L. C. Woo (1979). The ovalbumin gene: organization, structure, transcription, and regulation. *Recent Progr. Horm. Res.* **35**:1–46.

28. Peter, R. E., and L. W. Crim (1979). Reproductive endocrinology of fishes: gonadal cycles and gonadotropin in teleosts. *Ann. Rev. Physiol.* **41**:323–335.

29. Prasad, M. R. N., M. Rajalakshmi, G. Gupta, and T. Karkun (1973). Control of epididymal function. *J. Reprod. Fertil.* Suppl. 18:215–222.

30. Richards, J. S. (1979). Hormonal control of ovarian follicular development: a 1978 perspective. *Recent Progr. Horm. Res.* **35**:343–373.

31. Schams, D., E. Schallenberger, B. Hoffman, and H. Karg (1977). The oestrous cycle of the cow: hormonal parameters and time relationships concerning oestrus, ovulation and electrical resistance of the vaginal mucus. *Acta Endocrinol.* **86**:180–192.

32. Sherman, B. M., and S. G. Korenman (1975). Hormonal characteristics of the human menstrual cycle throughout reproductive life. *J. Clin. Invest.* **55**:699–706.

33. Short, R. V. (1970). The bovine freemartin: a new look at an old problem. *Phil. Trans. R. Soc. London* **B259**:141–147.

34. Steiner, R. A., D. C. Clifton, H. G. Spies, and J. A. Resko (1976). Sexual differentiation and feedback control of luteinizing hormone secretion in the rhesus monkey. *Biol. Reprod.* **15**:206–212.

35. Tata, J. R., and D. F. Smith (1979). Vitellogenesis: a versatile model for hormonal regulation of gene expression. *Recent Progr. Horm. Res.* **35**:47–95.

36. Tyndale-Biscoe, C. H., J. P. Hearn, and M. B. Renfree (1974). Control of reproduction in macropodid marsupials. *J. Endocrinol.* **63**:589–614.

37. Wu, C., and L. M. Prazak (1974). Endocrine basis for ovulation induction. *Clin. Obstet. Gynecol.* **17**:65–78.

14

The Pineal Gland

The term *pineal organ* is used here to mean any epiphyseal structure derived from the roof of the brain diencephalon. The term *pineal gland* is restricted here to those cases where a secretory function has been demonstrated or where indirect information (such as cytological appearance) indicates a secretory process. In cases where there is more than one structure developed in the epithalamic region (e.g., an epiphyseal structure and a parapineal device), the term *pineal complex* is appropriate.

Ectothermic vertebrates commonly have pineal complexes consisting of the pineal organ proper (*epipysis cerebri*) and a more superficial parietal or parapineal organ (sometimes known as the "third eye") (Fig. 14.1, Fig. 14.2 *A–D*). Birds and mammals (Fig. 14.2 *E, F*) have only a glandular pineal organ and lack a parapineal organ.

Pineal organs are so strikingly varied in morphology, cytology, and innervation as to suggest a diversity of functions. Indeed, it appears that pineal organs may have rather different roles among the vertebrate classes or even among orders of some classes. In all animals investigated, the pineal organ appears to have characteristics of an endocrine gland but, in addition, in many groups it also has sensory functions. Indeed, the pineals of fishes and amphibians appear to be involved predominantly with photoreception and secondarily with secretion.

The relative size of the pineal gland in birds and mammals varies remarkably, from quite small (e.g., owls, shearwaters, opossums, shrews, whales, and bats) to very large (e.g., penguins, emus, sea lions, and seals). It has been rather astounding to discover that a few species lack a pineal organ altogether. This clearly is the case in crocodilians and armadillos and seems to be so also in hagfishes, dugongs, sloths, and anteaters. Thus pineal organs are probably the most variable of vertebrate structures. Correspond-

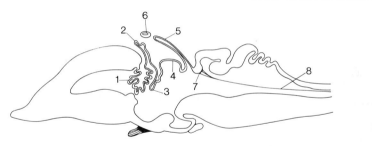

FIGURE 14.1. Diagrammatic sagittal section of the brain of a lower vertebrate. *1,* Choroid plexus; *2,* paraphysis; *3,* velum transversum; *4,* dorsal sac; *5,* epiphysis cerebri; *6,* parietal eye (parapineal organ); *7,* subcommissural organ; *8,* Reissner's fiber. [After W. Bargmann, *Handbuch der Mikroskopischen Anatomie des Menschen,* Vol. 6, No. 4, Springer, Berlin, 1943.]

ingly, the endocrine mechanisms of the glandular pineal organs have proven to be intriguingly elusive, but appear to be astonishingly pervasive.

ANATOMY AND DEVELOPMENT OF THE EPIPHYSIS

In all vertebrates the pineal organ arises as a vesicular evagination or compact bud from the dorsal wall of the diencephalon. This is also the case for the parapineal organ, when present. The lumina of these early primordia communicate with the third ventricle. The open ventricular connection persists among some teleosts, but there tends to be a progessive phylogenetic reduction of the lumen of the pineal body, leading to the compact, glandlike pineal organ of birds and mammals.

The parapineal organ may develop quite independently of the pineal organ, as in lizards, or the two may arise in close association with one another. In some fishes and anurans the pineal and parapineal primordia commonly fuse to form a united complex.

The pineal organs of most cyclostomes, fishes, amphibians, and lizards have sensory elements. Photoreception has been electrophysiologically demonstrated in a number of species of lower vertebrates, and cells with the characteristics of photoreceptors have been observed by electron microscopy in the pineal complex. Indeed, eyelike differentiations of the pineal or parapineal organ have been demonstrated in lampreys, frogs and lizards. Thus it appears that the more primitive pineal organ is, fundamentally, a photosensory organ. J.-P. Collin has proposed that the pineal organ of lower vertebrates gradually lost its sensory role but retained and enhanced its endocrine function as it evolved in the higher groups. He suggests that a line of photoreceptive cells, present in pineal systems of Anamniota, evolved into "regressed photorecepter cells"—a prominant cell type in reptiles and birds—and finally into the exclusively secretory pinealocytes that are characteristic of snakes and mammals (Fig. 14.3).

Concomitant changes in innervation accompany the changes from photoreceptor cell to secretory pinealocyte. In fishes and amphibians the pineal photoreceptors convey transduced light information to sensory neurons. The axons of the sensory neurons coalesce into a pineal tract that extends to the epithalamic region of the brain, where most of the neurons join fibers of the posterior commissure. The site of eventual termination of these fibers is presently unknown. Among lizards and turtles, in which the typical photoreceptor cell is rare (Fig. 14.3), there is a corresponding reduction in sensory neurons, and the number of fibers running in the pineal tract is reduced. However, there are signs of sympathetic innervation, which is, as we shall see, a feature of the secretory pineals of birds and mammals.

In birds pineal tract fibers have occasionally been found in the pineal organ, and synaptic junctions between nerve cells and "regressed photoreceptor cells" have been seen, although rarely. Sympathetic, aminergic fibers originating in the superior cervical ganglia are the dominant type of innervation. There also may be cholinergic fibers in the avian pineal, as suggested by histochemical studies, but their origin and function is presently unknown.

The pineal gland of most mammals so far examined appears to have no afferent or efferent neural connections with the brain proper. Commonly, there are fibers that pass up the pineal stalk from the habenula and posterior commissural regions, but these appear to return without synapsing in the pineal gland. It has been reported that the pineal gland of the ferret contains a collection of ganglion cells that send axons to the brain through the epiphyseal stalk. In a few other species a nervous connection between the pineal organ and brain is indicated, but not well proven. It is generally agreed that the mammalian pineal gland is primarily innervated by the peripheral autonomic nervous system. The major set of fibers are sympathetic postganglionic fibers originating in the superior cervical ganglia. They enter the pineal gland either along with the vasculature, and terminate in the pineal parenchyma of the pericapillary space, or via two nervi conarii, which course over the brain and enter the gland at its caudal pole. These fibers also branch extensively to terminate in the pineal parenchyma. This pattern of a single, peripheral innervation is observed in many mammalian species, including the well-studied rodents. However, in other mammals, in addition to the sympathetic innervation, there are parasympathetic fibers which probably originate in the superior salivatory nuclei and run with the greater superior petrosal nerve after leaving the brain stem in the facial nerves. The distribution of the postganglionic parasympathetic fibers is similar to that of the sympathetics, with many terminating in the pericapillary spaces. The sympathetic innervation of the pineal gland of mammals regulates indoleamine metabolism (see below). The functional role of the parasympathetic innervation is not known.

It is well established in mammals (but not in other vertebrate classes) that the eyes are responsible for mediating the effects of light on indoleamine

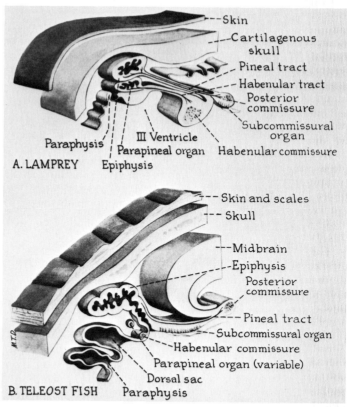

A. LAMPREY

Skin
Cartilagenous skull
Pineal tract
Habenular tract
Posterior commissure
Subcommissural organ
Paraphysis
III Ventricle
Parapineal organ
Epiphysis
Habenular commissure

B. TELEOST FISH

Skin and scales
Skull
Midbrain
Epiphysis
Posterior commissure
Pineal tract
Subcommissural organ
Habenular commissure
Parapineal organ (variable)
Dorsal sac
Paraphysis

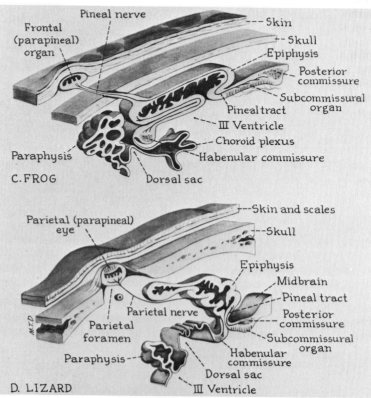

C. FROG

Pineal nerve
Frontal (parapineal) organ
Skin
Skull
Epiphysis
Posterior commissure
Subcommissural organ
Pineal tract
III Ventricle
Choroid plexus
Habenular commissure
Paraphysis
Dorsal sac

D. LIZARD

Parietal (parapineal) eye
Skin and scales
Skull
Epiphysis
Midbrain
Pineal tract
Posterior commissure
Subcommissural organ
Parietal nerve
Parietal foramen
Habenular commissure
Paraphysis
Dorsal sac
III Ventricle

520

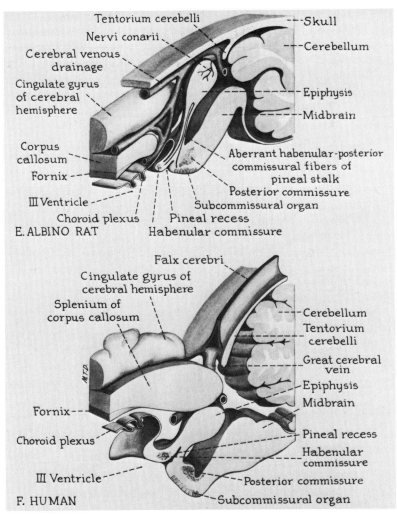

E. ALBINO RAT

Tentorium cerebelli

Nervi conarii

Cerebral venous drainage

Cingulate gyrus of cerebral hemisphere

Corpus callosum

Fornix

III Ventricle

Choroid plexus

Skull

Cerebellum

Epiphysis

Midbrain

Aberrant habenular-posterior commissural fibers of pineal stalk

Posterior commissure

Subcommissural organ

Pineal recess

Habenular commissure

F. HUMAN

Falx cerebri

Cingulate gyrus of cerebral hemisphere

Splenium of corpus callosum

Fornix

Choroid plexus

III Ventricle

Cerebellum

Tentorium cerebelli

Great cerebral vein

Epiphysis

Midbrain

Pineal recess

Habenular commissure

Posterior commissure

Subcommissural organ

FIGURE 14.2. *A through F*: diagrammatic representations depicting longitudinal slices from the diencephalic roof region of the brains of several vertebrates. The facing surface of each slice has been taken at or near the median saggital plane of the brain. Overlying cranial and/or integumental components are shown, particularly in relation to several pineal derivatives. These diagrams serve to illustrate the various pineal components as they appear in different species, their innervation, their vascularization, and their relationship to other diencephalic circumventricular organs. [From R. J. Wurtman et al., *The Pineal*, Academic, New York, 1968.]

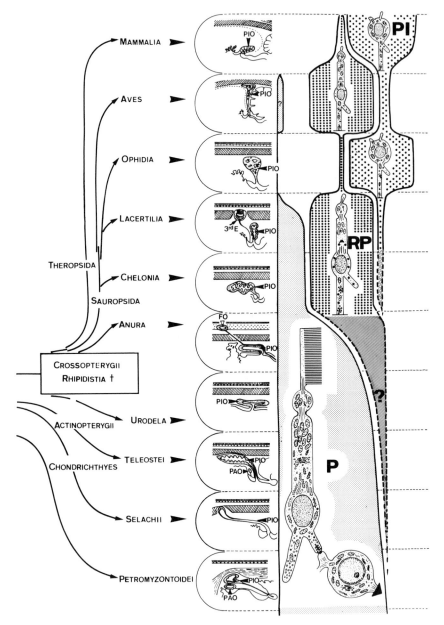

FIGURE 14.3. Phylogeny and possible multiplicities of sensory-line cells in the pineal organ of vertebrates. *Center:* diagrammatic representation showing sagittal sections through the diencephalic roof of vertebrates; *on the right:* gradual transformation of the photoreceptor cell during phylogeny, and the plurality of cells of the receptor line in a given pineal organ. Since in Anamniota (fishes and amphibians) our knowledge of the process of rudimentation is only fragmentary, no details are indicated for these groups of vertebrates. Three types of pineal cells (*PI, RP,* and *P*) are shown within shaded areas on the right side of the figure. The widths of these shaded areas opposite each vertebrate group indicate the extent to which that cell type is represented in the pineal apparatus of that vertebrate group. *FO,* frontal organ; *P,* photoreceptor; *PAO,* parapineal organ; *PI,* pinealocyte; *PIO,* pineal organ; *RP,* rudimentary photoreceptor cell; *3rd E,* third (or parietal) eye [Courtesy of J.-P. Collin.]

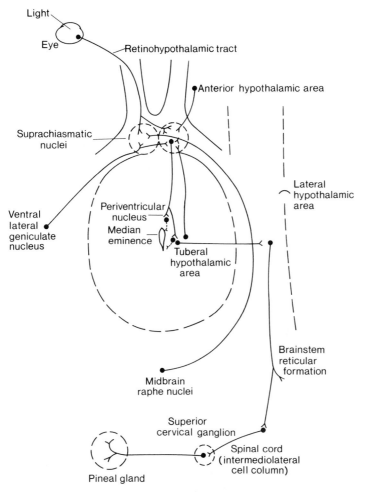

FIGURE 14.4. Diagrammatic representation of the functional innervation of the pineal, including the connections of the suprachiasmatic nuclei, as they are known in the rat. See text for description. [After R. Y. Moore, *The Pineal Gland* (I. Nir, R. J. Reiter, and R. J. Wurtman, eds.) Springer-Verlag, Wien, 1978.]

metabolism in the pineal gland. The neural pathway from the eyes to the sympathetic fibers that terminate in the pineal gland has been rather well defined, largely through the work of Moore (Fig. 14.4).

PINEAL GLAND CYTOLOGY

Because the subject of this book is endocrinology, the remainder of the chapter will focus on the secretory aspects of pineal organs. Obviously,

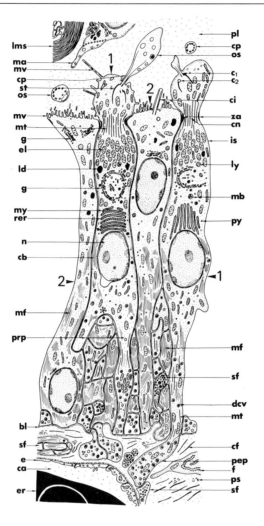

FIGURE 14.5. Cellular types in the follicular epithelium of the pineal organ of the magpie (*Pica pica* L.). *1*, Rudimentary photoreceptor cell; *2*, ependymal (supportive, interstitial) cell. *bl*, Basal lamina; c_1, axial centriole; c_2, oblique centriole; *ca*, lumen of a capillary; *cb*, cellular body; *cf*, collagen fibrils; *ci*, cilium; *cn*, cellular neck; *cp*, connecting piece; *dcv*, dense-core vesicle; *e*, endothelium; *el*, mitochondria of the ellipsoid; *er*, erythrocyte; *f*, fibroblast; *g*, Golgi complex; *is*, inner segment; *ld*, lipid droplet; *lms*, lamellated membranous structures (lamellar body); *ly*, lysosome; *ma*, macrophage; *mb*, multivesicular body; *mf*, microfilament; *mt*, microtubule; *mv*, microvilli; *my*, myoid; *n*, nucleus; *os*, outer segment; *pep*, perivascular process; *pl*, pineal lumen; *prp*, processes of a rudimentary photoreceptor cell; *ps*, perivascular space; *py*, polysomes; *rer*, rough endoplasmic reticulum; *sf*, orthosympathetic fibers; *st*, striated ciliary rootlet; *za*, zonula adhaerens. [From J.-P. Collin, *The Pineal Gland* (G. E. W. Wolstenholme and J. Knight, eds.), Churchill Livingstone, Edinburgh, 1971.]

then, it is the pineal glands of birds and mammals that become the organs of primary interest, because they are secretory organs (probably exclusively so, and not photosensory). Also, there is little that can be said about pineal secretions in other classes simply because we know very little about the secretory aspects of their pineal organs.

Avian Pineal Glands

The epiphysis is the only component of the pineal system in birds. It extends dorsally from the roof of the diencephalon, between the cerebrum and the cerebellum, to the meninges. In general form, it varies from saccular in passerine birds to parenchymal in gallinaceous species. There are two classes of cells: the chief cell, or regressed photoreceptor cell (RP) of Collin, and supportive cells (Fig. 14.5). The RPs retain some of the features of photoreceptors, but are considered to be secretory and not photosensory. The outer segment is represented by clublike, whorled, lamellar structures. The ciliated connecting structure has lost the two central filaments, as in other sensory cells, but the nine pairs of circumferential filaments terminate in one of the typical centrioles located within their striated rootlets in the inner segments. A well-developed Golgi apparatus is present in the inner segment, and many dense-cored vesicles and aggregations of mitochondria are found in the cytoplasm. The RPs terminate either on the basement membrane or, in some species, may penetrate into the pericapillary space (Fig. 14.5). Although "synaptic ribbons" are seen in the terminals as well as throughout the cytoplasm, there is some question as to whether those are true synaptic junctions. However, in sparrows (*Zonotrichia* and *Passer*) typical synaptic junctions with pre- and postsynaptic membrane specialization have been observed.

Supportive cells appear to correspond to glial cells of other nervous tissue. They are characterized by microvilli and, sometimes, by cilia. Numerous microfilaments, mitochondria, and glycogen particles are present in the cytoplasm.

Unmyelinated nerve fibers are found in the stalk of the pineal gland of *Passer*, but the termination of these fibers is unknown, and nothing is known of their function. Ganglion cells have been observed in *Passer*, but they are very rare. As noted above, the avian epiphysis is well innervated by sympathetic (noradrenergic) fibers. Bilateral superior cervical sympathectomy results in complete degeneration of these fibers.

Mammalian Pineal Glands

The pinealocyte is the chief cell type of mammalian pineal glands (and of ophidians, also; see Fig. 14.3). The evolution of the photoreceptor cell into a typical secretory cell is culminated in the pineal gland of mammals and snakes. Adult pinealocytes retain no evidence of an outer segment or lamellar structure, although they do retain the 9 + 0 centriolar apparatus. The cytoplasm of the cell body contains the usual organelles: centriolar apparatus, mitochondria, smooth and rough endoplasmic reticulum, Golgi complex, lysosomes, and lipid droplets. Pinealocytes make contact with other pinealocytes, but processes or pedicles also terminate close to the basement membrane of the epithelium or enter the perivascular space (Fig. 14.6).

Both clear and dense-cored vesicles are found throughout the cytoplasm of the pinealocyte, and some of these are aggregated around electron-dense rodlets to form bodies that resemble synaptic ribbons of photoreceptors. However, they are scattered throughout the cytoplasm and are not grouped near bounding membranes, so that pre- and postsynaptic arrangements are not suggested. Nonetheless, these structures may not be merely vestiges of a photoreceptive heritage but, perhaps, are functional organelles of the pinealocytes. One sort of evidence supporting this idea is that, in guinea pigs, synaptic ribbons are more numerous during nighttime than during daytime.

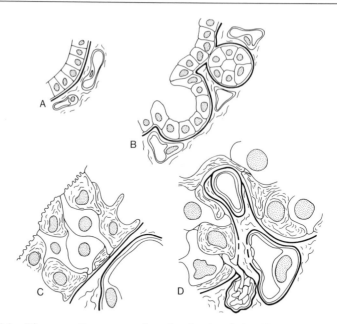

FIGURE 14.6. Diagrammatic representations showing the relationship between mesenchymally derived connective tissue components and neuroepithelially derived pineal parenchymal constituents during development of a mammalian pineal system. Epithelial evaginations into a vascularized mesenchymal stroma carry with them their underlying basal lamina (heavy dark line) and form partially or completely isolated rosettes or follicles (*A* and *B*). The walls of such follicles (*C*) differentiate mainly into pinealocytes (light) or astrocytes (filamentous supporting cells). Astrocytes seem, in some species, to line the basal surface or, in the majority, are adjacent to the epithelial basal lamina. Vessels within the connective tissue compartment meanwhile have acquired a perivascular basal lamina. The epithelial wall is gradually converted into characteristic pineal parenchyma as continued cell differentiation, diverticulation, and rearrangement take place. Still, in final form (*D*), the basic relationships between the parenchyma, vessels, and the connective tissue compartment are largely retained. [After R. J. Wurtman et al., *The Pineal,* Academic Press, New York, 1968.]

PINEAL SUBSTANCES

Indoleamines

The modern era of pineal research was opened when Aaron Lerner and his co-workers at Yale University decided to attempt to isolate and identify the substance in pineal extracts that blanched the skin of frogs. Lerner, who was a pioneer in the study of melanin formation and regulation, was intrigued by reports—especially that of McCord and Allen in 1917—demonstrating that extracts of beef pineals cause blanching in frog tadpoles. McCord and Allen had concluded that the pineal organ "contains within itself an active principle capable of inducing pigment changes independent and wholly apart from environmental conditions." Lerner and colleagues employed a frog skin bioassay to detect the elusive lightening agent, since there was no clue as to its chemical nature. After many discouraging and frustrating attempts to isolate the active principle from about 250,000 bovine pineal glands, they finally purified, by countercurrent distribution from an ethyl acetate extract, an indolic compound that was identified as 5-methoxy-N-acetyltryptamine. From its action of causing melanophone melanosomes to aggregate, it was named *melatonin* by Lerner in 1958.

Melatonin can be measured chemically by extraction into organic solvents, such as chloroform or p-cymene, and then assayed fluorometrically in $3N$ HCL. However, fluorometric methods usually are not sufficiently sensitive or specific to measure the minute amounts of melatonin normally present in the pineal glands of most species. Hence in the earlier work on melatonin, bioassays were often employed because of their relatively greater sensitivity and specificity than the chemical or physical methods then available. The isolated frog skin bioassay, developed by Lerner's group, was an essential key to the identification of melatonin, since they never had more than 100 µg of melatonin available for analysis. Later, other workers developed bioassays—including Ralph and Lynch, who used tadpoles of *Rana*, and Lynch and co-workers, who used *Xenopus* tadpoles—to detect melatonin in solutions into which the animals were placed. These methods can measure as little as 0.0001 µg of the indole.

Soon after the discovery of melatonin, investigations were initiated to determine the manner in which the compound is synthesized in pineal glands. Julius Axelrod, at the National Institutes of Health in Bethesda, Maryland, became a leader in this effort, bringing to the task his familiarity with catecholamine synthesis. Since he had shown that the enzymatic O-methylation of catecholamines required S-adenosylmethionine as the methyl donor, Axelrod incubated an extract of bovine pineal gland with a likely precursor of melatonin, N-acetylserotonin, and added ^{14}C-methyl-S-adenosylmethionine. He obtained a radioactive compound that had the same R_f value on paper chromatograms as authentic melatonin. This result, reported in 1960, indicated that the pineal gland contains an enzyme that can transfer the methyl group of S-adenosylmethionine to the hydroxyl group of N-acetylserotonin. This enzyme, subsequently purified from bovine pineal glands and characterized by Axelrod and Weissbach, was named hydroxyindole-O-methyltransferase (HIOMT).

HIOMT was found to methylate a wide variety of hydroxyindoles. However, of all the substrates examined, N-acetylserotonin was shown to be the most preferred. The distribution of the enzyme appeared to be restricted to the pineal gland in the several mammalian species that were examined by Axelrod and colleagues. Later work, as detailed in the last section of this chapter, was to reveal that this is not the case, but that the enzyme is found in other sites as well. However, the discovery and characterization of HIOMT as a unique pineal enzyme gave impetus to other investigators to try to determine the physiological function of the pineal gland and to define the role of the special pineal product, melatonin.

Now that HIOMT was characterized, the principal method for obtaining information about melatonin production in pineal glands became measuring the activity of this enzyme. This is an appropriately sensitive assay method. Subsequently, the activity of a second enzyme, serotonin-*N*-acetyltransferase (NAT), mainly characterized by Richard Wurtman and colleagues and by David Klein and colleagues, also came to be used as an indicator of melatonin synthesis (Fig. 14.7). More recently still, radioimmunoassay (RIA) methods have become strong favorites for directly measuring melatonin, because the indole can be detected in extremely low concentrations and in tissues where it is present but not synthesized, such as in blood or cerebrospinal fluid. There also have been significant advances in the use of gas chromatography coupled to mass spectrometry for measuring melatonin.

The biosynthesis of melatonin begins in a conventional fashion with the uptake of the essential amino acid tryptophan into pineal parenchymal cells. Tryptophan is then converted to 5-hydroxytryptophan by tryptophan hydroxylase and then to 5-hydroxytryptamine (serotonin) by aromatic L-amino acid decarboxylase. Serotonin was shown by W. B. Quay, using fluorometry, to be in higher concentration in the pineal gland than in any other region of the brain or in any other organ. Also, Quay revealed that there is

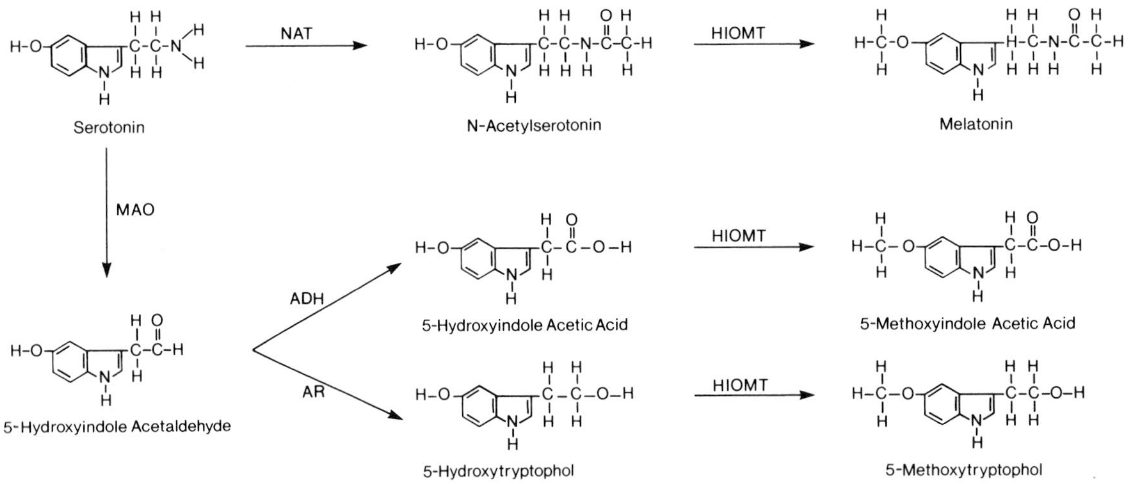

FIGURE 14.7. Biosynthesis of pineal methoxyindoles from serotonin. Serotonin may be either acetylated to form *N*-acetylserotonin, through the action of the enzyme serotonin-*N*-acetyltransferase (NAT), or oxidatively deaminated by monoamine oxidase (MAO) to yield an unstable aldehyde. This compound is then either oxidized to 5-hydroxyindoleacetic acid, by the enzyme aldehyde dehydrogenase (ADH), or reduced to form 5-hydroxytryptophol, by aldehyde reductase (AR). Each of these 5-hydroxyindole derivatives of serotonin is a substrate for hydroxyindole-*O*-methyltransferase (HIOMT); the enzymatic transfer of a methyl group (from *S*-adenosylmethionine) to these hydroxyindoles yields melatonin (5-methoxy-*N*-acetyltryptamine), 5-methoxyindoleacetic acid, and 5-methoxytryptophol, respectively. Pineal serotonin is synthesized from the essential amino acid tryptophan by 5-hydroxylation followed by decarboxylation. The first step is catalyzed by tryptophan hydroxylase; the second by aromatic L-amino acid decarboxylase.

a striking diurnal rhythm of serotonin content in the rat pineal gland, with the highest levels during daylight and very low levels during darkness. It was later proven that most of the serotonin is converted—primarily during nighttime—to melatonin by the actions of NAT and HIOMT. The activity of NAT increases dramatically with the onset of darkness, apparently enhanced (in mammalian pineal glands) by the release of norepinephine from the sympathetic neurons that terminate on the pineal parenchymal cells. This effect can be readily duplicated *in vitro* with intact, cultured pineal glands to which norepinephine is added.

Some of the pineal serotonin is deaminated by monoamine oxidase (MAO) and then either oxidized to form 5-hydroxyindoleacetic acid or reduced to form 5-hydroxytryptophol. Both of these products are also substrates for HIOMT and are converted to 5-methoxyindoleacetic acid and 5-methoxytryptophol, respectively (Fig. 14.7). According to Wurtman, the level of the latter indole, like that of melatonin, rises markedly in the rat pineal gland with the onset of darkness.

Circulating melatonin is thought to be loosely bound to albumin. It is almost entirely metabolized in the liver by 6-hydroxylation, followed by conjugation with sulfate or glucuronic acid, and excreted in the urine. No more than 2% of administered melatonin appears in the urine as 5-methoxyindoleacetic acid. In all the species of vertebrates so far examined, melatonin is present in the pineal gland—as well as in the blood, cerebrospinal fluid, brain and other tissues—in greater quantities during darkness than in light. As noted above, the nighttime elevation of melatonin is paralleled by the remarkable changes in pineal NAT activity (Fig. 14.8). Furthermore, as Ralph and co-workers first demonstrated in 1971 with rats, the diurnal cycle of melatonin production persists as a free running, circadian rhythm under constant lighting conditions (no light-dark changes), and the phase of the rhythm can be predicted from the animal's persistent activity rhythm.

The nighttime rise in NAT activity in chickens is under the control of an entrained endogenous circadian system, as demonstrated by Sue Binkley and colleagues in 1973–1975. When chickens are exposed to four hours of darkness during normal light-time, there is no change in NAT activity. However, during the anticipated dark-time, darkness increases NAT activity, whereas exposure to light during normal dark-time causes a rapid decrease in NAT activity. Furthermore, when chickens that were previously exposed to standard 24-hours cycles of light and dark are held in continuous darkness, the pineal NAT activity decreases in "anticipation" of the expected onset of light. Thus the enzyme rhythm has circadian features.

It is commonly agreed that the pineal secretes melatonin into the blood. There appears to be little storage of melatonin within the pineal gland; thus, as melatonin synthesis is increased, so also is release into the blood increased. Thus determinations of melatonin content of the pineal gland or its rate of melatonin synthesis correlate rather closely with the levels of me-

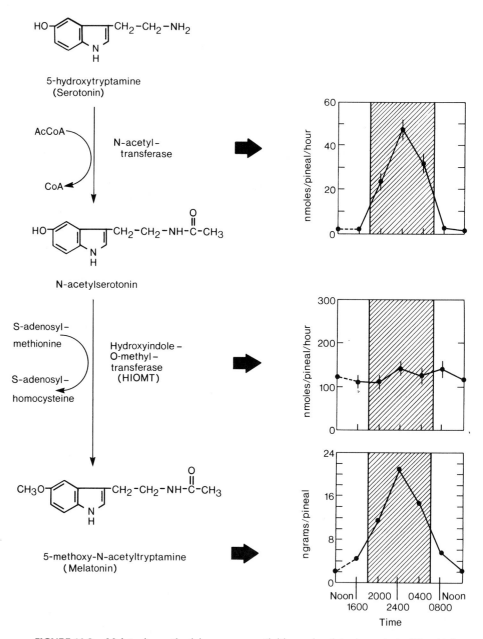

FIGURE 14.8. Melatonin-synthesizing enzyme activities and melatonin content of the chicken pineal gland. The period of darkness is indicated by shaded areas. *N*-acetyltransferase activity and melatonin content are greater at night than during the day. HIOMT activity remains fairly constant at all times. [After S. Binkley, et al., *Science,* **181**:274, 1963. Copyright 1963 by The American Association for the Advancement of Science.]

latonin found in body fluids, at least in chickens and some rodents, the most extensively studied animals in this regard.

Binkley has pointed to some possible differences among various species in regard to melatonin production. For instance, whereas norepinephrine stimulates NAT activity of rat pineal glands *in vitro*, it does not stimulate the enzyme of chickens (*Gallus domesticus*), sparrows (*Passer domesticus*), or hamsters (*Mesocricetus auratus*). Also, the rat pineal gland clearly depends upon the eyes and the superior cervical ganglion pathway for control of pineal enzyme activity. Chickens are different in this regard, for blinding or superior cervical ganglionectomy does not abolish the light–dark effects on melatonin synthesis. Thus direct photosensitivity of the pineal gland in birds is suggested. Indeed, *in vitro* studies of the chick pineal gland demonstrate such photosensitivity. However, the locus of receptivity and the mode of light transduction in the pineal gland are unknown. A recent report by Takeo Deguchi indicates that dispersed cells from chicken pineal glands are sensitive to illumination and exhibit circadian changes. Thus the endogenous oscillator, the photoreceptor, and the melatonin-synthesizing machinery may reside in a single cell of the chicken pineal gland.

To conclude this section on indolic substances of the pineal gland, it is appropriate to point out that in addition to melatonin, 5-methoxytryptophol, 5-hydroxytryptophol, and other pineal indoles have been shown to have biological actions in certain bioassay systems. However, at the present time it is not possible to claim that any one of them is a hormone in the classical sense.

Proteinaceous Substances

In addition to the methoxyindoles that are found in all vertebrate pineals, mammalian (and perphaps avian) pineals contain low–molecular weight peptidic or polypeptidic compounds that have been alleged to be pineal hormones. The octapeptides arginine vasotocin, lysine vasotocin, and arginine vasopressin, as well as neurophysinlike proteins, have been reported to be present in pineal glands. To one or more of the octapeptides some workers have ascribed the so-called antigonadotropic activity of the pineal gland. Additionally, hypophysiotropic hormones—including TRH, LHRH, and prolactin-releasing and inhibiting factors, as well as renin and vasoactive peptide—have been localized in the rat pineal gland. Large amounts of taurine also have been found in bovine pineal glands. It remains, however, to be proven that these substances are actually synthesized by the pineal gland. The evidence at the time of this writing is fairly persuasive that the particular cell type in the pineal glands of all vertebrates that synthesizes melatonin also engages in secretory protein synthesis. Collin has argued that the regressed photoreceptor cell (RP) of reptiles and birds and the pinealocytes (Pi) of snakes (and probably mammals) engage in both indoleamine and protein secretory processes. Whereas an enzymatic mechanism pro-

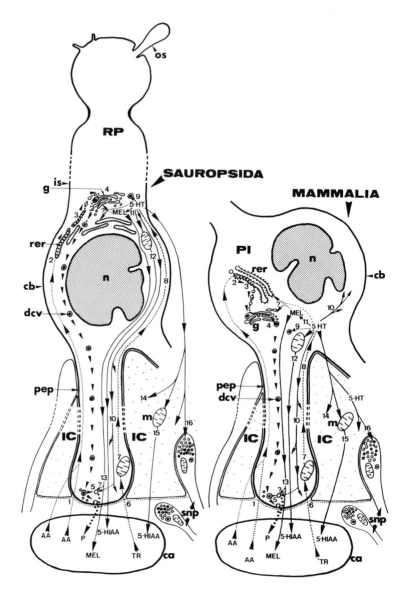

FIGURE 14.9. Secretory processes in the rudimentary photoreceptor cell (*RP*) of Sauropsida (chelonians, lacertilians, birds) and in the pinealocyte (*PI*) of Mammalia and ophidians; hypothetical relationships between indoles and protein secretion. os, outer segment; is, inner segment, n, nucleus. *Protein secretion*: (*1*) uptake of amino acids (AA) by *RP, PI*, and interstitial cells (*IC*); (*2*) biosynthesis of proteins by a ribosomal mechanism and segregation in the cisternal space of the rough endoplasmic reticulum (*rer*); (*3*) intracisternal transport of the proteins; (*4*) concentration in the Golgi complex (*g*) and formation of dense-cored vesicles (*dcv*). The dense-cored vesicles, storing a proteinaceous compound, migrate (arrowheads) from the cell body (*cb*) to the endings of the perivascular processes (*pep*). (*5*) Accumulation and possible sites of release of the protein secretion in the terminals of the perivascular processes, and passage of this secretory product into the capillaries (*ca*). *Indoleamine secretion*: (*6*) uptake of circulating tryptophan (*TR*) by *RP, PI*, and *IC*. (*7*) TR is hydroxylated by tryptophan-5-monooxygenase, located in mitochondria, to 5-hydroxytryptophan, which is converted to *5-HT* by an aromatic

duces indoleamines, the classical ribosomal mechanism is postulated to produce the protein secretion (Fig. 14.9).

Collin's proposal is based upon his own work and that of other investigators employing combined microspectrofluorometric, fluorescence histochemical, immunocytochemical, radioautographic, and ultracytological data. They clearly suggest that anabolism, catabolism, and storage of indoleamines take place in the RP cells and Pi. In the supporting cells (interstitial or glialike cells), storage of serotonin and membranous sites for oxidative deamination are indicated.

Collin proposed in 1979 that the dense-cored vesicles, originating from the Golgi zone of the perikaryon of RP cells and Pi, may contain a specific, complex peptidergic neurohormone carrier (neurophysinlike?) to which a more or less considerable portion of the indoleaminergic pool may be facultatively bound. Such an association conforms to the hypothesized amine precursor uptake and decarboxylation (APUD) cells of Pearse, which constitute the so-called diffuse neuroendocrine system (DNES). Indeed, Leong and Matthews, in 1979, hypothesized that the pineal gland is an APUD organ. (See Chapter 8 for an explanation of the APUD hypothesis.)

FUNCTIONS OF PINEAL GLANDS

It would be pleasing to address the subject of pineal function by starting with the basic mode of action of pineal gland hormones. However, this simply is not possible at present because (1) no mechanism of central action has been adequately characterized, (2) it is not certain that melatonin is the only hormone of the pineal gland (as noted above), and (3) melatonin and other pineal-characteristic substances are not produced exclusively by pineal glands (as will be explained later in the chapter). Thus the current state of understanding of pineal function is comparatively superficial, allowing a description of certain manifestations that ensue following such manipulations as pineal gland removal or melatonin administration.

Most of what is known about the physiology of pineal glands is derived from the study of mammalian species, primarily rats and hamsters, plus a

---

L-amino acid decarboxylase (8). Then 5-HT may be facultatively taken up by dense-cored vesicles (dcv) (9) and/or, depending on the species, stored in the cytosol and in some organelles of RP (10), PI (10), and IC (14), or metabolized via several pathways. A small fraction of 5-HT is converted (11) into melatonin (MEL) by N-acetylation and O-methylation. MEL gains access (13) to the capillaries (ca). An important fraction of 5-HT is deaminated by a monoamine oxidase located in the outer membrane of the mitochondria (m) (12) of RP, PI, and IC (15), to give 5-hydroxyindoleacetic acid (5-HIAA), which is excreted. Another part of 5-HT may enter (16) the sympathetic nerve terminals (snp). *Relationships between the two secretory processes*: MEL (and perhaps 5-HT) may act locally on the formation and/or storage and/or release of the protein secretion—peptidic or polypeptidic neurohormone(s)—stored in dense-cored vesicles (dcv). [From J.-P. Collin, *The Pineal Gland of Vertebrates Including Man* (J. Ariëns Kappers and P. Pévet, eds.), Elsevier/North-Holland, Amsterdam, 1979.]

few birds, mainly chickens. It is doubtful that the functional view obtained from the study of a few representative mammals or birds provides an adequate, comprehensive, panvertebrate explanation of pineal mechanisms. For one thing, the majority of vertebrate species (fishes, amphibians, and many reptiles) have a photoreceptive pineal organ, quite unlike the glandular pineal organ of birds and mammals. The vast differences in morphological arrangement, innervation, and cytological composition, as noted above, suggest a possible diversity in function. Indeed, it can be safely asserted that *the* function of the pineal body is not established. However, it is also possible to state that pineal organs have been clearly implicated in several regulatory processes, including stress responses and homeostasis. Exactly how the pineal gland might be involved with such diffuse, general mechanisms is not established as yet. Other, better-documented functions attributed to pineal glands are the control of (1) color change, (2) reproduction, (3) rhythmicity, and (4) body temperature.

Color Change

Among some fishes and amphibians, the pineal gland has been implicated in color change. In 1911 von Frisch noted that the pineal region of the teleost *Phoxinus laevis* (*Phoxinus phoxinus*) was sensitive to light and influential in controlling melanophore responses. Young, in 1935, reported that the pallor that occurs in larval lampreys on transference from light to darkness is abolished after removal of the pineal complex. Other investigators, including McCord and Allen, observed that mammalian pineal extracts induce melanosome aggregation in larval and adult amphibians. Cautery of the diencephalic roof (pineal region) of *Xenopus* larvae, by Bagnara, resulted in their failure to show the normal blanching response when placed in darkness. These and other observations provide strong evidence that melatonin may play a role in the control of chromatic changes. However, this is best supported only for young larval amphibians. No such physiological role has been demonstrated for adult amphibians. Although exogenous melatonin does act directly on the dermal melanophores of adult amphibians and fishes, there is no good evidence that it does so naturally. Color change in the adults of these two classes of vertebrates can be accounted for by the exclusive action of MSH in amphibians and by neuroendocrine control mechanisms in fishes. Melatonin may influence pituitary MSH and thus have some indirect effect on color change. Indeed, pinealectomy increases the MSH content of the rat pituitary, whereas melatonin decreases it, according to Kastin. However, there are no chromatic changes known to be associated with these hormones in rats. Implants of melatonin were found by Rust and Meyer to induce the differentiation of a winter-type, white pelage in male weasels (*Mustela erminea bangsi*), and Lynch and Epstein induced pelage changes in the white-footed mouse (*Peromyscus leucopus*) with melatonin, but, in general, even massive doses of melatonin are without effect on most of the mammals in which it has been tested. Furthermore, there is no evidence that pineal organs are involved in the color changes of the skins of reptiles or the plumages of birds. Thus pineal glands and melatonin appear to have only very restricted involvement with color change.

Reproduction

The pineal gland has been characterized as a neuroendocrine transducer that responds to light either directly (the photoreceptive pineal organ of ectotherms) or indirectly via autonomic pathways (the pineal gland of mammals) by releasing pineal hormone(s). (As noted above, although sympathetically innervated, the avian pineal gland appears not to be dependent upon sympathetic input for responding to light or darkness, but, instead, may be directly sensitive.) Pineal hormones, in turn, are presumed to act on the hypothalamus, higher brain centers, the pituitary, the gonads, or some combination of these sites. Thus the influence of photoperiod on reproduction, which is well known among virtually all vertebrates, is considered by several investigators to be, in part at least, mediated by the pineal gland.

The applicability of the above scheme to vertebrates in general is questionable, in part because of limited experimentation with an adequate sampling of the different classes, but also because it seems to be a poor fit for some groups—especially for birds, in which the photoperiodic control of reproduction has been extensively studied. The literature on pineal involvement with reproduction in birds, reviewed thoroughly by Ralph in 1970 and 1981, is not clearly supportive of such a role. For example, the some three dozen reports on the effects of pinealectomy in birds (mostly Japanese quail and domestic chickens) indicate that the pineal gland may be (1) antigonadal, (2) progonadal, (3) antigonadal during one developmental period but progonadal during another, or (4) without influence on the gonads. Likewise, implantation of pineal glands and administration of pineal extracts or pineal-characteristic substances, including melatonin, have produced mixed results. Mostly such treatments have been ineffective in influencing the gonadal state in birds. Furthermore, although bilateral superior cervical ganglionectomy deprives the pineal gland of sympathetic innervation, this surgical procedure has no detectable effect on ovarian function (as evidenced by egg laying) in Japanese quail. Remarkably, pinealectomy plus blinding is reported to have no effect on patterns of gonadal responses to changing photoperiods in male Japanese quail.

There is little or no information from many vertebrate groups about a possible role for the pineal gland in reproduction. This is the case for Cyclostomata, Chondrichthyes, Amphibia, and most Reptilia (except lizards). There is a small body of evidence suggesting that the pineal complex of lizards is involved with reproductive conditions, but the details remain largely to be discovered, and the data support only a tenuous connection. Indeed, it is possible that the effects induced by pinealectomy or melatonin administration could be primarily upon thermoregulation and only secondarily upon reproduction. Normal thermoregulatory precision is essential for reproductive processes of lizards. For example, successful gamete formation and reproductive synchronization of the sexes are thermally dependent (and dependent on the photoperiod as well). Until thermal and photic conditions are adequately considered in experimental designs, the reality of pineal–gonadal interaction in lizards remains equivocal.

There is substantial evidence to support the contention that the pineal organ plays a reproductive role in bony fishes (Osteichthyes). Water temperature and photoperiod, as well as season, interact to influence the gonadal state in fish. Most investigators have astutely taken these variables into account. Pinealectomy commonly leads to acceleration of gonadal development in fishes, and melatonin inhibits gonadal growth. However, there is a confusing variety of responses that have been reported, some of which probably reflect species differences as well as differences in experimental design. Additionally, the observed effects are season dependent. The variable results that have been obtained from fish studies are so numerous and diverse that it would be inappropriate to summarize them here.

The pineal gland has been particularly implicated in the reproduction of mammals. In general, the pineal gland is considered to exert a suppressive action on gonadal maturation and function. Most of what is known concerning this role is derived from experiments employing laboratory rats (*Rattus norvegicus*) and, especially, golden hamsters (*Mesocricetus auratus*).

It has proven rather difficult to demonstrate a role for the pineal gland in regulating the reproductive system of rats by the use of pinealectomy. Extirpation of the pineal gland of prepubertal rats results in only slight increases in gonadal size. Pinealectomy of adult rats has been found to cause slight hypertrophy in some studies and no effect in others. When blinding is combined with olfactory bulb removal (anosmic condition), however, the gonads are dramatically reduced in size. (Olfactory bulb removal alone only slightly retards gonadal growth.) When pinealectomy, too, is performed, the gonads of the rats are grossly and histologically near normal. The morning values of pituitary LH are elevated and plasma LH is depressed in blinded, anosmic female rats; these hormonal alterations also are prevented by pinealectomy.

Darkness, when imposed early in the life of female prepubertal rats, delays the day of vaginal rupture and retards ovarian development. Pinealectomy prevents these dark-induced effects. Furthermore, neonatal pinealectomy advances the time of opening of the vaginal membrane by eight to nine days and accelerates the rate of sexual maturation. These effects are exaggerated if neonatal rats are blinded and made anosmic. The combined surgeries increase the mean age of vaginal opening from 40 to 51 days; pinealectomy prevents this effect. Blinding of male rats impedes development of testes and accessory structures; pinealectomy counters this effect.

In contrast to the rat, the reproductive system of the golden hamster, especially that of the male, is extremely sensitive to the influence of the pineal gland, as fully documented by Russel Reiter. Blinding causes, after about nine weeks, the testes and accessory organs to atrophy to about one-sixth the normal size. If blinded animals are simultaneously pinealectomized, atrophy is prevented. Correspondingly, pituitary LH is subnormal nine weeks after blinding and this depression is prevented by pinealectomy.

Surgical procedures that denervate the pineal gland are as effective as pinealectomy in preventing dark-induced gonadal atrophy in hamsters. Indeed, in every species in which it has been examined, interference with the sympathetic innervation to the pineal gland renders it nonfunctional in terms of antigonadotropic activity (Fig. 14.10). It should be noted, however, that superior cervical ganglionectomy, the procedure commonly employed to

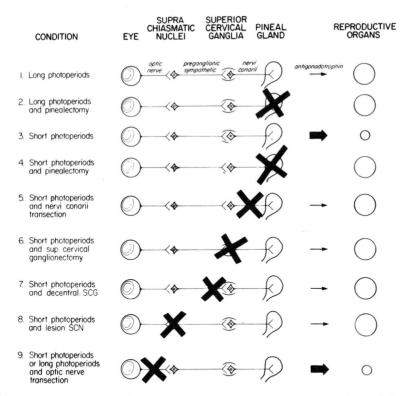

FIGURE 14.10. Diagrammatic summary of the surgical procedures that either eliminate or exaggerate pineal antigonadotrophic activity in mammals. The bold *X*'s represent removal of the organ or surgical transection of a fiber tract. The thickness of arrows indicates the antigonadotrophic capability of the pineal gland. In the portrayal, *preganglionic sympathetic fibers* refers to a multitude of neurons that intervene between the suprachiasmatic nuclei (SCN) and the superior cervical ganglia (SCG). *Decentral. SCG* refers to decentralization of the SCG, i.e., separating the SCG from their connections with the central nervous system. [From R. J. Reiter, *The Pineal and Reproduction* (R. J. Reiter, ed.), S. Karger, Basel, 1978.]

denervate the pineal gland, also denervates other head structures, including the Harderian gland and portions of the eye. These are melatonin-producing structures, as will be explained later, and thus superior cervical ganglio-nectomy should not be equated with pinealectomy.

Curiously, blinding in hamsters does not effect permanent inhibition of gonadal function. If hamsters are maintained for 27 weeks after blinding, the gonads and accessory reproductive organs regenerate to the normal, adult condition even though the pineal gland remains *in situ*. This inertial feature may relate to the biological advantage afforded a species that enters hibernation in the fall, when the photoperiod is shortening, with regressed gonads and emerges in the spring with reproductively competent gonads. Reiter has speculated that the spontaneous regeneration of the gonads may be attributed to (1) the hypothalamic–hypophyseal–gonadal axis becoming refractory to the pineal inhibitory substance or (2) the cessation of secretion of the pineal antigonadotropic hormone (Fig. 14.11).

A few other species of mammals, in addition to rats and hamsters, have been successfully used to demonstrate a pineal-mediated suppression of

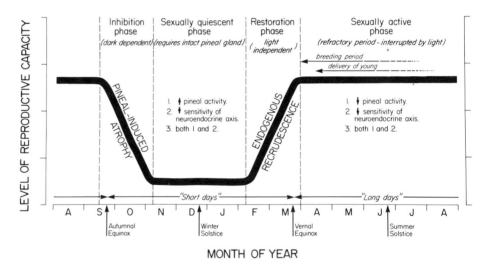

Pineal and Annual Reproductive Cycle in a Long Day Breeder

FIGURE 14.11. Schematic representation of the supposed relationships between the pineal gland and seasonal reproductive capability in a long-day breeder. The data on which the figure is based were derived primarily from experiments with the golden hamster. The annual repro-ductive cycle has been divided into four phases: inhibition phase, sexually quiescent phase, restoration phase, and sexually active phase. The cycle depends on the photoperiod acting by way of the pineal gland. The quiescent phase may be attributed to (1) increased pineal secretion of antigonadotropin, or (2) increased sensitivity of the neuroendocrine axis to pineal antigon-adotropin, or both (1) and (2). The sexually active phase would be explained by the opposite conditions. [Modified from R. J. Reiter, *Chronobiologica*, **1**:365, 1974.]

gonadal function. Pinealectomy (or superior cervical ganglionectomy) prevents the gonadal atrophy that would normally be occasioned by short photoperiods in voles (*Microtus agrestis*) and gerbils (*Meriones unguiculatus*). Rather surprisingly, pinealectomy of Djungarian hamsters (*Phodopus sungorus*) with involuted testes inhibits the acceleration of gonadal development that would normally be expected in animals exposed to long photoperiods. However, somewhat parallel findings are described by Herbert for the ferret. The onset of estrus is advanced by several weeks in ferrets that are exposed to long photoperiods during autumn and winter; this effect is eliminated by pinealectomy or superior cervical ganglionectomy. Thus the pineal gland, in these last two instances, appears to have a progonadal effect that is stimulated by light. However, estrous ferrets can be made anestrous prematurely by exposure to short photoperiods, and this effect is also prevented by pinealectomy. Melatonin may be involved in this response, since exogenous melatonin duplicates the effect of short days; it does not, however, duplicate the effects of long days in advancing estrus.

Melatonin, in many investigators' experiments, has been a rather poor antigonadal agent. This is especially the situation in studies employing rats. The earlier attempts to demonstrate its antigonadal action in hamsters also were quite disappointing. However, as Tamarkin and collegues discovered, the *pattern* of melatonin administration is all-important in demonstrating an effect. If melatonin is injected into hamsters during the morning (when in a light–dark cycle of 14:10; lights on at 6 A.M.), there is no effect on the gonads. However, similar injections given daily at 4 P.M. induce total regression of the sexual organs. Intriguingly, if the hamsters are first pinealectomized or if the pineal gland is denervated, the afternoon injections of melatonin are without effect on the gonadal state.

The dependence of melatonin's antigonadotropic action on the intact pineal gland may suggest, according to Reiter, that melatonin acts on the pineal gland to induce the release of another substance (peptide?), which then inhibits the neuroendocrine–reproductive axis. Alternatively, melatonin injected in the late afternoon may inhibit the gonads only because it supplements the nighttime elevation of endogenously produced melatonin.

Further complicating matters are the more recent demonstrations by both Klaus Hoffman and by Reiter that melatonin can act as a "counterantigonadotropic" agent. When melatonin is delivered to hamsters in a continuous manner—by placing melatonin in pellets of beeswax or into silastic capsules, which are then implanted subcutaneously into experimental animals—the expected dark-induced gonadal regression is prevented. Thus, paradoxically, both pinealectomy and chronic melatonin availability prevent darkness from inducing gonadal involution! Furthermore, subcutaneous depots of melatonin also prevent acute afternoon melatonin injections from causing gonadal atrophy. That is, melatonin appears to be capable of preventing its own action!

One possible explanation for these confounding findings is that when melatonin is chronically available, it binds all available melatonin receptors, making the animal permanently refractory to the action of additional melatonin. Under these conditions, melatonin cannot act as an inhibitor of the reproductive state. However, the particular mode of action of melatonin in normal reproductive physiology obviously remains to be revealed. Furthermore, the functional roles of the other pineal indoleamines and the peptides have not been adequately investigated. Several workers have shown vasoactive octapeptides and various fractions of pineal extracts that contain uncharacterized peptides to be effective antigonadal agents in particular assay systems. Obviously, many interesting investigations of the pineal gland as a regulator of reproduction remain to be done.

Rhythmicity

The pineal gland may play a central role in the circadian organization of fishes, lizards, and some species of birds. However, such a role has been demonstrated in only a few kinds of these animals, and there is even negative evidence from other species. The most convincing data for involvement of the pineal gland in rhythmicity have been derived by Michael Menaker and his associates in studies with the house sparrow (*Passer domesticus*).

Removal of the pineal gland from house sparrows abolishes free-running circadian rhythms of locomotion. Also, pinealectomy eliminates the circadian rhythm of body temperature. Surgical interruption of the sympathetic fibers extending from the surperior cervical ganglia to the pineal, as well as of the acetylcholinesterase-positive fibers that leave the pineal gland through the stalk, does not eliminate free-running circadian rhythmicity. This finding suggests that neural connections are not necessary for the sparrow pineal gland to perform its circadian function. Indeed, when the pineal gland was transplanted by Menaker and Zimmerman to the anterior chamber of the eye of arrhythmic recipient sparrows, they assumed a free-running circadian rhythm, and, furthermore, the phase of the restored rhythm was like that of the donor!

When melatonin is administered continuously to sparrows, low doses shorten the period length of the free-running locomotor activity rhythm, and high doses induce continuous activity. Additionally, daily injection of melatonin appears to synchronize the activity of pinealectomized starlings (*Sturnus vulgaris*).

A circadian rhythm of NAT activity persists for at least a few cycles in chick pineal glands that are cultured *in vitro* in darkness. This rhythm entrains to light cycles and damps out in bright, continuous light. As mentioned earlier, the chicken pineal gland is directly photosensitive. In other words, the behavior of the isolated pineal gland is similar to that of the pineal gland *in situ*. It is rather astonishing, then, that pinealectomy of chickens does not abolish their free-running circadian rhythmicity, as it does in sparrows. In fact, only in two other species of sparrows—the white-crowned *Zonotrichia leucophrys gambelii* and the white-throated *Z. albicollis*—has a clear-cut abolishment of rhythmicity following pinealectomy been demonstrated.

When house finches (*Caprodacus mexicanus*) are pinealectomized, most—but not all—exhibit abolishment of rhythms. For starlings, rhythmicity is affected in only a minor way by pinealectomy, and in the Japanese quail (*Coturnix coturnix coturnix*) it is not affected at all. Thus the involvement of the pineal gland with rhythmic functions among species of birds appears to be variable and, indeed, may be peculiar to only passerine species.

Pinealectomy of a lizard (*Anolis carolinensis*) has been shown by Underwood to modify the pattern of locomotor activity or, in some cases, to abolish it. Additionally, implants of melatonin cause aberrations of the lizard's activity rhythm. In the killifish (*Fundulus heteroclitus*), Kavaliers found that pinealectomy eliminated the circadian rhythm of color change but did not affect its ability to show background adaptation. Pinealectomy of rats was shown by Quay to have only a very small affect on the rate of resetting of locomotor rhythms by phase-shifted light cycles.

As is evident, the concept of the pineal gland as an essential component in circadian organization in vertebrates in general simply cannot be supported. The ultimate proof of this contention is found in the report of Harlow and co-workers that the armadillo (*Dasypus novemcinctus*), a mammal completely lacking a pineal organ, is typically rhythmic in all normal respects. It shows circadian rhythm of locomotor activity, body temperature, and oxygen consumption under prolonged, constant conditions. It also shifts the phase of these rhythms in response to altered photoperiods. Interestingly, in this animal melatonin implants cause a lengthening of the free-running period of activity and body temperature. Thus it is sensitive to melatonin. Also, the alligator (*Alligator mississippiensis*), as shown by Kavaliers, has rhythmic, circadian locomotor activity, and it also does not have a pineal organ. (As explained later, the armadillo and alligator both have circulating melatonin of extrapineal origin.)

Thermoregulation

Although a thermoregulatory role for pineal organs has not been as well publicized as their involvement in reproduction or rhythmicity, a strong case can be made for pineal involvement in body-temperature regulation. In fact, such a role is more readily demonstrated in more classes of vertebrates than any of the other ascribed pineal functions.

A few studies have reported minor cytological changes in pineal glands of animals exposed to cold (rats, hamsters) or to hot (lizard) temperatures. Also, changes in NAT activity have been demonstrated in rats exposed to chronically high or low temperatures; generally, the activity was lowered by both extremes. Changes in HIOMT activity in response to temperature also have been noted in lizards and frogs, but the correlations are variable and difficult to interpret.

Removal of the parietal eye of lizards elevates their behaviorally selected body temperature. Parietalectomy also lowers the critical thermal maximum of *Anolis carolinensis*. Pinealectomy, in contrast, lowers body temperature in *Sceloperus occidentalis* and *Crotaphytus collaris*. Also, pinealectomized *C. collaris* exhibit elevation of heart rate at higher head temperatures, suggesting that the pineal organ somehow is involved in a physiological mechanism of temperature regulation in lizards. However, because parietalectomy and pinealectomy have been done on different species of lizards under different experimental conditions (e.g., incandescent illumination versus sunlight), a proper understanding of how the components of the pineal complex may relate to thermoregulation is lacking. To date, a thorough study of the specific effects of extirpating the extracranial parietal organ *and* of removing the intracranial pineal gland has not been conducted on a particular species of lizard.

Incidentally, the parietal eye is not present in all lizards. Its distribution has been phylogenetically determined by Gundy, who observed that those families of lizards having centers of abundance at higher latitudes tended to bear parietal eyes, whereas those at lower latitudes tended not to have parietal eyes. Thus the implication was drawn that temperature tolerence and thermoregulative capacity, which are more critical at higher latitudes, are somehow related to possession of the pineal accessory component.

Administration of melatonin to *Amphibolurus muricatus* by Firth and Heatwole lowered the panting threshold. Injection of chlorpromazine, an agent known to elevate blood melatonin, had a similar effect in lowering the panting threshold.

Ralph, Firth, and Turner, in a review of the role of pineal bodies in ectotherm thermoregulation, developed a hypothetical scheme for the central interactions of the components that relate to the pineal complex (Fig. 14.12). They propose that the parietal eye may exert an influence on behavioral thermoregulation through an action on the limbic system, possibly via the habenular nuclei. The area pretectalis may be a locus for parietal eye–pineal–lateral eye interaction, since it receives numerous projections from both the lateral eyes and the pineal organ and is concerned with coordinating visual and motor information between the optic tectum, the cerebral cortex, and the thalamus. The pineal tract may also project directly onto thermoregulatory centers such as the preoptic nucleus, and the parietal eye may connect with this nucleus via the habenula. The possibilty that these two components of the pineal complex (which are known to interact with each other) send separate tracts to the preoptic nucleus may account for the divergent thermoregulatory effects observed following their removal. The suprachiasmatic nucleus may also participate in this scheme, in view of its known thermoregulatory action and its connection in mammals with the pineal gland. Finally, hypothalamic mechanisms for sensing and regulating body fluid osmolality and, in turn, body temperature may be influenced by the pineal complex. Whether the proposed pathways between pineal

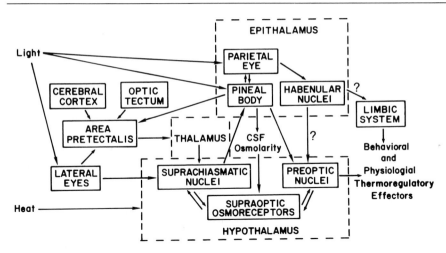

FIGURE 14.12. Hypothetical scheme depicting the neuroanatomic components influencing thermoregulation with which the pineal complex interacts. See text for explanation. [From C. L. Ralph et al., *Am. Zool.*, **19**:287, 1979.]

components and other parts of the brain are linked neurally or humorally is largely unknown. The parietal eye and pineal body are known to have two-way neural connections. The pineal body may communicate with the brain mainly or exclusively through secretion (melatonin?).

Binkley demonstrated that pinealectomy of house sparrows abolished their circadian rhythm of body temperature when they were in continuous darkness. A body-temperature rhythm was maintained in pinealectomized sparrows under alternating light–dark cycles, although the nocturnal minimum was invariably higher than that of intact control birds. Pinealectomized pigeons, according to John and colleagues, have abnormally high temperatures. Pinealectomized chickens, as shown by Cogburn, exhibit thermal dysfunctions at night, but not during the day. Binkley injected house sparrows with melatonin and depressed their body temperature by 4.7°C. John counteracted pinealectomy-induced hyperthermia of pigeons by implantation of melatonin in beeswax pellets.

Melatonin appears to have variable effects on the body temperature among mammalian species. It induces hyperthermia in rats, hypothermia in mice, and has no effect in rabbits (according to a few, scattered reports). The effects of pinealectomy on body temperature also appear to be varied among species of mammals. It has been reported that pinealectomy elevates the temperature of sheep and rabbits, and either lowers the temperature of rats or has no effect.

Brown adipose tissue (BAT), which is associated with the thermogenic responses of many mammals, may be regulated by the pineal gland. Heldmaier and Hoffman demonstrated a weight increase of the BAT in Djungarian hamsters that were implanted with melatonin in beeswax. Lynch and Epstein reported a similar increase in BAT following melatonin treatment in the white-footed mouse (*P. leucopus*). Additionally, Reiter and colleagues found a reduction in the weight of the interscapular BAT of golden hamsters after pinealectomy.

It should be noted that pineal involvement in the hibernation of mammals is suggested by a few studies. Thus perhaps additional clues as to how the pineal gland influences thermoregulation might be derived from studies of seasonal cycles of body-temperature changes in hibernators. Also, it should be of great interest to carefully examine thermoregulation in animals lacking a pineal gland, particularly to see how they cope with extremes of environmental temperature changes.

The persistent difficulty that investigators have encountered in defining a specific role for the pineal gland probably stems from its very basic involvement with the regulatory centers of the brain. Because pineal organs are part of the diencephalon, it seems likely that they have maintained an intimate association with this ancient part of the brain which is involved with an amazingly varied and fundamental set of functions, including thermoregulation, reproduction, and sexual behavior, as well as daily rhythmicity and color change.

MELATONIN PRODUCTION BY EXTRAPINEAL TISSUE

When HIOMT was discovered by Axelrod and Weissbach in 1960, as noted above, they believed that the enzyme was unique to the pineal gland because they failed to find it in several other tissues of a variety of species of mammals. However, five years later, HIOMT was found by Axelrod, Baker, and Quay in the brain and eyes of anuran amphibian larvae. Quay, additionally, demonstrated HIOMT activity in the retinas of several species of fishes, amphibians, reptiles, and birds. Subsequent research by a number of workers, especially Cardinali, Wurtman, Pang, Bubenik, Pévet, and Binkley, has demonstrated HIOMT, NAT, and melatonin in numerous sites, including the brain, Harderian gland, and gut.

The melatonin that is found in certain tissues could be, theoretically, of pineal gland origin and acquired through the blood. However, it has been shown that the HIOMT of the rat retina is active as early as the 17th day of gestation, whereas HIOMT is detected in the pineal gland no earlier than the 12th postnatal day. Melatonin per se has been detected in the retina of rats as young as 2 days of age. Thus the eye clearly seems to be synthesizing melatonin several days before the pineal gland does. Furthermore, melatonin has been detected in the retinas of pinealectomized chickens and trout and in the hypothalamus of pinealectomized rats.

Some of the melatonin that is synthesized in extrapineal sites appears to find its way into the blood, for the plasmà of rats, sheep, trout, and green sea turtles that have been pinealectomized still carries melatonin, as demonstrated by radioimmunoassay. The amount present is reduced in some cases by pinealectomy. A common consequence of pinealectomy seems to be that the normal nighttime rise in melatonin content of the blood no longer is seen. This is a reported effect in rats and sheep. Thus in mammals the pineal gland may uniquely contribute the nighttime surge of plasma melatonin. In trout, however, Gern found the nightly elevation of plasma melatonin to persist following pinealectomy.

To find melatonin in the blood of animals lacking pineal organs is to offer the best proof that the melatonin produced in extrapineal sites can find its way into the circulation. This was accomplished when Roth and colleagues showed that the blood of alligators contained melatonin. However, no day–night rhythm was evident. The second demonstration—and a more dramatic one still—was that of Harlow and co-workers, who showed that melatonin was present in the blood of the armadillo, a mammal totally lacking a pineal gland. The levels found were within the normal range for other mammals. Surprisingly, the amount varied in a diurnal cycle, with higher nighttime levels, as in other animals.

Binkley found the NAT activity of the retinae of chickens to have a daily rhythm, with peak activity during the night. Also, like pineal NAT, the retinal NAT rhythm persists for at least a few days in continuous darkness. Exposure to light during nighttime dramatically drives down NAT activity. The total amount of NAT in both eyes together is about equal to that in the pineal gland. Binkley also reported that while blocking the pineal region to exclude light had no effect on retinal NAT, blocking light from the eyes prevented the expected suppression of pineal NAT activity.

Pévet found that HIOMT in the eyes of the mole (*Talpa europae*) is 2 to 10 times more active than pineal HIOMT. Thus in this species the pineal gland may not be the primary gland for melatonin secretion. In larval *Xenopus laevis*, Baker and Hoff found that 75 to 90% of the total melatonin was present in the eyes, with only minor amounts in the brain and pineal region. The trout retina has also been shown, by Gern, to be a very active site for melatonin synthesis.

Melatonin synthesized in the eyes and in the gut may serve as a hormone in the tissue of origin. The distribution of melatonin appears to correspond to the localization of serotonin-producing argentaffin cells. Indeed, the widely dispersed production of melatonin may be explained by Pearse's concept of a diffuse neuroendocrine system. As noted above, the pineal gland may be an APUD organ. Perhaps cells in the retina, gut, brain, and Harderian gland also are APUD types in the dispersed endocrine system.

Obviously, melatonin is a molecule that must command some attention from endocrinologists. However, frustratingly little is known with certainty about the function of melatonin, either of pineal or extrapineal origin.

ADDITIONAL READING

1. Ariëns Kappers, J., and P. Pévet, eds. (1979). *The Pineal Gland of Vertebrates Including Man*. Elsevier/North-Holland, Amsterdam.

2. Birau, N., and W. Schloot, eds. (1981). *Melatonin: Current Status and Perspectives*. Pergamon, Oxford.

3. Nir, I., R. J. Reiter, and R. J. Wurtman, eds. (1978). *The Pineal Gland. J. Neur. Trans.*, Suppl. 13, Springer-Verlag, Wien.

4. Ralph, C. L., B. T. Firth, W. A. Gern, and D. W. Owens (1979). The pineal complex and thermoregulation. *Biol. Rev.* **54**:41–72.

5. Reiter, R. J. (1977). *The Pineal*. Eden, Montreal (A continuing series of annual reviews; the first was assembled by R. Relkin in 1976.)

6. Reiter, R. J. (1978). *The Pineal and Reproduction, Progress in Reproductive Biology*, Vol. 4. S. Karger, Basel.

7. Various authors (1976). *Endocrine Role of the Pineal Gland. Am. Zool.* **16**(1):1–101. (A symposium.)

8. Wolstenholme, G. E. W., and J. Knight (1971). *The Pineal Gland*. Ciba Foundation Symposium, Churchill Livingstone, Edinburgh.

15

Multihormonal Regulation of Physiological Adjustments

ENDOCRINE REGULATION OF INTERMEDIARY METABOLISM

In the introductory chapter in this book, the living organism was compared to a machine—a contrived device in which a series of parts are made to operate together by linkages and gears in order to achieve a particular function. This analogy is nowhere clearer than in the phenomenon of intermediary metabolism and its regulation. In the largest sense, intermediary metabolism is all of the chemical reactions that occur within the organism between the intake of chemical foods and respiratory oxygen and the ultimate elimination of chemical wastes, water, and carbon dioxide. These chemical reactions are linked sequentially, the products of one reaction becoming the interacting components of another, and the directions of the reactions are guided by the presence of enzymes or other catalysts that favor one alternative chemical reaction over another. The roles of hormones in intermediary metabolism are to regulate the intensity, or the timing, or the direction of intermediary metabolic steps in several ways, most often by affecting the synthesis of appropriate enzymes.

It is helpful, before becoming engrossed in the complex details of intermediary metabolism, to consider it, as well as its hormonal regulation, from a teleological point of view. After all, it is only to the extent that metabolism achieves certain purposes or functions that its adaptiveness or usefulness to an organism or to a species can be judged.

Generally, metabolism is oriented toward two important goals: provision of chemical energy and synthesis of complex chemical units in the organisms. Synthetic metabolism—anabolism—produces the important structural proteins and enzymes that are characteristic of a particular species; in addition, it produces complex molecular forms of carbohydrate and fat in which chemical energy is stored for later needs. Catabolism, or destructive metabolism, provides the chemical energy that makes anabolism possible; it also produces regulated heat in warm-blooded animals.

Hormones can influence metabolism in several ways. The most obvious mechanism, direct intervention and control over synthesis of enzymes, has already been mentioned, and it is the most common. However, there are other possible mechanisms, such as regulation of transport of metabolite chemicals through the plasma membrane and alteration of the intracellular concentrations of ions and enzyme cofactors, which affect the intensity or direction of certain metabolic steps. However, the latter mechanisms, which activate or inhibit certain enzyme-mediated metabolic steps, are themselves the result of direct enzymatic changes mediated by the hormone. For example, it is clear that insulin can influence protein synthesis in a cell by stimulating the rate of transport of amino acids into the cell, making them available for coupling in the endoplasmic reticulum. However, the active transport of the amino acids into cells is itself mediated by protein carriers, and the activity of the protein carriers and enzymes involved in active transport is directly affected by insulin.

Figure 15.1 presents in broad outline the general patterns of metabolic flow of the three major types of organic constituents in food. It shows how these substrates are moved into the cell and their fate within the vertebrate animal cell: anabolic (conversion to protein, neutral fat, and glycogen) or catabolic. In their simpler forms all three food types are interconvertible. That is, although only glucose formation from amino acids or glycerol is shown, fat may be derived from the other two food classes as well. Not all of these processes occur in all cells. That is, the enzymes that govern the directions of alternative metabolic pathways are localized in different cell types, to give these cells a differentiated and characteristic pattern of intermediary metabolism. Furthermore, in vertebrate species, intermediary metabolism even in the same cell types is adapted to radical variations of diet, life style, environmental requirements, body size, and other factors. Within species other metabolic adaptive features correspond to stages of development and to life cycles. For example, migrating birds flying long distances face different problems and metabolic demands than birds protecting a nest and feeding their young. When mammals hibernate, they require different properties of heat generation and general energy yield than they do during activity and feeding. An aquatic, vegetarian tadpole faces metabolic problems different from those of a terrestrial, carnivorous frog.

Many of these adaptive metabolic differences are built into the genome-controlled differentiation of tissues and their constituent array of intracellular enzymes. However, many metabolic specializations are also regulated by endocrine influences. Since the number of regulated enzyme systems and the number of hormones regulating them are large, the comparative

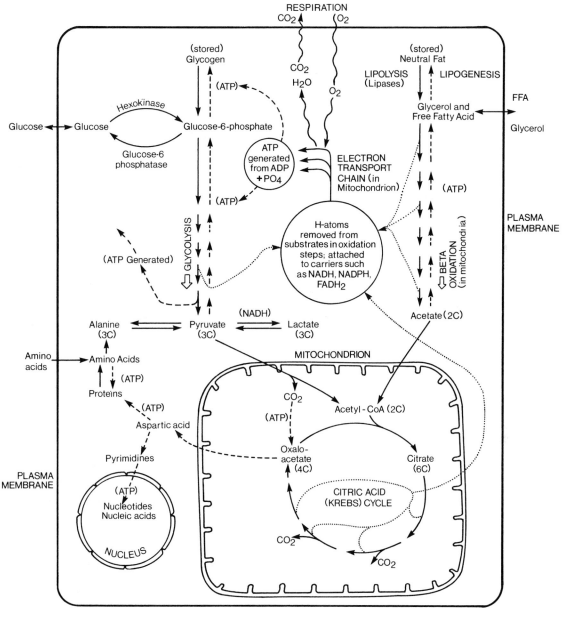

RESPIRATION
CO_2 ↑   (O_2)

(stored)
Glycogen

CO_2
H_2O
O_2

(stored)
Neutral Fat

LIPOLYSIS   LIPOGENESIS
(Lipases)

FFA

Glucose ⇄ Glucose   Glucose-6-phosphate

Hexokinase

Glucose-6
phosphatase

(ATP)

ATP
generated
from ADP
+PO_4

ELECTRON
TRANSPORT
CHAIN (in
Mitochondrion)

Glycerol and
Free Fatty Acid

Glycerol

PLASMA
MEMBRANE

(ATP)

(ATP)

GLYCOLYSIS

(ATP Generated)

H-atoms
removed from
substrates in oxidation
steps; attached
to carriers such
as NADH, NADPH,
$FADH_2$

(ATP)

BETA
OXIDATION
(in mitochondria)

Alanine
(3C)

(NADH)

Pyruvate
(3C)

Lactate
(3C)

Acetate (2C)

Amino
acids

Amino Acids

(ATP)

Proteins

(ATP)

Aspartic acid

Pyrimidines

(ATP)

Nucleotides
Nucleic acids

NUCLEUS

MITOCHONDRION

CO_2

(ATP)

Oxalo-
acetate
(4C)

Acetyl-CoA (2C)

Citrate
(6C)

CITRIC ACID
(KREBS) CYCLE

CO_2

CO_2

PLASMA
MEMBRANE

Solid lines ———— Catabolic and reversible reactions
Dashed lines - - - Anabolic reactions
Dotted lines ········ Movement of H-atoms on carriers to electron transport chain
(ATP)   ATP in parentheses = ATP utilized in a reaction
(3C)   C in parentheses indicates size of molecule in terms of number of carbon atoms

FIGURE 15.1. Diagrammatic outline of the pathways of intermediary metabolism. See text for discussion.

endocrinology of metabolic control becomes too complex a subject to consider in detail. Accordingly, we will consider here only some of the better-known information concerning endocrine-influenced metabolic phenomena in mammals, including humans.

The principal metabolic hormones are insulin, glucagon, adrenaline (epinephrine), corticosteroids (particularly the glucocorticoids), growth hormone (STH), thyroxine (or triiodothyronine), and the sex steroids. Strictly speaking, virtually all hormones affect intermediary metabolism in some way. For example, thyrotropic hormone (TSH) specifically stimulates protein synthesis (enzymes concerned with thyroid hormone synthesis and synthesis of thyroid structural proteins) in the thyroid gland, and ACTH does the same in the adrenal cortex. However, in this chapter we consider only the more general endocrine regulation of the metabolic pathways outlined in Figs. 15.1 and 15.2. Since intermediary metabolism is a continuum of interconnected biochemical reactions, the influences of a hormone at any step must necessarily support or oppose those of other hormones that act at other points in the continuum.

In the next section teleological thinking is employed frequently. That is, the pattern or "purpose" of the actions of individual hormones in metabolism, when they can be recognized, is indicated. However, such rationalization is often difficult. Since we must assume that the actions of hormones on any process are adaptive and serve a real purpose, in those instances in which the teleology is not clear or appears to be contradictory, we should conclude that our information is faulty or incomplete.

Actions of Insulin

The most obvious overall action of insulin is the reduction of glucose and amino acid levels in the blood. Further analysis shows that insulin increases all storage forms of the basic biological constituents—carbohydrates, fats, and amino acids—stimulating their deposition in the form of glycogen, neutral fat (triglycerides), and protein. Obviously, insulin is a "growth hormone," favoring anabolism generally. In this metabolic role it interacts with and is supported by the insulinlike factors whose secretion is stimulated by growth hormone.

The actions of insulin begin by stimulation in muscle and several other organs (but not in liver) of the inward cellular transport of glucose and amino acids. Insulin stimulates intracellular accumulation of nonmetabolizable sugars and amino acids (e.g., xylose, α-aminobutyric acid), so that the cellular entry of these substances is due to specific coupled transport; thus the cellular entry of glucose is not due merely to a more efficient metabolic disposal after it has penetrated the cell membrane.

Immediately after cellular entry, glucose is phosphorylated through the mediation of hexokinase (or glucokinase). Insulin has been shown to stim-

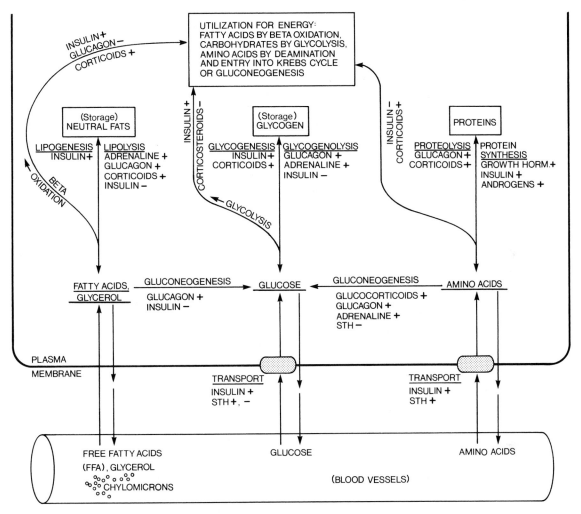

FIGURE 15.2. Schematic diagram of the intracellular actions of the major metabolic hormones on intermediary metabolism. Movement of the transport forms of the three principal organic metabolites between the blood and the cell are shown in the lower part of the figure. Intracellular interconversion of these simpler metabolites (e.g., gluconeogenesis) is represented in the middle. Storage forms and metabolic utilization of these substances are depicted in the upper part of the diagram. The actions of particular hormones on these various processes and their directions is indicated next to the arrows that represent them. +, stimulation; −, inhibition. These metabolic processes and their endocrine regulation are discussed further in the text.

ulate the synthesis of this enzyme, as well as the synthesis and activity of glycogen synthetase, the enzyme that promotes glycogenesis.

Other actions of insulin are consistent with its anabolic role (Fig. 15.2). It increases the activity and/or synthesis of all enzyme systems for lipogenesis, glycogenesis, and protein synthesis.

Another interesting direction of metabolism promoted by insulin is the breakdown (to yield energy) of fatty acids and glucose entering the cell by enzymes of the β-oxidation and glycolytic pathways. However, insulin has no such action on amino acids and, in fact, inhibits enzymes involved in amino acid deamination and catabolism. Furthermore, insulin inhibits the utilization of amino acids in gluconeogenesis.

Thus the metabolic actions of insulin are directed toward two clear ends: (1) the reduction of plasma glucose levels and (2) the promotion of protein synthesis. The energy for protein synthesis is provided in part by insulin's actions on glycolysis and β-oxidation of fatty acids.

The cellular receptors for insulin are located in the plasma membrane. However, the typical actions of insulin are not mediated by cAMP formation. In fact, insulin action generally is accompanied by a reduction in cAMP. It has been proposed that insulin attachment to its receptor generates the production of a yet unknown second messenger, which, through stimulation of protein kinases, leads to the transcriptive and translational events that result in the characteristic enzyme actions.

That it is not necessary for insulin to enter its target cell was proven by testing the effects of the hormone attached to macromolecular particles, which permitted insulin interaction with membrane receptors, but prevented the hormone from entering the cell. On the other hand, recent immunocytochemical data have shown that insulin can be found within the cytoplasm of target cells. A recent model has been proposed by Jameson and others to explain how insulin and other protein hormones can enter cells. They suggest that insulin–receptor complexes in the plasma membrane tend to flow together, forming aggregations on the cell surface. These aggregations so alter the membrane's properties that it sinks inward and, by a type of pinocytosis, forms intracellular, "coated" microvesicles.

Clinical diabetes mellitus is really a complex of conditions with different causative features, but all presenting a common property: hyperglycemia, and usually glycosuria. One type of diabetes involves a primary failure of insulin production, and its treatment requires lifelong injection of exogenous insulin. The most common form of diabetes mellitus, the so-called mature-onset diabetes, occurs principally in older persons. In such individuals there is a tissue insensitivity to insulin, and plasma insulin levels may, in fact, be elevated, together with supernormal levels of plasma glucose. It has been found that the insulin insensitivity in these individuals is due to reduced target cell receptor function. Very often in such patients dietary caloric restriction alone will reduce plasma glucose levels to normal values. It is interesting that when the blood glucose levels are restored to the normal range, the cell receptor activity also increases, while immunoreactive insulin in the blood falls. Mature-onset diabetes is frequently associated with obesity. In experimental animals obesity alone leads to loss of insulin receptor activity. Thus it would seem that both hyperglycemia and obesity contribute to the insulin insensitivity of mature-onset diabetes.

Actions of Adrenaline, Noradrenaline, and Glucagon

Catecholamines, secreted by the adrenal medulla and by adrenergic nerve fibers, and glucagon oppose the anabolic actions of insulin. That is, these hormones activate enzyme systems for lipolysis and glycogenolysis. It should be remembered that mammalian glucagon is limited in its actions largely to the liver because (1) a large fraction of glucagon is destroyed during its first passage through the liver, and (2) while there are glucagon receptors in liver cells, there are few or no glucagon receptors in muscle or other possible cellular targets. Thus glucagon is the only hormone in this group that appears to stimulate proteolysis, and this action is limited to the liver. The binding of both catecholamines and glucagon is followed by an increase in the level of cAMP, which acts as a second messenger in target cells. Furthermore, cAMP in *in vitro* experiments has the lipolytic and glycogenolytic actions of the hormones themselves.

These hormones also promote gluconeogenesis from amino acids and glycerol. Glucagon also favors the production of glucose in the liver by inhibiting the β-oxidation pathway, encouraging the release of fatty acids, and promoting gluconeogenesis from glycerol. Finally, glucagon (and possibly the catecholamines) stimulates the entry of newly formed glucose into the blood by activating the glucose-6-phosphatase enzyme system (in the liver only).

The latter is a "logical" action for glucagon, since its own secretion is triggered by low blood glucose levels. The liver, after all, is a storage organ for carbohydrate energy, and it is appropriate for glucagon to oversee glucose release and distribution from the liver via the blood when it is needed peripherally, especially in the brain. Adrenaline (epinephrine) and noradrenaline (norepinephrine) are more important as mobilizers of stored energy (lipid from adipose cells and glucose from extrahepatic glycogen stores, where there is no action by glucagon). It is "logical" that the catecholamines do not promote the loss of muscle glucose (as glucagon does in the liver by activation of glucose-6-phosphatase) after its release from the relatively small store of muscle glycogen. Unlike the liver, muscle tissue is a "user" of glucose as an energy source, not a distributor.

It may be noted in Fig. 15.2 that glucagon inhibits the oxidative utilization by the liver of fatty acid fragments after lipolysis. This, too, makes sense if the role of the liver in energy metabolism is largely the storage of foods (after their absorption from the gut) for later use by more peripheral tissues. It will be remembered that in the intact animal catecholamines inhibit insulin secretion by stimulating alpha-adrenergic receptors. This tends to accentuate the metabolic actions of catecholamines, since insulin is the chief counteracting endocrine agent for the catecholamines.

Actions of Glucocorticoids

Figure 15.2 indicates that glucocorticoids in the intermediary metabolism of humans and laboratory mammals follow their own characteristic "scenario." Their influence on the cellular enzyme systems results in the breakdown of stored fat and of protein, while carbohydrate stores are protected. That is, lipolysis and stimulation of β-oxidation result in the use of fatty acid fragments for energy. Proteins also undergo breakdown in the presence of higher levels of corticosteroids, and the amino acids, derived from intracellular proteolysis as well as from dietary sources form glucose in relatively large proportions (by gluconeogenesis). Glucocorticoids favor the utilization of amino acids as an energy source. The use of glucose as an energy source is inhibited by glucocorticoids in most tissues, but not in the brain.

Glucocorticoids, like glucagon, stimulate glucose-6-phosphatase activity, resulting in the release of significant amounts of glucose into the blood. Glucose release after administration of large doses of glucocorticoids can be so extensive that the resulting hyperglycemia is referred to as *steroid diabetes*.

It is difficult to rationalize the pattern of glucocorticoid action on intermediary metabolism unless we place it in the context of adaptation to stress. As we have learned in Chapter 2, one of the primary stimuli of ACTH secretion is physiological or traumatic stress. Typical stresses can be starvation, disease, or other harmful states during which feeding and the nutritional status of the organism are seriously compromised. Under such circumstances ACTH-stimulated glucocorticoid secretion first draws upon stored fat, the most efficient source of physiological energy. As this source becomes depleted, and in the absence of additional food, hydrolysis of endogenous proteins under continued influence of glucocorticoids, supplies the next energy source (through gluconeogenesis). The action on glucose-6-phosphatase ensures the distribution of glucose to such organs as the brain, which depends largely on carbohydrate for energy and has little or no stored energy of its own. Glucocorticoids protect the organism against glycogen breakdown until protein wastage is so far advanced that hypoglycemia ensues. At this point glucagon and the catecholamines stimulate glycogenolysis, assuring some metabolic support for the brain and central nervous system until the end of the period of depletion and stress.

The danger of prolonged hypoglycemia to the brain is real. In clinical observations it has been found that starvation hypoglycemia or "insulin-shock" therapy of schizophrenic patients produce degenerative changes, and even necrosis, in certain parts of the brain.

Actions of Growth Hormone

While pituitary growth hormone undoubtedly has a role in metabolic regulation, this role defies a rational overall definition. In part this may be due to the fact that some, if not most, of the actions of growth hormone (STH) are mediated by the insulinlike factors (including somatomedin) that appear in the blood when STH is secreted. Another source of confusion is that STH treatment stimulates insulin secretion and may affect insulin target cell receptor activity. Furthermore, although we might expect an insulinlike metabolic response to STH, sometimes the actual response is just the opposite.

The primary "objective" of STH action is the stimulation of somatic growth. Its general stimulation of amino acid transport into cells, of the incorporation of these amino acids into proteins, and its inhibition of gluconeogenesis (which uses up amino acids)—all are consistent with its role in growth. However, the role (or roles) of STH in the metabolism of carbohydrates and fat remains relatively enigmatic and cannot be rationalized at this time.

STH at first stimulates lipogenesis in adipose cells of laboratory mammals and of humans, but this is followed (after several hours) by lipolysis. Similarly, STH at first accelerates intracellular utilization of glucose in energy-yielding pathways, but this is followed by a period of decreased glucose utilization. Transport of glucose into cells, again, is at first stimulated (insulinlike action), followed by a period of decreased glucose transport. In the animal as a whole the first action of STH is an insulinlike, hypoglycemic response, followed by a longer-lasting hyperglycemia.

Other interactions, relationships, and comparisons with insulin secretion yield additional puzzles. For example, insulin secretion is stimulated by high blood glucose levels (hyperglycemia), or by abnormally high plasma amino acid levels (or by STH). STH secretion, on the other hand, is keyed to hypoglycemia. The hypoglycemic release of STH operates through the hypothalamus, as has been confirmed by experiments involving hypothalamic lesions. Furthermore, there is a circadian (early morning maximum) rhythm of STH secretion, which would indicate a hypothalamic influence as well.

People with STH deficiency have a *hypersensitivity* to insulin. This hypersensitivity can be reduced by giving a small dose of STH. Higher STH doses (or clinical acromegaly) can lead to a relative insulin resistance. Thus there is an inverse relationship between insulin responsiveness and STH levels. One possibility is that STH-evoked somatomedins, because of their molecular similarity to insulin, may occupy cell membrane insulin receptors, thus competing with insulin for these sites. However, somatomedins may be less effective, or even ineffective compared to insulin, in evoking postbinding, second-messenger formation. This is, perhaps, the most rational explanation that can be offered for the apparent inconsistencies mentioned above. This possibility is real, since antibodies prepared against insulin or against somatomedins will interact with both types of hormones. If the antibodies are "confused" by their molecular similarities, it is possible that the target cell insulin receptors similarly may be unable to distinguish between the two kinds of proteins.

Actions of the Thyroid Hormones: T_3 and T_4

The metabolic actions of the thyroid hormones were considered at some length in Chapter 6. They are considered here again, briefly, in connection with their influence on intermediary metabolism. Although thyroid hormones (principally T_3) have important actions upon metabolism, there is no clear understanding of how these actions are exerted. In the organism as a whole, thyroid hormones affect growth; oxygen consumption; plasma levels of glucose, lipids, minerals, and water; and the transport of some of these substances across target cell membranes. Thyroid hormones broadly influence nervous function, presumably through membrane polarization and effects on neuronal intermediary metabolism. All of these actions are in addition to the numerous morphological actions of thyroid hormones.

Most attention has focused on the stimulation of respiratory oxygen consumption and calorigenesis by thyroid hormones. Since relatively low doses of T_3 and T_4 lead to increases in cytochrome oxidase activity (upper middle portion of Fig. 15.1) in the mitochondrial electron transport chain (where respiratory oxygen is consumed), mitochondrial biochemical phenomena have seemed a likely place for further experimental analysis and study. However, in most experiments with isolated mitochondria and in analyses of mitochondrial generation of ATP, the concentrations of T_3 that must be used to produce an effect are far in excess of physiological levels. One of the clearest enzymatic effects of thyroid hormone treatment is a 20-fold increase in α-glycerophosphate dehydrogenase activity in tissues that respond to thyroid hormone treatment by increasing oxygen consumption. This enzyme is involved in an exchange between α-glycerophosphate and dihydroxyacetone (in the glycolysis pathway) in which a shuttling of substrates into and out of the mitochondrion occurs. The net effect of these movements is the transport of hydrogen atoms into the mitochondrion for utilization in the electron transport chain.

Currently there is a tendency to attribute to T_3, at *physiological* levels, a role in regulating oxygen consumption indirectly by stimulating the active outward transport of sodium ions (the sodium pump). Such transport is continuous, since the cell membrane must maintain a lower inner concentration of sodium ions against a concentration gradient. When this transport is depressed or abolished by reduction of Na^+ in the fluids bathing the cell or by use of the drug ouabain, which "poisons' the sodium pump, T_3 is relatively less effective (by about 50%) in raising the oxygen consumption of responsive tissues. Furthermore, T_3 treatment increases the *in vitro* outward movement of Na^+. Thyroid hormones can influence the activity and, presumably, the synthesis of the enzyme (Na, K-ATPase) principally involved in releasing ATP energy, which fuels the sodium pump. Also, it has been shown that physiological doses of T_3 increase the number of "pump units," that is, the protein constituents of the cell membrane that participate in sodium transport. Heat would be generated in this system from the continuous dissociation of ATP to ADP, especially when no net change in sodium ion concentration is achieved. This reveals a rational difficulty in the otherwise attractive concept of sodium pump control of oxygen consumption and thermogenesis. If resting oxygen consumption (nonmuscular) is adjustable according to need through changes in the amount of sodium pumped, then how can the cell protect itself against T_3-influenced excessive or insufficient sodium pumping? To accommodate this problem it has been proposed that when excessive sodium pumping occurs, the plasma membrane becomes more "leaky" and permits more Na^+ to reenter by increased diffusion. The control over the amount of sodium pumped, according to those who champion this concept, would occur through T_3-stimulated synthesis of protein pump units, including the synthesis of Na,K-ATPase. Left unexplained by the sodium pump hypothesis is how Na^+ leakiness of the plasma membrane might be regulated, and to what extent ATP generation would also be regulated by T_3 to support the energy requirements of the pump.

Table 6.8 contains a list of cellular enzymes whose activity and/or synthesis may be influenced by thyroid hormone levels. It will be recognized that in this list are components of the mitochondrial ATP-generating systems, mitochondrial citric acid cycle enzymes, and enzymes involved in the glycolytic and β-oxidative pathways. Furthermore, T_3 stimulates the synthesis and activity of hexokinase, an enzyme that favors entry of glucose from the blood and its metabolic utilization. Considering this large list, it becomes clear that thyroid hormones would have to interact with all of the other hormones that influence intermediary metabolism, supplementing some and countering others.

Within this multiplicity of possible metabolic actions of T_3, as interpreted from studies of its effects on the activity of individual enzyme systems, some are predominantly anabolic and some catabolic. The net effects must be judged against the observed overall actions of thyroid hormone in intact organisms. First, it should be mentioned that the general hormonal effects are dose-dependent, and can be biphasic. That is, at lower dose levels T_3 can favor growth, lipogenesis, and protein synthesis. However, at higher doses T_3 can be predominantly catabolic, leading in homoiothermic animals (birds, mammals) to increased heat production, increased ATP generation, and depletion of cellular stored forms of energy (fat, protein, glycogen). There is at this time no acceptable explanation of this reversal of metabolic roles at different dosage levels of thyroid hormone. The consistent features at all doses are stimulation of ATP production and thermogenesis. It is possible that at lower levels of ATP production anabolism is favored, because sufficient ATP for anabolic steps is thus provided without wastage of metabolites. These metabolites, using the ATP energy so provided, can then be incorporated into proteins or neutral fat stores. At higher levels of ATP production and utilization, as during excessive stimulation by T_3 of Na^+-pumping against a leaky membrane, metabolites are channeled away from anabolic pathways and utilized more or less exclusively to support these higher levels of ATP production.

In addition to growth and the intermediary metabolic actions of thyroid hormones, other physiological actions of T_3 and T_4 are also biphasic. For example, the heart contraction rate in mammals increases with increasing doses of T_3 or T_4 up to a point. Beyond that, further increases in thyroid hormones *decrease* the heart rate.

CALCIUM REGULATION

It must be clear by now that only rarely is a physiological adjustment regulated by a single hormone. This fact has led some writers of endocrinology textbooks to organize their books around phenomena (e.g., growth, metamorphosis, thermoregulation, lactation, etc.) rather than around individual glands and hormones. Actually, the "phenomenological" presentation, though it more accurately reflects real physiological events, generally is not practical for the student who begins without a basic knowledge of the functional properties of the individual hormones.

In this book a compromise has been attempted for pedagogical purposes. If the reader will review the material that has been presented, he will see that it begins with an emphasis on the structural organization and enumeration of the glands involved in endocrine regulation and on the chemical nature of their hormones. However, phenomenological endocrine analysis was introduced in depth in Chapter 7 in which the actions of parathyroid hormone, calcitonin, and vitamin D were discussed with respect to calcium metabolism.

However, even an apparently simple phenomenon such as calcium regulation cannot be exhaustively dealt with in terms of these three primary hormones. Since their major regulatory actions involve bone metabolism, kidney transport phenomena, and calcium absorption from the gut, and since these actions involve metabolic regulations of phosphate as well as of calcium, a variety of other hormones exert influences as well. At the level of bone metabolism, for example, both growth hormone (and somatomedins) and thyroid hormones are involved, as has been pointed out. Thyroid hormones in certain species have a strong maturational influence on differentiation of bone tissues and affect calcium deposition in a complex way. Estrogens also have a strong influence on calcium metabolism and distribution. A primary action of estrogens is oriented toward hepatic synthesis of yolk proteins and calcium-carrying proteins. These proteins enrich the nutritive content of the egg and cover it (in birds) with a calcified shell. However, even in mammalian species, which lack a yolky or shelled egg, estrogens still have some action on hepatic protein synthesis, and in some species (rodents) they strongly stimulate endosteal bone formation. It is tempting to consider these effects of estrogens on calcium metabolism in mammals to be evolutionary remainders of an earlier physiological role. We should remember that, after all, there are mammals (monotremes) that lay a yolky, shelled egg.

In bony fishes there is an additional hypocalcemic hormone, hypocalcin, from the corpuscles of Stannius, the nature of whose action still must be adequately explored. There is a further comparative endocrinological puzzle in the fact that fishes manufacture calcitonin in their ultimobranchial glands but that calcitonin has little calcium action in fishes (though fish calcitonin is extremely potent in mammals).

As was pointed out in Chapter 7, a second order of control of calcium metabolism is exerted by hormones or nervous influences that affect the release or action of the primary controllers: parathyroid hormone and calcitonin. There is evidence that vitamin D has such an influence; the gut hormones gastrin and CCK may also act in this way.

Beyond the metabolic regulation of calcium levels in the blood, there are cellular phenomena involving calcium that are even more complex. These include calcium regulation of cell membrane permeability (nerve, muscle, and others) and intracellular distribution of calcium. The list of hormones that affect these intracellular events is so long that it is obvious that these hormones are related only in a general way, and it is not useful to discuss them together. Factors affecting the intracellular movement of calcium— some of them through the calcium-binding protein calmodulin—are also numerous. The nature of hormonal regulations of cellular events through calmodulin and associated protein kinases is just now being defined and should be better understood in the near future.

HORMONES IN OSMOREGULATION

The principal hormones that regulate concentrations of osmotically active substances in the blood have been discussed separately in preceding chapters. They are the neurohypophyseal hormones (Chapter 3) and the adrenal corticosteroids (Chapter 12). However, if we include under this heading other hormones with important effects on the concentration of osmotically active substances in blood plasma (salts, water, and protein), we must also list prolactin, thyroid hormone, noradrenaline, angiotensin, and probably urotensin as well. As in the case of calcium regulation, there are numerous mechanisms whereby movement of salts and water between body tissues and blood or between blood and the organism's exterior is accomplished. Some of these mechanisms are localized in the somatic cells themselves;

they affect the inward or outward transport of salts and/or water through the plasma membrane and the rates of metabolic production or utilization of osmotically active substances. Other, more obvious mechanisms affect the inward or outward movement of salts and/or water through membranes that mediate such exchanges between the blood and the organism's external medium. Such membranes are located in the skin, kidney tubules, gut, gills, urinary bladder, rectal glands (some fishes), and nasal salt glands (certain birds).

The multiplicity of tissue sites at which osmoregulatory phenomena can occur is indicative of the fact that evolutionary adaptation has produced an array of different patterns in vertebrates according to the special osmoregulatory problems each faces. For example, in maintaining constancy of salt and water in the vascular system, it is clear that a freshwater fish, living in a medium that is hypotonic to its blood, has a different problem from the seawater fish whose environment is hypertonic to its blood plasma. Furthermore, since their environment is always aquatic (regardless of its salt content), all fishes face a problem of water supply that is different from that of terrestrial animals, which must consume water or, in a few instances, can even generate it metabolically from dry food. In this sense, desert animals in a generally waterless environment have a more severe osmoregulatory problem than animals with free access to drinking water.

With so many kinds of osmoregulatory problems in different vertebrates, and with so many tissue sites at which salt and water regulation can be effected, it is not surprising that different hormones assume different degrees of importance in different vertebrate groups. However, it is possible to draw a few generalizations. Thus in fishes, adrenal corticosteroids (e.g., cortisol) are important regulators in the seawater environment largely because they stimulate salt secretion by certain cells (the so-called chloride cells) in the gills. In seawater, fishes acquire water through the gut by swallowing. Since salt is absorbed into blood along with the water, cortisol regulation at the level of the gill activates the primary mechanism for ridding the blood of excess salt. In fresh water, on the other hand, water is in excess, and salt must be retained for survival. The hormone most active in this respect is prolactin. Hypophysectomized teleosts can be kept alive in fresh water only by giving them prolactin, and for this reason the hormone has been called *freshwater survival factor*. The primary—but not exclusive—sites of action of prolactin are the gut epithelium (selective uptake of salt) and the kidney (reabsorption of salt and water excretion). Unfortunately, exceptions in particular species of fishes make it impossible to generalize on the cortisol–prolactin interplay in freshwater–saltwater adaptation. In the hypophysectomized trout, growth hormone rather than prolactin promotes freshwater survival. In the European eel the same hormone (cortisol) has opposite actions upon plasma salt concentrations in freshwater-adapted versus saltwater-adapted fishes.

Not all fishes have both hyper- and hypotonic adaptive mechanisms.

Some species cannot survive in fresh water, some will not tolerate seawater, while still others (eels) easily range between the two. In Pacific salmon born in fresh water, tolerance to seawater (hence the necessary endocrine and other mechanisms) does not appear until a particular stage of development (the smolt). The cortisol-mediated seawater tolerance seems to require thyroid hormone action before it appears.

In amphibians and other terrestrial vertebrates sensitive to dehydration, lack of water leads to hemoconcentration of electrolytes (various ions in the blood). As mentioned in Chapter 3, such hemoconcentration appears to be more or less directly sensed by hypothalamic neurons, probably the octapeptide-secreting neurons themselves. The neurohypophyseal octapeptides alter the permeability of renal tubules (as well as the bladder epithelium and skin) to water, permitting it to be absorbed into the blood along the osmotic gradient. This water-conservation mechanism is quite general among terrestrial vertebrates.

An interesting hormone-mediated behavioral response to dehydration has recently been characterized: the action of angiotensin II. This hormone has been found to stimulate drinking behavior (thirst) in a variety of vertebrates. It is of further interest that in animals inhabiting arid, desert environments, the drinking response to angiotensin II usually is lost. It clearly is not useful in such an animal to stimulate drinking behavior, since the dry environment offers no means to satisfy it.

Other examples of endocrine involvement in physiological phenomena affecting salt and water concentration in the blood can be given. However, the student by now should be aware that osmoregulation is too broad a topic to pursue in detail, since there are so many adaptive variants in it. The student is referred to the chapters on the individual osmoactive hormones for a deeper understanding of the appropriate actions of each of them.

ADDITIONAL READING

1. Ball, J. N., and D. M. Ensor (1967). Specific action of prolactin on plasma sodium levels in hypophysectomized *Poecilia latipinna* (Teleostei). *Gen. Comp. Endocrinol.* **8**:432–440.

2. Ball, J. N., and P. M. Ingleton (1973). Adaptive variations in prolactin secretion in relation to external salinity in the teleost *Poecilia latipinna*. *Gen. Comp. Endocrinol.* **20**:312–325.

3. Bentley, P. J. (1976). *Comparative Vertebrate Endocrinology.* Cambridge University Press, Cambridge. (Chapter 5: Hormones and nutrition; Chapter 6: Hormones and calcium metabolism; Chapter 8: Hormones and osmoregulation.)

4. Butler, D. G. (1966). Effect of hypophysectomy on osmoregulation in the European eel (*Anguilla anguilla* L.). *Comp. Biochem. Physiol.* **18**:773–781.

5. Chan, D. K. O., I. Chester Jones, I. W. Henderson, and J. C. Rankin (1967). Studies on the experimental alteration of water and electrolyte composition of the eel (*Anguilla anguilla* L.). *J. Endocrinol.* **37**:297–317.

6. Cheung, W. Y. (1981). Discovery and recognition of calmodulin: a personal account. *J. Cyclic Nucleotide Res.* **7**:71–84.

7. Clarke, W. C. (1973). Sodium-retaining bioassay of prolactin in the intact teleost *Tilapia mossambica* acclimated to sea water. *Gen. Comp. Endocrinol.* **21:**498–513.

8. De Luca, H. F. (1981). Recent advances in the metabolism of vitamin D. *Ann. Rev. Physiol.* **43:**199–210.

9. Dharmamba, M., N. Mayer-Goston, J. Maetz, and H. A. Bern (1973). Effect of prolactin on sodium movement in *Tilapia mossambica* adapted to sea water. *Gen. Comp. Endocrinol.* **21:**179–187.

10. Doneen, B. A. (1976). Water and ion movements in the urinary bladder of the gobiid teleost *Gillichthyes mirabilis* in response to prolactins and to cortisol. *Gen. Comp. Endocrinol.* **28:**33–41.

11. Ensor, D. M., and J. N. Ball (1972). Prolactin and osmoregulation in fishes. *Fed. Proc.* **6:**1615–1623.

12. Gaillard, P. J., and H. H. Boer, eds. (1978). *Comparative Endocrinology*. Elsevier/North-Holland, Amsterdam. (Contains sections by numerous authors under the following section titles: Endocrine control of hydromineral regulation, pp. 197–272; Endocrine control of calcium metabolism, pp. 243–286; Endocrine control of intermediary metabolism, pp. 423–464.)

13. Gaitskell, R. E., and I. Chester Jones (1970). Effects of adrenalectomy and cortisol injection on the *in vitro* movement of water by the intestine of the freshwater European eel (*Anguilla anguilla* L.). *Gen. Comp. Endocrinol.* **15:**491–493.

14. Handler, J. S., and J. Orloff (1981). Antidiuretic hormone. *Ann. Rev. Physiol.* **43:**611–624.

15. Henderson, I. W., and N. A. M. Wales (1974). Renal diuresis and antidiuresis after injections of arginine vasotocin in the freshwater eel (*Anguilla anguilla* L.). *J. Endocrinol.* **41:**487–500.

16. Hirano, T., D. W. Johnson, H. A. Bern, and S. Utida (1973). Studies on water and ion movement in the isolated urinary bladder of selected freshwater, marine and euryhaline teleosts. *Comp. Biochem. Physiol.* **45A:**529–540.

17. Holmes, W. N., and I. M. Stanier (1966). Studies on the renal excretion of electrolytes by the trout (*Salmo gairdneri*). *J. Exp. Biol.* **44:**33–46.

18. Johnson, D. W. (1973). Endocrine control of hydromineral balance in teleosts. *Am. Zool.* **13:**799–818.

19. Kochakian, C. D. (1976). *Anabolic-Androgenic Steroids*. Springer-Verlag, Berlin (*Handbuch der Experimentellen Pharmakologie*, Vol. 43.)

20. Leatherland, J. F., and B. A. McKeown (1974). Effect of ambient salinity on prolactin and growth hormone secretion and on hydro-mineral regulation in Kokanee salmon smolts (*Oncorhynchus nerka*). *J. Comp. Physiol.* **89:**215–226.

21. McKerns, K. W. (1969). *Steroid Hormones and Metabolism*. Appleton-Century-Crofts, New York.

22. Maetz, J., and E. Skadhauge (1968). Drinking rates and gill ionic turnover in relation to external salinities in the eel. *Nature* **217:**371–373.

23. Meister, A. (1965). *Biochemistry of the Amino Acids*, Vols. 1 and 2. Academic, New York.

24. Oduleye, S. O. (1975). The effect of hypophysectomy and prolactin therapy on water balance of the brown trout, *Salmo trutta*. *J. Exp. Biol.* **63:**357–366.

25. Oguro, C., and M. Uchiyama (1980). Comparative endocrinology of hypocalcemic regulation in lower vertebrates. In *Hormones, Adaptation and Evolution* (S. Ishii, T. Hirano, and M. Wada, eds.). Springer, Berlin.

26. Pang, P. K. T., and J. A. Yee (1980). Evolution of the endocrine control of vertebrate hypercalcemic regulation. In *Hormones, Adaptation and Evolution* (S. Ishii, T. Hirano, and M. Wada, eds.). Springer, Berlin.

27. Pastan, I. H., and M. C. Willingham (1981). Receptor mediated endocytosis of hormones in cultured cells. *Ann. Rev. Physiol.* **43:**239–250.

28. Raisz, L. G., and B. E. Kream (1981). Hormonal control of skeletal growth. *Ann. Rev. Physiol.* **43:**225–238.

29. Sawyer, W. H. (1972). Neurohypophysial hormones and water and sodium excretion in African lungfish. *Gen. Comp. Endocrinol.* Suppl. 3:345–349.

30. Young, J. B., and L. Landsberg (1979). Catecholamines and the sympathoadrenal system: the regulation of metabolism. In *Contemporary Endocrinology*, Vol. 1 (S. Ingbar, ed.). Plenum, New York, pp. 245–304.

Index